S0-AIN-126

FOURTH EDITION

Principles of Community Health

Jack Smolensky, M.P.H., Ed.D.
San Jose State University

1977
W. B. SAUNDERS COMPANY
Philadelphia, London, Toronto

W. B. Saunders Company: West Washington Square
Philadelphia, PA 19105

1 St. Anne's Road
Eastbourne, East Sussex BN21 3UN, England

1 Goldthorne Avenue
Toronto, Ontario M8Z 5T9, Canada

Library of Congress Cataloging in Publication Data

Smolensky, Jack.

Principles of community health.

Includes bibliographical references and index.

1. Public health. I. Title. [DNLM: 1. Community health services. WA100 S666p]

RA425.S643 1977 362.1 75-44607

ISBN 0-7216-8428-9

Principles of Community Health ISBN 0-7216-8428-9

Last digit is the print number: 9 8 7 6 5 4 3 2 1

PREFACE

The dominant concern of the late 70's and early 80's will continue to be the quality of human life. We must strive to achieve environmental quality without sacrificing our way of life and our aspirations. A plan for health progress must be based on improvement in the quality of life for all people. This involves placing human needs above the protection of economic interest in our value systems. This book stresses these human needs.

There is little doubt that social and medical problems have become the main focus of tomorrow's public health programs. The entire spectrum of "social ailments," such as drug abuse, venereal disease, mental illness, alcoholism, suicide, and accidents, includes problems appropriate to public health activity. Participation in mass screening and medical care programs, the utilization of existing health facilities, and community support for public health measures are only some of the problems facing public health today that require a knowledge of social action. Social action and social change as they affect health programs are stressed throughout the book.

The greatest potential for improving the health of the American people is to be found in what they do and don't do to and for themselves. Individual decisions about diet, exercise, stress, and smoking are of critical importance, and collective decisions regarding pollution and other aspects of the environment are also relevant.

Increased demand for health services means careful planning by community agencies, more efficient utilization of present health professionals, recruitment and training of paramedical personnel, and coordination among health and welfare agencies. Poverty, malnutrition, minority health problems, ecology, population control, genetic counseling, health department reorganization, necessary legislation, and international health are but a few of the complex areas confronting us.

Important new and expanded areas covered in this text include mental health (emphasizing guidelines for the early childhood years), alcoholism, geriatrics, women's health issues, maternal and child health, and voluntary health agencies. Review questions for test purposes have been added to the discussion questions at the end of each chapter.

This edition of the text has been fully revised and rewritten to incorporate new and relevant material on all of the aforementioned topics. The book was written primarily for college and university students who are preparing to assume some degree of responsibility in community health programs. Useful materials were carefully selected from each of the 50 states. Current reference lists were chosen with care and designed to stimulate further interest. New text has been added throughout. New illustrations, charts, graphs, and national and local programs are included. The theme throughout is successful and effective public health programs through greater cooperation among all groups and members of the community.

Valuable critical assistance and helpful suggestions were received from Henry M. Bockrath, M.D., M.P.H., Psychiatrist; Merle Cosand, M.D., M.P.H., Former Health Officer, San Bernardino County Health Department, California; Franklin Haar, Ph.D.,

Eugene, Oregon; Franz Rosa, M.D., Division of Family Health, World Health Organization, Geneva, Switzerland; Bradley Greenblatt, M.D., Psychiatrist; Lawrence Schwartz, M.D.; Robert Truitt, M.D., Neurologist; Virginia Lindsay, M.S.W., Psychiatric Social Worker; and Jack Dunigan, D.D.S., M.P.H.

Thanks to Nadine Pokorski for typing the manuscript and to Deborah Pokorski for organizing and coordinating all the materials. "Warm fuzzies" to Norma C. for her countless suggestions, assistance, and "true grit."

JACK SMOLENSKY

CONTENTS

CHAPTER 1

Basic Health Problems

CRISIS IN PUBLIC HEALTH

The crisis in public health is, of course, only part of the larger crisis in American life, reflected in the energy crisis, ghettos, and pollution. Health is inextricably linked with all aspects of life. Fundamental progress in health depends on solving the major issues that challenge our entire national life. The health dimension is most varied and important.

Although man has adapted to his environment, he has destroyed the quality of his life. One example would be the high frequency and severity of emphysema and chronic bronchitis due to air pollution—and the automobile, which is here to stay, continues to emit poison gases, which are insidiously choking us to death. Man has adapted so that noise levels that were once offensive to the ear are now tolerable. As "progress" continues apace, concrete replaces flowers and orchards, oil spills destroy fish and wildlife, and garbage fills in marshes, and it becomes increasingly difficult to remember "the corn fields and the distant mountains."

Habituation to overcrowding may inevitably lead to an increasingly organized and regimented world. Overpopulation and regimentation are likely to generate stress, social disorder, and violence. Morris states, in the *Human Zoo,* that under natural conditions, wild animals do not mutilate themselves, masturbate, attack their offspring, develop stomach ulcers, become fetishists, suffer from obesity, form homosexual pair-bonds, or commit murder. But, confined in the unnatural conditions of captivity, they exhibit the same neurotic behavior patterns as those common to urban man caged in his crowded cities. Clearly, then, the city is not a "concrete jungle"—it is a human zoo.

Basically, man is still a primitive tribal hunter, ill-equipped to cope with the social hazards of a vast, impersonal community. Many of his cultural enterprises can best be interpreted as a desperate attempt to recreate a reassuring pseudo-tribal condition. Yet, balanced against the dangers and disadvantages of city life are its considerable rewards, the exhilarating opportunities it offers to man's insatiable curiosity and his intellectual ability. It remains to be seen whether man will turn his human zoo into a magnificent human game preserve or into an insane asylum reminiscent of the cramped animal menageries of the last century.

One element which led to the current health dilemma was failure to comprehend that long-term adverse health effects can result from the application of certain technological innovations, such as cars, aerosol sprays, nuclear energy, insecticides, cigarettes, thalidomide, and color TV sets (radiation). We did not, for example, recognize the total consequences of cigarette smoking until four decades had passed, and it has taken us another three decades to reach the point of taking action.

Another element which has added to our problem involves inadequate testing of new foods and drugs. Testing has been based upon the premise, "innocent until proven guilty." Today, however, with an increasing number of consumer guardians and a more organized and efficient Federal Drug Administration, this axiom is being reevaluated. Of course, it is most difficult to accurately correlate test results with animals, since there are so many variables. In addition, food and drug manufacturers will challenge any questions about the safety of their product with their own research statistics. Production and profits, in our society, must continue, whatever the cost in health.

We cannot achieve environmental quality without changing our ways of life and even our aspirations. A strategy for achieving health progress must be based on improvement in the quality of life for all people. This involves placing human needs above protection of economic interest in our value system. For example, the great interest and action taken by the public had a direct affect on the legislature's decision to cancel production of the SST (Supersonic transport). René Dubos, winner of a Lasker Award in Public Health and a Pulitzer Prize, stated:

> We shall have to limit the amount of energy introduced into ecological systems, the kinds of industrial goods produced, the extent of our aimless mobility and our population size. All these limitations can be achieved without causing economic stagnation or stopping real progress. Indeed, a change in social structure and goals can enrich our lives, by opening the way for a social renaissance.
>
> The colossal inertia and rigidity—if not indifference—of social and academic institutions make it unlikely that they will develop effective programs of action or research focused on environmental problems. Two kinds of events, however, may catalyze and accelerate the process. One is some ecological catastrophe that will alarm the public and thus bring pressure on the social, economic, and academic establishments. Another, more attractive, possibility is the emergence of a grass-roots movement, powered by romantic emotion as much as by factual knowledge, that will give form and strength to the latent public concern with environmental quality.[1]

Another contributor to our health crisis is pollution. Government and business will be forced to spend ever-increasing sums to control pollution of air and water and to prevent the destruction of natural beauty. Already, the young seem to be turning their protest to problems of the environment, organizing demonstrations against irresponsible corporations and municipalities. In the next few years, increasing attention will be paid to inadequate development and the infamous urban sprawl; it will be widely recognized that like most forms of pollution, defilement of the landscape, whether it be with shopping centers or expressways, is hard to reverse. In the interests of preserving their open spaces—not to mention domestic tranquility—some nations may bar or limit tourism. International relations will certainly be affected by the cause of conservation, since air and water pollution observes no boundaries. Nations will discover that sovereignty can be threatened by pollutants just as much as by invasion.

> Much more is involved than putting filters on chimneys and car exhausts and building new sewage plants. As the decade advances, it will become clear that if the ecological effort is to succeed, much of today's existing technology will have to be scrapped and something new developed in its place. The gasoline-powered automobile, at present the chief polluter of the air, will be made clean or it will be banned from many urban areas—a threat that some car makers already recognize. Alternatives are electric or gas-turbine-powered autos. Increasingly, it will be seen that any kind of mass transportation, however powered, is more efficient than the family car. Some, however, cynically argue that the revolt against the car may not take place until a thermal inversion, combined with a traffic pile-up, asphyxiates thousands on a freeway to nowhere. In addition, factories will have to be built as "closed systems," operated so that there is no waste; everything, in effect, that goes in one end must come out the other as a usable, non-polluting product. Man's own body wastes will have to find use as fertilizer—the cheapest and most efficient means of disposal. Planning will have to be a much greater concern.
>
> Popular though the cause is, it is by no means clear that the struggle to save the environment will be won. The attitude, central to the modern mind, that all technology is good technology will have to be radically changed. "Our society is trained to accept all new technology as progress, or to look upon it as an aspect of fate," says George Wald, Harvard's Nobel-laureate biologist. "Should one do everything one can? The usual answer is 'Of course'; but the right answer is 'Of course not.'"[2]

CHANGING PATTERNS

Dramatic ecological changes during the past few years have made it necessary to regroup our forces in planning and providing community health services. These changes include the following:

1. Nearly 50 per cent of our population is under 25 years of age. This means that we must be ready and able to cope with the increasing problems of this group, including drug abuse, suicide, venereal disease, and accidents.

2. Since more people are living to old age, more senior citizens are being faced with problems of economic security, of being needed, and of needing something to do. Older people are more subject to chronic and debilitating illnesses. Some of the special needs for the older citizen are (1) periodic health checkups as a means of detecting disease while it is easier to control or cure, (2) health education programs, particularly to counteract the information of mass media regarding unnecessary use of vitamins, laxatives, and worthless arthritis and chronic disease cures, (3) provisions for worthwhile activities so that they can feel liked and be constructive citizens within the limits of their capabilities, (4) available facilities for custodial, nursing, and medical care for those who are partially or completely disabled, and (5) recruitment of health personnel into the field of gerontology.

3. Because of improved health conditions and medical technology, the number of infants surviving the first year of life is continuing to increase. This means that we are keeping alive many children with physical and mental defects who will require special care. It also means that we must learn more about child growth and development and must educate parents and prospective parents.

4. Movement from rural to urban and suburban areas has increased mobility. This means that decentralization of health services is necessary to make them "closer to the people." Also, many agencies have eligibility requirements of an economic, residential, or geographic nature. Availability of health services and facilities will require the removal of these artificial barriers which are no longer practical in a mobile society.

5. There are changing patterns of illness due to (1) resistance to antibiotics (gonorrhea, tuberculosis), (2) stress and emotional problems (increase in population; complex, crowded, permissive society), (3) heart disease (older people living longer, obesity, stress, smoking, lack of exercise), and (4) insidious idiopathic health problems (due to chemicals in food, water, and air) that we are only beginning to understand.

6. Increased demand for health services means careful planning by community agencies, more efficient utilization of present health professionals, recruitment and training of paramedical personnel, and coordination among health and welfare agencies. The demand for health services will continue to grow for many reasons. The Governor's Committee on the Study of Medical Aid and Health cites the following:

Rising income levels and the spread of prepayment enable more people to afford better care, rising levels of education create greater awareness of the value of medical care. New health education programs reinforce public concern with matters of personal health. The achievement of medical science increases the importance of health care as the successful treatment of a growing number of diseases and conditions becomes possible.

These changing patterns are inextricably linked to the major problems confronting us *now*.

PROBLEMS AND CHOICES

The promises of today's health planners and politicians need to be seen against the reality of difficult choices. The most basic

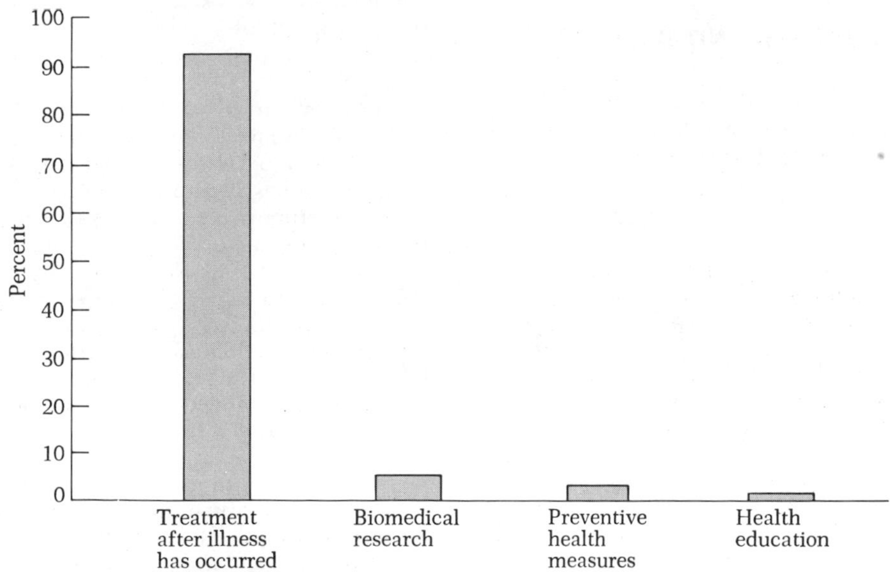

Figure 1–1 Percentage allotments of the approximately $90 billion currently spent each year for medical, hospital, and other health care. (Adapted from *The Report of the President's Committee on Health Education, 1973.* U.S.P.H.S., U.S. Government Printing Office, 1973.)

level of choice is between health and other goals. Although social reformers tell us that "health is a right," the realization of that "right" is always less than complete because some of the resources that could be used for health are allocated to other purposes. Figure 1–1 shows how the money allocated for health care in the United States is spent.

Discussion of the choices that face our society helps put the major problems of health and medical care in proper perspective. These problems, as perceived by the public, are high cost, poor access, and inadequate health levels. In order to attack them intelligently, we must recognize the scarcity of resources and the need to allocate the resources we have as efficiently as possible. We must recognize that we can't have everything.

The greatest current potential for improving the health of the American people is to be found in what they do and don't do to and for themselves. Individual decisions about diet, exercise, and smoking are of critical importance, and collective decisions affecting pollution and other aspects of the environment are also relevant.

These conclusions notwithstanding, the demand for medical care is very great and growing rapidly. As René Dubos has acutely observed, "To ward off disease or recover health, men as a rule find it easier to depend on the healers than to attempt the more difficult task of living wisely."

LOCAL NEEDS AND DEMANDS

Emphasis in public health has changed from sanitation to the whole patient and his entire biological and psychosocial environment. As the Governing Council of the American Public Health Association stated:

> Past roles no longer provide an adequate basis for determining what future roles should be. With rapid changes in social needs, environmental problems and programs, and the organization and financing of health care, official health agencies must be ready to act swiftly to solve new problems. Local circumstances will weigh heavily in determining priorities for new activities. In one area, a health maintenance organization or its successor may seek help in forming the necessary preventive and early detection measures which its consumers need and desire. In a second area, national health insurance may produce unforeseen imbalances in the health care system, demanding rapid and expert evaluation for speedy correction. In a third, a large elderly population may feel neglected by the existing system of health care, and seek both guidance and services to narrow the gaps between demand and supply. In a fourth, a new industrial development may cause serious social malaise which consumers wish the official health agency to correct, even when the health implications are not clear. Each of these situations, and many other unique events, will occur in some localities but not in all.[3]

Comprehensive health services fall into four general categories: Community Health Services, Environmental Health Services, Mental Health Services, and Personal Health Services. The optimum population and geographic unit to be covered by these services varies. Population size and geographic area served by local governments also vary enormously, as do established customs of government operations. Some local governments already provide many services directly, others purchase them on contract, and still others are part of larger regional programs.

Economic, political, and social upheaval lead to reevaluation of program objectives, priorities, and organization. Without conflict, there is no growth. Conflict and crises have made people more aware of consumer involvement, revenue sharing, comprehensive health planning, conservation, interdisciplinary and paramedical involvement and support, and the importance of ensuring equal consideration for *all* members of a community. The strength of local health agencies can best be assured by fostering in them a spirit of flexibility, adaptiveness, innovation, and responsiveness to local needs:

> Changes in demand for both health services and delivery techniques are requiring health agencies to modify their programs. The federal government has attempted to decrease categorical program support, and expects that local governments will assume greater responsibility for the financing and delivery of health services. These changes will have great impact on program organization and financing. The disciplines of economics, public administration, and public finance have added much to the practice of public administration in general, and to methods of financing and delivering human services. Thus, it is likely that existing programs, and existing ways of doing business within many health agencies, will be put in new organizational, institutional, and personal settings. How health agencies adjust to these changes, and how aggressive they become in terms of moving ahead with comprehensive health services for their constituent populations within this context, will to a large degree deter-

mine the future of public support for health programs.[4]

While striving to eliminate factors that lower the quality of life, we must nonetheless recognize that complete freedom from disease, stress, frustration, and struggle is incompatible with the process of living and evolution. As Dubos states:

Life is an adventure in a world where nothing is static, where unpredictable and ill-understood events constitute dangers that must be overcome, often blindly and at great cost; where man himself, like the sorcerer's apprentice, has set in motion forces that are potentially destructive and may someday escape his control. Every manifestation of existence is a response to stimuli and challenges, each of which constitutes a threat if not adequately dealt with. The very process of living is a continual interplay between the individual and his environment, often taking the form of a struggle resulting in injury or disease.[5]

DEFINING PUBLIC HEALTH

Winslow probably has the best known and most widely accepted definition of public health and of its relationship to other fields. For analytic purposes it is presented in the following manner:

Public Health is the Science and Art of (1) preventing disease, (2) prolonging life, and (3) promoting health and efficiency through organized community effort for

(a) the sanitation of the environment,
(b) the control of communicable infections,
(c) the education of the individual in personal hygiene,
(d) the organization of medical and nursing services for the early diagnosis and preventive treatment of disease, and
(e) the development of the social machinery to insure everyone a standard of living adequate for the maintenance of health,

so organizing these benefits as to enable every citizen to realize his birthright of health and longevity.[5a]

John J. Hanlon considered the multifaceted relationships of health and public health in the following terms:

Health is a state of total effective physiologic functioning; it has both a relative and an absolute meaning, varying through time and space, both in the individual and in the group; it is the result of the combination of many forces, intrinsic and extrinsic, inherited and contrived, individual and collective, private and public, medical, environmental, and social; and it is conditioned by culture, economy, law, and government.

Accordingly,

Public health is dedicated to the common attainment of the highest level of physical, mental, and social well-being and longevity consistent with available knowledge and resources at a given time and place. It holds this goal as its contribution to the most effective total development and life of the individual and his society.[6]

The official statement of the House of Delegates of the American Medical Association, formulated in 1948, defined public health as:

The art and science of maintaining, protecting and improving the health of the people through organized community efforts. It includes those arrangements whereby the community provides medical services for special groups of persons and is concerned with prevention or control of disease, with persons requiring hospitalization to protect the community and with the medically indigent.

From its inception, the protection and promotion of public health has been one of several stated concerns of the American Medical Association. This definition of public health is of particular interest and significance in view of subsequent social and legislative trends.

The most widely accepted definition of individual health is that of the World Health Organization: "Health is a state of complete physical, mental, and social well-being and not merely the absence of disease or infirmity." Although this definition is positive and includes more than physical health, it infers that health is an absolute or ultimate state. However, because of innate differences, all individuals cannot achieve the same level of health; some of us are born with severe physical and mental limitations. Bauer defines health as:

. . . a state of feeling well in body, mind, and spirit, together with a sense of reserve power. It is based on normal functioning of tissues and organs of the body . . . and a harmonious adjustment to the physical and psychological environment, together with an attitude which regards health not as an end in itself, but as a means to a richer life as measured in constructive service to mankind.[7]

The term "good health," then, has a relative meaning. It is based upon an individual's physical, mental, and emotional capacity, and takes into account what the individual does during his life. Oberteuffer aptly expresses why attention to physical and emotional well-being is of value:

The more man can learn how to use the knowledge he has and the knowledge he is steadily accumulating from scientific investigation, the greater facility he will have for understanding and solving his problems. His worlds of economics, production, religion, homemaking, or politics will become easier to control, his objectives more easily attainable, and his life safer but more complicated. . . . [Science] can be a great liberator and a protector. From laboratories all over the world have come discoveries which have been so useful to civilization – discoveries of surgical techniques, protective vaccines, ways to preserve food, to heat houses, to purify water, to promote growth, and to do hundreds of other things.[8]

The President's Commission on Health Needs of the Nation states that

Health reflects dynamically the measure of man's control over his environment and his ever-changing adjustment to it. Health makes possible the maximum self-expression and self-development of man. It is the first prerequisite for leading a full life. The degree to which individuals, voluntary groups, and the State cooperate successfully in providing for the health of all represents the maturity and level of civilization of the Nation.[9]

NATIONAL HEALTH CARE

History of Organization

More than 40 years have passed since the Committee on the Costs of Medical Care, established by a group of foundations, undertook the first and so far the only thorough attempt to create a national health policy for the United States. Among other things, the committee recommended a change in the financing of health services, so that prepayment for a regime of care would replace payment by the patient at the time of service, and a change in the structure of the delivery of medical service whereby the payment mechanism would be combined with group practice. Movement in these directions has been so slow that today this organized type of medical care is available to only a small fraction of the American people.

The cause of change is seldom simple. The structure of medical care is not an isolated phenomenon but a reflection of the social and cultural values of the society. In this century the general trend in the United States has been toward greater social equity, although the changes are now so much an accepted part of life that one forgets how many of them there have been. Antitrust and labor laws, personal and corporate income taxes, and the Social Security system all reflect the trend. Until about 10 years ago, however, legislative initiatives affecting the organization and provision of medical care lagged conspicuously.

The structure of medical care involves not only the attitudes of society but also the attitude of the medical profession. In the United States the profession has had a consistent record. It opposed workmen's compensation laws, social security, and voluntary health insurance when they were in their formative stages; it vigorously opposed hospitalization for the aged under the Medicare amendment to the Social Security Act. The profession currently opposes legislation that would facilitate the formation of Health Maintenance Organizations. For years the profession opposed proposals for national health insurance; when it appeared that the adoption of some such plan was inevitable, organized medicine came forward with a limited and preemptory plan of its own.[10]

However, the American Medical Association, which has in the past been a fortress of reactionary conservatism, vigorously opposing any form of control over the fee-setting prerogative of physicians, especially in the form of medical insurance plans, is slowly gaining a new image. As Malcolm C. Todd, president of the AMA for 1975, stated:

. . . But we've changed our position on national health insurance regarding mandatory participation. The AMA now feels that it is proper, in the area of employer-employee contributions made towards payroll tax deductions. But we remain vehemently opposed to Social Security financing and Social Security administration because it has been proven time and time again that the Social Security administration is very inefficient.[11]

In the past 15 years, the ultra-conservative stand of this organization of over 170,000 doctors has made it lose the position of prestige and power it once enjoyed. Today the AMA finds itself fighting hard before legislative committees on most major issues, losing almost as many times as it wins. In addition, the rising cost of malpractice insurance has paralyzed health services in many areas.

Health as a priority is seldom high on the list of society's demands until other basic requirements have been met. This order of affairs is characteristic of underdeveloped societies, and it is equally true for the underdeveloped segments of our own society.

By the early 1960's it had become clear to almost every element of American society, with the notable exceptions of organized medicine and the private insurance industry, that private health insurance had failed for the poor and the elderly. A great struggle ensued, culminating in the Medicaid and Medicare modifications of the Social Security Act in 1965. These modifications are not generally regarded as ideal legislation for health but rather as a compromise reflecting what was politically possible as a major departure from previous federal policy. The changes that Medicare and Medicaid brought about in public attitudes and expectations and in the costs of medical care were more rapid than most people had anticipated. They marked the arrival in the public consciousness of what is widely described as a health crisis in the United States.

Health Maintenance Organizations (HMOs)

Early in 1971, President Nixon sent to Congress a health message in which he related that:

> In recent years a new method for delivering health services has achieved growing respect. This new approach has two essential attributes. It brings together a comprehensive range of medical services in a single organization so that a patient is assured of convenient access to all of the services, and it provides needed services for a fixed-contract fee which is paid in advance by all subscribers.

Such an organization can have a variety of forms and names and sponsors. One of the strengths of this new concept, in fact, is its great flexibility. The general term which has been applied to all of these units is HMO—Health Maintenance Organization. The most important advantage of Health Maintenance Organizations is the services a consumer receives for each health dollar. This happens first because such organizations provide a strong financial incentive for better preventive care and for greater efficiency.

Under traditional systems, doctors and hospitals are paid, in effect, on a piecework basis. The more illnesses they treat—and the more service they render—the more their income rises. This does not mean, of course, that they do any less than their very best to make people well. But it does mean that there is no economic incentive for them to concentrate on keeping people healthy. A fixed-price contract for comprehensive care reverses this illogical incentive. Under this arrangement, income grows not with the number of days a person is sick but with the number of days he is well. HMOs therefore have a strong financial interest in preventing illness, or, failing that, in treating it in its early stages, promoting a thorough recovery and preventing any reoccurrence. Like doctors in ancient China, they are paid to keep their clients healthy. For them, economic interests work to reinforce their professional interests.

The centralized form of Health Maintenance Organization usually goes by the name of prepaid group practice. In a typical arrangement the subscriber pays monthly premiums for comprehensive health care services, which are provided by an organized medical group. Many groups of this kind have been organized; the largest and probably best-known one is the Kaiser-Permanente program (Fig. 1–2). Prepaid group practice freed doctors in this program to do what they do best—treat patients—and administrators have taken over the paperwork. Meanwhile doctors in the cottage industry fee-for-service system are still supervising their administrative staff, attending to financial affairs, and completing government and insurance forms. This is a waste of their much needed healing talents. Another major advantage to prepaid group practice is that patients are no longer passed from doctor to doctor and specialist to specialist for treatment of their often complex illnesses. They get comprehensive care through one source.

The decentralized form of Health Maintenance Organization is encompassed by the term Foundation for Medical Care. Participating physicians agree in advance on a schedule of fees, and they accept review of their work by peers, but they continue to practice individually. Again the subscriber pays an annual fee for health care, and when he needs to see a physician, he chooses one from a list of the physicians participating in the foundation. The San Joaquin Foundation in California is an early example of a group organized along these lines.

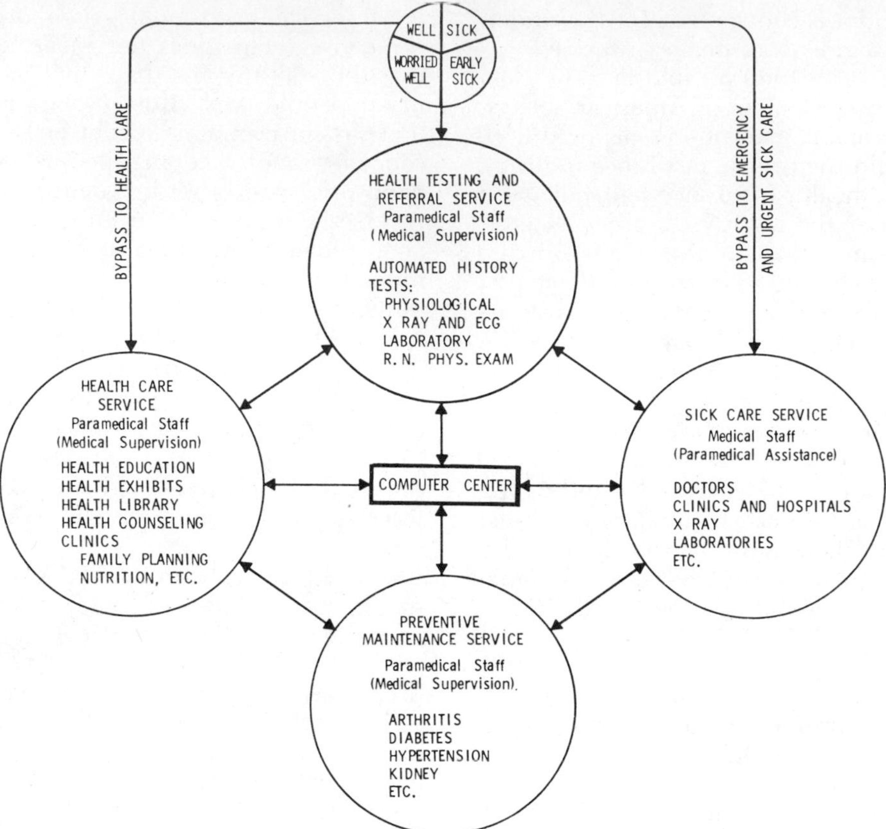

Figure 1–2 Triage system used in Kaiser-Permanente Medical Care Program, Oakland, Calif. (From Collen, F. B., and Soghikian, K.: A health education library for patients. Health Services Reports, *89*(3):237, May–June, 1974.)

Increasing Need for Expanded Health Care

At no time in modern history has there been a greater need for expanding and coordinating the existing elements of the health care system in America. The demands on this system have been created by a number of factors which can be expected to continue to increase for the foreseeable future. Two obvious reasons for the increase in demand for care are an increased population and an increase in services available. Other less apparent trends also influence the demand:

1. Rising income levels which result in increased capacity to pay for medical care, either directly or through insurance.
2. Rising educational levels leading to greater awareness of the need for and value of medical care.
3. Increased longevity with its increased susceptibility to chronic conditions requiring extensive medical care.
4. Large segments of population with poverty-level incomes making heavy demands upon a system poorly suited to their needs, and greater expectations for increased and more equitable availability of quality health care to all segments of the population.
5. Increased population mobility requiring repeated diagnostic services as people move from place to place.
6. Extension of existing voluntary and legislated prepayment plans and the creation of new systems for purchasing health care for the entire population.
7. Increased amount and scope of social legislation.
8. Changing age distribution of population, with increasing numbers at both ends of the age spectrum.
9. Ever-increasing need for continuing education of the health professions and the public for the appropriate and efficient utilization of health care knowledge and resources.

Paralleling these trends, sometimes prompting them, have been the significant changes in the science and technology of medicine. A bewildering number of new drugs currently in use were unknown a decade ago. The use of tissue and organ transplant procedures, artificial organs, and radioactive isotopes are now accepted practices in saving and prolonging life. The number of physicians has been increasing faster than the population, but not fast enough to supply the demand.

If past experience is any guide, the increase in the number of doctors will not increase the doctor-people ratio in rural areas and city ghettos, where the ratio is lowest. Nor is there any promise of increase in the number of primary doctors, the category in shortest supply. It is evident that the present and future health care needs of all the people cannot be met without improving the delivery systems. In view of this, it is inevitable that some form of national health care program will be adopted soon to meet this need. This will further increase the demands on the system, and exert increasing pressures on the existing resources and those that can be developed in the immediate future. (See Fig. 1–3.)

Significant Components

The delivery of health services is a complex situation of many interrelated factors. Significant components of the delivery of health care include a knowledge of the population to be served, the needs among that population, the availability and accessibility of the needed services, and the conjoining of the population and medical community as represented by the utilization of health services.

If all persons are to receive the maximum benefits from the increasing knowledge of health maintenance and disease, a health care system must be devised which will work in a coordinated manner. By definition, a comprehensive health care system is a viable formal or informal dynamic, cooperative, cohesive, and coordinated organization of health care agencies, facilities, and staff designed to render a full spectrum of health care, ranging from primary prevention to extended care for all segments of a geographically defined population. A creatively developed health care delivery system must meet certain professional and economic requirments:

1. A functional integration of the health services and resources of any region and their effective utilization for the transmission and encouragement of new knowledge and techniques in order to provide high quality care, and make optimal use of all health manpower.

2. Comprehensive health care services that are available, accessible, and economically feasible for all United States citizens, with participation by

By 1976, patients will be paying about a third of total physicians' fees out of their own pockets--even with no Federal health plan. Though their share of the cost keeps on shrinking, patients now pay twice as much in dollars as they did in 1960. That dollar increase is a major argument advanced by proponents of national health insurance plans.

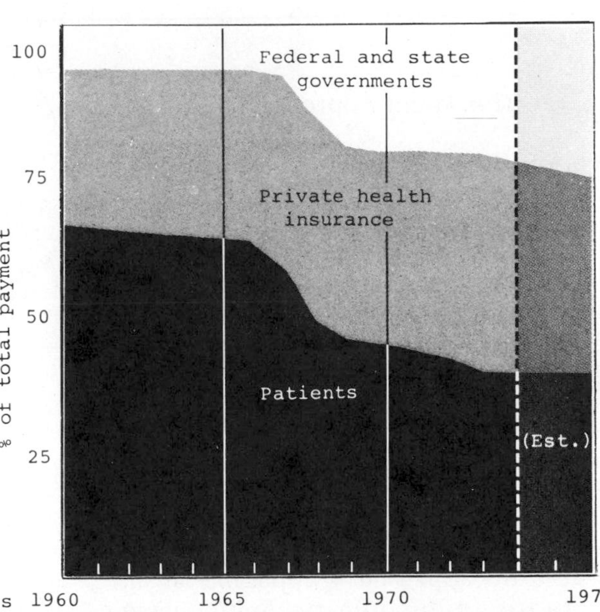

Figure 1–3 Patients' shrinking share of the doctor bill. (From Medical Economics, May 12, 1975, p. 233; based on data from Office of Research and Statistics, Social Security Administration.)

the recipient in the financing of the service, depending on his ability to pay.

3. Maintenance of choice in selection of the type of service and the professional providing the service.

4. Maintenance of the quality of health services through peer review, continuing education, and continuing professional evaluation of all health professionals.

5. Built-in tangible and scaled incentives for both professionals and institutions for effecting economy of operation.

6. Built-in mechanisms for protection of the necessary traditional types and for the creation of new types of health manpower and facilities, and for continuous evaluation and improvements in the system for health care and delivery.

7. Built-in mechanisms for maintaining a steady progress in the state of the art and science of health through research.

8. Improved awareness by those who use the system of where and how services are available, and assurance that the services will be available and continue as long as needed.

9. Provision of health services by a method that not only enhances the dignity and self-respect of the individual, but contributes to the total society of which he is a part.

A vigorous effort is needed to accomplish these objectives. Some health care systems already exist that meet some of these requirements and have potential for improving the delivery of health care. One such system is that operated by the Department of Medicine and Surgery of the Veterans' Administration.

The Team Approach

Various kinds of health care teams are being used to bridge the manpower gap in primary medical care. The team concept for medical care should be based on a "hierarchy of enablers" that includes both highly specialized technical and medical personnel and multipurpose workers who maintain direct patient contact. In some areas, particularly those made up of the lower socioeconomic groups, an additional level in the hierarchy would include the indigenous worker who, as part of the community itself, enables it to understand and gain access to the medical care system.

The team approach is applicable at all levels of care. At the primary level the team may consist of a physician (usually a generalist, internist, or pediatrician), a public health nurse, and a social worker. This kind of team has been used in a prepaid group practice plan to emphasize the family health approach to medical care rather than the specialized patient-disease approach. Patients assigned to the health team may call upon any member of the team for care. Generally the patient finds himself relating to the team as a whole for his total care, while at the same time receiving discrete services from individual members of the team. In other instances, one member of the team may be the primary contact point operating under directions from the team as a whole.

Neighborhood Health Centers

Many clinics have been developed by members of the community to fill a long-standing need. These include neighborhood health centers, women's clinics, senior citizens' clinics, and teenage clinics. Health education, disease prevention, and promotion of general well-being are of prime importance to each of these centers. Neighborhood health centers should have the following characteristics:

—Accessibility to a population concentration;
—Open 24 hours a day, 7 days a week;
—Family-centered care by a team of internists, pediatricians, clinic and public health nurses, and social workers;
—Availability of frequently required specialists in such fields as psychiatry, obstetrics, gynecology, and surgery;
—Continuity of doctor-patient relationship;
—Family records with social and medical summaries of relevant information about each family member;
—Availability of basic diagnostic laboratory and x-ray facilities, drugs, and biologicals;
—Direct link (by center-controlled ambulance when necessary) to a teaching hospital for diagnostic and therapeutic services requiring the facilities and personnel of the hospital;
—Patient-centered and community-oriented care.

The interdisciplinary relationships within the center have a unique potential because neither the hospital nor group practice has been able to prevent the dominance of the physician from becoming an effective barrier to the development of an optimal and essentially equal role for such disciplines as nursing and social work. The neighborhood health center permits patients to have direct access to these professionals without physician referral and provides for shared responsibility in patient management in a flexible, nonauthoritarian setting.

The Office of Educational Opportunity neighborhood health centers have now been established in more than 30 neighborhoods throughout the United States with concentrations of low income populations. They are required to be sensitive to the community they serve by giving their consumers a voice in policy matters and by employing indigenous personnel in a variety of subprofessional and paramedical jobs.

As these centers develop further, they may well represent a new entry point into the medical care system which can replace for some patients the present haphazard use of hospital emergency and outpatient clinics and restore these latter to the role and functions they are best equipped to perform. There is evidence that such experimental delivery systems can make better use of existing resources. Substantial reductions have been demonstrated in the number of admissions to hospitals and the total number of bed days utilized when ambulatory health

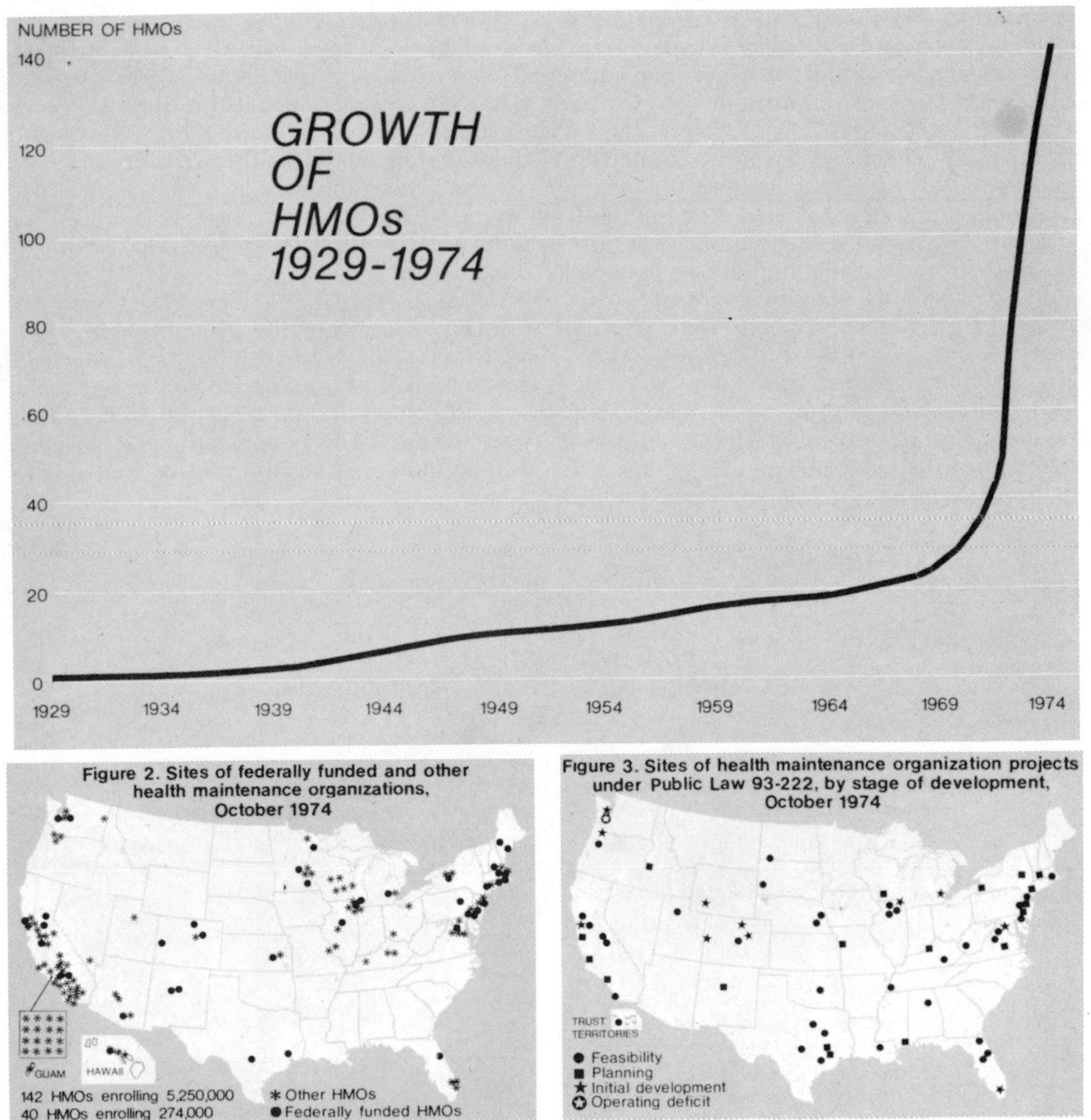

Figure 1–4 Growth of HMOs from 1929 to 1974. (From Seubold, F. H.: HMOs—the view from the program. Public Health Reports, *90*(2):101, March–April, 1975.)

care services for preventing and treating illness are available. Similar findings have been reported when health coverage is received in group practice rather than Blue Cross–Blue Shield plans.

Problems and Future of National Health Care

A key issue in current discussions of improved health delivery systems is the effective use of new health manpower. For example, registered nurses perform many of the routine screening and treatment tasks which take much of a physician's time but do not require medical judgment based on clinical experience. Administration of mass screening tests and prenatal care are only two of many functions recently allocated to many nurses. The organization of the health care delivery system in the United States cannot be based on a single model, no matter how promising the preliminary results. Generalizations are extremely hazardous because of the diversity of community life and structure in a nation as large and as complex as the United States. Systematic planning and evaluation of alternatives is necessary if increasing health costs are to be brought under control. Important goals to aim for include the establishment of a cooperative, coordinated program involving people and health workers; equitable taxation (including a review of the present tax structure); providing patients with a sense of dignity and self-respect; and building democratic profit-free institutions.

Current programs (such as Medicaid) have been plagued by complaints of fraudulent practices, inadequate services, high-pressure and deceptive patient recruitment practices, inadequate funds invested by groups of doctors signing prepaid health plan contracts, inadequate funds appropriated by state legislators, and money expended on administrative costs rather than services.

Figure 1–4 illustrates the growth of HMOs in the United States from 1929 to 1974. However, with all the optimism concerning the contribution that successful HMOs can make to the health care industry—their ability to provide quality care with cost containment and efficiency, and to improve the accessibility and availability of health care—HMOs do not solve *all* health care problems. Rather the HMO was advanced as an *option* for those providers and consumers who wished to take advantage of its benefits. It is intended to be just one more valuable alternative among the choices that the citizens of this nation can make in determining how they wish to receive their health care.

SHORT SUMMARY NATIONAL HEALTH PLANNING AND RESOURCES DEVELOPMENT ACT OF 1974 (P.L. 93–641)

President Ford has signed into law the National Health Planning and Development Act of 1974, authorizing a three-year health planning and facilities program. The measure adds two new titles to the Public Health Service Act. Title XV establishes national, state, and local organizations for health planning and revises and combines existing health planning programs. Title XVI revises and extends the medical facilities construction (Hill-Burton) program and authorizes funds for developing health resources.

The act creates a network of Health Systems Agencies (HSAs) responsible for areawide health planning and development throughout the country in health services areas to be designated by State Governors.

The health systems agency shall:

- Establish and implement health systems plans
- Review and approve federal funding for health services.
- Review and approve capital expenditures and appropriateness of health facilities.
- Provide technical and limited financial assistance to implement area health systems plans.

The HSAs are to be non-profit private corporations, public regional planning agencies, or single units of local government. The governing body is to be representative of the total community. Half the members plus one must be health care consumers. Of the remainder, not less than one-third must be direct providers—that is, persons whose primary activity is the provision of health care and who have received professional training and are licensed or certified.

The act also provides for State Health Planning and Development Agencies to be selected by the Governor in each State and designated by the Secretary of Health, Education, and Welfare.

The State Health Planning and Development Agencies are to prepare long-range and short-term State Health Plans, serve as designated planning agencies for administering Section 1122 of the Social Security Act or administer the State Certificate of Need Program, review all existing institutional health services being offered and health facilities and HMOs located in the State periodically, and administer the State medical facilities construction plan.

The State agency is to be advised by a State Health Coordinating Council which includes representatives of each Health Systems Agency within the State.

The establishment of at least five Centers for Health Planning is authorized to provide Health Systems Agencies and State agencies with technical and consulting assistance and to conduct research, studies and analyses of health planning and resource development.

Title XVI authorizes allotments and loan guarantees and interest subsidies for modernization of medical facilities, construction of new outpatient medical facilities, construction of new inpatient facilities in areas of recent rapid population growth, and conversion of existing facilities for providing new health services.

HOLISTIC HEALTH

The American health care system faces a tremendous challenge in fully meeting the needs of the very diverse population it serves. In an effort to better meet this challenge, recent federal legislation, Public Law 93–641, has mandated that health planning and administrative systems be restructured so that the consumer will be represented and will be able to participate in planning processes. The hope is that involvement of the consumer public will allow health planning to become a truly effective mechanism for change and bring new perspectives to determining what it is that people really need to create and maintain their health. Public Law 93–641 expresses special concern for low-income, minority, and what is generally termed the medically underserved consumer. Unfortunately it is often the case that the "underserved" consumers are those whose beliefs, background, culture, or language would cause them to choose not to use the services of the modern technological medical systems as they are.

In order for all consumers to be truly represented in the planning and future structure of health care services, it will be necessary to develop new concepts of health care—new concepts that incorporate ancient traditions, world cultural teachings, and the accumulated knowledge of centruies past into a whole and total view of humanity. "Holistic health" is a perspective on health care that views all persons as whole beings whose individual psycho-physio-cultural-spiritual relationships with the environment directly affect their state of health. The holistic perspective takes into account the particular patterns manifested by all of the internal and external factors influencing a person's behavior and physical reactions; these patterns are viewed as highly instrumental in determining each individual's health needs. Methods used to determine, assess, and manage these patterns may be in some part derived from modern technological medicine; however, there is a tremendous wealth of information to be derived from the teachings and traditions of both Eastern and Western ethnic groups, as well as from the cultures of ancient civilizations. It is from these world cultural sources that the holistic perspective draws its practical data and develops concepts and skills of life-style modification that allow individuals to confront and deal with their health needs.

WOMEN'S LIBERATION

Today's woman wants considerate, respectful treatment from her physician, wants complete information about her bodily condition, and wants a voice in the medical decisions that affect her. Refusing any longer to regard doctors as awesome gods, she comes armed with a list of what she expects, including prompt explanation of the results and meaning of tests or examinations; discussion of alternative treatments and their pros and cons; full information about the purpose and possible risks of any prescribed drugs; and respect for her right to request that an examination or procedure be stopped at any time and to seek a second opinion.

The demand for improved medical care for women goes far beyond the activist movement. Women who don't regard themselves as liberationists are embracing the new health care goals much as they have the right to equal pay. And many of the demands are equally applicable to male patients.

The women's health movement is a blend of consumerism and feminism. To women's rights advocates, the predominantly male-dominated medical profession and its institutions represent classic examples of the male authority structure they seek to change. But, along with changes in the attitudes of doctors toward female patients, they demand basic changes in clinical care and its quality.

Out of the protests has come the self-help movement, a loose network of hundreds of informal do-it-yourself groups located mostly in major cities and on college campuses. Some are connected with clinic facilities, while others serve mainly as information centers where women can get advice and directions to medical services.

What kind of self-help do the women undertake? Primarily they conduct courses and study projects on their own body functions, on birth control, abortion, VD, pregnancy, childbirth, breast-feeding, food and nutrition, cancer, and menopause. Some groups go a step further, the women performing their own gynecological examinations on themselves and on each other. They also conduct surveys of clinic and medical care facilities and compile evaluations of doctors, services, and fees.

Some doctors view the self-help trend with alarm, others with hostility. But there are a growing number who see the movement as a constructive step toward developing better public health and preventive medicine, more informed patients, and improved doctor-patient relations.

Some of the women's groups also widely promote and use do-it-yourself Pap tests and VD tests. Although they interpret opposition by doctors as an effort to retain control of health care, again there are sound medical grounds for criticism. One physician says: "Some groups do their own testing by taking a smear from a tampon, a procedure that carries too great a risk of false negatives. Falsely reassuring results from self-taken Pap smears or gonorrhea tests are dangerous because they delay treatment." Another inadequacy of self-testing is the inability of cytology to pick up ovarian cancer. Its detection requires a bimanual pelvic examination, which can only be performed with accuracy by highly trained and experienced people. Some nurses are trained for about six months just to do Pap tests properly. For the women's self-help groups, a more practical approach would be to have a physician, nurse, or allied health person do their Pap tests.

Many feel that the new generation of sexually liberated women needs a generation of sexually educated gynecologists. The gynecologist today has the added job of teaching women how to be comfortable with their sexuality and their body functions. Women's Liberation has imposed a new—often unattainable—standard of normalcy. As a consequence of new expectations, which not all women feel they can live up to, some gynecologists are finding an increase in complaints with a psychosomatic etiology. When women are feeling insecure, anxious, or guilty, they may project these feelings toward their pelvic organs.

Certainly, an organized sisterhood of women consumers of medicine cannot be ignored. After all, as is pointed out in the book, *Our Bodies, Ourselves,*[12] women "consume" the largest proportion of health services, average 100 per cent more visits each year to the doctor than men (when visits with children are counted), take 50 per cent more prescription drugs than men, and are admitted to hospitals much more frequently. Women also make up 70 per cent of all health workers in the U.S., 75 per cent of all hospital workers, and 60 per cent of all medical workers in the world. In stark contrast to these figures is the fact that only about 8 per cent of the physicians in the U.S are women.

Our Bodies, Ourselves sharply challenges the old relationship between doctor and patient. The book warns women: "The myth still persists that we meet the doctor as parent and child, and that you as patient must both obey and pay for the privilege. . . . If you cannot present yourself with conviction as an adult, and if you don't really feel fully entitled to argue or protest or get information and open communication, you will probably be treated accordingly." It adds, "Knowledge is power."*

POPULATION AND FAMILY PLANNING

The simplistic view of the population problem as a Malthusian race between the food supply and a rapidly growing population has given way to a widespread awareness that the issue is not quantity but the quality of life. According to this more comprehensive view, food and population growth rates are important but they are intertwined with legal, moral, ethical, and technological questions that concern man's relation to man, both present and yet to be born, and his relation to other living species and to his environment in general. In expanding from a limited, two-dimensional plane to a complex, value-laden, multidimensional model, the population problem is raising profound new issues concerning human rights, the status of women and minority groups, the moral responsibility of the rich for the poor, and, in the developed countries, the ethos of unrestricted economic growth. The significance of all this for family planning is a trend toward the promotion of its practice as a human right, in the interests of freedom of choice, and on the grounds of health, quite apart from or indeed in spite of any antinatalist effect. Nevertheless, in the developing countries with family planning programs, the antinatalist effect is more often welcome than not and is in fact the chief reason for government sponsorship of national programs.[13]

Conservative traditions and cultural modes have been in constant flux since the dawning of history, as individuals, tribes, and nations were in turn buffeted by new factors of modernization and development. Varying population growth rates are the product of the dynamic reaction between traditional cultural patterns and factors of modernization. In one era of history, or within a circumscribed geographic space, an extremely rapid population growth rate may have been desirable or even vital to the continuation and well-being of the species. Yet during another stage in man's history, or within another geographic area, the quality of life may require that the population grow at a slower pace.

Latin America

A brief assessment of current population problems (including a historical review) facing Latin Americans may help us to un-

*For further reading, see Sprague, Jane B.: Women and health bookshelf. American Journal of Public Health, *65*(7):741–746, July, 1975.

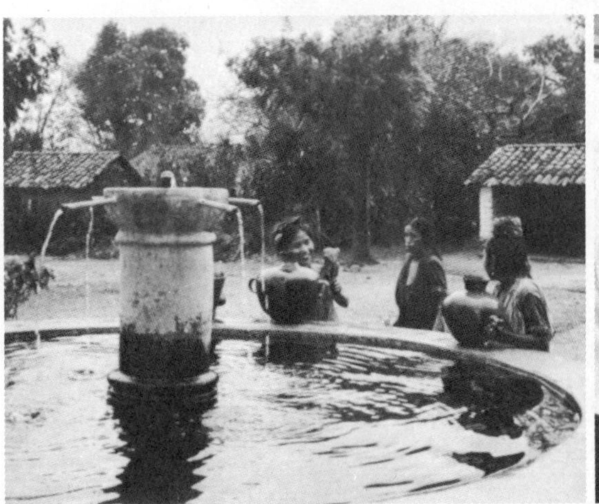

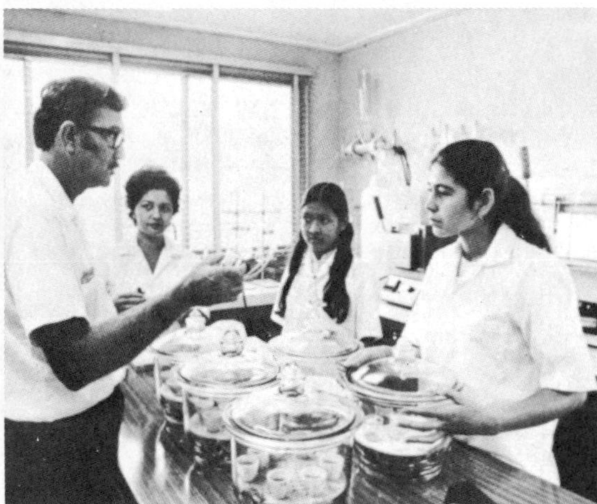

Figure 1–5 Improving the status of women in underdeveloped countries is essential to reduction of fertility rates. (From Ball, R.: Venezuelan family planning: winning government support. Population and Family Planning in Latin America, Report #17, Fall, 1973, p. 33. Victor Bostrom Fund for International Planned Parenthood Federation, 810 7th Ave., New York, N.Y.)

derstand similar problems existing in countries throughout the world.

The contact between Conquistador and Indian in Latin America wrought a frightful mortality on the latter. New diseases, against which the indigenous population had no immunity, decimated their numbers so that in Mexico, for example, within 80 years, the native population plummeted from 20 million to one 1 million. The same tragedy must have occurred elsewhere in the continent. Noting this decimation of the native population, the Conquistador, anxious to bring the land he had won into production and desperate for the labor to help him in both agriculture and mining, turned to two policies: a massive immigration of African peoples through the slave trade and a vigorous pronatalist policy for each inhabitant already in the region. The fertility of women was deliberately exploited to provide the labor that the newly discovered continent required.

The situation was not greatly affected by the long and bloody Wars of Independence. The defeat of the Spaniards failed to bring peace, since the wars had produced the warriors. To the demand for workers was added the demand for service in the armies that were fighting to slice up the continent. Men learned "machismo," and the ideal life for a man was to wander with the armies, changing women from day to day, and feeling no responsibility for whatever children might be engendered. If this pro-natalist policy, which for centuries maintained natality at a level above 50 per 1000 inhabitants, nevertheless seemed incapable of producing a substantial population growth, it is because adverse conditions maintained the death rates at an equally high level, especially for the first five

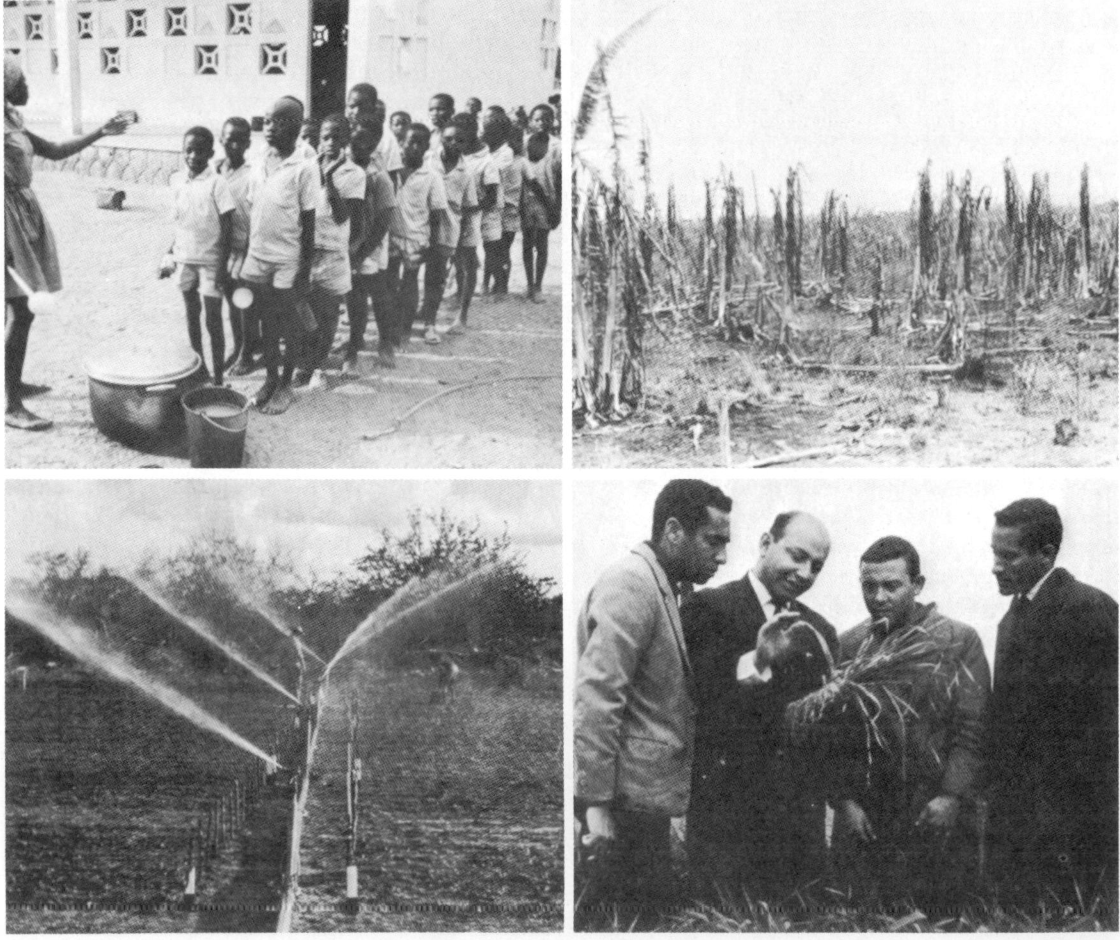

Figure 1–6 Rapidly growing populations with unmet nutritional needs, inefficient patterns of agricultural production, and the long-term energy crisis present a world challenge that can be surmounted only by cooperative international action. (From Harrar, J. G.: Nutrition and numbers. Food and Population, Report #19, Summer–Fall, 1974, pg. 5. Victor Bostrom Fund for International Planned Parenthood Federation, 810 7th Ave., New York, N.Y.)

years of life. Of every 100 children born, not more than 50 survived to the age of 5, and not more than 20 reached adulthood.

At the end of the 19th century, Latin America began to industrialize. This occurred first in those countries that had attained political peace and had important raw materials to be exploited. Argentina and Uruguay, for example, received a massive influx of European immigrants who arrived in Latin America with European technology and culture. These immigrants created in both countries conditions that were different from the rest of the continent.

The effects of the mortality decline which began in 1930 and continues right up to the present have been dramatically felt in the last decade. Infant mortality, which once killed 4 out of every 10 children before they reached the age of 1, declined so much that it has resulted in meager meals being divided among many mouths. Ignorant of any contraceptive method, many Latin American women have resorted to illegal abortion, a practice that has reached epidemic proportions. One-third of the hospital beds intended for obstetrical services are now used to care for women suffering from complications of illegal abortions, which often are performed by people with little medical education, using rudimentary techniques and paying little or no attention to antiseptic procedures.

The children suffer too. Not all children who survive to the age of 6 will find room in the schools. Educational systems expanding at the rate of only 1 per cent per year are incapable of meeting the educational needs of a population growing at a rate of 3 per cent per year. As a result, only 60 out of every 100 children of school age find room in the schools. The remaining 40 are condemned to illiteracy or to an incomplete education which will fit them only for unproductive work. For those who reach age 18, the prospects are even more somber. No economy possesses a growth rate that would enable it to create an annual 3 per cent increase in gainful employment. Many young men and women can expect only unemployment or part-time employment. The continual growth of an unemployed and underemployed population creates conditions that stimulate political instability and delinquency.

Food production, which the United Nations Food and Agricultural Organization reports as having increased considerably in the past decade, has still proved incapable of increasing the per-capita supplies in Latin America. Furthermore, evidence indicates that the per-capita consumption of animal protein is less today that it was 10 years ago. The increase in food production, although extraordinary, has not kept up with the population increase.

Reasons for Pro-Natalist Attidues in Various Countries

COUNTRIES	REASONS FOR PRO-NATALIST ATTITUDE
Philippines	More family members to work the land.
Latin America	Children will eventually care for the aged; Many children needed because some children will die at an early age; Religion (Catholic Church); Male machismo (masculinity and virility).
Bulgaria Hungary Romania Czechoslovakia	Declining birth rates, resulting in strict abortion regulations; increased birth grants and family allowances.
Afghanistan Burma	Emphasis on healthy children (Moslem country); Vast untapped resources and bountiful supplies of food; Children are regarded as priceless gems.
rural India	Belief that large families are the "happiest";

	Lack of knowledge, misinformation; Every male child means an extra pair of working hands—the law relates a family's land holdings to its size; High infant death rate (therefore necessary to have more children); Child marriage and dowry system for brides (tradition); Political attitudes and issues involving Hindus and Moslems do not emphasize family planning; Although India's birth rate is down, India's population is rising at a rate of 2.3 per cent a year, owing to a substantial reduction in the death rate during the same period.
Ecuador	Embarrassment and modesty of the women makes them reluctant to discuss family planning.
Canada	Tax laws favor "baby Canadians."
Africa, India, Latin America	Only a small number of women have access to family planning information and services; Family planning clinics are few and generally located only in urban areas; It is estimated that in the total developing world, population programs reach only 10 to 15 per cent of the women of childbearing age; Lack of trained personnel and facilities.
Nigeria	Fear of diminishing rural class.
Attitudes in other countries	Poor countries cannot be expected to reduce their population growth so that the richer ones can maintain a higher standard of living; Important condition for the fight against imperialism—by decreasing population, countries might succeed only in distributing their poverty among fewer and fewer people; Family planning campaigns are implied plots; Concentrate first on reducing maternal and child mortality.

Church and State

A pro-natalist tradition of 400 years, however, cannot be changed in one decade. Opposition groups have emerged in some countries against those who advance the cause of family planning. These include the Catholic Church, Marxists, and nationalists of an extreme conservative stripe. In spite of promoting responsible parenthood, the Catholic Church was initially opposed to the use of modern contraceptives. Today, this opposition is tending to disappear. Many pastoral letters from bishops to their parishioners emphasize responsible parenthood together with freedom of conscience in selecting methods for reducing fertility.

Marxist political groups, anticipating that the unemployment caused by excessive population growth will produce the revolution that will bring them to power, have accused the family planning movement of genocidal purposes encouraged by imperialist powers. But each day it becomes more difficult for them to maintain this position. At the present time, the socialist world includes the most successful family planning program known—that of the People's Republic of China. The birth rate in the Soviet Union is even lower than that in the United States.

The Chinese program promotes all recognized contraceptive methods. Legalized abortion by vacuum aspiration, a Chinese invention, is now spreading throughout the world.

Women's Desire for Family Planning

Conservative nationalist movements continue to argue that the strength of a country lies in the numbers rather than in the quality of its inhabitants. Against these movements which oppose family planning is a great and sympathetic force – the *women* of Latin America. Opinion surveys carried out in recent years demonstrate that 80 per cent of Latin American women are in favor of family planning and want no more than three children. The women of fertile age, who today number an estimated 70 million, will determine whether demographic catastrophe can be avoided, a catastrophe that would bring back death at a young age as the ultimate check on population growth.

The population growth rate is also being affected by cultural changes, particularly in the status for women. Many women in Latin America are being freed from purely domestic tasks and are being integrated into public life. Women are being offered a wider range of possibilities and options, so that they may combine their domestic duties with other occupational activities.

While the educational level among older women tends to be low, among the younger population the differences between the educational levels of men and women tend to diminish. Many countries in Latin America have shown an increase in the participation of women in productive employment. The liberation of women of middle and gradually of lower urban economic groups has been influential in transforming the traditional concepts of motherhood. This transformation has definite implications for population growth in the region, because education, social mobility, participation of women in the labor force, and access to the market place combine to depress the rate of growth of the population.

The number of governments that have issued proclamations favoring family planning is steadily increasing. Mexico in 1972 joined Colombia, Chile, and a number of Central American nations in endorsing family planning for health and other reasons. Mexico is establishing a broad family planning program for which it has sought the support of the United Nations Fund of Population Activities and the International Planned Parenthood Federation. Today few Latin American countries continue to cling to the traditional pro-natalist policies that were common under Spanish rule. Not every Latin American nation has openly endorsed family planning, but most of them do not usually interfere with family planning programs.

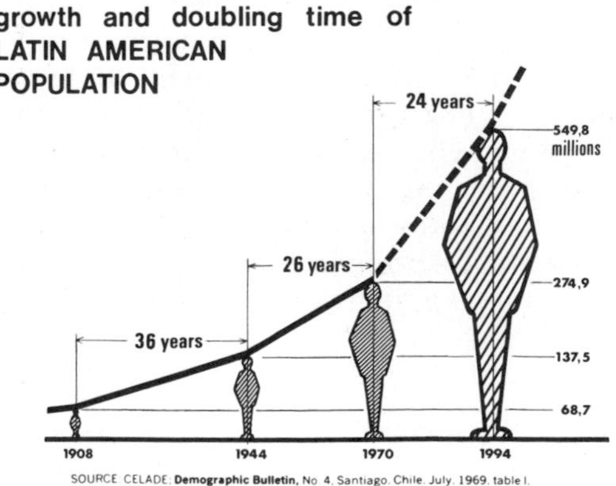

Figure 1–7 Growth and doubling time of Latin American population. (From Viel, B.: The demographic explosion in Latin America. Population and Family Planning in Latin America, Report #17, Fall, 1973, p. 14. Victor Bostrom Fund for International Planned Parenthood Federation, 810 7th Ave., New York, N.Y.)

Other Factors

Nevertheless, despite the favorable opinion of women of fertile age toward family planning and ebbing resistance from opponents of birth control, Latin America does not yet exhibit a clear tendency toward declining natality. The answer is obvious – of the 70 million women of fertile age, no more than 10 million are able to pay for the costs of contraceptive services. The other 60 million, although convinced of the advantages of contraception, are too poor to pay for such services. Governments in countries of low productivity, confronting immense expenditures for other services in health and education, lack the financial capacity to meet the total demand.

The ultimate determining factor of the changes in population growth is the individual judgment, conscience, and aspirations expressed collectively through the successive social organizations that comprise man's environment: the family, the extended family, the local and national communities. But the individual's responsibility is paramount. This fundamental principle, respecting the individual's beliefs and personal values, is reflected in the Declaration of Human Rights of the United Nations.

An equally basic human right is that of knowledge—of access to information that will enable the individual, within the family unit, to make responsible decisions concerning what family size will assure its members access to health, employment, and security. The desires and aspirations of all families define the social goals of the community: overall improvement in the quality of life and the well-being of the human family.

Emphasis on family planning to the exclusion or neglect of other programs of preventive medicine and public health in a developing country is unwise and generally ineffective. Because a reduction of the high mortality among young children is an important prerequisite for the success of family planning, there is a strong argument for combining family planning efforts with those health measures that will reduce such mortality. There are other reasons why maternal and child health, nutrition, and family planning programs should be brought together. Attendance at family planning clinics and the acceptance of family planning workers are often improved by such a policy. Also, there can be a significant increase in efficiency and a saving of time if the same health center staff can serve the multiple purpose of promoting nutrition, health, and family planning in women of child-bearing age, whether in the hospital, clinic, or home. In addition, maternal and child malnutrition can be reduced or avoided entirely by effective spacing of pregnancies combined with measures to control infections and assure adequate food supplies to vulnerable groups.

High birth rates, poor social and environmental conditions, low-birthweight babies, and high infant mortality and morbidity are all common and related in most poor countries. All the available evidence suggests that a necessary prerequisite for lowering birth rates is a decrease in infant and early childhood mortality rates. In areas where many children die, birth rates will remain high, but a fall in fertility follows within a few years after a visible decline in mortality. Thus, in many countries, preventing deaths in infancy and childhood deserves the highest possible priority as part of any effort to reduce birth rates and prevent excessive population growth.

The survival of infants and young children is determined more by their nutritional status than by any other single factor. Attempts to reduce mortality by extensive and expensive improvements in medical care alone, or even by broad-scale application of public health and sanitation measures, have had minimal results. Improved nutrition has been shown to be the most effective means for lowering deaths among infants and young children. Thus, the success of efforts to promote willingness to limit family size in underprivileged populations depends at least as much on improving nutrition of mothers and children as it does on making available sophisticated techniques for contraception. Moreover, success in efforts to promote family planning will have important favorable repercussions on the health of mothers and children in developing countries and on the adequacy of food supplies.

Package programs which include such mutually reinforcing components as nutrition, health education, sex education, family planning, immunization, and improvement of sanitation are needed. Social changes, aimed at raising the marriage age and providing increased opportunities for employment and education of women, and social security measures that will guarantee minimum living wages for families will, in the long run, produce greater impact on nutrition and wider acceptance of family planning than crash-feeding programs and family planning campaigns.

PLANNED PARENTHOOD . . . A BASIC HUMAN RIGHT

Planned parenthood works in the community to make the public aware of problems related to growth of population and to enable women to successfully plan their families so that there will be no unwanted births.

Clinical service:

Birth control service to all regardless of income.

Cancer detection test (Pap smear) for all patients.
Instruction in birth control methods.

Counseling:
Individual interview during clinic sessions.
Referrals and follow-up.
Unplanned pregnancy counseling program.

Community education:
Printed materials, media publicity, and exhibits.
Speaker's bureau.
Library of resource materials.
Information to the public on the population crisis.

Research:
To find better methods of conception control.

WORLD POPULATION PLAN OF ACTION[14]

A. The principal aim of development is to improve levels of living and the quality of life;

B. True development cannot take place in the absence of national independence; it also requires international cooperation, recognition of individual dignity, elimination of the consequences of natural disasters and elimination of discrimination in all its forms;

C. Population and development are interrelated;

D. Population policies are constituent elements of socioeconomic objectives;

E. Independent of these objectives, respect for human life is basic to all societies;

F. All couples and individuals have the right to decide freely and responsibly the number and spacing of their children and to have the education, information and means to do so;

G. The family is the basic unit of society and should be protected by legislation and policy;

H. Women have the right to complete integration in development, particularly by equal participation in educational, social, economic, cultural and political life;

I. Recommendations in the plan recognize the diversity of conditions within and among countries;

J. In forming population policies, consideration must be given to natural resources, the environment and all aspects of food supply; attention must be directed to the just distribution of resources and minimization of wastage;

K. It is increasingly important that international measures be adopted to deal with development and population problems, but they will not succeed unless the underprivileged can improve their living conditions;

L. The plan must be sufficiently flexible to take account of changing circumstances;

M. The objectives of the plan should be consistent with the United Nations Charter, the Declaration of Human Rights and the objectives of the Second United Nations Development Decade.

Population Trends in the United States

For the first time in history, American women are having only 1.9 children each, an insufficient number to replace the present population. (To do that, each woman in the United States would have to have an average of 2.11 children.) This does not mean instant Zero Population Growth (ZPG). Although young parents are not having enough babies to replace themselves, there are still more births than deaths in any given year. Unless the number of deaths increases drastically because of some catastrophe, the birth rate must stay down for a sustained period, 50 years or so, before a stationary population can be reached.

Long before ZPG is achieved, which some experts predict will happen around 2025, when they expect the population to be over 260 million, the United States may be a considerably different country than it is today. Reasons why the United States birth rate continues to fall include:

1. The development of an industrialized, mobile, affluent, educated, and urban society that led to the nuclear family;
2. Availability and dissemination of information regarding the Pill and other contraceptives; acceptance of sterilization procedures; and legalized abortion;
3. Radical decline of moral objections to birth control in the United States since World War II;
4. The increasing number of Roman Catholics and Orthodox Jews who do not consider contraception morally wrong;
5. The new wave of feminism, which helped keep birth rates down by encouraging women to challenge their traditional roles as mother and homemaker;
6. Growing concern over increased population and food, energy, and environmental crises,* quality of international life, and well-being of future children and the community;
7. Greater education and rapid increases in the number of working women;
8. Proliferation of services such as planned parenthood and free community clinics;
9. Economic causes such as inflation and recession;
10. Increasing number of family-life education courses in elementary and high schools.

Demographers, economists, and scientists are far from unanimous on whether ZPG is a good thing or not. Some fear that an end to population growth will produce social and economic stagnation; they stress that major American institutions, including the government and the free economy, require constant expansion. But most agree that the United States would be better off if its rate of expansion could be considerably slowed.

The most dramatic effect of a sustained low birth rate will be the aging of America. With a falling birth rate, the proportion of the young declines, while that of the elderly increases. Today the proportion of youths under 15 (about 30 per cent) to the whole population is almost 3 times as great as the proportion of people 65 and over (10 per cent). At ZPG, those under 15 and those over 65 would account for 20 per cent of the population each if the average American's life expectancy remains unchanged. If the expectancy goes up a few years, as it probably will, the proportion of older people will be even larger. Thus in the next 50 years the number of people over 65 will at least double. This phenomenon will have a profound effect on our way of life.

ZPG and the Future of the United States. While continuously expanding, the United States has been too caught up in responding to the ever-changing challenges of growth itself to effectively deal with such problems as mass transportation, housing, race relations, conservation, and the search for new sources of energy. The achievement of a stable population will not automatically provide solutions to these problems. In the next decade, perhaps children will be physically healthier, since wanted children generally receive better pre- and postnatal care than unwanted ones. Parents will be likely to take more interest in those children they decide to have. Demands upon the cities and the country's natural resources will be even greater than they are today, but perhaps ZPG can at least give the nation breathing space to meet its old challenges even as it faces its new ones.

FOOD AND POPULATION

The soaring demand for food, spurred by continued population growth and rising affluence, has begun to outrun the productive capacity of the world's farmers and fishermen. The result has been declining food reserves, increased food prices, intense international competition for exportable food supplies, and export controls on major foodstuffs by the world's principal food supplier—the United States.

The nutritional status of developing countries has many complicated interrelationships with the total development prob-

*With only 6 per cent of the world's population, Americans use one-third of its natural resources.

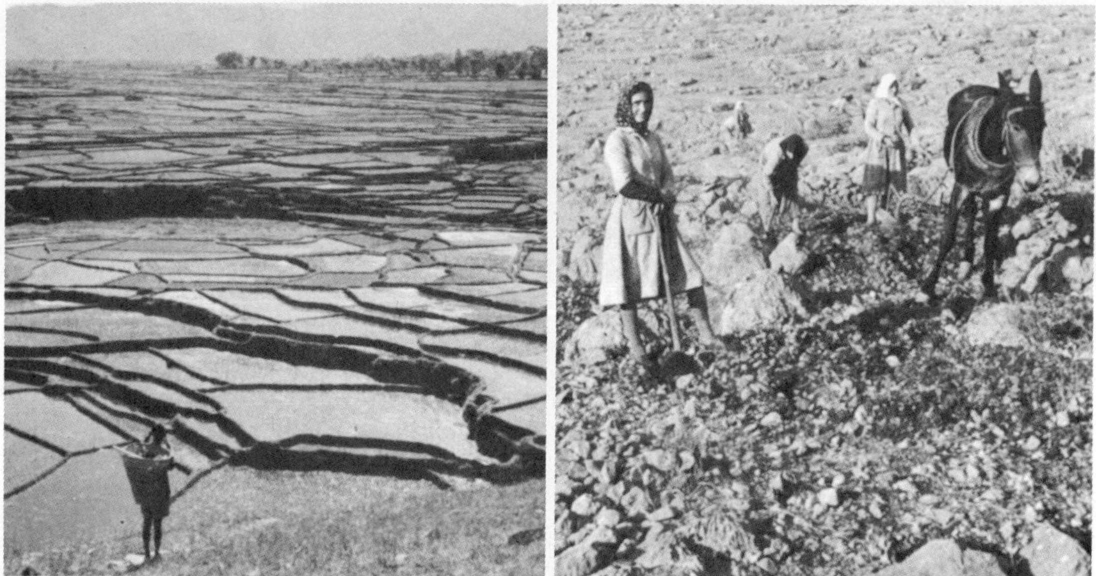

Figure 1–8 In many developing countries there is little additional available land that can be easily brought into production. (From Boerma, A. H.: The case for world food security. Food and Population, Report #19, Summer–Fall, 1974, p. 11. Victor Bostrom Fund for International Planned Parenthood Federation, 810 7th Ave., New York, N.Y.)

lems of these countries. The major source of difficulty is food production. Agricultural development is very slow in many developing countries because the methods used are largely elementary and very inefficient. There is a low level of capital inputs and low fertilizer usage. The fuel crisis has affected the fertilizer industry, thus increasing the cost of food production. In many places, the food crop production is entirely dependent on climatic and weather conditions. Whenever these conditions become adverse, man is exposed to the ravages of nature.

In addition to actual food production, storage and processing difficulties are immense. In tropical Africa, for example, between 10 and 30 per cent of all the grain is destroyed by insects and vermin. There is much waste also during the distribution and marketing of the food. The disproportionate investment by governments in cash crops has helped to aggravate the situation.

Education affects nutrition and food choice of an individual both directly and indirectly—indirectly, because the better educated a person is, the more likely he is to get a well-paying job and therefore be able to afford a variety of foods. With a good income, the percentage of a salary spent on foods is small and permits flexibility in times of rising food prices. The poorly paid do not have this flexibility and, as costs rise, tend to buy only the cheapest and least nutritious foods. More educated people are freer from taboos and have a better understanding of the reasons for the choices in food. Even the methods of food preparation used by those ignorant of nutrition can diminish the food values.

There is also the question of the "pecking order" of those who consume the food. In many homes in developing countries, for instance, the father has first choice of the more nutritious part of the food; the women and children come last. Where there is plenty of food and a wide variety of it, this hierarchy has very little influence on family nutrition and health, but where the food available is only marginally adequate for the family, then the distribution of that food within the home becomes a matter of some considerable importance. The women and children who need the most may get the least of the protein-rich sauces that generally accompany the staple rice or grain.

U.N. Declaration on Food and Population

The following Declaration on Food and Population, signed by over 2,200 distinguished citizens from over 100 countries, was presented to United Nations Secretary-General Kurt Waldheim on April 25, 1974:

1. Stocks of grain have hit an all-time low since the end of World War II. Surplus stocks formerly held in reserve have nearly been exhausted and no longer offer security against widespread hunger and starvation.

2. Food prices have reached new highs. Last year, despite a record world harvest, escalating demand nearly doubled grain prices. The increasing cost of food threatens to cause serious hardship for many people already spending most of what they have on food.

3. Less of the cheaper protein foods, which normally supplement grain diets, is available. The world's fish catch and per caput production of protein-rich legumes, the staple diet in many countries, have declined.

4. Food shortages have created serious social unrest in many parts of the world and are particularly severe in countries where hunger and the diseases that thrive on undernourished bodies are prevalent. This security has been aggravated by the consumption of more and more grain to produce meat, eggs and milk.

5. Mounting fertilizer and energy shortages are reducing food production in certain areas and increasing food prices. In this new and threatening situation, a bad monsoon in Asia (which could occur in any year), or a drought in North America (like those in the 1930's and 1950's), could mean severe malnutrition for hundreds of millions and death for many millions.[15]

This dangerously unstable world food picture, when seen against an unprecedented population increase, has created a great sense of urgency. The dangers of food shortages could remain a threat for the rest of this century, even if bumper crops in some years create temporary surpluses and even if the trend toward reduced birth rates becomes general throughout the world.

World food production in the years ahead must rise at least 2 per cent a year to keep pace with the present rate of population growth. But it must rise a good deal more if the world's people are to be provided with an adequate diet. This required annual increase in food production is considerably greater than that which occurred during recent decades—and seems to be increasingly harder to achieve each year. But unless there is this necessary and continuous increase in food production, there will be even more hunger and malnutrition and soaring food prices.

Plan of Action

It has been estimated that an organized, integrated plan of action involving all nations could, through improvements in conventional agriculture, at least double annual world food production within a reasonable period of years. If, during the same period, substantial progress is made toward zero population growth, then the lamentable and unreasonable gap between the affluent and disadvantaged nations could be substantially narrowed, with enormous benefits to all. In an organized world food plan, all of the nations concerned would have to accept the rationale of balanced production worldwide. Thus, decisions would have to be made as to where individual crops could be most efficiently and economically produced and how they could be appropriately distributed in exchange for other commodities produced elsewhere.

Americans, along with citizens of other affluent countries, can commit themselves, as many already have, to eating one really restricted meal a week and faithfully sending the money saved to UNICEF (the United Nations Children's Fund), CARE, Oxfam (an international famine relief agency), or to their church or community famine fund. With money, food can be bought and help given to the starving. Expanding voluntary efforts to feed the hungry will be a signal to the government to do more research in this area and to take a stronger position.

We also can radically and immediately reduce our consumption of meat. Cattle are very inefficient converters of grain into protein, and when range-fed cattle are moved onto feed lots, it takes 7 or 8 pounds of grain to add each pound of meat. In this way we turn cattle into competitors with humans for food. This is also true, to a lesser extent, of pigs and chickens. It has been estimated that reducing meat consumption by 10 per cent would release 12 million tons of grain a year for other uses. There isn't much grain in the world to feed people or animals. The United States and Canada at present possess the only massive grain reserves in the world.

We learn most about nutrition in times when food is costly or scarce. During the Second World War, millions of persons learned how to produce balanced meals that gave natural protection even with scarce and rationed foods. Research and health education will help us learn about sources of good protein other than meat, and perhaps help *prevent* conditions such as heart disease. It is urgent that we change our basic food habits and patterns. We shall have to devise new ways of eating more economically and at the same time more nutritiously, for the sake of children everywhere. A spirit of commitment, sharing, caring, and concern must pervade the people of all nations.

RELATIONSHIP BETWEEN POVERTY AND HEALTH

The relationship between family income and the health status of family members is well documented. For example, poverty reflects many unfavorable conditions associated with childbirth which affect survival of the infant. Women in the lower income classes become pregnant younger, are pregnant more frequently, and therefore have shorter intervals between pregnancies. They also continue childbearing in their late 30's and 40's, longer than do most middle class women. Poor women are more likely to have either late or no prenatal care. They have more complications of pregnancy and a great number of spontaneous abortions, premature babies, and stillbirths. They are also likely to have a higher maternal mortality rate. Infant and perinatal mortality rates are higher among the poor. An infant born in a poor family has only half the chance of a middle class baby of reaching his first birthday.

Children and youth in low-income families—as compared with those in middle income families—have a higher incidence of gastrointestinal infections, tuberculosis, venereal disease, speech disorders, and behavioral or learning disorders. They also have more mental illness, more dental disease, and a greater incidence of rheumatic fever. They have lower immunization rates against the common communicable diseases of childhood. Children in low-income families make fewer visits to a physician or a dentist, and a smaller percentage of children under 15 years old see a physician or a dentist within a year.

Poor families have little money for adequate nutrition. The diet of many pregnant or lactating women, of infants, and of children is inadequate because these families need various kinds of help: assistance in budgeting, food stamps, supplemental foods, and education in nutrition. Preschool children in low-income families have poor diets that are especially low in iron and vitamin C. These children are shorter than middle and upper class children and weigh less.

Families with low income are less likely to have health insurance. Low-income families frequently do not use health services, especially prenatal care, supervisory health care of seemingly well children, and family planning. This underutilization of services results from differences in perceptions and expectations of illness and health care.

Concomitantly, less health care is accessible to low-income families: factors such as distance from a clinic or hospital and transportation are important. Health care for low-income families is likely to be episodic rather than continuous, and these families are more likely to use hospital emergency rooms. Also, the delivery of care to low-income families is more likely to be fragmented—supplied through many kinds of clinics, with long periods of waiting for each clinic and loss of work because of the long waiting periods, which poor families can ill afford.

PROBLEM: ENVIRONMENT

Ecology

For every American, environmental decay has become a personal experience—a glass of water bitter with impurities, a mountain view obscured by haze, the acrid smell of industrial smoke or automobile exhaust, the boom of jets or the rumble of trucks piercing the 85-decibel level beyond which noise can do damage to the ear. Every nation, large and small, is confronted with environmental hazards. The Rhine River may be even more polluted than the Ohio. The archipelagos of the South Pacific are threatened by a plague of starfish that consume their vital barrier reefs.

The word "ecology" derives from the Greek *oikos,* meaning house. Ecology, therefore, really means the study of houses, or, in a broader sense, of environments. Ecologists examine the precarious relationships between living things and their surroundings.

To understand ecology—and the present dilemma that man has created for himself—one must first understand the concept of "ecosystem." An ecosystem is the sum total of all of the living and nonliving parts that support a chain of life within a selected area. The four primary links in the chain are: (1) *Nonliving matter,* the sunlight, water, oxygen, carbon dioxide, organic compounds and other nutrients used by plants for their growth. (2) *The plants,* ranging in size from the microscopic phytoplankton in water up through grass and shrubs to trees. Those organisms convert carbon dioxide and water, in a process called photosynthesis, into carbohydrates required both by themselves and by other organisms in the ecosystem. (3) *The consumers,* higher organisms that feed on the producers. Herbivores, such as cows and sheep, are primary consumers. Carnivorous man and such animals as the wolf feed upon the herbivores and are secondary consumers. (4) *The decomposers.* These tiny creatures—bacteria, fungi and insects—close the circle of the ecosystem when they break down the dead producers and consumers and return their chemical compounds to the ecosystem for reuse by the plants.

Although growth and decay are going on simultaneously and continuously in an ecosystem, they tend to balance each other over the long run, and thus the chain is said to be in equilibrium. Nonhuman environments have a remarkable resiliency; as many as 25 or even 50 per cent of a certain fish or rodent population might be lost in a habitat during a plague or disaster, yet the species will recover its original strength within one or two years. It's man-made interference or pollution that can profoundly disturb the ecosystem and its equilibrium.

An example: In the shallow waters of the Pacific Ocean off Los Angeles, sea urchins—small sea animals—are enjoying a population boom, thanks to the organic materials in sewage being washed out to sea. Normally, the sea urchins' population levels are tied to the quantity of kelp on the ocean bottoms; the animals die off when they have eaten all the kelp, thus allowing new crops of the seaweed to grow. But now that the sewage is available to nourish the sea urchins, the kelp beds have not had a chance to recover. In many places, the kelp, for which man has found hundreds of uses, has disappeared altogether.

There is, of course, no way of calculating the exact effects of the loss of kelp on its particular ecosystem. This has been one of the disadvantages of ecology; there have been precious few quantitative measurements to support the ecologists' empirical observations. But this is rapidly changing. At scores of universities across the nation, there are projects under way to determine just what happens in a fresh-water ecosystem or a coastal estuary. Perhaps the most comprehensive and exhaustive of these is the International Biological Program, a 57-nation cooperative effort to study distinctly different environments (for example, grassland, three types of forest, desert, and arctic tundra) and the life web of each. The scientists, working at instrumented field sites, are trying not only to determine who eats what and with what effect, but also to measure the total energy flow in each system, starting with the sunlight and rain falling on the designated site and ending with the total amounts of herbage and animal weight growth.

American ecologists also are conducting a series of studies of environmental programs that focus on man—Eskimos, migrant people, American Indians—and nutritional adaptations to specific climatic zones.[16]

Highly technological societies such as the United States, of course, feel a powerful temptation to call upon new technology to cure the ills wrought by the old. Many scientists are hopeful of finding technical solutions for many pollution problems. Examples are cleaner fuels for automobiles, with more efficient engines to make up for the loss in volatility, and recycling systems to make use of the wastes that are currently pumped into streams or thrust into the sky. But there is a danger here. Often these technological solutions have a way of creating new environmental problems of their own: nuclear power plants avoid smoke pollution but cause heat pollution (temperature rises that upset the balance of life) in the rivers they use for coolants; detergents used to disperse oil slicks do more damage to marine life than does the oil itself.

For this reason, a number of today's environmental reformers conclude that mankind's main hope lies not in technology but in abstinence—fewer births and less gadgetry.

Environment and Population

Environmental problems are a product of population growth, the demands popula-

ECOLOGY

Ecology is a field that has to do with the relationships between living things and their environment.

An ecological point of view is a new way of looking at the world, with man inseparable from his surroundings. This way does not come easily to us, for throughout most of Western civilization the emphasis has been on man against nature. This old way of looking at things no longer works. Our past mistakes have caught up with us.

A new age has come and our survival depends upon creating a balanced ecological system for ourselves on the Earth.

SOME POPULATION-RELATED PROBLEMS

Pollution:
- Air: smog, noise, fallout
- Water: sewage, thermal, industrial
- Land: garbage, litter, junkyards, mining, roads
- Biological systems: pesticides, bioactive chemicals, radioactivity

Crowding:
- Tension
- Indifference – cheapening of life
- Traffic jams, crowding of airways
- Blight – slums
- Crime
- Congested parks

Shortages:
- Minerals
- Energy – oil, gas, coal, uranium
- Water
- Land – open space, forests, agriculture, recreation

Facilities:
- Food
- Housing
- Schools
- Hospitals, medical care
- Services – fire, police, courts
- Cultural
- Transportation – highways, mass transit, airports

Quality of Life:
- Space – hiking, thinking
- Quiet
- Wilderness, wildlife
- Individuality

tion makes on natural resources, and the availability of those resources. Each government must examine its population policies in relation to its environmental carrying capacity, in order to effectively plan how to achieve the standards and quality of life to which its citizens aspire.

Urban areas, particularly in the developing world, are growing at approximately double the rates of overall population growth, which is producing a fundamental transformation in the structure of human society. A largely rural world will by the end of the century have been converted into a largely urbanized world. The implications of this are enormous and have not been fully appreciated or taken into account either by people or by their governments. Most of the growth is taking place in the existing urban areas, where the pressures on the resource base are intensifying at a rate that clearly cannot continue in many cases.

The prospect of large-scale eco-catastrophes in the urban areas of the developing world is a very real and imminent one, because current rates of urban growth are going beyond anything ever experienced in the industrialized world, and are straining the ability of governments with limited resources to provide even the most basic services.

In the developing countries, environmental problems can to some extent be seen as resulting from the lack of development itself. The contamination of water supplies by sewage, the degradation of soil through overgrazing and misuse, rampant urbanization, and the mushroom growth of shanty towns are some of the serious problems that rapid population growth poses for the development process.

In the more developed countries, population growth combined with affluence and technology has led to environmental problems which, though often different from those experienced in the developing world, are not less serious.

The energy crisis has dramatically

shown that we cannot continue our careless and wasteful practices of exploitation and use of natural resources. We must move from an ethic of high consumption and abundance to one of scarcity and conservation. The energy shortages and high prices will reduce the rate of growth of fossil fuels, limit the size of automobile engines, and require more prudent and safe use of the automobile. The scarcity factor will also lead to development of alternative sources of energy, some of which might be kinder to the environment.

Many advisors agree that we do not need any further manifestations of the tendency of the industrialized world to proselytize the developing world on the need for them to limit their populations in the interest of the world community, while the affluent continue to use a disproportionate share of the world's resources and produce a disproportionate share of its pollution. We do need an awareness by all nations of the importance of population policies designed to limit growth and a series of practical ideas as to how they can do this; mobilization of greater resources to provide assistance to those who want it; and development of new technologies and sociological approaches that sound population policies require.

What Can One Person Do?

To understand the complexity of the problem, ask yourself the following questions:

Am I willing to—

1. Adopt if I want more than two children?
2. Use public transportation, share car rides, and ride bicycles?
3. Educate myself about pesticides I am using in my garden?
4. Use returnable containers to decrease the refuse problem?
5. Use my consumer power to apply pressure for constructive change?
6. Become aware of conservation activities?
7. Take the time to write my opinions to legislators, television stations, newspapers, educators, and industry?
8. Read *The Population Bomb* and related books?
9. Encourage the government to examine its priorities of goals?
10. Look at my personal goals freshly in terms of this crisis?

QUESTIONS FOR DISCUSSION

1. What are some of the problems in your community related to public health services?
2. What advancements have occurred in public health medicine in the past 10 years?
3. List the 10 leading causes of death in (a) your community, (b) your state, (c) the United States.
4. What factors have been responsible for lowering the death rate from tuberculosis? Polio?
5. What are some of the problems of population control in the U.S. and other countries? What are some of the suggested population control methods?
6. What are the major community health problems in the eastern United States? The South? The West?
7. Discuss the major health problems on your campus. What preventive steps could be taken?
8. What are some of the things that medical research has done for our health today? Does research need to continue?
9. What do you consider to be the leading health problems of today?
10. What is the average lifespan in the United States? How has it changed since the 1600's, and what has brought about this change? How does it compare with that in other countries?
11. What are the leading causes of death in the U.S. for these age groups: 1–6, 7–14, 15–21, 22–35, and over 35?
12. Interest in physical fitness has increased markedly the past 10 years. Give instances of research in the field and discuss a couple of good programs.
13. What epidemics have occurred in your community in the past 50 years?
14. How would you define health? Public health? Preventive medicine?
15. Discuss the growing interest in ecology, both pro and con.
16. Why do many people ignore the basic principles of good health and public health? What can be done about this attitude?
17. What can be done to meet the challenge of attaining good health for all the people in the U.S.?

QUESTIONS FOR REVIEW

1. How long has it taken us to recognize the total consequences of cigarette smoking and how much longer to take action?
2. What other two elements besides our failure to

comprehend long-term and adverse health effects of innovations have led to the current health dilemma?

3. What must be done to our health services on account of the increased mobility caused by movement from rural to suburban and urban areas?
4. List three services that come under the heading of clinical service for planned parenthood.
5. What are the four primary links in the chain of life of an ecosystem?
6. What is an alternative solution to technology in alleviating our pollution problems?
7. Why are technological solutions not always a good answer to the pollution problems of today?

REFERENCES

1. Dubos, R.: Five who care. Look, *34*:34, April 21, 1970. © Look Magazine.
2. Wald, G.: Man and the environment. Time, the Weekly Newsmagazine, May, 1969, p. 22. © Time, Inc., 1969.
3. Governing Council of the American Public Health Association: Resolutions and position papers adopted October 23, 1974, New Orleans, La.
4. Ibid.
5. Dubos, R.: *Mirage of Health.* Garden City, N.Y., Doubleday & Co., 1960, p. 24.

5a. Winslow, C. E. A.: *The Evolution and Significance of the Modern Public Health Campaign.* New Haven, Yale University Press, 1923.

6. Hanlon, J. J.: *Public Health Administration and Practice.* St. Louis, C. V. Mosby Co., 1974, p. 4.
7. Bauer, W. W.: *Your Health Today.* New York, Harper & Row, 1960, p. 4.
8. Oberteuffer, D.: *School Health Education.* New York, Harper & Row, 1960, p. 4.
9. Report of the President's Commission on the Health Needs of the Nation. Vol. 1. Washington, D.C., Superintendent of Documents, 1951, p. 1.
10. Saward, E.: The organization of medical care. Scientific American, *229*(3):169, September, 1973.
11. A conversation with Malcolm Todd. Healthnews (California Department of Health), *2*(8):4, February, 1975.
12. The Boston Women's Health Book Collective: *Our Bodies, Ourselves.* New York, Simon & Schuster, 1973.
13. Nortman, D., and Hofstarter, E.: *Report on Population/Family Planning, #2.* 5th ed. Population Council, September, 1973, p. 3.
14. United Nations: *Declaration on Food and Population,* 1974.
15. Ibid.
16. Odum, E. P.: Dawn for the age of ecology. Newsweek, *75*:35, January 26, 1970. © Newsweek, Inc., 1970.

SUGGESTED READING

A bookshelf on family planning. Amer. J. Publ. Health, *64*(7):666–673, July, 1974.

Bennet, J. P.: *Chemical Contraception.* London & New York, Macmillan, 1975.

Berelson, B. (ed.): *Population Policy in Developed Countries.* New York, McGraw-Hill, 1975.

Berg, A.: *The Nutrition Factor.* Boston, The Brookings Institution, 1974.

Borgstrom, G.: *The Food and People Dilemma.* N. Scituate, Mass.: Duxbury Press, 1975.

Brooks, S. M.: *Ptomaine: The Story of Food Poisoning.* Cranbury, N.J., A. S. Barnes & Co., 1974.

Brown, L. R., and Eckholm, P.: *By Bread Alone.* New York, Praeger (for Overseas Development Council), 1974.

Curtin, S.: *Nobody Ever Died of Old Age.* Boston, Little, Brown & Co., 1972.

Elliott, K., and Knight, J.: *Human Rights in Health.* Ciba Foundation Symposium 23. New York, American Elsevier Publishing Co., 1974.

Ford Foundation: *A Time to Choose: America's Energy Future.* Final report by the Energy Policy Project. Cambridge, Mass., Ballinger, 1975.

Freedman, R.: *The Sociology of Human Fertility: A Bibliography.* New York, Holt, Rinehart & Winston, 1974.

Frejka, T.: Reference tables to "The Future of Population Growth." Washington, D.C., Population Council, 1974.

Gubrium, J. F. (ed.): *Times, Roles, and Self in Old Age.* New York, Behavioral Publications, 1975.

Hobson, W. (ed.): *The Theory and Practice of Public Health.* 4th ed. New York, Oxford University Press, 1975.

Hollingsworth, D., and Russel, M. (eds.): *Nutritional Problems in a Changing World.* New York, Halsted Press, 1974.

Hunter, J. M. (ed.): *The Geography of Health and Human Disease.* Chapel Hill, University of North Carolina Press, 1974.

International Planned Parenthood Federation (England): People, *1*(1):40, October, 1973; *1*(2):16, January, 1974.

Jaco, E. G. (ed.): *Patients, Physicians and Illness.* 2nd ed. New York, Macmillan, 1972.

Kent, D. P., Sherwood, S., and Kastenbaum, R. (eds.): *Research Planning and Action for the Elderly.* New York, Behavioral Publications, 1972.

Libby, J. A.: *Meat Hygiene.* 4th ed. Philadelphia, Lea & Febiger, 1975.

Magnuson, W. G., and Segal, E. A.: *How Much for Health?* Washington and New York, Robert B. Luce, 1974.

Manocha, S. L.: *Nutrition and Our Overpopulated Planet.* Springfield, Ill., Charles C Thomas, 1975.

McCoy, T. L. (ed.): *The Dynamics of Population Policy in Latin America.* Cambridge, Mass., Ballinger, 1974.

The Medicine Show. Revised edition by the editors of Consumer Reports. New York, Pantheon, 1974.

Osborne, B. M., et al.: *Foundations of Health Science.* Boston, Allyn & Bacon, 1968.

Percy, C. H.: *Growing Old in the Country of the Young.* New York, McGraw-Hill, 1974.

Pfeiffer, E. (ed.): *Successful Aging.* Durham, N.C.: Duke University Center for the Study of Aging and Human Development, 1974.

Piotrow, P. T.: *World Population Crisis: The U.S. Response.* New York, Praeger, 1973.

Planned Parenthood Federation of America: *Contraceptive Technology 1974–75.* New York, 1975.

Poleman, T., and Freebairn, D. (eds.): *Food, Population and Employment.* New York, Praeger, 1974.

Rosow, I.: *Socialization to Old Age.* Berkeley, University of California Press, 1975.

Schulberg, H. C., Sheldon, A., and Baker, F.: *Program Evaluation in the Health Fields.* New York, Behavioral Publications, 1970.

Shima, M. E. (ed.): *Advances in Voluntary Sterilization.* New York, American Elsevier Publishing Co., 1974.

Sipple, H. L., and McNutt, K. W. (eds.): *Sugars in Nutrition.* Conference, Nashville, Tenn., November 8–11, 1972. New York, Academic Press, 1974.

Smolensky, J.: *A Guide to Child Growth and Development.* Dubuque, Iowa, Kendall/Hunt, 1974.

Stein, Z., et al.: *Famine and Human Development.* New York, Oxford University Press, 1975.

Wilner, D. M., Walkley, R. P., and Goerle, L. S.: Introduction to Public Health. 6th ed. New York, Macmillan, 1973.

You and Your Health; 12 articles published by Council on Family Health, 633 Third Ave., New York, N.Y. 10017.

CHAPTER 2

Historical Aspects of Community Health in the United States

During the middle of the nineteenth century, major health problems confronted citizens of growing states and cities throughout America. Many of these problems, such as water pollution and smallpox epidemics, were prevalent at approximately the same time throughout the entire United States. With the discovery of the causes of certain diseases; the production of vaccines, serums, and antibiotics; the organization and cooperation of official, voluntary, and community health agencies; and the application of the principles of sanitation and health education, the number of communicable disease cases and deaths declined. This decline was slow, but it appeared uniformly throughout the country. As one epidemic subsided, however, there was usually another of a different nature to take its place.

EARLY HEALTH LEGISLATION

Health measures in towns and communities were slow to develop; early settlers were primarily interested in building their homes and developing land. Woods Hutchinson, M.D., Secretary of the first Oregon State Board of Health, reflected the situation when he stated:

> . . . it was rather hard to stir up popular interest in public hygiene or to secure adequate appropriations for its promotion. . . . This of course was only natural, . . . because our people were so closely engaged in building the railroads, clearing the forests, breaking the prairies and providing housing and shelter in a wild, new country, that there seemed to be no time for consideration of "doctors' fussiness" about sewage and ventilation and food inspection and quarantine. . . .[1]

The population of cities and states was small, and regulations concerning public health were not demanding at that time. For example, the original city charter of Portland, Oregon, adopted in 1851, made no provisions regarding public health except to empower the city council to enact ordinances and bylaws concerning the "good government of said corporation, and the health, morals, and safety of its citizens."[2] In 1853 the council was given additional authority "to make regulations to prevent the introduction of contagious and other diseases into the city; to establish hospitals and make regulations for the government of the same; and to secure the general health of the inhabitants."[3] Furthermore, citizens were reluctant to accept public health reforms, and public health legislation was difficult to establish.

The first state health department was organized in Louisiana in 1855. Massachusetts organized the second state health department in 1869.[4] Shortly after, other state health departments were established in rapid succession. It is interesting to note that the fear of importation of specific diseases was directly responsible for the creation of many state and local health departments. For example, the Louisiana State Board of Health was founded to prevent the further inroads of yellow fever. An epidemic of the same

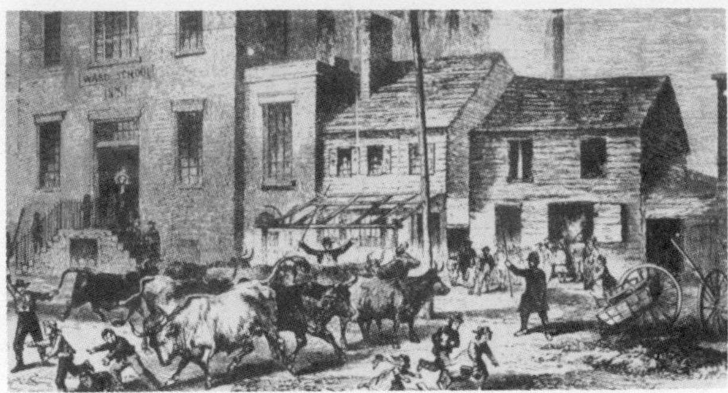

Figure 2–1 Protesting unsanitary conditions, an indignant 1865 report on New York City included this print showing a slaughterhouse next to a public school. In these slaughterhouses, the accompanying text said, "Large collections of offal are allowed to accumulate... constantly undergoing decomposition." The report, which also complained about fearful overcrowding and neglected sewers, led to the formation of the Metropolitan Board of Health in 1866. (From Dubos, R., and Pines, M.: *Health and Disease*. New York, Time-Life, 1971.)

disease in the southern states prompted Congress to create a National Board of Health in 1878 in order to combat the disease. The Board was unorganized and ineffective, however, and was discontinued in 1888. Fear of the importation of cholera from Europe was directly responsible for the National Quarantine Act of 1893.[5] Importation of diseases by steamers arriving from Europe and the Orient constantly threatened the coastal states, especially during the periods of heavy immigration from 1880 to 1910. In addition, a new manner of disease importation occurred in 1883 when cross-country rail communication was completed.

COMMUNICABLE DISEASE CONTROL

The major activities of local and state health departments from 1850 to 1920 involved communicable disease control and sanitation.[6] The chief methods of controlling communicable diseases included escorting diseased persons to the town pesthouse (i o-lation), quarantine, and fumigation to destroy bacteria. However, quarantine failed as the major measure of communicable disease protection because health officials and others did not understand the epidemiological principles of the disease carrier in relation to the spread of infection. Furthermore, the modes of transmission and periods of incubation and communicability of infection were not well understood. Because pride and business interests were involved, citizens in most communities falsely denied that diseases existed in their midst.

Although tuberculosis and typhoid fever claimed many lives, smallpox was the most dreaded disease ever to invade the country. Smallpox instilled fear and terror in the public mind because of its loathsome appearance and disfiguring consequences, its extreme communicability, and its high fatality rate. Smallpox vaccine had been introduced as early as 1796, but mass vaccination programs were not conducted in the United States until the 1920's because many individuals were slow to accept the preventive measure. With the application of measures for community sanitation and health education, and with an increasing proportion of the population protected by immunization against typhoid fever, diphtheria, and smallpox, the number of cases and deaths from these communicable diseases gradually decreased.

THE PLAGUE AND THE SQUIRREL SQUAD

When plague first appeared in San Francisco at the beginning of the twentieth century, merchants were paralyzed by fear that the commercial interests of the port would be irreparably damaged, and the governor and even the State Board of Health refused to admit that the disease did, in fact, exist.

But after the entire State was threatened with a quarantine by the U.S. Public Health Service, opposition by those who contended no plague existed died out. In 1902, a new governor appointed a new secretary of the Board of Health. He had no offices, no other paid staff, and a total budget of $1,500.

Californians driven by fear of the plague began to demand a stronger State Public Health organization (121 cases of plague with 113 deaths were reported between 1900 and 1904). Plague struck Los Angeles in 1923, the last such epidemic in the state. Occasional cases now reflect the endemic nature of the disease in California. The Board, working with the USPHS and the San Francisco Board of Health, undertook systematic rate extermination and sanitary measures.

Plague control, including mass shooting of the ground squirrel host, continued through the thirties and is still practiced today.

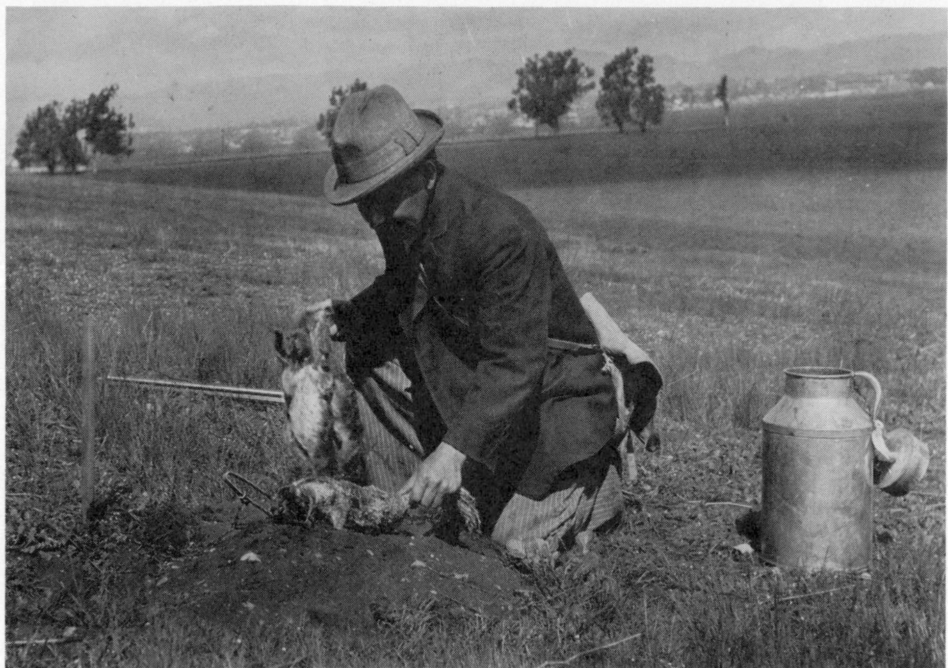

Figure 2–2 Plague trapper. (From California's Health, Centennial Issue, 1870–1970, State Dept. of Public Health, Vol. 28, December, 1970.)

During the next six years, fundamental legislation setting the general pattern of the present organization was passed. Emphasis was placed on local health departments and the forerunner of the California Conference of Local Health Officers was formed. The State bureau of vital statistics, the State hygienic laboratory and the State food and drug laboratory were authorized by legislation.[7]

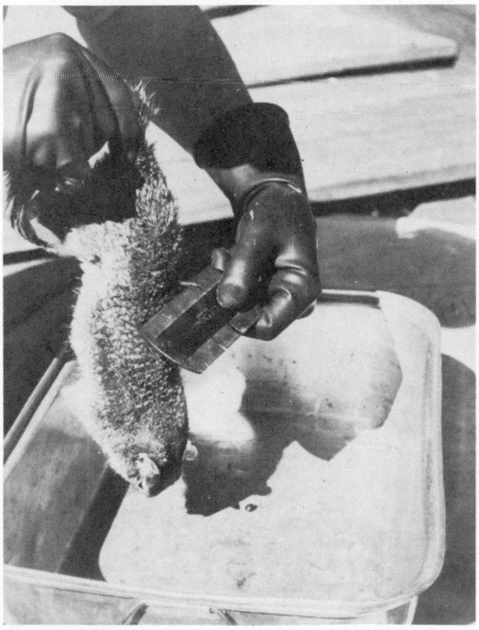

Figure 2–3 Fleas carry plague and squirrels carry fleas. (From California's Health, Centennial Issue, 1870–1970, State Dept. of Public Health, Vol. 28, December, 1970.)

CHOLERA

Cholera was the classic epidemic disease of the nineteenth century, as plague had been of the fourteenth. When cholera first appeared in the United States in 1832, yellow fever and smallpox, the great epidemic diseases of the previous two centuries, were no longer truly national problems. Yellow fever had disappeared from the North, and vaccination had deprived smallpox of much of its menace. Cholera, on the other hand, appeared in almost every part of the country in the course of the century. It flourished in the great cities, New York, Cincinnati, Chicago; it crossed the continent with the forty-niners; its victims included Iowa dirt farmers and New York longshoremen, Wisconsin lead miners and Negro field hands.

It was not until 1883 that Robert Koch, directing a German scientific commission in Egypt, isolated the organism that causes cholera—*Vibrio comma,* a motile, comma-shaped bacterium. Once they find their way into the human intestine, these vibrios are capable of producing an acute disease which, if untreated, kills roughly a half of those unfortunate enough to contract it. Cholera, like typhoid, can be spread along the

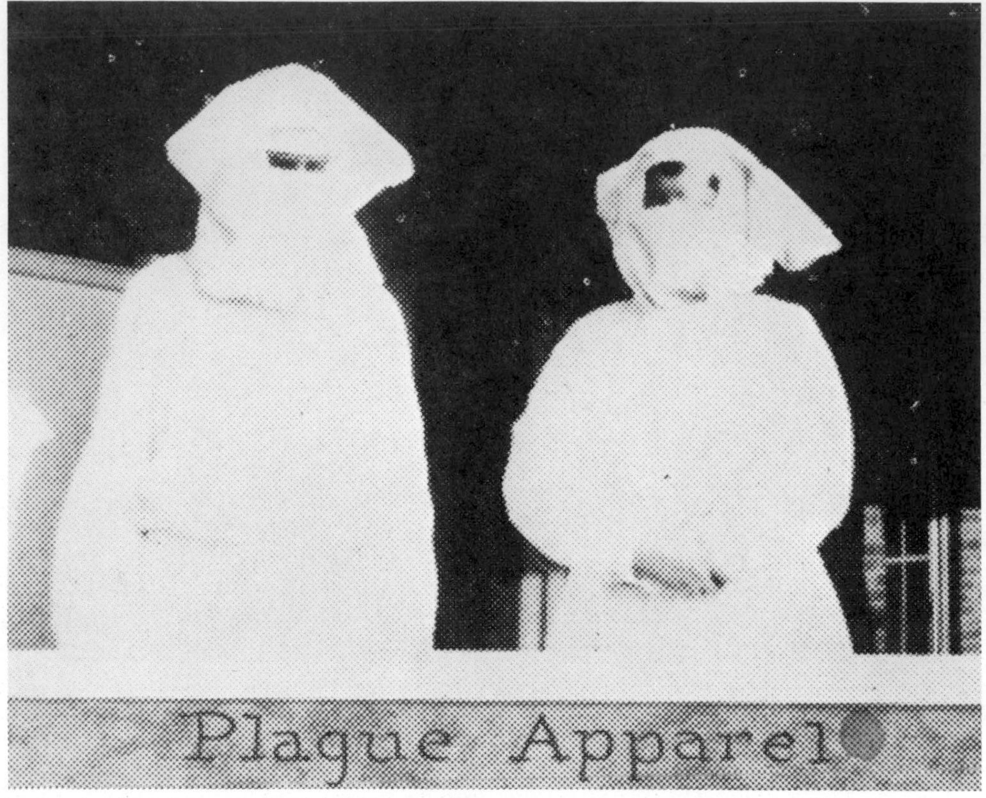

Figure 2–4 Plague apparel. (From California's Health, Centennial Issue, 1870–1970. State Dept. of Public Health, Vol. 28, December, 1970.)

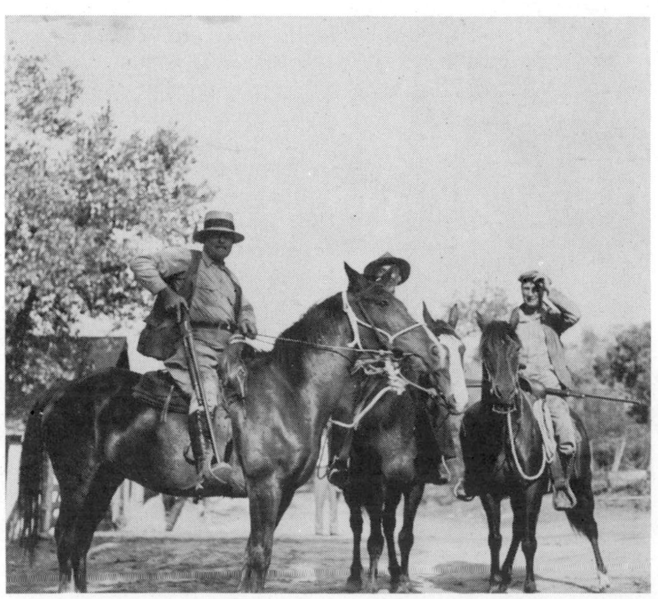

Figure 2–5 The Squirrel Squad. (From California's Health, Centennial Issue, 1870–1970, State Dept. of Public Health, Vol. 28, December, 1970.)

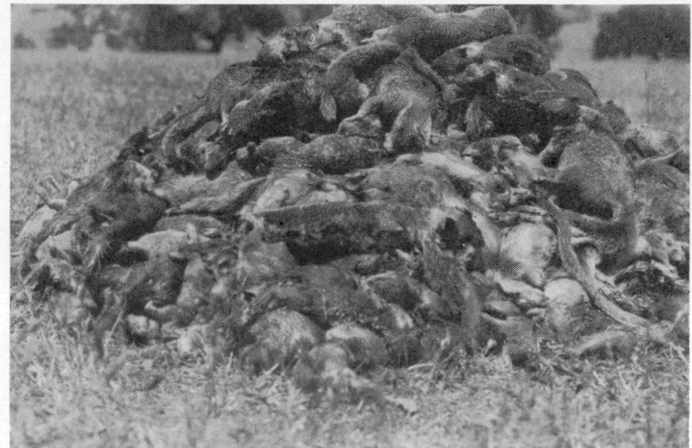

Figure 2-6 Dead squirrels. (From California's Health, Centennial Issue 1870–1970, State Dept. of Public Health, Vol. 28, December, 1970.)

pathway leading to the human digestive tract. Unwashed hands or uncooked fruits and vegetables, for example, are frequently responsible for the transmission of the disease, though sewage-contaminated water supplies have been the cause of the most severe, widespread, and explosive cholera epidemics.

Though never endemic in this country, cholera returned to the United States four times after its initial appearance in 1832–34. After this two-year visit, North America was free of the disease until the winter of 1848–49. Between 1849 and 1854, however, no 12-month period passed without cholera appearing in some part of the United States. Then the disease disappeared as abruptly as it had in 1834; it was not to return until 1866.

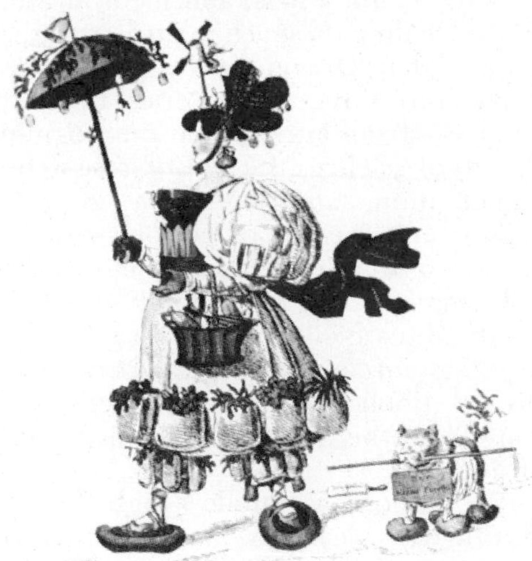

Figure 2-7 A cholera costume, this attire appeared in a Viennese cartoon during a serious cholera outbreak in the 19th century. It simply exaggerated the many desperate notions people had about how the disease was transmitted and how best to ward it off: outsized shoes to avoid contamination from the ground, bottles of medicine in a basket, bags of aromatic herbs to overcome toxic vapors, a windmill to dispel evil air. Even the lady's dog wore shoes and carried a syringe. (From Dubos, R., and Pines, M.: *Health and Disease.* New York, Time-Life, 1971.)

The means of improving the public health seemed clear enough. Clean streets, airy apartments, a pure supply of water, were certain safeguards against epidemic disease. And by 1866, advocates of sanitary reform could in justification of their programs point to the discovery of John Snow, a London physician, that cholera was spread through a contaminated water supply. The matter-of-fact, empirical approach to epidemiology which enabled Snow to confirm his theory of the disease's transmission would have been rare a century before. He had, as well, new theories of disease causation, of the very nature of disease, available to him. Cholera in 1849, for example, was assumed by the great majority of physicians to be a specific disease, whereas in 1832, most practitioners had still regarded cholera as a vague atmospheric malaise and had vigorously disavowed the very existence of specific disease entities.[8]

POPULATION CHANGES

The rapid change of population from a rural to an urban economy was a major factor in molding the pattern of public health organization, administration, and services in the United States. From 1880 to 1910, many cities grew rapidly as a result of heavy immigration and a high birth rate. Urbanization of cities without proper understanding of the problems and hazards of crowded community life was one of the most important problems at that time. Hygienic measures that were quite adequate in sparsely settled areas were completely unsuited to the city dweller. Thus, sickness and the communicable disease death rate increased to such a degree that specific sanitary problems were eventually recognized, faced, and finally solved. Another key to the high communicable disease fatality rate in the United States from 1880 to 1910 related to the age distribution of population. At that time, epidemics were most fatal to children and young adults, and over 40 per cent of the nation's population was under 20 years of age.[9]

MILK AND WATER CONTROL

Impure milk and water accounted for a large number of communicable disease cases and deaths from 1850 to 1915. Epidemics of typhoid fever, diphtheria, scarlet fever, diarrhea and enteritis, tuberculosis, and other diseases were traced directly to impure milk or water supplies. Although state and city health officials devoted a great deal of time to those major public health problems, it was not until the period from 1910 to 1915 that legislation was enacted and organized campaigns were conducted to remedy this situation. Education, scientific advances, chlorination, pasteurization, and sanitary improvements also contributed to pure milk and water supplies. A sharp decrease in the number of communicable disease cases and deaths resulted.

EXPANSION OF STATE AND LOCAL HEALTH DEPARTMENTS

Although the states as sovereign powers had the responsibility and authority to guard the health of their citizens, they granted permission to separate local communities to establish local public health laws and to solve their own public health problems. In 1797, for instance, Massachusetts granted state-wide authority to towns and cities to establish local health services, but the state itself assumed no responsibility for public health affairs. Even such matters as maritime quarantine were carried out by the local community.[10] The creation of state boards of health, however, brought about a great improvement of public health within the state. The boards, originally designed to control communicable diseases by interstate and intrastate quarantine methods, rapidly expanded their services and personnel in an effort to prevent disease and prolong life. Bacteriology laboratories were established to aid in the diagnosis of communicable diseases. More efficient systems of reporting and recording vital statistics were introduced. In addition, county health boards were organized, health officers were appointed, and each county was required to meet certain minimum public health standards and regulations. Funds granted by private health foundations and the United States Government enabled the state boards of health to expand their services, activities, and programs. Through the years, prevention of disease and prolonging of life were stressed.

The growth of public health is also closely linked to the disease patterns of different historical periods and the success with which medical science was able to cope with these threats to the community. In an excellent analysis of the concept of preventive medicine, Anderson and Rosen delineated five patterns of disease over the past one thousand years: leprosy and plague, louse-borne disease and syphilis, gastrointestinal diseases, tuberculosis and the communicable diseases of childhood, and cardiovascular-renal diseases, malignant neoplasms, and accidents. They conclude this list by predicting a sixth pattern—the psychosomatic diseases—characterized by the emergence of social and psychological factors as major forces in health, illness, and medical care.

Paralleling these changing patterns of disease, Alan Gregg divides public health history into three major eras: the era of authority—from antiquity to the beginnings of medical science; the era of research, experimentation, and treatment of specific diseases; and the era of ecology—the modern era, now just beginning, in which the whole patient and the community, rather than the disease entity, becomes the focus of medical attention. Many of the current problems in public health and medical care spring from the difficulties of this period of transition.

For tomorrow, public health has set itself a further ideal proclaimed by the World Health Organization in its declaration of the goal of public health as "a state of complete physical, mental and social well-being and not merely the absence of disease or infirmity." This is admittedly an ideal, which like any statement of a creed would be difficult to define in exact terms, but it does set the standard for the basic philosophy of the modern public health movement.[11]

Pestilence and plague have had dra-

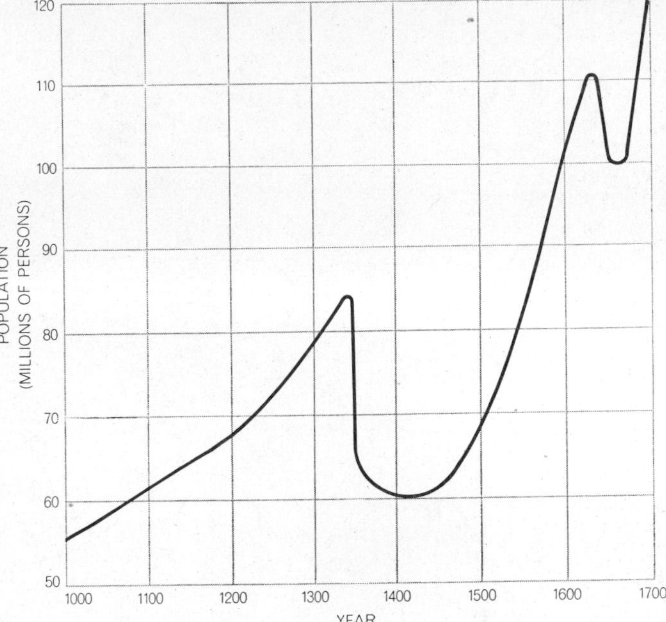

Figure 2–8 The impact on population from recurrent plagues in Europe. For more than 300 years after 1347 the plagues checked the normal rise in population; sometimes, as in the 14th and 17th centuries, they resulted in sharp reductions. The figures are derived from estimates by students of population; actual data for the period are scarce. (From The Black Death, by W. L. Langer. Copyright © 1964 by Scientific American, Inc. All rights reserved.)

matic effects on the course of history. As Zinsser points out, typhus fever was largely responsible for Charles V's becoming ruler of the Holy Roman Empire. The decline of early European civilization may be traced to the advent of the malaria mosquito in Greece in 400 B.C. Yellow fever defeated France's attempt to build the Panama Canal. The tsetse fly helped to shape the political division of southern Africa in the late nineteenth century. To a large extent, the prosperity and security of modern nations continue to depend upon the health and physical well-being of their citizens.

Bubonic plague, or Black Death, had demographic, economic, psychological, moral, and religious effects on the people of Europe. Before the Black Death ravaged Europe in 1348–1350, the continent had enjoyed a period of rapid population growth, territorial expansion, and general prosperity (Figs. 2–8 and 2–9). After the pandemic, Europe sank into a century or more of economic stagnation and decline. The most serious disruption took place in agriculture.

The English Catholic prelate and historian, Francis Gasquet, in a study entitled *The Great Pestilence,* tried to demonstrate that the Black Death set the stage for the Protestant Reformation by killing off the clergy and upsetting the entire religious life of Europe. This no doubt is too simple a theory. On the other hand, it is hard to deny that the catastrophic epidemics at the close of the Middle Ages must have been a powerful force for religious revolution. The failure of the Church and of prayer to ward off the pandemic, the flight of priests who deserted their parishes in the face of danger, and the shortage of religious leaders after the Great Dying left the people eager for new kinds of leadership. And it is worth noting that most if not all of the Reformation leaders—Wycliffe, Zwingli, Luther, Calvin, and others—were men who sought a more intimate relation of man to God because they were deeply affected by mankind's unprecedented ordeal by disease. The profound disturbance of men's minds by the universal chronic grief and by the immediacy of death brought fundamental and long-lasting changes in religious outlook. In the moral and religious life of Europe, as well as in the economic sphere, the forces that make for change were undoubtedly strengthened and given added impetus by the Black Death.[12]

Thus, we see that the history and philosophy of public health are an inherent part of the growth of civilization. This history has had its periods of enlightenment and darkness, of humanity and inhumanity; and public health's prevailing norms and values reflect both this historical background and current social, economic, political, and medical forces. With its roots in medical science, public health is dedicated to the use of the scientific approach, both for the discovery of new knowledge and for the evaluation of ex-

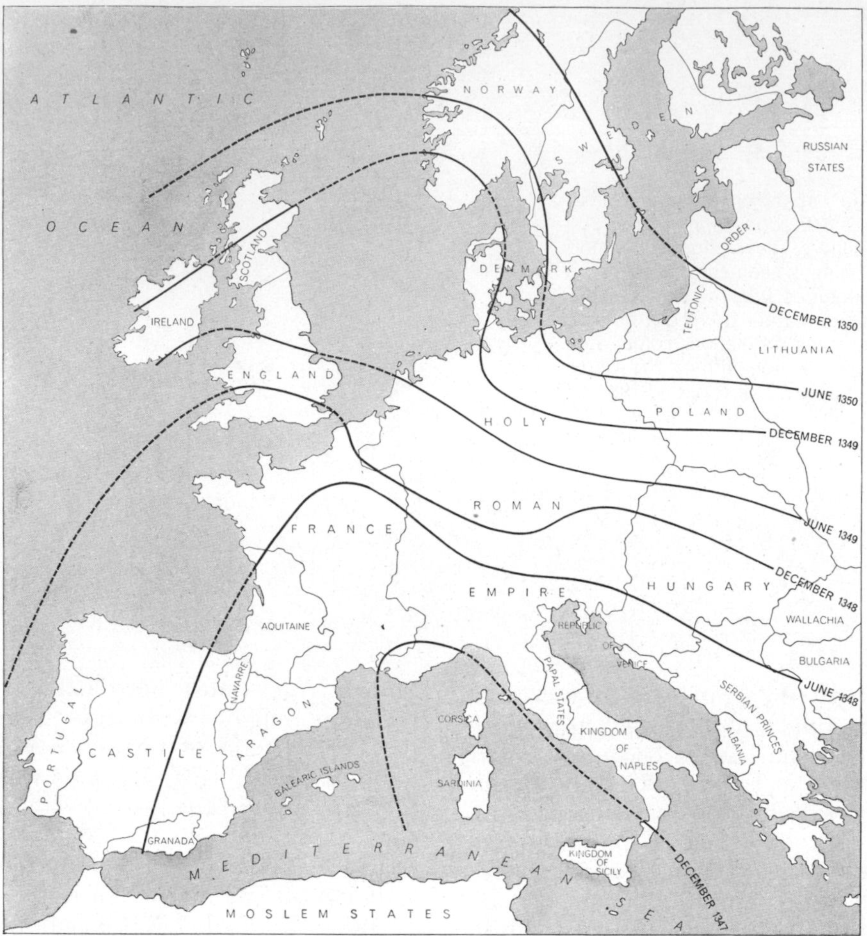

Figure 2–9 Approximate chronology of the Black Death's rapid sweep through Europe in the middle of the 14th century is indicated on this map, which shows the political divisions as they existed at the time. The plague, which was apparently brought from Asia by ships, obtained a European foothold in the Mediterranean in 1347; during the succeeding three years only a few small areas escaped. (From The Black Death, by W. L. Langer. Copyright © 1964 by Scientific American, Inc. All rights reserved.)

isting programs. Men in public health believe that research is basic to progress and they constantly seek to advance the frontiers of new knowledge by means of medical, epidemiological, and more recently, behavioral science research. As a field of action, they are imbued with a strong sense of public service and are highly aware of their professional and moral responsibilities to improve the health of the public. Public health workers approach this task with a value system that presupposes the ability of man to control himself and his environment and, through planning, to attain a state of better physical and mental well-being.[13]

MAJOR CONTRIBUTIONS TO PUBLIC HEALTH

Eighteenth Century—The Beginning of Public Health

The rising industrialization during the eighteenth century was reflected in medicine by the work of *Bernardino Ramazzini* (1633–1714), who studied epidemics and wrote on trade diseases and industrial hygiene. *Johan Peter Frank* (1745–1821) wrote a treatise on public health, covering sewerage, water supply, sex hygiene, and food and drug inspection. This was the beginning of public

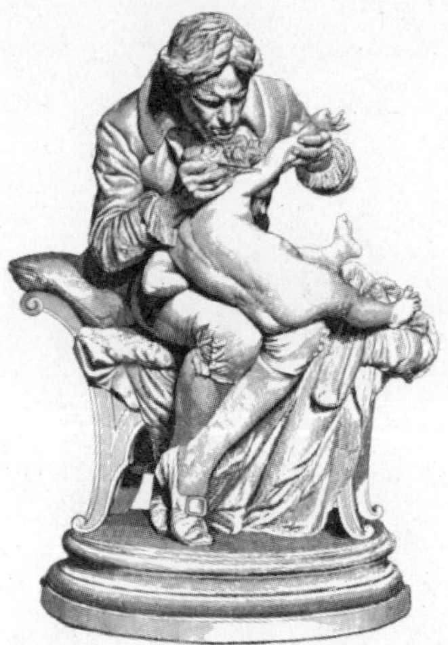

Figure 2–10 Vaccination of a boy by Dr. Edward Jenner marked his discovery of a smallpox preventive, and catapulted him from the obscurity of a rural British practice into international fame. The sculpture above commemorates the day in 1796 when Jenner took cowpox pus from the sore on a milkmaid's hand and smeared it on scratches on a healthy boy's arm, and found a safe method of immunization against the long-feared disease. (From Dubos, R., and Pines, M.: *Health and Disease.* New York, Time-Life, 1971.)

health. *Edward Jenner* (1749–1823) observed that milkmaids who frequently had a mild skin rash (cowpox) were free of smallpox. He undertook the vaccination of patients, using material from the arms of the milkmaids. He demonstrated that vaccination with material from the sore of cowpox protects against smallpox (Fig. 2–10). This idea was accepted in Europe and in America, and the incidence of smallpox declined. Although there was opposition to the idea, it established the principle of immunity, and made preventive medicine a possiblity.

The greatest American physician of the period was *Benjamin Rush* (1745–1813), a signer of the Declaration of Independence. He gave careful accounts of disease, described dengue fever, and prepared a monograph on insanity. He was particularly interested in yellow fever. He showed that focal infection might cause severe sickness, finding that the extraction of decayed teeth sometimes would relieve distressing symptoms. *Benjamin Franklin* (1706–1790) also pursued medical interests, inventing bifocal lenses and a flexible catheter, and proposing the treatment of paralysis by electricity. In addition he founded the Pennsylvania Hospital and made observations on gout, sleep, deafness, and the death rate among infants.

Nineteenth and Twentieth Centuries

Louis Pasteur. The greatest name in French medicine was *Louis Pasteur* (1822–1895), a chemist who was shocked by the horrors of rabies. Pasteur found that the spoilage of wine was caused by microorganisms that grow in the wine. Similarly, he found that beer spoils as a result of contamination with microorganisms. In both cases he observed that heating destroys the organisms. His work resulted in the "germ theory" of disease and the famous process of "pasteurization," which is now used everywhere to assist in preventing disease. Pasteur made an extensive study of diseases of silkworms in southern France. He found that these diseases could be controlled by keeping the silkworms in a sanitary environment, which inhibited the growth of microorganisms.

Pasteur's first clinical demonstration was concerned with anthrax of sheep. He discovered a motile organism in the blood of diseased sheep and prepared from it a material for vaccination. He predicted that his vaccine would prevent the disease in sheep. The test was completely successful. Pasteur's success in preventing rabies was dramatic. His most famous case was that of an Alsatian boy, Joseph Meister, who had been bitten by a mad dog. Pasteur undertook the preparation of a vaccine from the brain of the rabid dog. Although filled with fear at the possibility of failure, he injected the vaccine. The child did not develop rabies. He stayed and worked with Pasteur and became his lifelong servant and technician. After this spectacular success, institutes for the preparation of antirabies vaccine were established all over the world. The bacterial origin of infectious disease was universally accepted, and a new science, bacteriology, was born.

Bacteriology. The field of bacteriology was investigated widely by the Germans. *Robert Koch* (1843–1910) found methods for the isolation of specific microorganisms, so they could be grown in pure culture. Koch introduced the technical methods of bacteriology, and discovered the tuberculosis organism. His vaccine for tuberculosis, however, was not successful. Meanwhile *Armauer Hansen* (1841–1912) discovered the organism causing leprosy, and *Edwin Klebs* (1834–1913) found the club-shaped bacillus which causes diphtheria. *Joseph Leidy* (1823–1891) of Philadelphia described intestinal parasites and began the study of their life cycles. His discovery of *Trichina spiralis* in the muscles of pigs made possible prevention of trichinosis by cooking all pork products.

Yellow Fever. The conquest of yellow fever was the most significant event in American medicine during the latter period of the nineteenth century. Yellow fever had been brought to the Americas by shiploads of infected African slaves. For many years it devastated coastal cities of the United States and made pest-holes of the seaports of Central and South America. During the Spanish-American War, yellow fever was a serious problem among American troops in Cuba. A special commission of the army medical corps was appointed, with *Walter Reed* (1851–1902) as chairman. Reed studied the theories of the Cuban physician, *Carlos Finaly de Barres* (1833–1915), who insisted that yellow fever was transmitted by mosquito bites. This theory was tested and proved to be correct. Immediate methods were instituted to control the spread of mosquitoes. The results were impressively effective.

Large-scale methods of mosquito control, by draining swamps and removing places where mosquitoes breed, resulted in the eradication of yellow fever from the New World. Under the direction of *William Gorgas* (1854–1920), a Surgeon General of the United States Army, mosquito control and the prevention of yellow fever made possible the building of the Panama Canal. Methods of sanitation introduced by Gorgas were based on the accumulated knowledge of the prevention of infectious diseases acquired during the nineteenth century.

Malaria. The close of the century also was marked by the beginning of the conquest of malaria (Fig. 2–11), which had taken a heavy toll of life all over the world for centuries. There is evidence that it may have contributed to the decline of some of the powerful Mediterranean civilizations. Medical writers have discussed this possibility frequently, and various theories have been developed. The introduction of cinchona bark in the seventeenth century, and the isolation of quinine from the bark in the nineteenth, had provided a semblance of control. However, such measures were effective only as a cure, not as a preventive. Little was known of the cause of the disease until *Ronald Ross* (1857–1932) found malaria organisms in the red blood cells. He traced the course of the parasite, and confirmed its

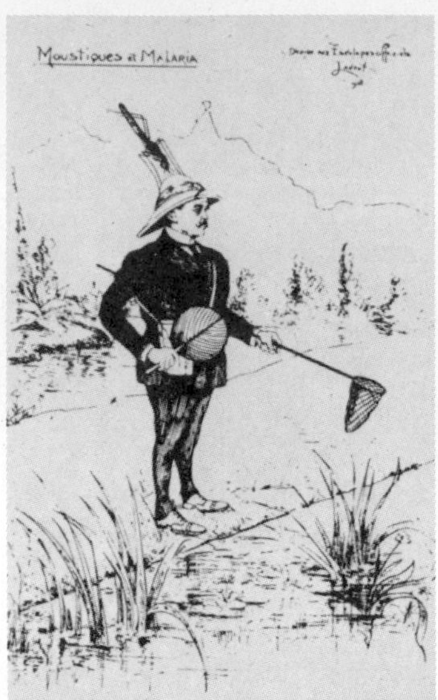

Figure 2–11 Malaria's conqueror and the mosquito he defeated are affectionately caricatured in a 1908 cartoon published by a newspaper in the British colony of Mauritius. The colony's hero was Sir Ronald Ross, a British Army surgeon, who had proved nine years earlier that malaria was transmitted by the bite of the *Anopheles* mosquito, and not by *mal aria* (Italian for "bad air"). Invited to Mauritius in the Indian Ocean, where malaria had spread with increasing ferocity for 40 years, Ross ordered the mosquito-breeding swamps to be drained, and thus halted the epidemic. (From Dubos, R., and Pines, M.: *Health and Disease.* New York, Time-Life, 1971.)

transmission by mosquitoes. Thus, mosquito eradication became one of the most important measures in the field of preventive medicine during the twentieth century.

PUBLIC HEALTH AND MEDICAL ADVANCES

An infant born in 1900 had a life expectancy of 50 years. Today, because of tremendous strides made in public health and medicine, an infant has before him a life span of more than 72 years. When the early state boards of health were created, epidemics of typhoid fever, smallpox, diphtheria, and bubonic plague threatened the country. Tuberculosis and typhoid fever were leading causes of death at that time. Today, smallpox has also disappeared from the country, plague is an extremely rare disease, and significant reductions have been made in the incidence of and deaths from typhoid fever, diphtheria, whooping cough, measles, scarlet fever, tuberculosis, the dysenteries, and the tick-borne diseases. The period from 1900 to the present has revealed a steady

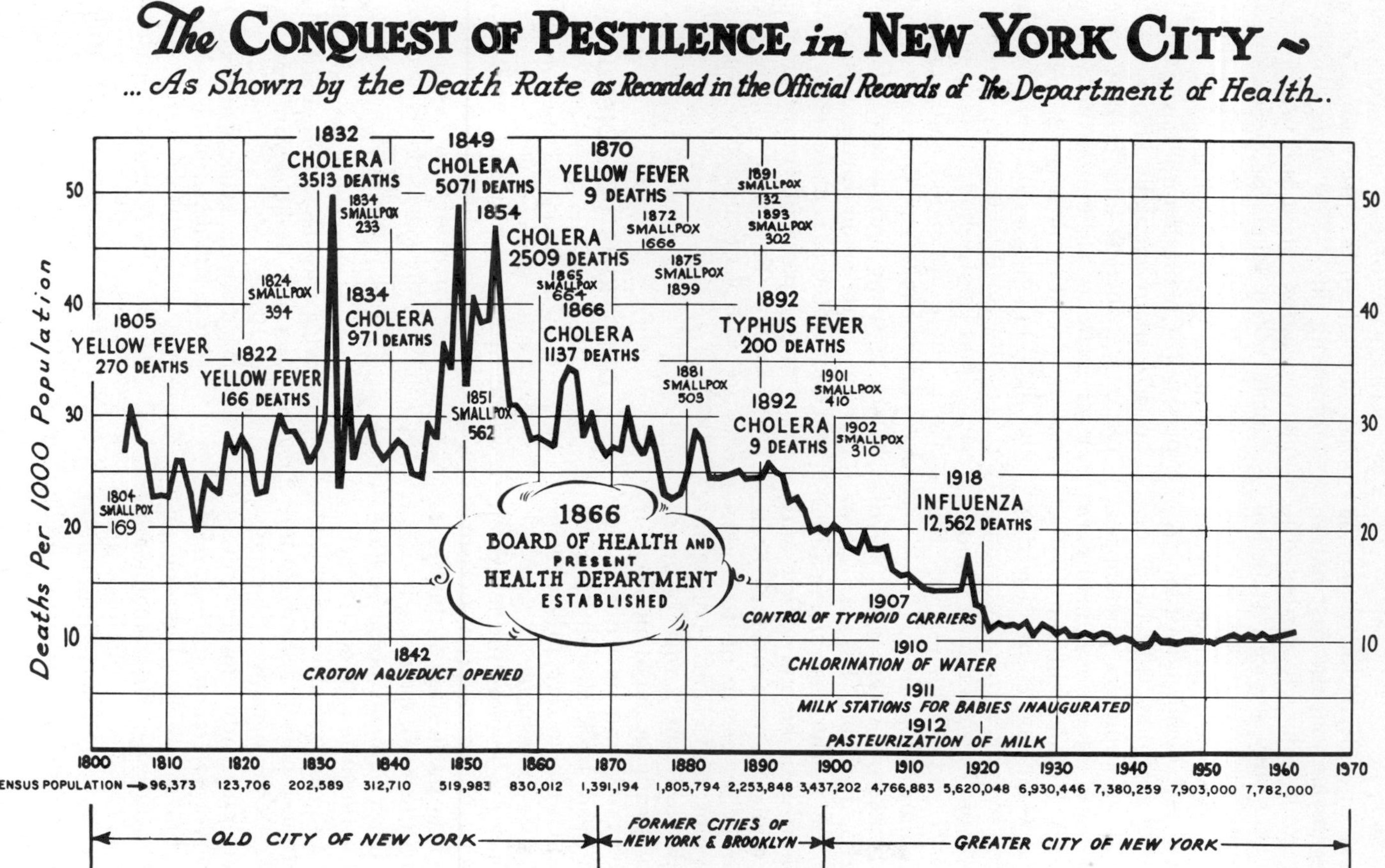

Figure 2–12 The conquest of pestilence in New York City. (From Baumgartner, L.: *Report of the Department of Health, the City of New York, for the years 1959–1960*, p. 177.)

decline in the communicable disease morbidity and mortality rates. Maternal mortality has been reduced to a great extent, and infant deaths have been cut from 99.9 per thousand in 1915 to 16.8 per thousand today.

The success of official and voluntary health agencies throughout the first half of the twentieth century is largely attributed to public health laboratory services, statistical services, environmental sanitation services, immunizations, antibiotics, public health nursing services, and health education. Although communicable diseases have decreased, tuberculosis, influenza pneumonia, venereal diseases, and infectious hepatitis are among those still prevalent in the 1970's. Therefore, health officials emphasize that continued success in the control of communicable diseases cannot be maintained without continued effort and evaluation of the effectiveness of control measures.

Medical advances in recent years have been rapid and remarkable. Physicians are trying to solve the mysterious interrelation between the mind and the body. New and ingenious devices and instruments have been developed to probe the secrets of the body's cells, tissues, organs, and glands. For example, we can now study the nature of genes and chromosomes with the aid of an electron microscope. Reflecting and recording tapes attached to the head, neck, shoulders, arms and legs of a walking man reveal the precise pattern of muscular movement.

Other devices probe more hidden body activities. Modern electronics can measure minute variations in the beating of the heart, (even before birth), which makes early diagnosis of many heart ailments possible. Electrodes attached to the head can record fluctuations in the brain's electical activity and thus detect certain brain tumors or lesions. Radioactive isotopes, mammography, thermography, and brain and body scanners reveal tumors and abnormal chemical changes taking place within the body. High voltage x-ray machines can destroy these malignant tumors. Ultrasonic waves, radium, and electric currents can also destroy unwanted cells or tissues. Devices like the heart-lung machine can take over a patient's entire circulation while the heart is immobilized. During the operation, accessory devices monitor the patient's pulse and blood volume, add coagulants or anticoagulants as needed, and maintain a complex state of anesthesia that can be altered instantly. Slender bladelike rods can scrape diseased or clogged blood vessels and thereby add years to the life of the patient with atherosclerosis.

Discovery of new antibiotics and drugs has also aided in preventing disease and prolonging life. New drugs have helped many persons defeat and prevent such previously noted killers as pernicious anemia, subacute bacterial endocarditis, tuberculosis, rheumatic fever, syphilis, and high blood pressure. Chemotherapy has given a ray of hope to many mentally ill patients, needle-plagued diabetics, and certain cancer and heart patients. Rheumatism and arthritis may be cured or at least alleviated to allow our aged to enjoy a fuller and happier life.

As longevity increases, people require more and more body replacement parts. Today there are blood banks, bone banks, eye cornea banks, cartilage banks, and artery banks, to name only a few. There replacement parts are taken during autopsy, frozen, and then stored as replacements for diseased or damaged parts of future patients. Surgeons believe that they will eventually be able to transplant most types of tissue and organs.

QUESTIONS FOR DISCUSSION

1. (a) Name five leading causes of death in the United States in 1900.
   (b) Name in order four leading causes of death in the United States today.
   (c) Give five reasons for this change, if any.
   (d) What effect does this change have upon community health programs?
2. What major factors led to the establishment of local and state health departments?
3. (a) What were the two major activities of local and state health departments from 1850 to 1920?
   (b) What are the major activities of local and state health departments today?
4. "Despite major public health gains in the United States, new health problems have appeared." Discuss this statement.
5. Name four leading causes of death in your community today.
6. Name four leading causes of death in your state today.
7. Is there a possible link between the epidemics of the late Middle Ages and the Reformation?
8. Trace the history of the Tuberculosis Association and of the American Cancer Society.

9. What are the outstanding achievements of the American Public Health Association? When was it founded?
10. Report on the history of public health in your community and in your state.

QUESTIONS FOR REVIEW

1. Why were so few health measures taken in the early settler days of towns?
2. What was one of the major reasons for the development of the first state health departments (especially in the coastal states)?
3. What were the two major activities of local and state health departments from 1850–1920?
4. What was the most dreaded disease ever to come into the country? How long did it take for a mass vaccination program against this disease to come into effect?
5. From the years 1850–1960, what was the major cause of the epidemics of typhoid fever, diphtheria, scarlet fever, diarrhea, enteritis, tuberculosis, and other infectious diseases?
6. Besides the fact that the population was moving into more crowded urban areas, what was another reason for the high communicable disease fatality rate in the U.S. from 1880–1910?
7. Explain how the state boards of health improved and expanded their services.
8. What is the sixth pattern of disease predicted by Anderson and Rosen in their analysis of the concept of preventive medicine?
9. List the three major eras into which Alan Gregg divides public health history.
10. What other effects besides physical ones did the bubonic plague or Black Death have on the people of Europe?
11. Public health is dedicated to the use of the scientific approach in what two areas?
12. What was the life expectany of an infant in 1900? What is the life expectancy of an infant born today?
13. Name four communicable diseases that are still prevalent today.

REFERENCES

1. Oregon State Board of Health: *Fourteenth Biennial Report to the Governor.* Salem, 1931, pp. 5, 6.
2. Oregon Laws, 1851, p. 18.
3. Oregon Laws, 1853, p. 9.
4. Smillie, W. G.: *Public Health: Its Promise for the Future.* New York, Macmillan, 1955, p. 319.
5. Mountain, J. W.: The history and function of the United States Public Health Service. *In* Simmons, J. S. (ed.): *Public Health in the World Today.* Massachusetts, Harvard University Press, 1949.
6. Chapin, C. V.: *A Report on State Public Health Work Based on a Survey of State Boards of Health.* Chicago, American Medical Association, 1916.
7. *California Health, Centennial Issue, 1870–1970.* California Department of Public Health, *28*:22, 1970.
8. Rosenberg, C. E.: *The Cholera Years.* Chicago: University of Chicago Press, 1962, pp. 22–26.
9. Dublin, L. I.: *The Facts of Life From Birth to Death.* New York, Macmillan, 1951.
10. Blake, J. B.: *Public Health in the Town of Boston, 1630–1822.* Unpublished Ph.D. dissertation, Harvard University, 1953.
11. Suchman, E. A.: *Sociology and the Field of Public Health.* Philadelphia, W. F. Fell Co., 1963, pp. 17, 18.
12. Langer, W. L.: The Black Death. Scientific American, *210*:121, February, 1964.
13. Suchman, E. A.: *Sociology and the Field of Public Health.* Philadelphia, W. F. Fell Co., 1963, p. 18.

SUGGESTED READING

Abbott, E., and Breckinridge, S. P.: *The Family and Social Service in the 1920's.* An original Arno Press compilation. New York, Arno Press, 1972.

American Academy of Pediatrics: *Child Health Services and Pediatric Education: Report of the Committee for the Study of Child Health Services.* New York, Arno Press, 1949.

Bernstein, N. R.: *History of the American Public Health Association.* Washington, D.C., American Public Health Association, 1972.

Bremner, R. H. (ed.): *Care of Handicapped Children.* Vol. 7. An original anthology. New York, Arno Press, 1974.

Bremner, R. H. (ed.): *Care of Dependent Children in the Late Nineteenth and Early Twentieth Century.* An original anthology. New York, Arno Press, 1974.

Budd, W.: *Typhoid Fever, Its Nature, Mode of Spread and Prevention.* New York, George Grady Press, 1931.

Chapin, C. V.: *The Papers of C. V. Chapin.* New York, Commonwealth Fund, 1934.

Curry, H. B., et al.: *Twenty Years of Community Medicine.* Hunterdon Medical Center symposium, Flemington, N.J. Frenchtown, N.J.: Columbia Publishing Co., 1974.

Debus, A. G. (ed.): *Medicine in 17th Century England.* Berkeley, University of California Press, 1974.

Disease and Society in Provincial Massachusetts: Collected Accounts, 1736–1939. An original Arno Press compilation. New York, Arno Press, 1972.

Duffy, J.: *History of Public Health in New York City, 1866–1966.* New York, Russell Sage Foundation, 1974.

Egeland, J. A.: *Final Report of the Community Health Survey.* Milton S. Hershey Medical Center, Pennsylvania State University, 1974.

Eliot, M. M.: The Children's Bureau, fifty years of public responsibility for action in behalf of children. Amer. J. Publ. Health, *52*:576, 1962.

Fertility Controlled! The British Argument for Family Limitation. An original anthology. New York, Arno Press, 1974.

Gauldie, E.: *Cruel Habitations: A History of Working-Class Housing 1780–1918.* New York, Barnes & Noble, 1974.

Hanlon, J. J., Rogers, F. B., and Rosen, G.: A bookshelf on the history of philosophy of public health. Amer. J. Publ. Health, *50*:445, 1960.

Havemann, E.: *Birth Control: A Special Time-Life Report.* New York, Time-Life, 1967.

Hobson, W.: *World Health and History.* Baltimore, Williams & Wilkins, 1963.

Knowlton, C., and Owen, R. D.: *Birth Control and Morality in Nineteenth Century America: Two Discussions.* An original Arno Press compilation. New York, Arno Press, 1972.

Larsell, O.: *The Doctor in Oregon.* Portland, Binfords & Mort, 1947.

Lerner, M., and Anderson, O. W.: *Health Progress in the United States, 1900–1960.* University of Chicago Press, 1963.

Lifton, R. J., and Olson, E. (eds.): *Explorations in Psychohistory: The Wellfleet Papers.* New York, Simon & Schuster, 1974.

Means, R.: *A History of Health Education in the United States.* Philadelphia, Lea & Febiger, 1962.

Miller, G.: *Bibliography of the History of Medicine in the United States and Canada 1939–1960.* Baltimore, Johns Hopkins Press, 1964.

Origins of Public Health in America: Selected Essays, 1820–1855. An original Arno Press compilation. New York, Arno Press, 1972.

Rosen, G.: *A History of Public Health.* New York, MD Publications, 1958.

Rosen, G.: *From Medical Police to Social Medicine: Essays on the History of Health Care.* New York, Science History Publications, 1974.

Rosoff, J.: *Medicaid, Past and Future.* New York, Planned Parenthood Federation of America, 1972.

Rusk, H.: Congress and medicine. New York Times, November 20, 1965.

Schneider, M. G.: *The Aged and the Depression: Two Reports.* An original Arno Press compilation. New York, Arno Press, 1972.

Shapter, T.: *The History of Cholera in Exeter in 1832.* New York, British Book Centre, 1974.

Silverman, M., and Lee, P. R.: *Pills, Profits, and Politics.* Berkeley, University of California Press, 1974.

Smillie, W. G.: *Public Health: Its Promise for the Future.* New York, Macmillan, 1955.

Smolensky, J.: *A History of Public Health in Oregon.* Doctoral dissertation, Oregon, University of Oregon Press, 1956 (microcard).

Symonds, R., and Carder, M.: *The United Nations and the Population Question.* New York, McGraw-Hill, 1973.

Turner, C. E.: *I Remember.* New York, Vantage Press, 1974.

Uiseltear, A. J.: *Emergence of the Medical Care Section of the American Public Health Association, 1926–1948.* Washington, D.C., American Public Health Association, 1972.

Wain, H.: *A History of Preventive Medicine.* Springfield, Ill., Charles C Thomas, 1970.

Weinberg, D.: *State Adminstration and Financing of Family Planning Services.* New York, Planned Parenthood Federation of America, 1972.

Winslow, C. E. A.: *The Conquest of Epidemic Diseases.* Princeton, N.J., Princeton University Press, 1944.

Zinsser, H.: *Rats, Lice and History.* Boston, Little, Brown, 1945.

CHAPTER 3

Sociological Aspects of Community Health

In public health, as in all fields, there is a cultural lag between yesterday's traditional activities and today's needs. There can be little doubt that these sociomedical problems will become the target of tomorrow's public health programs. Social ailments, such as alcoholism, venereal disease, juvenile delinquency, drug abuse, suicide, and accidents, are problems appropriate to public health activity. The etiology of these problems has its basis in the family, the neighborhood, the community, and the total society. The treatment and prevention of the problems can come about only through control of these social forces.

The public health profession, by virtue of its orientation, techniques, and specialties, is uniquely suited to deal with sociomedical problems, and should assume responsibility for coping with them. One of the difficulties encountered in trying to deal with these problems through health agencies is the public's reluctance to view them as medical problems. The social stigma attached to these diseases creates serious problems in case-finding and prevention. Conversely, the reluctance of public health agencies to view these health problems as associated social problems has often resulted in the failure of public health programs aimed at their control. The increasing prevalence of mental illness in America also suggests need for a careful reappraisal of the facilities and methods available to cope with it, as well as increased cooperation with social scientists. The growing concern of public health with international health programs offers fertile ground for development of the comparative or cross-cultural method. Local population laboratories for the study of community health problems can help to advance sociological techniques for the study of community structure and action.

The shift in control and treatment from communicable diseases to chronic and degenerative diseases has led to a need for new voluntary programs requiring community support and individual motivation. People must now be persuaded, rather than compelled, to take advantages of preventive measures. The chronically ill do not present the same threat to the health of the general public as do individuals with communicable diseases. The formal authority and legal sanctions so crucial in the fight against communicable disease have been displaced by appeals for community support and education of the individual concerning the advantages of public health programs and facilities. The health of the individual has become largely a personal rather than a public matter. Thus, public health personnel today must seek out and utilize information relating to social organization, occupational structure, community action, individual behavior, and communication. In addition, the value system of a society helps to shape the public's attitudes, beliefs, and behavior in regard to health and illness.

Public health officials must necessarily be concerned with social process and social change, because these affect health action. Research in these areas may be expected to advance current theory on such problems as individual and community decision-making processes; the relationship of perception to fact, of knowledge to attitude, and of attitude to behavior; the principles of communication and public opinion; and structural-functional relationships in health organizations. Participation in mass screening programs, the utilization of existing health facilities, and community support for public health measures are only some of the problems facing public health today that require a knowledge of social action. Special groups such as the disabled and aged are already demanding new public health services. Medical care is already closely related to the economic problems of health and malpractice insurance and organizational problems in administrative medicine. Legislation such as Medicare, antipoverty, and civil rights cannot but expand the already heavily burdened treatment aspects of public health practice.

In an effort to persuade and motivate individuals and families to change their health habits, public health has entered an era of new competition—competition with other community interests opposed to health measures that can no longer be justified by the threat of epidemics; competition with business interests that have found the health field financially profitable (such as manufacturers of drugs and vitamins) and that have powerful economic interests in activities that may prove harmful to the public's health (such as tobacco, food additive, and insecticide industries); and competition with private medicine over the quantity and quality of health care. As public health assumes a role less dramatic than that of preventing major epidemics, it must take its place alongside other necessary public services, such as urban redevelopment and education, in competing for the increasingly scarce tax dollar.

Public health must accept the responsibility for meeting these complex problems even if this means introducing fundamental changes in its current values, objectives, and modes of operation. In any case, the problems of the future will have to be met by a reallocation of financial and personnel resources.

THE COMMUNITY AND HEALTH

The phrase *community health* is composed of two words: community and health. In order to conduct a successful community health program, health workers must consider the significance and implication of both words. We are dealing with a product, *health,* and a recipient, *the community.* Complete knowledge and understanding of both are necessary. We must understand and deal with the health problem; we must also understand and treat the social or public phase of the situation.

Health is a social responsibility in and of the community. In order to formulate ways of meeting and solving health needs by the democratic process, a community must have groups of interrelating and interacting individuals functioning for a common purpose. This demands recognition of differing groups in the community and appreciation of the fact that their goals or values may not be totally in accord with our own. We cannot have adequate motivation for health or develop adequate participation by these groups unless we are willing to accept people, whoever they are and wherever they may live, and work with them toward sharing goals, aspirations, and tasks.[1]

Concepts and Obstacles

There are many obstacles to be overcome and certain concepts to be understood before a community can organize and successfully solve its health problems. As a result of urbanization, relationships among individuals in the community have become less effective. Some authorities believe that there has been a corresponding decrease in the effectiveness of channels of communication.[1] Another obstacle presents itself when "mod" children and "old-fashioned" parents disagree upon the objectives and philosophies behind certain health programs. In each community the family represents the most powerful example of social cohesion. Therefore, if conflicting opinions, objectives, and philosophies cause families throughout the community to become separated, community health programs are weakened and often defeated. On the other hand, certain members of the family may disseminate factual health information that, in turn, may lead to strengthened family support for certain controversial health programs. For example, many parents may be undecided concerning fluoridation of water supplies. Their high school or college boy or girl, however, may have learned that fluoridation is beneficial, and he or she may have an opportunity to discuss the problem with other members of the family. As a result, more of these informed parents may join the campaign for fluoridation. However, we must remember that in many families the parents' attitudes and prejudices are instilled in the children from early childhood, and although the child is exposed to new ideas and concepts in school, more concentrated effort and education is needed to erase unfavorable prejudices and attitudes.[2]

Present economic, sociologic, and technologic conditions have caused the family to be less closely knit than in the past, and this must be considered when organizing and planning health programs. Members of the family have barely enough time to speak to each other, and certainly haven't time to discuss community health problems. Often the young adult members of the family marry or leave for college; in addition, many families do not stay in one community long enough to learn of or to concern themselves with the health problems and needs of the community. Because Americans are migrating from state to state at such a rapid pace, many new health problems are being created every day. An insecure and fast pace of living, pressure and interest groups, racial integration in schools and communities, increased chronic disease and accident fatalities, longer life expectancy, population explosion, increased mental illness, and swift methods of travel that bring cities, states, and countries closer together are other factors to consider when a community attempts to organize and promote health programs today.

Community organization involves recognition of the fact that there are definite separations among upper, middle, and lower classes, and that these separations are on the increase.[3] Communities are also divided into racial, religious, and national minority groups, age groups, and occupation groups, to mention but a few. The college graduate is separated from the high school graduate, the factory worker from the store owner, and the owner of a Rolls-Royce is separated from the owner of a Pinto or Mustang. Correspondingly, poor housing projects develop in one section of a town and larger, more modern homes are found in another section. As a result, small, nucleated groups develop; these groups have little in common and in some ways may be antagonistic. A strong and united community is composed of groups of cooperative individuals who are functionally related in meeting common needs. Although each group may have different values, the health priority rating of each group and of the total community must be determined and understood. How high does health really rank in the value systems of the people? Each community must ask this question.

Often a community is divided into many different kinds of areas or tracts, resulting in many and varied neighborhoods. These neighborhoods or zones gradually overlap, and sometimes social problems follow such changes. A master plan formulated by an official city planning board could greatly alleviate the results of these changes in land-use patterns. Furthermore, artificial city and county boundaries tend to promote factionalism, which lessens active cooperation and participation for better health and vitiates the appeal for popular support.

Interest in many community health programs often wanes because only a small percentage of the people in any community are members of organized groups (in rural communities, the percentage is especially small). Active participation by a cross-section of all the people in the community is not accomplished if representatives are chosen only from the various agencies and groups. Instead, *all* members of the community should be considered when representatives are being chosen. Certain members within a group or community are assumed to be leaders and are therefore assigned leadership positions; community programs would be much more effective if the real or natural leaders were elected by their respective groups. Many times majority groups choose leaders or representatives from certain minority groups without consulting minority members. If members of the minority groups were asked, they would readily confess that the real or natural leaders had not been chosen.

Although there are 25 to 100 organized health groups and established health agencies operating in many communities in the United States, there is usually a lack of cooperation, coordination, and planning. Health workers and other professional personnel often forget that health interests are only one aspect among many in the community. Some agencies are interested in organizing the community for their own ends, and those ends are determined in the national headquarters, not in the community. Pressure and interest groups may hinder or halt certain health programs; vested interests, ignorance, and lack of the facts are a few contributing factors. The cooperative efforts of many agencies enable communities to produce citizens with complete physical, mental, and social well-being. An effective program includes group-defined philosophy, objectives, fact finding, education, decision making, community action, and evaluation. This democratic process is of the community, for the community, and by the community.

Effect of Cultural Patterns on Health

A society is any community of individuals drawn together by a common bond of nearness and interaction—a group of people who act together for the achievement of certain common goals. A person's culture determines how he thinks, feels, acts, speaks, worships, dresses, marries, eats, prepares food, treats the sick, and disposes of the dead.[3] There are usually a great many cultures in each community. Each culture respects and accepts certain values, attitudes, and beliefs. Public health programs necessarily involve the introduction of new practices and changes in values and beliefs into the culture of the society. If such programs are to be constructive rather than destructive forces, the social structure and the traditional cultural way of life of the community must be taken into account and utilized. The accepted value systems of a culture are deeply ingrained, and people adhere strongly to their attitudes and beliefs. Crowded living conditions, low economic status, and discrimination have made certain cultures look upon change or suggested change with misgivings and suspicion. Community health programs involve time, patience, sincerity, planning, and understanding.

One example of the effect of culture on health is acceptance or rejection of birth control. Resistance to taking the Pill is inextricably linked to many social and ethnic considerations. In many countries in Central America, a man's position is strengthened by an increase in the number of children in the family. Furthermore, having many children has been held in high esteem by his father and grandfather. It is not easy to convince men in this community that family planning is good. In India, motivation for acceptance of the Pill or vasectomy is linked to monetary reward.

Although religion is linked to large families in the Philippines, many farmers have many children in order to have nonsalaried help on the farm.

Even though cultural influences have a great effect upon our health attitudes and behavior, we find great variations within our own country. These variations are, to a large extent, due to two factors. First, immigrants from other countries brought with them their own original health cultures. Although these were modified or disappeared in subsequent generations, a few traits survived among descendants, particularly within those ethnic groups that have preserved some of their original national, racial, or ethnic characteristics. For example, an interesting study, done a few years ago in New York City, showed that when first- and second-generation Italians experience symptoms of illness, they tend to seek the quickest possible relief from the discomfort or pain when they go to see a physician. Jewish people, on the other hand, were found to be more concerned with learning about the causes of their symptoms and with seeking treatment for these causes. Although they, their parents, and perhaps even their grandparents were born in this country, people of Mexican, Chinese, Scandinavian, or any other national descent occasionally exhibit some modification of a health attitude or practice that has been passed on, with gradual changes, from their immigrant ancestors.

The second major factor that accounts for the existence of more or less distinct health subcultures within the more general health culture prevalent in this country is the existence of many large population groups in this country whose lives, physical environment, socioeconomic circumstances, and day-to-day problems of living set them apart from other population groups. Each group has developed certain cultural traits of its own, and these traits incorporate certain characteristic health attitudes and practices.

For example, the culture of the poorest segments of our population places relatively little value on personal cleanliness and sanitary living conditions. Many minor diseases of the skin or of the digestive system are so common among poor people that they are not even considered as abnormal and are rarely brought to a physician's attention. Venereal disease is also common and is often left untreated. A large proportion of pregnant women never obtain prenatal medical checkups and are not seen by a physician until the time of delivery, if they are seen at all. They often do not accept even medical services that are offered free of charge. Large numbers of the children of our poor never see a dentist or a physician until they go to school, and they do not obtain immunization for a number of diseases against which virtually all children among the more affluent social classes are protected.[4]

Public health programs must demonstrate to people that continuing improvement in their health, welfare, and level of living is their main purpose. A sincere and genuine interest in the people, individually and collectively, is a necessity. For example, residents of a Mexican settlement in San Bernardino County, California, were uncooperative and suspicious when asked to cooperate in a mass chest x-ray survey of that area. Fear, ignorance, and language difficulties barred all attempts. However, in time a Mexican public health nurse gained the people's confidence and acceptance. She helped them organize a community health council, which was composed of leading lay and professional citizens. Upon the satisfactory completion of a few successful health projects, the group decided to conduct the mass x-ray survey. Spanish literature was disseminated and films were shown. The successful x-ray survey program enabled health authorities to find and treat many early tuberculosis cases and precipitated a slum clearance project. The tuberculosis mortality and morbidity rates decreased accordingly in that area. It is interesting to note that certain groups have accepted many modern American health practices, such as immunization and x-ray, but often revert to traditional cultural patterns in relation to nutrition, home remedies, and family and marital problems.

Another example involves an American Indian health aide who helped the Los Angeles County Immunization Program raise immunization levels among the large Indian population in the county. Mrs. Carmella Coffer, member of the Paiute tribe, was a CEP (Concentrated Employment Project) aide, a "career-ladder" program. She bridged the cultural gap between the Indian community and the health district. The Indians are a sensitive and culturally isolated people. To reach them, the immunization project worked through their social, religious and athletic groups, which are organized on tribal lines. Immunization personnel distributed flyers through the Indian Welcome House and Indian Centers, and they also contacted Indian churches in the county. Mrs. Coffer also helped Indians in other health and welfare problems. She visited local Indian homes to tell the people about the services of the health department. She encouraged the increased use of available services and clinics and acted as a resource person to whom the Indians could turn in their attempts to solve their many other problems. Low income and education levels, high unemployment, large families, and cultural differences contribute to the severe disadvantage under which American Indians are forced to live.

There are many examples of the effect of cultural and social patterns on health. A few are included in Table 3–1, and a description of health care for Mexican-Americans is given in the following paragraphs.

Mexican-American Culture (One Example of an Ethnic Minority)

During the last 10 years many changes have occurred both within Mexican-American communities and between ethnic minorities and American society at large. Nevertheless, many still struggle with the same problems they faced 10 years ago—uncertain employment, low income, substandard housing, and inadequate medical care. Health and medical agencies have responded to some degree by adding Spanish-speaking professionals to their staffs and by attempting to establish new modalities of health care, but much more needs to be done. Mexican-American communities still do not have adequate medical facilities. Clinics are overcrowded and understaffed; most families do not have health insurance and can be bankrupted by soaring costs of hospital services and doctors' fees; crippling disabilities go untended; many children are inadequately fed and clothed; psychiatric care, except for the most seriously disturbed, is still largely unavailable to the poor; there are still far too few Spanish-speaking doctors, nurses, and other health professionals.

TABLE 3–1 Effect of Cultural and Social Patterns on Health.

SOCIAL FACTORS	DISEASE OR CONDITION
Ignorance or Lack of Knowledge	
Drinking unpasteurized milk	Brucellosis*
Drinking water from polluted stream	Dystentery, hepatitis
Visit to a "quack"	Cancer
Poor personal hygiene	Typhoid fever
Home canning, improper methods	Botulism
Economic Status	
Eating too many rich, fatty foods	Diabetes, atherosclerosis
Lack of balanced diet	Rickets, scurvy
Lack of shoes	Hookworm
Inadequate sanitary facilities	Typhoid fever
Inadequate prenatal care	Prematurity
Slum areas	Tuberculosis
Religious Beliefs	
Eating raw pork	Trichinosis
Worship of cows	Malnutrition
Medicine man or faith healer	Cancer
Stream rituals	Schistosomiasis
Heredity	
Race	Susceptible tendencies vary with certain diseases
Passed from parent to child	Diabetes, color blindness, feeblemindedness
Environment	
Mineral content: lack of	
(a) Iodine	Goiter
(b) Fluorine	Dental decay
Living in the tropics	Malaria
Living at South or North Pole	Freedom from and inactivity of certain germs
Activity	
Stress and strain	Cerebral hemorrhage, heart condition, mental illness
Lack of exercise	Heart condition
Occupation	
Atomic or radioactive plants	Radiation sickness, sterility
Sheep, goat herder	Anthrax
Paint sprayer	Encephalitis
Dairyman	Brucellosis*
Rabbit farmer	Tularemia
Working with parakeets or turkeys	Psittacosis
Hunter	Rocky Mountain spotted fever
Miner	Silicosis
Physician	Shorter life expectancy
Faulty or Negative Attitude	
"Good enough for my father"	Tuberculosis (unpasteurized milk)
"Why not overeat? Cancer or accidents will get me anyhow"	Heart disease
"Nothing's hurt me yet"	Dental decay
"An apple a day keeps the doctor away"	Cancer
"Let him learn by experience"	Childhood accident
"One more fast handball game, son"	Heart disease
"Have to work late"	Mental illness
"It always happens to the other fellow"	Auto accident
"I can't watch him every minute"	Childhood accident
"One for the road"	Alcoholism
"He likes me slim and trim"	Malnutrition

*The incidence of brucellosis is highest among farmers and packing plant workers.

Folk Beliefs vs. Scientific Medical Practice

Nonscientific concepts of disease from Mexico are an important influence in the lives of Mexican-Americans. Conflicts between beliefs and scientific medical practice can lead to fear and rejection of American health services. Many of these folk beliefs are persistent in second- and third-generation Mexican-Americans. Religious beliefs, prayers, and spells of Mexican origin are very important in the diagnosis and home treatment of disease. Barrio (neighborhood) people place considerable reliance on Mexican folk-curing practices such as herbal remedies, "cupping," topical applications of some sort, heat treatments, and massage. Patent medicines are also popular. Barrio people are sometimes afraid of taking strange medicines. It should be emphasized that folk syndromes are very real to barrio people. Health workers who flatly deny the existence of "evil eye," mal aire, empacho, "magical fright," or disease caused by witchcraft may expect to lose the confidence of many of their Mexican-American patients.[5]

Theory of Disease

Ideas about disease and its causes vary from culture to culture. Some concepts are clearly derived from folk beliefs and others are "scientific" syndromes. For purposes of organization, diseases are grouped into the following categories: diseases of "hot and cold" imbalance, diseases of dislocation of internal organs, diseases of magical origin, diseases of emotional origin, other folk-defined diseases, and "standard scientific" diseases. It is not always easy to place a disorder in a single category. For example, there are mechanical injuries such as burns which are clearly traumatic but which also are thought to cause an imbalance of body temperature. Other syndromes are thought to be primarily magical in origin, for example, *mal aire* ("bad air"; a folk disease attributed to sudden exposure to drafts or winds), but disturbances in "hot and cold" may make the victim particularly susceptible to the disorder. The etiology of even the "standard scientific" diseases may be misunderstood and the disorder attributed to magical causes.[6]

Diseases of "Hot and Cold" Imbalance

The "hot and cold" theory of disease is derived from the Hippocratic theory of pathology, which postulated that the human body in a state of health contained balanced quantities of the four "humours" (phlegm, blood, black bile, and yellow bile). Some of the four "humours" were thought to be innately "cold." A disproportion of hot and cold body essences was reflected in illness. This body of belief was brought to the New World by sixteenth-century Spanish explorers and colonists and was widely diffused among the native inhabitants of Spanish America. In parts of both Spain and America it is believed that illness results when real or imaginary parts of the body move from their normal positions.[7]

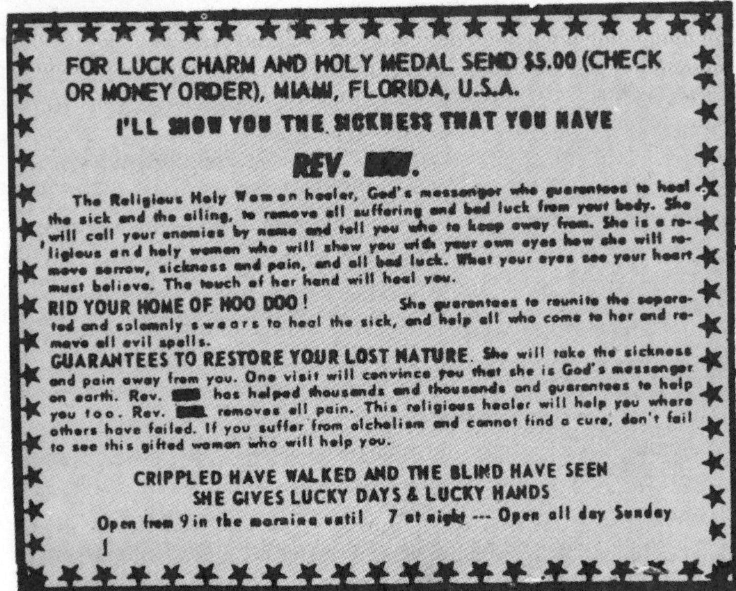

Figure 3–1 Recent ads in the *Miami Times* illustrate people's belief in faith healing and witchcraft. (From Scott, C. S.: Health and healing practices among five ethnic groups in Miami, Florida. Public Health Reports, *89*(6):524–532, November–December, 1974.)

GUIDE TO WORKING IN DEVELOPING COUNTRIES

1. Start with a belief that bringing better quality of life to the developing world is worthwhile.
2. Gain knowledge of local culture: language, taboos, superstitions, beliefs, slang terms.
3. Work with local leaders to better equip them to help their community. Help them to help themselves. Recognize that different areas in the same country work differently.
4. Have a desire to learn from the people you work with; encourage mutual sharing of knowledge.
5. Recognize that the health needs of any area must relate to the wants of the people. They decide *their* priorities.
6. Set goals at a realistic level. (A developing nation may want open heart surgery now—but must start with teaching about sterile equipment first.) Correlate *wants* with *needs*.
7. Adapt to available resources and limitations of the community.
8. Relate on a personal level, establishing mutual trust, friendship, and understanding.

Factors Responsible for Group Actions and Reactions

There are certain factors that determine the reactions of each community group to its health needs. One important factor involves the group's conception and meaning of the word *health*. There are many meanings of this particular word. For some, health means something related to pain, the abnormal, or "tired blood." Others may visualize health as a social, mental, physical, or emotional concept. Similarly, the phrase *community health* has about as many meanings as the number of people in each community. To some, community health means solving immediate, noticeable health problems, an adequate sewage treatment plant, or a pure water supply. To others, community health involves organization, long-range planning, leadership, needs, cooperation, coordination, and active involvement.

Another consideration revolves around the fact that different groups attach different values to their health needs. Alcoholic beverages and tobacco are much more important than periodic physical examinations to some groups; to others luxuries such as a new car or refrigerator may rank far above the value placed upon balanced diets or sanitary living conditions. A new park or highway may take precedence over needed health facilities in certain communities. Health as a value is always in competition with other values. The value system of a particular group must be recognized and understood for a community to organize and successfully solve its health problems.

A third factor determining group reaction to health needs involves past experiences and associations with health officials or agencies. Successful and rewarding experiences foster support; distasteful and negative experiences yield uncooperative, disinterested individuals and groups. Since active participation increases interest and support, the effective leadership of the natural groups in the community must be determined and utilized.

Faulty or negative attitudes account for many groups "playing the odds" on their health. To many, heavy smoking is favored over possible lung cancer, obesity is favored over possible heart disease, and heavy drinking is favored over possible accident. Members of this group rebel against health education with such remarks as, "It hasn't been proved," or "If I don't die from heart disease, I'll die from cancer," or "You have to go sometime." Positive health attitudes and practices must be instilled in individuals at an early age. Parents and educators must join in an effort to promote long life and prevent sickness through positive thinking, planning, and individual and community participation.

Barriers to Effective Community Health Programs

There are many reasons why community health organizations are difficult to maintain and community health agency or council suggestions fail to receive acceptance or adoption. Many of these reasons revolve around sociologocal or cultural problems. For example, the average American community, with its pioneer heritage of individualism and ever-changing group action, seems to be better prepared to cope with emergencies than to maintain an organization for planning and development. This requires a continuing, relatively stable structure.

Furthermore, studies reveal that the public is indifferent to health problems, surveys, and solutions.[8, 9] People remain passive as long as no serious health problem or large-scale fatalities occur. Although citizens are aware of health problems, they tend to view them as unpleasant conditions, but not particularly dangerous to the community. In fact, some people may regard certain health problems as a major threat to the prestige level of their community. Most local citizens feel that any existing health problems can be handled by the proper agencies, which in most cases is the health department. Some, however, still feel that health department services are limited to its historic functions: immunization and environmental sanitation.

Devoid of interest in many areas of public health, and caught in the grip of public health laws relating to sanitation, many persons resist the aims of those devoted to the prevention of disease. Since most preventive medicine cannot be instituted through legal enforcement, there is a need for a public that is informed, educated, and sympathetic to the goals of preventing disease and prolonging life. Health education thus becomes a very important tool in community health work.

Even when many persons are concerned and interested enough about a certain health problem to organize and plan as a group, disagreements, rebuttals, denials, postponements, repeated duplicate meetings, and lack of leadership, common objectives, and philosophy may be noticed. Since any one health problem may be splintered into many, it is necessary for the group to define the specific area with which it is most concerned. One well-planned, well-publicized, coordinated, cooperative meeting with well-defined objectives is sufficient for planning an action program. Each agency representative present must tell specifically what he can do, what he will do, and how his agency can work cooperatively with other agencies. Recommendations should be made by the group, a steering committee appointed, and recommendations by the steering committee submitted *in writing* to the city council or county board of supervisors for action. Action results in reaction, and this is necessary to propel motivation and interest.

Many well-meaning programs in community health have failed when they have been blanketed by generalizations in education. To educate is to form or change ideas and behavior, and some people are never clear about exactly what ideas or behavior should be formed or changed. They may not see how these changes can lead to improved individual, family, and community health. Many persons view health problems in either a curative or a contribute-to-the-Community-Chest sense.

A well-informed public is exceedingly important when one considers that community health funds are sharply controlled by a public which abhors increased taxation and may feel that other current city needs have greater priority. Some departments, whose functions are more easily recognized and on which the public has placed more value, find it easier to satisfy their needs. Contributions to voluntary agencies are viewed by many with mixed emotions. There is considerable confusion about which agencies belong to the United Fund, Community Chest, United Appeal, and others, and exactly how the money is apportioned. The situation is complicated by the fact that officials of certain large health agencies, such as the American Heart Association and the American Cancer Society, generally reject any suggestions for joining with the United Fund for fund-raising or any other purpose. These agencies contend that this procedure leads to administrative control, loss of identity, and elimination of the donor's choice of agency. More important, they contend that separate fund drives raise more money.

Public-spirited Americans, who contribute over $1,000,000,000 a year to organizations formed to combat health problems, are growing increasingly bewildered by the proliferation of health agencies and fund appeals. Many voluntary health agencies have developed during the past few years, and all of them are competing for public loyalty and financial support; jealousy prevails and services overlap. There are over 100 national fund drives today, as compared with only 15 in 1940. Duplication of effort is illustrated by the fact that 19 agencies compete nationally for money to aid the blind, at least three national groups compete for money to fight cancer, and three mental health agencies appeal for support. Besides increasing fund-raising costs, the keen competition for money sometimes appears to result in a haphazard distribution of available funds. One top official of a fund-raising group argues that allocations of funds "are decided almost entirely by such factors as which important citizens have which diseases, what agency can hire the best promoters and involve the most influential personalities, and which cause plucks hardest at the heartstrings of the public's emotions."[10]

Since the mark of success of many voluntary health agencies is determined by the success of the fund-raising campaign, such basic programs as education and research are often neglected or emphasized more before fund raising begins. If employees "volunteer" to contribute a certain amount of money each year to an agency of their choice, a feeling of employee resistance is noticed, and it seems to defeat the entire principle of giving.

Although there have been many public health advances in the past 50 years, desire for good health has not always been the motivating force in securing necessary action. We are extremely proud of the high percentage of our communities having approved water supplies. But how many of these public water supplies were demanded and supported because the public wanted a safe water supply, as compared to their desire for the comfort and convenience of an inside toilet and running water in the kitchen? Have Grade A milk programs spread from city to city because of the demands of the people for higher quality milk, or because of economic necessity and competition? Bovine tuberculosis in human beings in the United States is practically extinct. Was it the presence of bone and glandular tuberculosis in people that brought about this remarkable achievement, or the economics of the dairy and cattle industries? Legislation regarding feeding only cooked garbage to swine was prohibited in Indiana until many hogs died from a disease called vesicular exanthema. Legislators enacted a bill quickly when the hogs became ill.[11]

It is interesting and important to note here that health progress depends upon local, state, and federal regulations to a great degree. Since most local health officers and voluntary agency executive directors are *appointed* by the city council members, by county boards of supervisors, by boards of directors, or, in the case of most state health officers, by the governor, it is necessary for these members to exchange ideas and discuss program objectives and philosophy. Officials must be well informed on community health principles and must periodically review and evaluate the health needs, interests, and problems of the people in their area.

Community Health Progress—Real or Mirage?

Most people will agree that public health activities have made this country a healthier and happier place in which to live. Life expectancy has increased, and public health advances have had a beneficial effect on the cultural patterns of people, regardless of economic status, race, or religion. Elimination of certain diseases has given health workers more time to concentrate on mental health, chronic diseases, and geriatrics. These health fields have provided new occupations, activities, buildings, and even entire communities. These new avenues have led also to the current definition of and emphasis on health as a social and emotional aspect of an individual, community, or nation.

On the other hand public health activities may produce unexpected or undesirable results, and medicine's apparent triumphs may be mixed blessings. For example, an increase in leisure time may lead to an increase in the number of alcoholics, drug abusers, and delinquents. Increased leisure time, plus high-powered automobiles and other mechanized equipment, may lead to lack of exercise and increased auto accidents. Although a man past 45 years of age has little greater life expectancy than his grandfather had, he has the world's highest living standard; but a large share of his income today goes for medical care. Our greater ingenuity and inventiveness leads to a faster, less secure way of life and often results in more divorces, suicides, and mentally ill persons. Many of the new tranquilizing drugs encourage people to forget their worries. Industries release more smoke and hydrocarbons that may account for an increase in cancer and allergies. We live longer today only to wonder about obtaining a job after retirement and contemplate whether we will die from heart disease, cancer, intracranial lesions, or accidents.[3]

Although communicable diseases have decreased, they have not disappeared. Disease is an aspect of man's adaptation to his environment, and as his environment changes, so do his diseases. Disease has not surrendered unconditionally. The very sanitary techniques that did so much to control infections in the nineteenth century set the stage for the ravages of polio in the twentieth century. German measles, once universal in childhood, now skips many sanitized youngsters, but if a woman contracts the disease in the first three months of pregnancy, she may have a stillborn or malformed child. The effectiveness of insulin not only prolongs the diabetic's life but increases the risk of his passing on a diabetic tendency to his children. If this happens often enough, society may face medical, economic, and ethical problems for which it is not prepared.[12]

SOCIAL WORKERS IN PUBLIC HEALTH

The growing emphasis on the comprehensive approach to health and medical care, as well as the current concern with chronic diseases, has led to a greater need for and acceptance of social workers in public health and mental health programs. Medical social work together with other phases of social relief practice has long played a role in the development and improvement of health services. Public health and social welfare programs have the same broad goals. The functions of social work are complementary to those of public health. "Social work seeks to enhance the social functioning of individuals, singly or in groups, by activities focused upon the social relationships which constitute the interaction between man and his environment. These activities can be arranged into three functions: restoration of impaired capacity; provision of individual and social resources; and prevention of social dysfunction."[13] The recognition that society contributes to inadequate social functioning has increased the demand for social workers, who know how health influences and is influenced by social factors. For example, it is known that people in certain housing developments strive to raise their standards of living, and that in "keeping up with the Joneses" they may neglect their nutritional needs. Medical social workers, while generally interested in planning for improved housing, may make a unique contribution in pointing up this relationship between social and health factors. Of major concern to social workers in public health today are such problems as stresses arising from acute or chronic illness in the family; families with multiple health, financial, and housing difficulties; financial insecurity; social and emotional stresses contributing to dependency, disability, or delinquency; and children at risk because of family ill health.

Social workers employed in public health programs apply the social work methods of social case work, social group work, community organization, research, and administration to the removal, lessening, or prevention of social and personal obstacles to health evaluation and medical care. They help in the development of the varied services necessary for the maintenance and utilization of comprehensive health services. Adaptation in social work methods may be made to meet requirements of particular agencies. Further information relating to the specific objectives and activities of the social worker in health departments is presented in the following report from the Oklahoma State Department of Public Health:

> Social work has as its aim, assistance to human beings in their social relationships. Its objective is to enable individuals and groups to realize their maximum capacity and to work toward full and satisfactory living. Its concern is with potential or actual breakdown in social living due to social, psychological, cultural, economical, and physical factors.
>
> Social workers have been added to the Health Department staff in this biennium. They are responsible for the social work aspects of the public health programs as they relate to the prevention and alleviation of social problems associated with health care. They aided the health team in understanding the significance of these factors as they affect health, illness, and disability. Activities were carried out in collaboration with program directors, physicians, public health nurses, psychologists, nutritionists, health educators, and others.

Activities

The major activities of the social workers at the time of the report by the Oklahoma State Department of Public Health were:

1. Consultation regarding the social factors that influence the needs and treatment of patients served. They were concerned with problems of family breakdown, alcoholism, illegitimacy, children, mothers, youths, aging, and mental illness.

2. Help with program planning. This included the recognition of unmet needs and the development of services for meeting them.

3. Participation in community organization and planning related to the study of social, health, and medical needs. The social workers worked with local groups in considering homemaker, home care, and visiting nurse services.

4. Social case-work study, evaluation and counseling of individual patients, and parents who are using the health services, undergoing diagnostic study, or receiving medical care. This was done in one county health department.

5. Doing liaison work between the Health Department and health and welfare agencies. Specific help was given in individual situations where more than one agency was concerned.

6. Participation in studies, surveys, and projects concerned with health, disease, or disability. These included perinatal care and the social and nutritional needs of residents in nursing homes.

7. Teaching of social work concepts through lectures and by leading discussions, inservice training programs, and planning programs and workshops. Both formal and informal methods were used. The planning of field work placement for social work students in a county health center was begun.

Personnel

The social work staff consisted of three workers. A chief social worker was assigned to the Chronic Disease Division and one to the Maternal and Child Health Division. One worker gave both direct and consultative services in a county health department.

Needs

The most urgent need today is for an increasing number of trained *clinical* social workers in keeping with expanded mental health programs. These clinical social workers cooperate with physicians, school psychologists, parents, and other agencies in an effort to cope with problem children, educationally handicapped children, family problems, and emergency and crisis situations.

Furthermore, there is need for additional staff to work with local health departments on special social and community problems, such as the organization and use of health resources and the development of home care, homemaker, child care, and youth services.[14]

Services

The services of social workers in public health and mental health are directed toward the identification and modification of social, psychological, and environmental factors that contribute to health problems or influence the use of health services. The social worker in the health agency discharges his responsibilities as a member of an interprofessional group in close collaboration with other public health personnel. Concentration on social work practice depends on the scope and organization of the total public health agency and the level of operation. Emphasis shifts in relation to changing needs and priorities, the availability of social workers, and the changing goals of the health agency.

To help health personnel deal with public apathy and the social and behavioral phenomena that hamper execution of public health programs, the Pennsylvania State Department of Health employed an anthropologist and a psychologist. In addition to problem solving, the Division of Behavioral Science is alert to undesirable psychosocial or cultural side effects in programs and is responsible for assembling systematic and reliable information about significant populations in the state—those populations large in numbers or presenting significant public health problems. Specific activities of the new division have been:

1. Research into factors contributing to the loss by popular referendum of a county health department.

2. Setting up contracts of university-based studies of health behavior and felt needs in a rural vicinity and in a lower-class suburban population.

3. Delivering lectures before public audiences or as parts of educational programs arranged by other department units on such topics

as cultural contexts conducive to problem drinking.

4. Developing a short course designed to help beginning sanitarians to locate those community leaders and groups that enter into decisions affecting environment sanitation.

5. Providing consultation, and sometimes performing research, on such subjects as community organization, current social science knowledge about fluoridation controversies, beliefs and practices surrounding pregnancy and childbirth, maintenance of membership in voluntary organizations, and methods for evaluating a program in community sanitation.

The new unit is a behavioral science service rather than a division of research. With enlarged staff, this unit probably will become more active in research design and in continuing study of the sociocultural characteristics and thought and action patterns of several representative Pennsylvania populations.[15]

Major functions of social workers in public health and mental health are: social and consultation services; program planning, implementation, and policy formation; social work services to individuals and families and social case work; social work services to groups; social work services to the community; research, studies, and surveys; and educational responsibilities.*

Social workers are becoming more interested in the use of preventive methods as a further extension of their own services. Advances in psychiatric knowledge have resulted in an increased understanding of human behavior, and this knowledge and understanding are being utilized by the health professions for deeper insight into the individuals' or groups' behavior patterns in health. For example, it is now recognized that many alcoholics, many of the mentally ill, and many drug abusers are suffering from a form of social disorganization. This assumes that human behavior is in part characterized by a social factor, that the social group exists as a number of persons who have a set of perceived expectations in relation to one another, and that the expectations between individuals in a group specify or refer to a number of meanings and folkways or values, all of which together make up the culture or subculture of the group.*

Opportunities for prevention are limitless in the field of social work once we have the knowledge of the need, a clear understanding of the causes, and have developed skill in working at this level. For example, some of the areas in which social workers could be effective in presenting preventive measures are:

1. In cases of families facing crises, such as the birth of a congenitally handicapped child, acquired handicapping conditions due to trauma or disease, the birth of a premature baby, a patient newly diagnosed as having tuberculosis or cancer, a death, or a miscarriage. These all are family crises to which the individual members will react intensively. Knowing this and working with them at the time of crisis, or preferably in advance of an anticipated crisis, will help to lessen the impact on the individual and family.

2. During the years of marriage and in pregnancy at an early age.

3. During the separation of a child from the family or separation of the parent from a child. In recent studies it was found that the hospitalization of a parent often resulted in unfortunate experiences for the child.

4. When the individual is assuming a new responsibility, such as the role of becoming a spouse, a parent, or meeting the difficulties of widowhood.

5. When there are pressures on both mothers and children because mothers are working.

6. In counseling siblings of sick, disabled, or handicapped children.

7. In providing supportive services to adolescents who are trying to adjust to adult life.

8. With children who drop out of school, are without demand in the labor market, marry young, or who frequently become juvenile delinquents in a community.[16]

The increasing complexity of medical care illuminates and magnifies the need to describe, analyze, and solidify the role of medical social work in community health planning.

---

*For further discussion of general scope, functions, and qualifications, refer to Committee on Professional Education: Education qualifications of social workers in public health programs. Amer. J. Publ. Health, 52:317, 1962.

*For further discussion, refer to McGee and Reece: *Social Disorganization in America*. San Francisco, Chandler Publishing Co., 1962.

SOCIOLOGICAL IMPLICATIONS IN INTERNATIONAL COMMUNITY HEALTH

Since the advent of the United States bilateral technical assistance programs, many public health personnel have become involved in international cooperative health projects. The major long-range objectives of the programs are to strengthen the economy and the nation under assistance through health benefits, and to plan, develop, and share in cooperative efforts to resolve our common problems. In attempting to reach this goal, however, health personnel have learned the importance of understanding the way in which each level of a society interacts on every other level, and how the values and ideas of one group are related to those of all other groups. This is most clearly reflected in the following letter from a Peace Corps physician in Ethiopia:*

In truth, my mind constantly questions: Why did I ever leave the secure ivied walls of a university hospital to come to Dire Dawa, where a positive diagnosis can be confirmed only one twentieth of the time in the lab, where one's confreres speak a different tongue, where the x-ray technician cannot tell an anteroposterior chest from a right anterior oblique abdomen, where superstition dictates one third of the treatments. . . . Except that I also wonder why I did not come two years earlier.

What do I actually do? I am primarily a doctor for about 50 Peace Corps volunteers in my area, dealing with their medical and emotional problems, and handling some administrative details. The teachers are a fine group with a variety of, thus far, only minor medical problems. Actually, the volunteers have taken only a small part of my time. I am fortunate in having a well-localized group so I do not travel much. Five mornings a week I work in the outpatient clinic of the government hospital, a small, modern, but ill-equipped affair of about 90 beds. Infectious and preventable diseases make up the majority of cases. Dysenteries—bacillary, amoebic, and other forms—are the commonest complaints. Almost every day I see a fresh case of tuberculosis and malaria. . . . The children especially are infected with a variety of parasites. . . . Venereal disease is almost epidemic. Prostitution is seen in a very different light in this country; it is open and ubiquitous, and this is, no doubt, responsible for the very high incidence. All stages of syphilis, gonorrhea, balanitis, and venereal lymphogranuloma are the most frequent diseases.

. . . The health officer and I walked about three miles into the bush to see if we could locate the origin of an epidemic in a small town. There I saw my first cases of active small-pox as well as a little of the village life of these tiny isolated communities. Houses made of sticks and mud serve large families and the young animals, protecting them from the hyenas, baboons, and even occasional lions that trouble the herds at night. A month ago I helped treat a boy who had been slapped by a lion that had attacked his herd.

There is a great deal of trauma; some of it is self-induced, such as female circumcision, surgically induced chastity in young girls, uvulectomy in infants to keep away the bad spirits, and local application of red hot metal to the afflicted area for abdominal pain, chest pain, and backache. Surgeons are badly needed. Mental illness is truly an agonizing entity here, and when the afflicted are dangerous they are sent to prison. There are no inpatient facilities.

A few figures may help you to get a picture of the magnitude of the problem. Twenty million people are served by about 250 doctors. Something like one doctor for 100,000 people. Most of the doctors are in the big cities, most of the people are in the country, living in widely separated villages of around 60 inhabitants; the vast majority of these villages are totally inaccessible by road. The government approach to the problem has been made with the help of the USAID advisory group. Public health is the key, as universal curative medicine could not be obtained for probably a hundred years. The key unit is a self-sufficient health center staffed by an Ethiopian-trained health officer, a sanitarian, and two community nurses.

*Abstracted from two letters written by Dr. Hugh Clark in 1963.[17]

Resistance to Health Programs

There is little doubt that there still is a lack of understanding and acceptance of health care among the general populace of most underdeveloped nations. The three cardinal factors that must affect the planning of health services in developing nations are limited economic resources, scarce technological manpower, and population growth. No one method of approach to public health problems in these countries will suffice. The method to be followed is naturally dependent on the country and its circumstances. Some experts claim that the broad public health approach is dangerous because of the implication that it is possible to understand every man's ecology. Others suggest that the specific problem approach

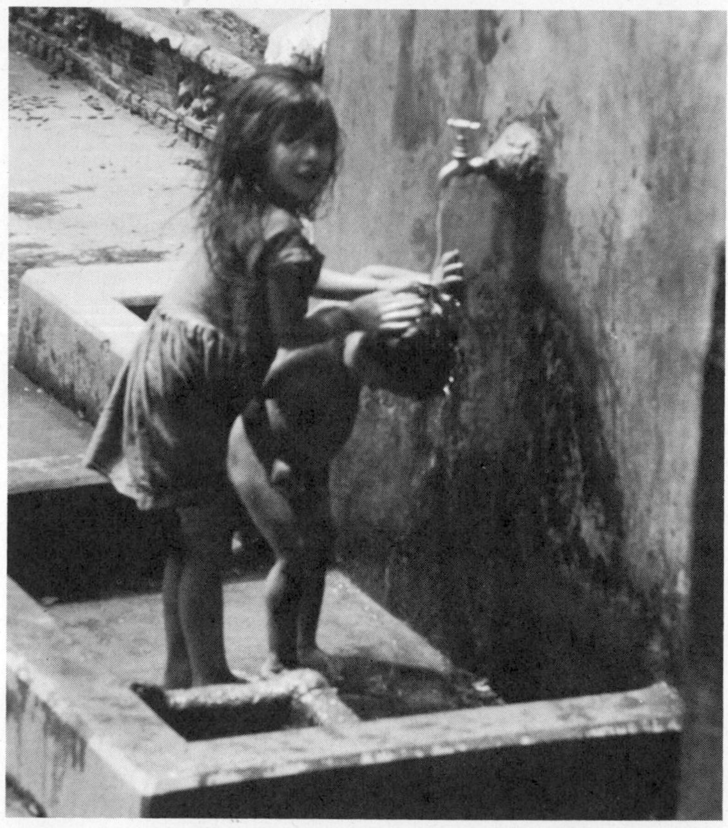

Figure 3–2 Poor sanitation can be seen even in capital city of Katmandu. (From Roche Laboratories: Medicine gains a foothold in the Himalayas. Medical Image and Commentary, April, 1969, p. 30. Courtesy of Mr. Joseph Breitenbach.)

may be the best. A broad attack on all traditional disease and the false concepts surrounding their cause and treatment, using the public primary school system as the battlefield, seems to be a promising approach. Kenya, for example, hosts a formidable range of diseases and health problems, and health personnel there were faced with many difficulties and divisions in planning and developing health services. Public health officials supported a broad ecological approach to health based on the concept of medicine as a liberal humanity and on serving the family's daily needs. The health services there regard the essential social unit as neither the individual nor the community, but the family. This approach has led to an integrated pyramidal structure of the services and the referral system. The rural health center, which serves as the basic community unit, is the foundation for the entire health service program.[18]

On the other hand, there was a surprising tide of resentment in Africa toward volunteers (in fact, toward Americans and whites in general) that made the continent the most troublesome area in the world for the Peace Corps. In fact, the Peace Corps was ousted from many African countries. Although the reasons are varied and complex, it is vitally important to review and analyze them if we expect to be successful in any international programs.

Young Africans often have a resentment against Europeans, against whites, and they resent having to depend on them so much. The Peace Corps was often the most visible evidence; Africans resented having outsiders doing a job that they feel they should have been doing themselves. So, an African leader, faced with mounting resentment and pressure, sometimes yielded to internal politics and asked the Peace Corps to leave, even when he knew it was doing a worthwhile or even vital job. The programs have been so large (Nigeria and Ethiopia, for instance, had more than 500 volunteers) that they became too obvious a target for young Africans resentful of outside help. Another problem was that the Peace Corps has put too much energy in one kind of work—teaching. Two thirds of the volunteers in Africa were teachers. It has always been that way. This puts too many volunteers into a sensitive, political area; African leaders are concerned about the indoctrination of their young.

Resistance to health programs and change is characteristic in all nations, including the United States. The *curandero,* or healer, treats tuberculosis, for example, with herbs and donkey milk in Texas, home of most of the country's two million or more citizens of Mexican origin. Because the disease does not respond, it is then rediagnosed as a supernatural disease, for treatment by a *brujo,* or witch doctor. When he fails, death is taken as God's will. Mental illness is always thought to be supernatural, and the hex must be eliminated by prayer or ritual. The brujos have a higher degree of success in treating these patients than do psychiatrists. Sociologists and anthropologists have suggested that modern preventive and scientific medicine can be most effective by adapting some of the curandero's methods and allowing persons to cling to their ancient customs and faith. Other recommendations include adding donkey milk to the tuberculosis treatment, injecting "holy water" during an epidemic, charging a token payment for each treatment (free treatment is refused as a despised form of charity), and enlisting curanderos as health aides.

The etiology of sickness and disease among nonwestern people has received insufficient attention. Many societies have their own special theory about disease; only through knowledge of the nature of their theory and its similarities and dissimilarities to modern theory can educators hope to be effective in inaugurating change through the teaching of scientific concepts and practices.

Etiology of Illness in Guinhangdan

One interesting study involves the etiology of illness in Guinhangdan, a village in

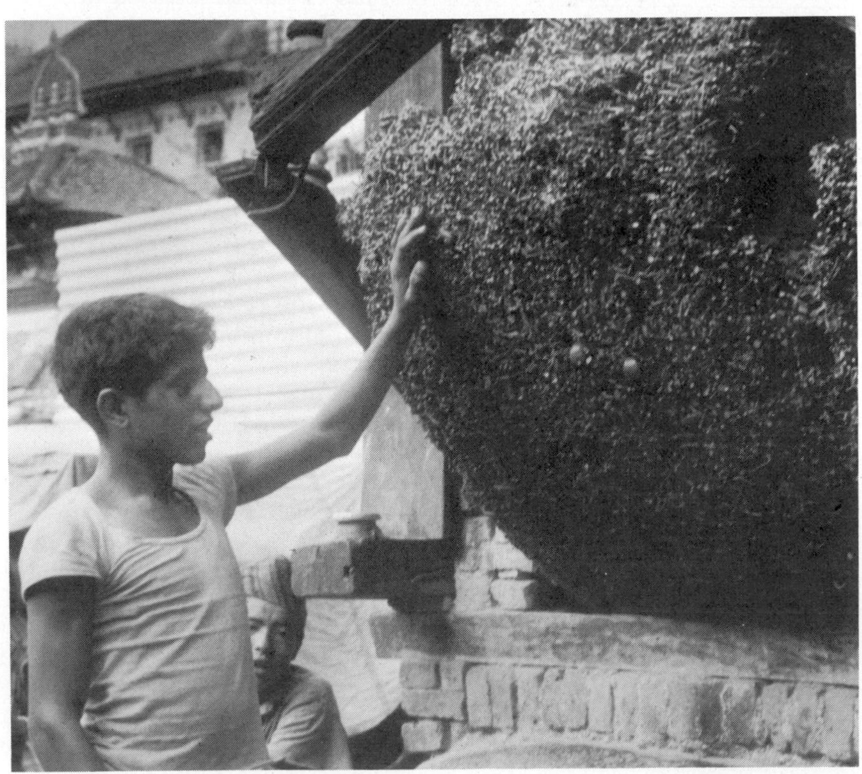

Figure 3–3 Nails hammered into a *bangae mudha* (crooked leg) are supposed to rid people of their toothaches In all Nepal there are only four dentists. (From Roche Laboratories: Medicine gains a foothold in the Himalayas. Medical Image and Commentary, April, 1969, p. 30. Courtesy of Mr. Joseph Breitenbach.)

eastern Leyte, the Philippine Islands, which is currently undergoing transition:*

The materials presented were gathered in a small agricultural-fishing village in eastern Leyte, Philippine Islands. The population, numbering 1,200, lives in houses which for the most part are made of bamboo and raised on stilts. The natives of Guinhangdan derive their subsistence from fishing in the ocean and, to a lesser degree, in the river which flanks the village on the west and north. Rice and coconuts are raised in fields west and south of the river, and a familiar part of the village picture is the pigs and chickens which wander freely around, in, and under the homes. The people are nominally Catholics, for the islands as a whole began to feel Catholic influence some 400 years ago. Individual commitment to the precepts and practices of Catholicism is tempered by allegiance to a pantheon of spirit-gods who are older in the area than are the supernaturals of the Catholic hierachy.

In the minds of the people, an important distinction as to the nature of illness has to do with the categorization of various afflictions, and this distinction is best understood in terms of the practitioner who treats the cases. Specialists among the curers and healers of the village include the midwife or partira who gives prenatal care when it is requested, assists at delivery, and routinely gives postnatal care. In most instances she will be called if the neonate becomes ill, and she will be consulted until the baby has passed the infant stage at about 1½ years of age. She is thus the obstetrician and pediatrician of the village. In addition, she treats painful menstrual cases. The masseuse or masseur, the hilot, attends to sprains, dislocations, and broken bones. His special province is the skeleton and such ills as the bones are heir to. If a person falls, twists an ankle, or has aches and pains near protuberant bones, he will call the hilot. The parasona, who may also be male or female, is consulted if one has been bitten by a centipede or a snake, or has been hurt by the spiny fins of a fish. There are two remaining classes of practitioners, the haplasan and tambalan; both treat skin diseases, infections, debilitating and fatal diseases, and the multitudinous vague aches and pains that are the lot of mankind. However, the haplasan treats only by anointing while the tambalan has a series of varied treatments. The tambalan is also reputed to be much more powerful, for his knowledge of agents of disease and treatment is more extensive.

Diagnosis, treatment, and patient education differ somewhat from specialist to specialist, but certain common notions are held by all. It is believed that treatment should be repeated three times, and preferably at the same time of day as during the first meeting. The most common forms of treatment are rubbing and massaging, ritual anointment with coconut oil accompanied by prayer, dry and wet poultices, and herbal additions to the drinking or bath water. No curer practices sucking or manual extraction. Nothing is injected into the body and pills are not prescribed. Dried roots, dried leaves, and scrapings of branches are popular medicinal ingredients, and coconut oil is ubiquitous. Specific leaves are required for specific ailments. For instance, a midwife treats constipation in children under five by placing tomato leaves on their stomachs; older children require "stronger" leaves. While the kind of leaf required is specific, the curer need not do the collecting. The parasona plants and tends a small patch of herbs which she uses in her therapy, a unique instance of a planned and conserved pharmacopoeia.

Diagnosis of malaise is arrived at by looking at the patient and by asking questions. A mother is guided by a fever or a dry tongue. The masseuse considers temperature and swelling. The paraphaplas has an exotic diagnostic technique. She ritually anoints the patients with coconut oil and has him lie down on large leaves, covers him with the same kind of leaves and lets him perspire for about an hour. When he is uncovered, the leaves are examined for the missiles which the annoyed encantos [gods] have presumably shot into him or at him. Bits of hair, sand, or part of insects are "proof" of the disease causation. The tambalan examines his patient and then awaits an inspirational diagnosis; the knowledge "just comes to him."

Little mention has been made of patent medicines, antibiotics, or any other paraphernalia of present-day therapy. The products of the pharmacist's shop and the services of an M.D. are not totally lacking in Guinhangdan, but they are accepted with but slight modifications of the old theories of disease. Some individuals who are both adherents to the old ways and timid advocates of the new show ingenuity in their resolution of conflicts between the two theories and the divergent practices. Some fail to effect a compromise and vacillate between the M.D. and the local curer. Some feel that the sphere of influence and competence of a local curer can be distinguished from the sphere of influence of a medical doctor, and this is a belief in which contemporary M.D.'s who were born and raised in a village are apt to concur. . . .[19]

*Reprinted from *Anthropology Today,* A. L. Kroeber, editor, by permission of the University of Chicago Press, excerpt from "Etiology of Illness in Guinhangdan" by Ethel Nurse. Copyright 1960 by the University of Chicago Press.

Other Points of View

Because the retaining of old mores and the development of new habits cause constant struggle throughout the world today, five points of view are presented that may be useful to persons seeking international assignments. They constitute an attitude that may affect the person's success and future:

1. In working in another country, one should understand what is already there—the physical, the mental, and the social—and these should be used as a foundation.

2. One should consider and recognize the relationship between the health programs and other developments in the region. Health and sickness are obviously not qualities that exist in a vacuum. A rise in the general level of a people's health usually means more production, but a sudden economic dip can wipe out the effects of a health program and even make the program itself grind to a stop.

3. One should handle the problems that the people themselves consider most important. Sometimes compromise is needed. Obviously, if we gain acceptance for none of our ideas, we shall have abdicated our role as experts. To be successful, we shall probably have to bend some of the heartfelt desires of the people with whom we work.

4. One should realize that transplants of whole technologies from one culture to another are not necessarily viable. For example, we pride ourselves on the success western medicine and public health have enjoyed. There is a natural temptation to attempt transplanting our know-how and technology, item by item, to the countries in which we serve. This often does not work. What is done in health in these less affluent lands must be tailored to local needs and local conditions. Because an approach to a problem is valid back home does not mean it is good somewhere else and the valid-back-home argument is seldom convincing.

5. It should be recognized that technical assistance is a two-way street. First of all, above all, let us be humble. Remember that we do not know it all. We have been wrong, and the people we seek to help have been right.[20]

Different as remote cultures may seem, they have their own strengths and resources. For example, in India it was found that latrines were more readily accepted by "spontaneously interested families, who were often the village leaders." If latrines were good enough for these leading families, they were good enough for the rest of the village population. Health workers coming from the West should be fully aware of the cultural blocks to health activities. In Latin America, belief in the power of the number three plays a big role: three pills for three days, or three injections, will have a "built-in acceptance."

Ritual days are also significant. In Indian villages, for instance, patients flock to health centers on Wednesdays, but few come on Thursdays. Unless the health worker pays heed to local practices and customs, he cannot meet with much success. Our Western ideas about rural-urban distinctions are not applicable to many of the newly developing countries. Many village areas in the East have a greater population density than urban areas have in the West. As a consequence, many "amenities of sanitation and other urban facilities can be supplied," although such areas are still psychologically and socially rural, with the customary cultural blocks to any change.[21] The following report on Malta Fever in Peru is just one example of cultural resistance to improvements in health care.

Malta Fever (Brucellosis) In Peru

Brucellosis is an infection of cattle, goats, and pigs that can be transmitted to man, usually through unpasteurized milk and cheese. Although rarely fatal, it is a serious disease that may last for several months, or even years, with recurrent episodes of fever accompanied by headache, weakness, profuse sweating, and chills.

In Peru, goats, rather than cattle or swine, are believed to be the primary source of the infection in humans. Goat milk is seldom drunk; it is mostly made into cheese, which is an important source of protein for many Peruvians. Those in the poorer sections of the population are in the habit of buying goat cheese sandwiches from peddlers, and prefer the cheese to be moist and fresh. Unfortunately, at that stage it usually still contains large numbers of bacteria, among them *Brucella melintensis,* the Malta fever organism.

All efforts to introduce pasteurization and chemical sterilization of milk and cheese have failed. Unsafe water supplies, lack of fuel for pasteurization or sterilization of utensils used in cheese-making, definite ideas about how goat cheese should taste, and the many persons involved in handling cheese add to the complexity of the problem.

A vaccine effective against brucellosis in goats has been developed and is suitable for mass operation.[22]

QUESTIONS FOR DISCUSSION

1. List and briefly discuss five obstacles that must be overcome before a community can

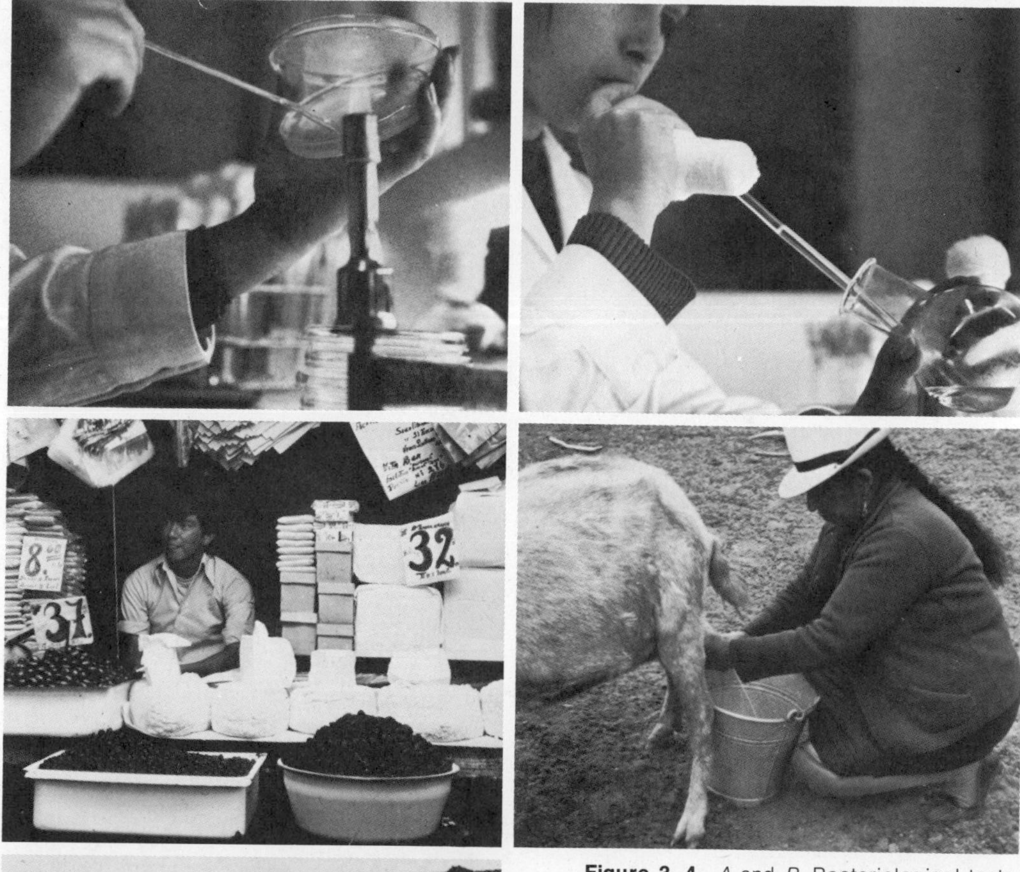

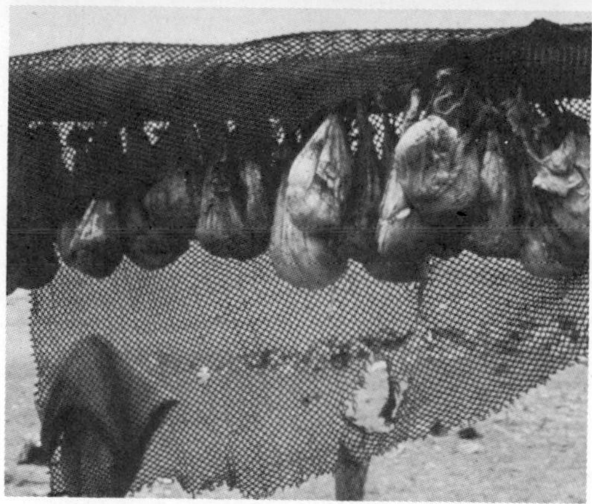

Figure 3–4 *A* and *B*, Bacteriological tests being carried out in a health laboratory in Lima. As part of the campaign against Malta fever, blood samples are taken from goats and tested for brucellosis infection. Analyses are also made of whey and milk during cheese-making. *C*, A stall in a Lima cheese market. The local people prefer the taste of fresh, unpasteurized goat cheese, but there is as yet no guarantee that it comes from one of the herds tested by the veterinary authorities. *D*, A worker milking one of a herd of goats that produce enough milk to make 25 kilograms of cheese every day. The most practical measure to guard against brucellosis is to vaccinate the goats and thus prevent the infection at its source. *E*, The rennet needed for cheese-making is obtained from the stomachs of young goats, first hung up to dry. (From Grinding, K.: Malta fever in Peru. World Health, September, 1973, pp. 8–10.)

organize and successfully solve its health problems.

2. What are some examples of the effect of cultural and social patterns on health? What are some examples in your community?
3. Name and briefly discuss three factors that may be responsible for group actions or reactions to community health programs.
4. "Public health activities may produce unexpected or undesirable results." Discuss this statement.
5. What are some major barriers to effective community health programs?
6. What is the purpose and function of a community health council?
7. How do the "social ailments" relate to public health programs?
8. "Public health must be concerned with disease prevention—*not* behavioral sciences." Discuss this statement.
9. Briefly discuss two changes in the nature of disease. How do these changes affect public health programs?
10. Briefly discuss two changes since 1900 in our social and environmental conditions. How do these affect public health programs?

11. Briefly discuss two recent changes in medical care practices and organization. How do these changes affect public health programs?
12. Briefly discuss two recent changes in public health practices. How do these changes affect public health programs?
13. Briefly discuss two recent changes in public opinion and behavior. How do these changes affect public health programs?
14. Why is there a greater emphasis on social workers in public health today?
15. Briefly discuss the philosophy behind public health social work.
16. List five general major activities of a public health social worker.
17. What major factors must affect the planning of health services in developing nations?
18. In Kenya, a broad ecological public health approach has been utilized. Briefly discuss the merits and weaknesses of this approach.
19. Why is there resistance to health programs and change in many countries?
20. List and briefly discuss five major points of view that may be useful to persons seeking international public health assignments.
21. How can students get involved in the social health problems of the community? The state? The country?
22. Discuss the implications of the population explosion. What is being done about it in the United States? In your state? In your city?

QUESTIONS FOR REVIEW

1. What different kinds of diseases are more prevalent today and have changed an individual's health into a private rather than a public matter?
2. Give some examples of three community interests with which public health has to compete.
3. Describe the full meaning of the term community health.
4. Which group represents the most powerful example of social cohesion in a community?
5. What are some of the reasons for a lack of community spirit in the health programs?
6. What disease is often caused by drinking unpasteurized milk? Among which group of people is this disease most prevalent?
7. What disease can be caused by eating raw pork?
8. List three factors that determine the reactions of each community group to its health needs.
9. Name some of the factors that mar the well-meant goals of health fund-raising agencies.
10. What two basic programs are often neglected as a result of the exaggeration of the money-raising aspect of a fund-raising agency?
11. What three kinds of regulations does health progress depend on?
12. Since the elimination of certain diseases, which aspects of community health are health workers now more able to concentrate on?
13. What is one of the future risks of a diabetic's prolonging his life by taking insulin?
14. Give two reasons for the greater need for and acceptance of social workers in public health and mental health programs.
15. According to a report by the Oklahoma State Department of Public Health, what specific kinds of social workers are urgently needed in mental health programs?
16. What are the major functions of social workers in public health and mental health?
17. What are the two major long-range goals of the new international cooperative health projects?
18. What are the important factors that affect the planning of health services in developing nations?
19. Why do many African countries resent the presence of the U.S. Peace Corps?
20. What is the first of the five points that a person seeking international assignments might find helpful?

REFERENCES

1. Koos, E. L.: New concepts in community organization for health. Amer. J. Publ. Health, *43*:466, 1953.
2. Paul, D. B.: *Respect for Cultural Differences.* Community Development Bulletin, University of London Institute of Education, *4*:42, 1953.
3. Hanlon, J. J.: *Principles of Public Health Administration,* 2nd ed. St. Louis, C. V. Mosby, 1955.
4. Hochbaum, G. M.: *Social Influences on Health Behavior.* Belmont, Calif., Wadsworth Publishing Co., 1970, pp. 45–47.
5. Clark, M.: Health in the Mexican-American Culture. Berkeley, University of California Press, 1970, pp. 1, 5.
6. Ibid., p. 164.
7. Horwood, A.: Hot and cold theory of disease. JAMA, *216*(7):1153, May 17, 1971.
8. Commission on Chronic Illness: *Chronic Illness in the United States: Prevention of Chronic Illness,* Vol. 1. Massachusetts, Harvard University Press, 1957, p. 43.
9. Sower, C., et al.: *Community Involvement.* New York, Free Press, 1957, p. 252.
10. Lancaster, P.: Donors' plight: health agencies grow in number with many offering same service. Wall Street Journal, October 11, 1960, pp. 1, 17.
11. Burney, L. E.: Community organization—an effective tool. Amer. J. Publ. Health, *44*:2, 1954.
12. Dubos, R. J.: *Mirage of Health.* New York, Harper & Brothers, 1959.
13. Boehm, W.: *The Curriculum Study.* Council on Social Work Education, 1959.
14. *Biennial Report, Oklahoma State Department of Public Health, July 1, 1960–June 30, 1962,* p. 17.
15. McCorkle, T.: The behavioral scientist in public health. a behavioral science service, Pub. Health Rep., *78*:431.
16. Rice, E. P.: Concepts of prevention as applied to the

practice of social work. Amer. J. Pub. Health, *52*:272, 1962.

17. Peace corps doctor (letter to the editor). JAMA, March 28, 1964, p. 1034.
18. Fendall, N. R. E.: Planning health services in developing countries. Publ. Health Rep., *78*:977, 1963.
19. Nurse, E.: Etiology of illness in Guinhangdan. *In* Kroeber, A. L. (ed.): *Anthropology Today.* Chicago, University of Chicago Press, 1960, pp. 1158–1171.
20. Baumgartner, L: Emerging adventure in world health. Amer. J. Publ. Health, *53*:549, 1963.
21. Taylor, C. E.: Medical care for developing countries (International Comments). JAMA, *188*:96, 1964.
22. Grinding, K.: Malta fever in Peru. World Health, September, 1973, pp. 8–10.

SUGGESTED READING

Abel-Smith, B.: *People Without Choice.* London, IPPF, 1975.

Alland, A.: *Adaptation in Cultural Evolution: An Approach to Medical Anthropology.* New York, Columbia University Press, 1970.

Christakis, G. (ed.): *Nutritional Assessment in Health Programs.* Washington, D.C., U.S. Department of Health, Education and Welfare, 1972.

Clark, M.: *Health in the Mexican-American Culture.* Berkeley, University of California Press, 1970.

Cooperstock, R. (ed.): *Social Aspects of the Medical Use of Psychotropic Drugs.* Symposium, Toronto, October 1973. Toronto, Addiction Research Foundation, 1974.

Elliott, K. M., and Knight, J.: *Human Rights in Health.* Amsterdam, Elsevier, 1975.

Fabrega, H., Jr., and Silver, D. B.: *Illness and Shamanistic Curing in Zinacantan: An Ethnomedical Analysis.* Stanford, Calif., Stanford University Press, 1973.

Frank, A., and Frank, S.: *The People's Handbook of Medical Care.* New York, Random House, 1972.

Gray, B. H.: *Human Subjects in Medical Experimentation: A Sociological Study of the Conduct and Regulation of Clinical Research.* New York, Wiley, 1975.

Gussow, Z.: A preliminary report of kayak-angst among the Eskimo of West Greenland: A study in sensory deprivation. Int. J. Soc. Psychiat., *9*(1), 1963.

Herskovits, M. J.: *Life in a Haitian Valley.* Garden City, N.Y., Doubleday & Co., 1971.

Insel, P. M., and Moss, R. H. (eds.): *Health and the Social Environment.* Lexington, Mass., D. C. Heath & Co., 1974.

Institute of Medicine: *Family Planning Training for Social Service.* Washington, D.C., 1975.

Judson, H. F.: *Heroin Addiction in Britain: What Americans Can Learn From the English Experience.* New York, Harcourt Brace Jovanovich, 1974.

Kohn, R., and White, K. L.: *Health Care: An International Study.* New York, Oxford University Press, 1975.

Lambo, T. A.: The concept and practice of mental health in African cultures. East African Med. J., *37*:464–472, 1960.

Lieberman, F., Caroff, P., and Gottesfeld, M.: *Before Addiction: How to Help Youth.* New York, Behavioral Publications, 1974.

Lynch, L. R. (ed.): *The Cross-Cultural Approach to Health Behavior.* Rutherford, N.J., Fairleigh Dickenson University Press, 1969.

McKeown, T., and Lowe, C. R.: *An Introduction to Social Medicine.* 2nd ed. Philadelphia, Blackwell Scientific Publications, 1974.

Morley, D.: *Paediatric Priorities in the Developing World.* London, Butterworth, 1973.

Nader, L., and Maretzki, T. (eds.): *Cultural Illness and Health.* Washington, D.C., American Anthropological Association, 1973.

National Clearinghouse for Alcohol Information: *Alcohol and Health Notes.* (Monthly newsletter.) Maryland, 1975.

National Health Forum (Chicago, 1973): *The Changing Role of the Public and Private Sector in Health Care.* New York, National Health Council, 1973.

National League for Nursing: *Response to Changing Needs.* Publication no. 15–1528, 1974.

Nolan, R. L., and Schwartz, J. L. (eds.): *Rural and Appalachian Health.* Springfield, Ill., Charles C Thomas, 1973.

Parker, A. W.: *The Team Approach to Primary Health Care.* Neighborhood Health Center Seminar Program, Monograph Series No. 3. Berkeley, University of California extension, 1973.

Quinn, J. R. (ed.): *China Medicine As We Saw It.* Department of Health, Education and Welfare Publication No. [NIH] 75-684. Bethesda, Md., National Institute of Health, 1974.

Read, M.: *Culture, Health and Disease.* London, Tavistock Publications, 1966.

Rin, H.: A study of the aetiology of koro in respect to the Chinese concept of illness. Int. J. Soc. Psychiat., *9*(1), 1965.

Risse, G. B. (ed.): *Modern China and Traditional Chinese Medicine: A Symposium Held at the University of Wisconsin, Madison.* Springfield, Ill., Charles C Thomas, 1973.

Rubel, A. J.: The epidemiology of a folk illness sustained in Hispanic America. Ethnology, *3*:268–283, 1964.

Sackheim, G.: *The Practice of Clinical Casework.* New York, Behavioral Publications, 1974.

Saltman, J.: *The New Alcoholics: Teenagers.* New York, Public Affairs Committee, 1974.

Selected bid on recent developments in medicine and public health; the People's Republic of China. Amer. J. Publ. Health, *64*(4): 406–410, April 1975.

Shanus, E.: *Making Services for the Elderly Work: Some Lessons From the British Experience.* Washington, D.C., U.S. Government Printing Office, 1971.

Shiloh, A., and Selaban, I. (eds.): *Ethnic Groups of America: Their Morbidity, Mortality, and Behavior Disorders.* Vol. 1—*The Jews;* Vol. 2—*The Blacks.* Springfield, Ill., Charles C Thomas, 1973, 1974.

Snow, L. F.: Folk medical beliefs and their implications for care of patients. A review based on studies among black Americans. Ann. Intern. Med., *81*:82–96, July, 1974.

Sprague, J. B.: Women and health bookshelf. Amer. J. Publ. Health, *65*(7):795–822, July, 1975.

Superintendent of Documents: *Multiple Source Funding and Management of Community Mental Health Facilities.* Washington, D.C., U.S. Government Printing Office, 1974.

Tancredi, L. R. (ed.): *Ethics of Health Care. Papers of the Conference on Health Care and Changing Values, November 27–29, 1973.* Washington, D.C., National Academy of Sciences, 1974.

Vogel, V. J.: *American Indian Medicine.* New York, Ballantine Books, 1975.

Whitten, N., Jr., and Szued, J. (eds.): *Afro-American Anthropology.* New York, The Free Press, 1970.

Wigley, R., and Cook, J.: *Community Health Concepts and Issues.* Chicago Eastern Illinois University, 1975.

CHAPTER 4

Solving Community Health Problems

Before we can attempt to solve community health problems, we must know a great deal about the community. A community may develop around such things as a church, a shopping center, a school, or common interests resulting from similar racial or national backgrounds. Communities may develop because of national or geographic boundaries which set them apart from other areas. They may be separated by man-made boundaries, such as railroads, main streets, and traffic arteries. They may exist simply because a group of similar people have elected to live near each other. The community, for our purpose, includes a group of people who have common health interests and needs which they can identify or be helped to identify. It includes among its residents enough people who have common interests and sufficiently similar backgrounds to work together toward common health goals.[1]

COMMUNITY ORGANIZATION

Community organization involves the neighborhood or other population unit in which there is common ground for action. Community organization also involves application of methods by which the people, the health services, and agencies of the community are brought together, usually through their chosen representatives, to identify their common health problems, to plan the kind of action needed to solve these problems, and to act together as a unit to solve them.[1] Knowledge of the neighborhoods, the people that constitute them, their interests, their needs, their cultural heritage and educational backgrounds is essential to successful community organization. All groups and all areas must have leaders if the program is to reach every home. A realistic understanding requires that we recognize the community as a power structure. Somewhere it has a point of authority. There are people in the community who decide what other people may or may not do, the best living and working conditions, and many other fundamental matters. Most citizens have good will and respect for their leaders, who, by virtue of past actions, are in a position to use this good will for the good of the community as a whole. Thus, the role of the community leader must be recognized as basically important in planning, organizing, and conducting community health programs.

Often the most successfully organized communities are those in which the planning is undertaken by the people themselves, with or without the aid of a professional worker. But a community can be guided in organizational techniques by many categories of professionally trained persons. If health is the prime incentive for organizing, then it is likely that the public health department or a voluntary health agency will provide the guidance or stimulus. Community population and area as well as available health resources and facilities must also be considered in community organization. In general, the more numerous the natural divisions of interest (racial and national groups, religions, shopping districts, etc.) in the community, the smaller will be the total number of people who can be brought together to work for common health goals.

For an effective program, the people themselves must become involved in determining and solving their health problems. They must determine their needs, set their goals, make their plans, and put those plans into action. They may accept some guidance, but they enjoy deciding for themselves what will be done about their needs. If the neighborhood health council is to have any longevity beyond the emergent need that prompts its establishment, then its members must continue to feel that it is *they* who make the decisions. Even if committee members decide to attack a health problem that may seem of little importance to health authorities, it is necessary that everyone cooperate in making the project a satisfying, successful experience for all. A successful program requires planning and active participation by community groups and health educators. For example, in Miami Beach, Florida, "Operation Re-entry" is a community-based center to help combat drug abuse. It has a comprehensive network of drug prevention, education, and treatment services. Community involvement combines community awareness groups and a professional advisory board.

Interested groups and individuals can study and plan together to improve the health of their community by carrying out the following six steps: recognizing health needs of the community, interesting others in community health needs, forming a community health council, conducting a community health survey to obtain the facts, educating the public and disseminating the facts, and evaluating the community health program.[2] *(Action* is the ultimate goal.) Following is a detailed discussion of each step.

Recognizing Health Needs

An organizational plan is essential to action and to the involvement of people from all parts of the community. The leaders must be identified and recruited as a first step in developing this plan. Finding leaders does not necessarily mean calling upon those who seem to be key people in a community. It means finding those persons who are acceptable to an entire group. The council must represent *all* community interests. Before a program can be developed, thorough knowledge of the community's health problems and resources is essential. This knowledge can be gained by:

1. Observation.
2. Comparing health services, activities, and facilities of the community with those of similar communities.
3. Ascertaining whether or not the community is served by a local health department.
4. Noting the size of population served by the health department.
5. Examining the health budget.
6. Comparing the health program with leading community health programs in other communities.
7. Studying the vital and communicable disease statistics of the community.

Interesting Others in Community Health Needs

Any organization or any individual can initiate action concerning a health problem by discussing it with others. After a number of people have been made aware of the problem, the interested individuals and organizations may be called together to plan for cooperative effort.

Community Health Council

The health service agency or comprehensive health planning council (as outlined in Chapter 1), mobilizing all the forces in a community willing to work for better health services, is the ideal instrument to achieve this goal. Objectives of the health council will include:

1. Bringing together medical, allied professional, and other interested groups for discussion and interchange of opinions. (The local health department, medical society, dental society, and other professional organizations must not be neglected.)
2. Serving as a clearing house for health and medical care problems and programs, facilitating joint planning where it is needed to speed up approved projects and to reduce duplication of efforts.
3. Encouraging, stimulating, fostering, and actively supporting the establishment of health and medical care programs designed to improve the health of the people in the community.
4. Gathering and analyzing information on medical care and health needs already obtained from surveys and initiating additional studies or surveys.

5. Devising means for reaching all the people, with particular attention to the extension of the projects into rural areas (theoretically, towns of less than 2500 people) and people living outside of cities and towns.[3]

The first task of the council is to prepare a constitution stating the council's objectives, membership, officers, funds, proceedings, bylaws, committees, and amendments. The composition of the council's membership is the key to success. The council must represent *all* community interests. There is nothing rigid about the operational chart, and each health council will need to vary its plan to meet local needs. Health council work should be an educational experience for the members and for the community. Also, there should be a good public information campaign so that the people may know the complete program, members, plans, and progress of the council. Although the success of a health council depends to a great extent upon leadership, a wise selection of activities is also of great importance. Each council will have to grow in a manner that best fits the needs of its own particular community. No general pattern can be applied equally to all councils. The concept of the health council implies that most of the existing health problems are created by the people, and therefore must be solved by the people. Working and planning together to solve health problems strengthens the group and the community.

The Group as a Medium of Change. The following eight principles represent a few of the basic propositions emerging from research in group dynamics. Since research is constantly going on and since it is the very nature of research to revise and reformulate our conceptions, we may be sure that these principles will have to be modified and improved as time goes by. In the meantime, they may serve as guides in our endeavors to develop a scientifically based technology of social management.

Principle No. 1. If the group is to be used effectively as a medium of change, those people who are to be changed and those who are to exert influence for change must have a strong sense of belonging to the same group.

Principle No. 2. The more attractive the group is to its members, the greater is the influence that the group can exert on its members.

Principle No. 3. The more relevant the changes that the group is trying to effect in attitudes, values, or behavior are to the basis of attraction to the group, the greater is the chance that the changes will be made.

Principle No. 4. The greater the prestige of a group member in the eyes of the other members, the greater the influence he can expect.

Principle No. 5. Efforts to change individuals or subparts of a group which, if successful, would have the result of making them deviate from the norms of the group will encounter strong resistance.

Principle No. 6. Strong pressure for changes in the group can be established by creating a shared perception by members of the need for change, thus making the source of pressure for change lie within the group.

Principle No. 7. Information relating to the need for change, plans for change, and consequences of change must be shared by all relevant people in the group.

Principle No. 8. Changes in one part of a group produce strain in other related parts, which can be reduced only by eliminating the changes or by bringing about readjustments in the related parts.

Conducting a Community Health Survey

The Health Service Agency or Health Planning Council or a cooperating group may undertake a health study in the community on a fact-finding level, with careful attention to community structure and function. A large proportion of social research in the field of public health has been devoted to community health surveys aimed at determining the health needs and resources of selected communities, the current patterns of utilization of health facilities and services, information and attitudes toward disease and public health programs, and social and psychological factors affecting health behavior. Most major public health departments and many voluntary health agencies have at some time conducted community studies to evaluate the state of public knowledge, attitudes, and behavior in regard to their programs. As might be expected, these surveys have shown great variation in health needs, resources, information, attitudes, and behavior according to demographic and social group characteristics.

Two of the more comprehensive of these community studies were conducted by Koos in the United States[4] and by Spence and associates in England.[5] These studies, conducted in widely varying geographic and social situations, have documented the relevance of community attitudes and values to the conduct of public health programs. Other community studies have been made in relation to specific public health problems, such as Leighton and associates in Canada[6] and Srole and associates in New York in their surveys of mental health.[7] In fact, most current social research studies on disease and health programs include an analysis of community factors as essential information for understanding the nature of the problem. A promising development in the field of public health is the establishment of community population laboratories in various schools of public health departments. These community laboratories are similar to the community laboratories attached to departments of sociology in many universities—for example, the Detroit Area Study of The University of Michigan. The idea of such community population laboratories is to set up a concentrated research study in a single community area. By studying one area in depth, a great deal of information is accumulated on various aspects of community structure, leadership, disease patterns, health resources, and needs.[8] Such information is then useful in all communities of similar character.

A survey is necessary to determine health *needs* and *resources* and to obtain facts. Once a health council has the facts, it is well on the way to better health services. Experience has proved that the people and their public servants are almost never opposed to establishing or improving local health services if only they can clearly see the need. The specific needs of the community may be determined through a professional survey or through a community self-survey. The second approach is one in which the citizens themselves, with the leadership of health authorities, make the study.

Method of Conducting a Community Health Survey. Either the self-survey or the professional survey method is useful in determining community needs. In assessing the needs of the nation, the United States Public Health Service staff, with cooperating agencies or a specially appointed commission that includes a number of staff members and field investigators, collect the data and report on their findings to officials at the executive level of the federal government. Direct federal action or federally supported local action is then undertaken where health needs are indicated.

A self-study of community health services is a useful way of informing community leaders and the public of health needs and the means for filling them. In any survey of community health services, motivation is needed that will lead to action. From studies sponsored by the Health Information Foundation, it is evident that community involvement in self-studies develops a core of persons who have a feeling of obligation to serve the community, community leaders who obtain additional information, and an increased knowledge of health in general and of health facilities available in the community. We have also learned from these studies that social scientists can be of assistance in the development of such studies, that it is necessary to have consultation from health experts, and that it is wise to have a community study tool or guide that can give direction to the marshalling of facts so that more of the people become aware of health needs and are thereby motivated to action.[9]

Self-study indicates involvement of community leaders, agency executives, and the public. The study must also consider the many aspects of our changing and developing communities. The *Guide to a Community Health Study* is a very useful and necessary document for persons engaged in evaluating the community health picture.

A community self-study should include:

1. Gathering of facts and opinions, and determination of interrelationships of agencies and individuals.
2. Determination of health needs.
3. Definition of specific objectives the community wishes to attain in order to solve needs or future health needs.
4. Consideration of alternative solutions to obtain these objectives.
5. Selection and development of a plan of action to attain the defined objectives.
6. Periodic evaluation of the program.[10]

The Springfield, Missouri community study of environmental health was a combined effort of city officials, county and state health officials, and the U.S. Public Health Service. The study encompassed the entire city area and that portion of the county included in concurrent studies being made for an area master plan. Detailed information on environmental health in both the city and the involved portion of the county was compiled, and recommendations were made for both areas.

A suggested outline for summarizing the results of this type of study is shown here:

1. Title of subject and area covered.
2. General statement on the subject including:
   (a) Importance in environmental planning.
   (b) Overall effects on the health, social, and economic factors in the community.
   (c) Interrelation with other environmental factors.
   (d) Description of acceptable standards for the subject.
3. Describe conditions in the community relating to this subject, including:
   (a) Conditions noted in study.
   (b) Areas where conditions do not meet accepted standards.
   (c) Governmental agency responsible for control of subject.
   (d) Present agency policies and activities relative to this subject.
   (e) Effectiveness of present policies and activities.
4. Recommendations for means of improvement to reach acceptable standards:
   (a) With existing resources: suggested policy changes, changed enforcement procedures, realignments of responsibility, additional enforcement authority, educational procedures, other means.
   (b) With expanded resources: additional funds; additional personnel; altered administration, such as transfer of responsibility or establishment of new department; with enabling legislation, either city, county, or state.
5. Recommendations of long-range goals (include necessity for, and means of, obtaining).
6. Establish priority of recommendations based on financial or other reasons.[11]

Some means of implementation, however, is needed if the full benefits of the study are to be realized.* The *Environmental Health Planning Guide* was used to provide guidance in the development of detailed information on each of the subjects analyzed in the study.[12]

*For further information refer to Kane, W. D.: Coordinating a community study of environmental health. Publ. Health Rep., 79:537, 1964.

Two other professional evaluative studies by Pyatt and Rogers[13] and by Wilner et al.[14] demonstrate the need and usefulness of surveys in helping to solve community health problems. Pyatt and Rogers estimated the benefit-cost ratios for water supply investments in Puerto Rico.[13] Such ratios have been used in the past for public works such as dams and highways, but seldom for public health. The investigators wanted to determine, in terms of mortality, morbidity, and decreased debility from water-borne diseases, the benefits of investing money in a municipal water supply. The methodology developed affords a formula for estimating the money value of man in relation to water supplies and for formulating policy decisions in developing areas.

Wilner et al. studied housing and its effect on family life.[14] They studied 1000 low-income families in Baltimore, Maryland. The test group had moved into new housing from ghettos. The control group had remained in the ghettos. The controls under 35 years of age had more serious episodes of illness and longer periods of disability than those in the new housing. Different housing did not appear to affect the outcome of pregnancies or the general morbidity of persons 35 to 39 years of age. Measurements of intelligence and school achievement of the test and control children were closely similar. However, the school promotion records were better for the test children than for the controls.

Six Kinds of Neighborhoods

Warren and Warren in a study on community interaction defined six kinds of neighborhoods, as described below:

To better understand and describe the variety of highly specialized roles that neighborhoods can play in the lives of their residents, a typology was developed based on three important principles of organization: interaction, identity, and connections. Research shows that these three factors are critical for understanding different situations people find themselves in when they want to take action at the neighborhood level. Taken together, these elements constitute a neighborhood's structural characteristics, the differences in neighborhood organization that cut across social-class, income, and ethnic lines.

In terms of specific questions to ask about a neighborhood, these dimensions can be put this way:

A. Interaction: During the year do people in the neighborhood get together quite often?

B. Identity: Do people in the neighborhood feel that they have a great deal in common?

C. Connections: Do many people in the neighborhood keep active in political parties and other forces outside the neighborhood?

Depending on how each question is answered, a specific neighborhood will fall into one of six types:

Integral. This is a neighborhood responding "yes" to the questions of identity, interaction, and linkage to the outside.

Parochial. Although people in a parochial neighborhood interact frequently, and feel very much a part of the area, they are isolated from the outside community; "we take care of our own" is the prevailing sentiment.

Diffuse. Neighbors have a good deal in common, but they share very little; most say they would go to their family, rather than their neighbors, for aid. Like most diffuse neighborhoods, people clearly identify with the community, but they have little interaction with each other, and feel little connection with the outside community.

Stepping-Stone. Close interaction between people and their ties to the larger community. The transient nature of the neighborhood, however, means that people often don't feel a strong connection to that particular area.

Transitory. There is neither interaction nor community identification in this type of neighborhood. Widespread distrust within the neighborhood.

Anomic. These neighborhoods are almost ephemeral, consisting of a lack of everything. There is little interaction between the residents, most of whom don't feel a part of the community, and few of whom engage in any activities outside the neighborhood. These communities are extreme.

Examination of neighborhood structure and process provides a useful, systematic description of neighborhood life in America's urban areas. It has been used over the years to study rioting patterns, alienation, energy conservation, response to mass-media influence, and mental health in many communities.[15]

Educating the Public

People in the lower socioeconomic segments of the population suffer from all of the major public health problems, but they are often ignorant of, or apathetic or resistant to, public health programs. They have many more immediate problems than those that are solved by the prevention of some distant and unknown disease or the lengthening of life. For most of these people, the rewards for participation in personal and family health are likely to appear unrealistic and remote. Studies are needed to aid in the planning of public health programs that are geared to the health needs of lower socioeconomic groups and that operate in accord with their values and behavioral patterns. A serious question may be raised as to whether it is members of these groups who are "disinterested and uninformed" about health services, or whether it is the public health worker who is "disinterested and uninformed" about the needs and cultural patterns of these groups.

Koos has investigated what the residents of a medium-size city in upstate New York thought and did about health and illness. In his study of "Regionville," a fictitious name for the community surveyed, a representative sample of the residents were interviewed regarding their process of identifying a given symptom as one that required medical attention, the reasons given for either seeking treatment or not seeking treatment, and their satisfaction or dissatisfaction with any medical care received. The respondents were grouped into three social classes, corresponding roughly to the upper, middle, and lower income levels.

A consistent difference in attitudes toward illness, the use of the physician and dentist, and in other aspects of health-related behavior was found in these three classes. In general, it was found that the lower an individual's social class, the less likely he was to identify a given symptom as one that indicated a need for professional treatment and, if identified, to seek treatment. Lower-class patients also tended to receive less psychological and physical satisfaction from the physician and from the treatment itself. This was felt to be partly a result of poor communication between the physician and his lower-class patient. Two factors appeared to be important in establishing a person's attitude toward personal health—the individual's estimate of what constituted acceptable behavior for a member of his social group, and the place of health in the value system of the individual and his family. The findings of Koos have been further substantiated by studies of the effectiveness of campaigns promoting free public polio vaccinations and chest x-rays. It was also found that more individuals in the higher-status groups tended to avail themselves of these health services when offered.[16]

The results of such research projects have demonstrated the effectiveness of community attitudes in blocking a public health measure despite its endorsement by professional health, dental, and medical associations. In general, these studies have shown that:

1. Appeals for public support through a referendum are not an effective way of introducing specific recommendations for health legislation, such as fluoridation.
2. The direct intervention of federal and state officials has not proved helpful in winning public support for obscurely defined health policies.
3. The issue of legal enforcement has largely shifted from one of medical protection to a violation of the rights of individuals.
4. Planting a "seed of doubt" is the most effective approach to opening new educational channels in the community.
5. The opponents of a program are often more vociferous than the proponents in their fight for a cause.
6. The opponents denounce the so-called medical experts and concentrate on weighted literature written by their allies.
7. The program meets with greater success if it is put into effect through community leaders and the enlisted support of strategic individuals.
8. Personal influence is a stronger factor than formal media of communication.
9. Most people are concerned and motivated by a threat to their life, not minor ills or discomforts.
10. Lower socioeconomic groups, in particular, find a way to strike back at status symbols, negative images, and authority.

Once the community health council has the facts, it is necessary to present them to *all* people in the community; the facts will often clearly reveal certain specific health needs. Council members will present definite workable plans for the solution of these needs, and action will begin. (See Fig. 4–2 for a community action plan.) Certain individuals and groups will always be opposed to suggested health reforms. This attitude reflects fear and ignorance, which may be overcome by revealing the facts. Dairy farmers, for example, often regard the phrase *public health* as a threat to their milk businesses. Yet countless experiences have proved that health department farm inspection and pasteurization programs have had exactly the opposite effect.

The Family

The family continues to be a basic natural unit in health education and health nursing, for the following reasons. The family monitors prevention, illness, health, and crisis. It is the family that decides whether an illness requires the attention of a health clinic or an M.D. or whether they should consult a health advisor, ask a druggist, seek a good friend's advice, institute home remedies, or "wait and see." In many instances public health workers can help maintain a home environment conducive to health maintenance and personnel development. Opportunities also exist for personnel to inform individuals and families about available community health agencies and resources and to distribute appropriate health education materials.

Other reasons why the family is the cogent unit of service include the following:

1. The family is considered the "natural and fundamental" unit of society.
2. The family as a group generates, prevents, tolerates, or corrects health problems within its membership. Health problems may be caused by family behavior or by family relationships.
3. The health problems of families are interlocking. The health of any one member of the family is highly likely to affect the health of others.
4. The family provides a crucial environmental force. Each individual member constantly interacts with the physical, social, and interpersonal milieu created by his family.
5. The family is the most frequent locus of health decision and action in personal care. In the long run it is most often the family unit, not the individual or the health professional, that decides whether or not to seek or to use health care.
6. The family is an effective and available channel for much of the community health education nursing effort. The community health nurse has the opportunity to develop sustained and close relationships with the families she serves.[17]

The community health worker's responsibility is not limited to using the family as a resource for health care; it also includes the provision of general support for family development. In planning service to families, community personnel must work within the framework of the whole structure of family health tasks. They must also understand that the resolution of many health problems will depend upon a family's skills in areas other than health. The family that utilizes health care services too late and too infrequently may be reflecting a general failure to relate to the community. Through efforts to solve a particular health problem, community health workers can help ameliorate other negative factors.

Community Heroes

It is interesting to note that community interest and support are sometimes stimulated or initiated by one individual. Upton Sinclair, Jessica Mitford, Dr. Frances Kelsey, Dr. Joseph Beasley, and Rachel Carson are only a few of these individuals. Public figures can have a great impact on health education and research. Consider the effect the following individuals have had on focusing the nation's attention on some very serious health problems: Franklin D. Roosevelt (polio); President Eisenhower (stroke); President Kennedy's sister (mental retardation); Arthur Godfrey (lung cancer); Richard Nixon (thrombophlebitis); and Shirley Temple Black, Betty Ford, and Happy Rockefeller (breast cancer).

Social Action

The free expression of the individual and group viewpoint on public policy plays an indispensable role in the functioning of practical democratic government. It is basic to such a government that there should be widespread acceptance of diversity in viewpoint and interest among differing economic, geographical, and social groups, a diffusion of political authority, and a free channel of communication between these diverse interests and the instruments of authority. This is especially true in the United States today, where explosive social changes are taking place and where there is an infinite variety of cultural backgrounds. Public interest groups can fulfill three important functions in support of these basic concepts: they can help those who make laws and policies to see current problems in total perspective, they can formulate useful proposals with respect to the mechanisms of carrying out legislation and public policy, and they can bring before the public the interests of those who are not articulate in their own right. Health workers can be particularly helpful in this last function because much of their work and knowledge is concerned with the nonproducers (such as the aged and children) and those who are ill or physically handicapped.

Programs are accepted and policies adopted only when the city council, the board of supervisors, or the legislature is convinced that such action is the logical and broadly accepted next step in the process of social evolution (Fig. 4–1). There must be evidence of general political and geographical boundary support, as well as local support. These three interrelated aspects of support can be well illustrated in the federal action for extension of coverage under the old age and survivors insurance program to farmers. To obtain congressional and senatorial support for this legislation, the following conditions were necessary: (1) there had to be the conviction that the country as a whole favored the contributory social insurance system and wished to see these workers brought under the system, (2) a majority of the members of Congress had to be convinced that their own constituencies were in favor of and would benefit by such a move, and (3) there had to be assurance that American agriculture – that is, a majority of farmers – was itself prepared to accept willingly such a move. Effective social action seeks to stimulate such support at all levels.[18]

It is doubtful that any single group or organization in this country possesses the power to bring about major legislative change without public support. This is one of the built-in safeguards protecting liberty in a multidimensional democratic society. Very large organizations do, however, often gain broad support for desired legislation by utilizing their own internal influence and voting power, and by seeking the active participation and cooperation of member agencies.

Mobilizing Support

Support of new or amended legislation at the community, state, or federal level must begin with the communication of information. Whether new legislation is sought by the individual, the group, or a major organization, information on the need for and purpose of such legislation must be communicated to the public and their support must be requested. In turn, the response of

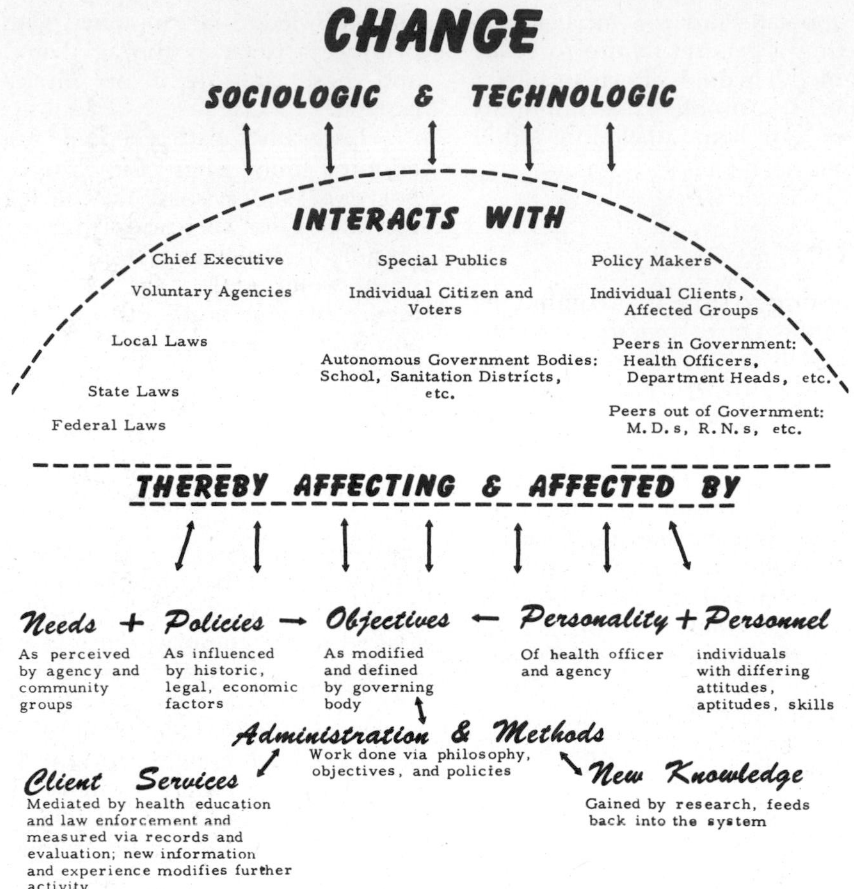

Figure 4–1 The ever-pressing climate of change and the spectrum of influences which shape administration and which, in turn, constantly respond to its activities. (From Blum, H. L., and Leonard, A. R.: *Public Administration—A Public Viewpoint.* New York, Macmillan, 1963.)

the public to such appeals must be communicated to persons in authority whose responsibility it is to carry out the will of the majority. How is such communication established? Obviously, direct communications of support are important evidences of opinion, whether in the form of letters, resolutions, or testimony. Often, a widely diverse series of communications is more indicative of a real climate of opinion than are concentrated policy declarations, because they seem to represent a broader cross-section of popular attitude.

Private public opinion polls are often carefully studied by policy makers, and some legislators conduct their own to analyze public attitude. Discussions in the press, on television, and on radio play an increasingly influential role in the development of this climate of support. It is often true that a multiplicity of diffused actions by a variety of groups, each acting independently in terms of its own particular interests, but moving in a common direction, is more persuasive than a single combined action by the same group of organizations. The simplest and most natural communication is often the most effective. For example, handwritten individual letters of obvious sincerity are sometimes more effective than the most elaborately formal resolution. Telegrams may be effective because they combine terseness and a sense of urgency. The conversational appeal is very effective since an exchange of ideas is present. In any case, specific reasons and facts for support or proposal are necessary. Councilmen or other officials need evidence of support and factual data with which to convince their still undecided colleagues. The most effective facts are those which a particular individual or group may have acquired through experience.

Public officials or leaders in business or in their community often command attention on public issues. Such individuals are accorded special consideration because of either their leadership abilities or their ability to influence public opinion (the editor of a local paper, for example). Leaders in organizations representing a major block of voters in a community also are especially influential—for example, labor leaders in a union town, Grange or Farm Bureau leaders in a rural community, and active members of registered political parties. Communications from all such persons are particularly helpful in gaining public support because their support infers support from the group they represent. Most effective of all, however, is evidence of a good cross-section of support from all elements—organizations, leaders, technicians, and average citizens.

Another important aspect of mobilizing support involves the minimizing of opposition to one's objectives. A major function of social action involves the analysis of the reasons for this opposition (for example, is the proposal considered a threat to present interests, is it regarded as competitive, is opposition based on ideological grounds?), the nature of its arguments, and the centers of its strength. In some cases, opposition can actually be converted to support by a proper presentation of facts. This is especially true when an organization is divided or has been persuaded to a position contrary to the best interests or full knowledge of most of its members by an aggressive campaign on the part of the opposition. When the opposition cannot be persuaded to change its position, its arguments can often be minimized and their effect with other groups limited by an effective presentation of a convincing rebuttal. Most important of all, naturally, is the aggressive mobilization of support for one's own cause to offset the opposition. Groups that do not take the trouble to offset the activities of their opponents are scarcely in a position to be indignant or surprised if the efforts of the opposition prove successful.

An important aspect of the art of advocacy in a democracy is acceptance of the existence of opposition. Opposition to most causes not only is inevitable and legitimate but can in many instances be most helpful. Causes that go unchallenged frequently stagnate; their proponents become lazy, their arguments cloudy, and the public increasingly indifferent. Public discussion and interest in the issues involved in a proposal are prerequisites to its achievement. Nothing so quickly creates this interest as a lively debate. Moreover, a challenge to a well-conceived program can often consolidate its support.

Directing expressions of support for a particular measure in a particular situation might be governed by three general objectives: the securing of a broad base of potential approval (as in a legislative body), specific action directed toward individuals who have a great deal of influence (doubtful members of a committee considering a bill, for example), and requests for secondary support from persons who might exert particular local influence (a request to local health officers and the local medical society that they indicate support for a particular proposal).

Any local group wishing to express support for a particular legislative proposal should always inform its own legislative representatives (city, county, state, or federal) of its position. When a bill is under committee consideration, the group should also let its views be known to the committee concerned, preferably (though not necessarily) through its own personal representative. If the group is a local affiliate of a national organization that has taken a position on a local or national issue, it may usefully express local endorsement of the position of the parent organization, especially in terms of local conditions. The more knowledge the group shows concerning the actual progress of such a measure through legislative process, the more respectfully its recommendations are apt to be treated. All elected representatives expect to be judged by their voting records and are sensitive to the views of local groups who follow and evaluate their actions.

Evaluating the Community Health Program

The council must periodically evaluate the program in terms of the objectives. A good program will change with the changing health needs and interests of the community. The following questions and answers may assist in evaluating the progress of a newly organized community health council:

1. Does the program enlist all groups? (All groups must be enlisted if the goal of reaching all people is to be attained.)
2. Do people understand the program? (No

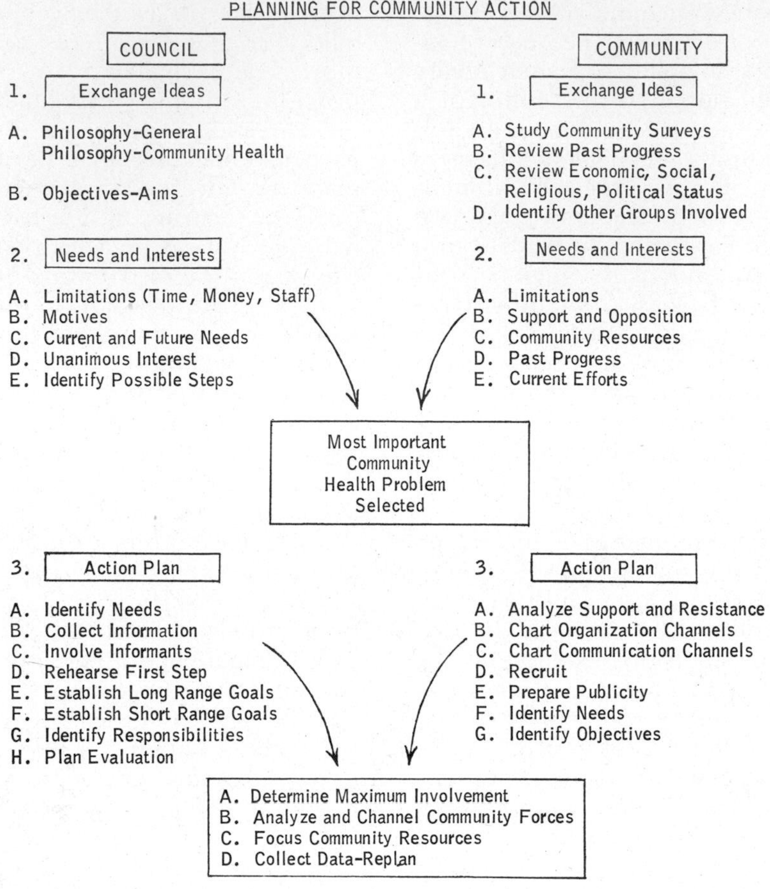

Figure 4–2 Community health councils must continually analyze and evaluate their objectives and actions in terms of their community as well as their groups.

program can succeed until the people fully understand it, become a part of its activities, and benefit from it.)

3. Do participating organizations and council committees assume responsibility for activities assigned to them?

4. Does the committee representing the professional groups properly support and provide stimulating guidance for the program? (The experience and training of the professional groups place them in a strategic position to perform this function to the end that sound and practical local health programs will be established.)

5. Are the people willing to give time and money when needed to support the activities of the local health council? (Greater success is assured and more lasting results can be expected when a large number of people take part in carrying out the approved program and participate in defraying its cost.)

6. Is it a genuine community effort? (For the sake of real progress and lasting benefits, all groups should work together in harmony with intelligently directed self-interest as a motivating force. Gains for the community as a whole should take precedence over individual and special group interests.)[19]

DELAYED COMMUNITY ACTION

Delay Through Minority Opposition

Pressure and special interest groups are always involved in any basic issue. Although issues should be aired and viewed from all sides, continued negative resistance by these groups against a statistically proven and accepted fact can seriously delay the community council's work. Certain religious beliefs and individual or group superstitions also tend to make the council's task tedious at times. However, the rights of these groups must be respected, and it is necessary to plan with representatives of these groups in an effort to reach satisfactory agreements and avoid delays in carrying out necessary programs.

Delay Through Procedure of Method

It seems obvious that any social action should always be directed toward an established goal. Yet it is extraordinary how much energy invested in social action is ineffectual because of the vagueness of such goals or because natural delays occur in their achievement.

The formulation of goals, to be effective, must be considered in three steps—long-range objectives, immediate next steps, and possible areas of compromise. An organization that has both long-range goals and intermediate objectives can usually make effective compromises in terms of maintaining forward progress. It is not enough, for example, to be for better housing, more security in old age, better oportunities for children, or a rising standard of living. Nearly everyone is for these objectives. The differences arise as to how they are to be achieved. Is better housing to be achieved by urging everyone to buy his own house, by government-insured apartment house construction, by public housing, by land subsidy, by subsidizing the rest of low-income families, by regulation of standards under the police power, or by some combination of these methods?

One of the biggest barriers to effective social action today is the complexity of these questions of method. Local groups, for example, inspired to action by the living conditions in ghettos or poverty pockets they see around them, are quickly discouraged in attempts to improve conditions by the complexities of the secondary mortgage market, lack of local financing, political influences, and property right. There is only one solution to these problems. Information and guidance in method must be obtained from some knowledgeable source whose judgment the local community committee can trust.

Organizations of national scope and affluence usually employ specialists to advise their leadership and their local affiliates on such questions. The policies of political parties evolve through national committees, which in turn are intended to guide their local affiliates on questions of procedure in solving local problems. Local, state, and federal governments make information and personnel available to assist public groups with planning on selected topics. Universities and colleges are excellent sources for research and for documentary information on social problems and methods for solution, and private research groups may be employed to evaluate the needs of the community and recommend the best method of action. In addition, community groups are obliged to rely heavily on each other for expert information on particular subjects. Thus, an organization devoted specifically to advancing the field of housing, health, social security, or welfare legislation will have to furnish technical information to other organizations whose interests are more broadly based.

Delay or failure of a community program may also occur where procedure has been legislated but individuals at the local level become discouraged in attempts to unravel the red tape caused by the many different levels and branches of government. Each branch has its own rules and regulations, and selected procedures must be followed in obtaining approval and appropriations. For example, a community may need a child guidance clinic. Obtaining the clinic involves initiation of the project in the local community and local approval, approval by a state agency, and probably federal review and approval of a grant of money. Unless an authority on legal and documentary procedure is consulted and state and federal interest obtained through support outside the community, the goal may not be attained.

Although communication of fact and verification of needs are basic to the establishment of community programs, current procedure in seeking public support for resolving social problems is often based on appeals to tradition, desires, prejudices, hatreds, and so on. So we have, on one hand, the rational and more ideal formation of public opinion, and on the other hand we have opinion formed in ways that deviate from such a pattern. Students of human motivation should understand how opinions are influenced and how support for programs is obtained in each case. These two procedures are shown in Table 4–1.

A classic example of how both the rational and nonrational patterns of public opinion may operate and how lengthy periods often associated with legislation of health measures can be is the history of the prohibition movement in the United States. Throughout early American history, isolated attempts were made to arouse public opinion against the sale and public consumption of alcoholic beverages. At first the problem was

TABLE 4–1 The Formation of Public Opinion.*

RATIONAL FORMATION OF PUBLIC OPINION	POSSIBLE DEVIATIONS FROM THE RATIONAL PATTERN
Locating and Defining the Problem	
Some problem begins to be defined by certain interested individuals or groups. A physical catastrophe such as a flood may pose the problem directly; the desire for a new community gymnasium may present and define the problem; rising prices may pose a very real problem to consumers; or a Pearl Harbor attack may raise the question of blame and begin an investigation. Whatever the problem, those who pose it must define it; they must determine its precise nature and location so that it can be discussed efficiently.	In modern mass society, social problems tend to be defined in vague and general terms. The complexity of modern society does not lend itself to clearly defined issues and simple solutions. If the expert outlines the facts of the problem sufficiently to provide a basis for its rational consideration, the layman often is smothered in a pile of complex data. Thus, the agitator or demagogue who simplifies the problem and offers an easy remedy may be given more support than that extended to the expert. In modern society, accurate and rational location and definition of a social problem are very difficult.
Analysis of the Problem	
Here an exploration is made of the problem. How serious is it? Is now the time to discuss it? How many of us does it affect? These and other questions are asked in our talks to our neighbors, in new stories and editorials, in radio discussions and speeches. Investigations are made to discover facts about the problem.	Persuaders for special interests may, by appeals to special interests, desires, group prejudices, and so on, prevent an objective analysis of the problem. Those who stand to benefit or lose personally from the solution of the problem may develop active systems of persuasion in an attempt to analyze the problem only from their particular point of view. Investigations are sometimes deliberately confused by special interests; censorship of certain facts may distort the analysis of the problem.
Examination of Possible Solutions	
After analysis of a problem, we look around for a possible solution. We examine various possibilities. The proponents of this or that solution begin to influence opinions. Radio and press, town hall, and	Special interest groups are very active during this stage of public opinion formation. Each group is attempting to win assent for its proposed solution. For example, industrial managers may contend that

*Adapted from Brembeck, W. L., and Howell, W. S.: *Persuasion, a Means of Social Control.* Englewood Cliffs, N.J., Prentice-Hall, 1963.

TABLE 4–1 The Formation of Public Opinion. ***(Continued)***

RATIONAL FORMATION OF PUBLIC OPINION	POSSIBLE DEVIATIONS FROM THE RATIONAL PATTERN
Examination of Possible Solutions	
church discuss the proposed solutions. The number of proposals gradually becomes reduced and the opposing camps of opinion become more clearly defined. In this step, investigative discussion usually changes to persuasive speaking in attempts to influence the direction of decision.	prosperity can come only through more production, and more production only by more rigid labor legislation; or contractors will favor a new gymnasium as the answer to the juvenile delinquency problem of the community. The systems of persuasion used by the special interest group may prevent the rational consideration of all the possible solutions, and focus attention on personal rather than the common welfare.
Selection of the Best Solution	
A preferred solution is tested in the crucible of debate. We examine its pros and cons. Some attempt is made to analyze the proposal carefully and objectively, organizing evidence to support each point at issue. Others choose to win the debate for their side by appealing to our needs, our desires, and our prejudices. In democratic organizations, a vote is taken to determine the winner, be it in political office, in a congressional debate over a bill, or in some local or community problem.	In the heat of public debate on a question of national concern, the use of irrational language, of slogans, stereotypes and legends comes in. Deep-seated emotional values are not readily changed by rational considerations. Skillful systems of propaganda, appealing to the old traditions and sentiments, may cause the direction of public debate to move toward a very irrational solution of a social problem.
Gaining Acceptance of the Chosen Solution	
In the previous step, usually a consensus is gained; seldom is there unanimous agreement. The majority may continue to legitimate its position by persuasion designed to get an ever-increasing acceptance of the winning proposal. The authors of a bill which has become law may continue to justify its existence; the political leader may continue a system of public relations "to keep himself in office"; or the proponents of the new gymnasium may conduct many community functions in the newly built building to enlist greater support.	Here the minority may continue to oppose in the hope that the majority opinion may be overthrown. Vast systems of propaganda may be established to render the majority legislation ineffective. On occasion, revolutionary groups attempt to arise at this point, defying the opinion of representative democracy and seeking to overthrow by force and violence that which they opposed earlier in a losing battle of persuasion.

attacked by only a few. Clergymen and such lay crusaders as Francis E. Willard aroused public discussion and support on the issue, whereas those personally engaged in the liquor industry attempted to minimize the public responsibility for, and the extent of, the problem. After 1900, the Anti-Saloon League was formed to voice the opinions of an ever-increasing number of "dry" sympathizers. Working through many of the churches, the League held numerous discussions regarding possible solutions to this health and social problem. It was decided that the mere teaching of temperance was not enough, but that prohibition laws must be established and enforced. The Drys then began chasing John Barleycorn in earnest. Their efforts were centered first on obtaining local option laws and next on passage of statewide prohibition laws. Soon it was apparent that state by state campaigns were slow, difficult to maintain, and in constant danger from as yet unreformed neighbors. At this point, persuasion was focused on Congress and a national program for support of prohibition.

The United States Brewers' Association was confronted by the weakness of their own methods of persuasion and the strength of their opponents' when in 1913 the Drys succeeded in gaining passage of the Webb-Kenyon bill. In 1916, a Congress favorable to the submission of a national prohibition amendment was elected, and in 1917 the Eighteenth Amendment to the Constitution was submitted to the individual states for ratification. By 1919, the necessary three-fourths of the states had ratified the amendment, which then became law. By 1922, 46 states had joined in supporting the law. An opinion that some years before had only the support of a few who felt a problem existed and needed a solution was now a public policy.

But today we know the story did not end here, for history has recorded how a minority persuaded its way back into majority rule. In the 1920's and early 1930's, the "Brewers' Big Wagon" began to roll again, and by 1933 the sneaking customer of the speak-easy gave way to the legal, respectable citizen consumer reinstated by public repeal of the hard-won law. Some have said that the failure of the prohibition movement simply demonstrates the fickleness of the public mind. Such an observation, however, overlooks the most obvious points—that public opinion is derived both rationally and irrationally, and that propaganda and other forms of modern persuasion have brought new elements into traditional methods of formulating public opinion and action.[20]

Other Factors That Delay Health Programs

Funds are necessary to conduct any program, and many times local, state, and federal funds for certain health programs are inadequate or even deleted from the budget. Fund-raising may cause a great deal of professional jealousy among community health agencies. Other factors causing jealousy include salaries, rank and status in the community, and professional training and preparation. These conditions lead only to uncoordinated, uncooperative, and unsuccessful programs.

In addition to the existence of these real problems in a community, there is also the problem of a time lag between new medical advances or discoveries and community action programs utilizing these advances. For example, Edward Jenner discovered smallpox vaccine in 1798, and yet it was not until 1920 that mass vaccination took place in the United States. Another illustration confronts many of our communities at the present time. Despite the fact that 25 years of research have proved that about one part per million of fluorine in community water supplies will reduce dental decay up to 65 per cent in children and will give life-long improved dental health, communities are slow to accept fluoridation. Also, consider the Salk polio vaccine. It has proved to be extremely effective, yet only about 60 per cent of the most susceptible age group have received vaccine. These are only a few examples of many such discouraging facts.

The reasons for this time lag are many and varied. Marred by the tragic occurrence of disease in 79 children as a result of faulty Salk polio vaccine administered at the start of its general use, many parents now cast a suspicious eye on all vaccines. The thalidomide tragedy compounded this distrust. Controversy and confusion among the "experts" about everything from the protection afforded by vitamins C and E to the effectiveness of the German measles vaccine leaves the public in an understandable state of uncertainty. Fear of doctors and needles, lack of funds, ignorance of the facts, indifference, adopting a "what was good enough for my father" attitude, and perhaps man's suspicious nature of anything with which he is not familiar and does not fully understand are all factors contributing to the time lag. For example, most persons realize that a major prevention of disease is periodic physical examination, yet many persons neglect these examinations because they are "too busy," "too thrifty," or "too healthy." Other persons do not recognize and accept the fact that they are either obese, alcoholic or in poor physical condition because they want to protect their ego.

Unexpected incidents sometimes do more to motivate or initiate the public to action than does a planned or organized health council. In 1959, the widespread publicity attending the illnesses of Secretary of State John Foster Dulles and of entertainer Arthur Godfrey probably did more to advance the crusade against cancer than any organized campaign. President Eisenhower's heart attack in 1955 and the health and medical publicity that followed alerted the nation to the cause and prevention of heart disease. President John F. Kennedy did a great deal to educate the public about mental retardation, as well as to promote physical fitness. Community epidemics that result in many fatalities, motor vehicle accidents resulting in deaths, and prominent community leaders committing suicide or being committed to a mental institution all leave their mark upon members of a community.

Our nation's competitive spirit weighs heavily in our favor. Americans do not like to be left behind in any field, whether it is science, education, physical fitness, medicine, or public health. Medical and public health advances of other nations certainly motivate many Americans to keep abreast and, if possible, ahead of them. In order to do this, community members have found that they must organize, plan, and work together in an effort to build a stronger and healthier nation.

Application of Established Methods

The following successful and effective community programs illustrate how different methods are utilized in obtaining greater active citizen participation in understanding and solving community health problems.

The first program involves creation of interest and use of community volunteers. Teenage volunteers were recruited and training for service in the Baltimore City Health Department during two summers. The first summer, 23 high school students and one college student contributed 2550 hours of volunteer service; the second summer 28 students gave 2070 hours of service. The supervisor of the volunteer program recruited the teenagers to meet two objectives: the students would supply manpower during the summer when clinics are crowded and full-time personnel are vacationing; and they would be working in areas of health and medicine, an exposure that might influence them to choose health careers. The students came from nine public high schools, one parochial school, one private school, and one college.

The second program involved community planning for special health needs. In Missoula, Montana, a group of physicians who treated most of the accident victims in the area became dissatisfied with the first aid given at accident sites and when the lack of planning in the community for medical coverage in multiple-victim accidents. Lack of organization seemed to be the chief obstacle to providing fast and adequate first aid and medical care to the community's accident victims. Ambulance services, hospitals, physicians, and surgeons were hampered by inefficient effort and delays, and the work of the police, the fire department, and military officials was hindered by confusion and ignorance. Three separate ambulance services, each from a different area, served the Missoula area with little or no coordination among them. The ambulances of all three services might be called to the scene of an accident when only one was needed, leaving none available for other calls that might occur. Sometimes the ambulances were manned with skilled first-aid personnel, sometimes with persons unskilled in first aid.

To promote better first aid service, a committee from the Western Montana Medical Society sought to persuade the three ambulance services to unite and to participate in planning a program for training ambulance personnel. However, the efforts at unification failed. During this period, the medical community, incensed at mismanagement of several accident cases, decided to assist a community telephone answering service in the establishment of a community ambulance service. The telephone service had been seeking financial aid for this purpose, and 36 local physicians signed a note for $3500 to get it started. Within two years of initiation of the new service, the caliber of Missoula's ambulance service had improved markedly, the time lapse in providing medical coverage at an accident and in delivery of victims to physician or hospital services was reduced, and the medical community and the general public have shown increasing confidence in the community's ambulance service. Following a review of the service by a group of local physicians, a revised course in first aid was offered to ambulance personnel to further improve the quality of emergency care in the area.[21]

The third program reveals that volunteers from community groups are vitally needed to help maintain and promote community health programs. For 10 years, the Santa Fe County Health Department in New Mexico had tried to conduct a community-wide tuberculin testing program. The tuberculosis association had carried out a yearly educational campaign, and the press, radio stations, and TV stations had assisted in the education and promotional appeal; but the important work of following up on persons with positive reactions had not been completed. The program was failing because public health and school nurses could not make the many home visits required to follow up those with positive reactions and at the same time keep up with their regular work. They just didn't have the time. As a result, the health department and the tuberculosis association had no records of the percentage of positive tuberculin reactors residing within the community. Without adequate records, how could the community possibly promote a progressive program for eradicating tuberculosis?

Representatives from the staffs of the tuberculosis association and the local health department met to discuss ways of conducting a tuberculin testing survey in which the follow-up phase could be successfully completed. The committee decided that if the incidence of positive reactors in the school-age population could be determined and followed, they would have an important basis for determining what the tuberculosis problem would be in the next 10, 20, and 30 years in Santa Fe County. In addition, because the county population is for the most part composed of large family units, an index of tuberculosis infection in the school-age group would provide a rather accurate index of tuberculosis in the community as a whole. Then, of course, it was expected that they would find some leads to additional active cases of tuberculosis, even though the tuberculosis register was kept up-to-date and all known contacts were investigated. They also sought to develop a successful and economical plan for operating a mass survey in the community that would not overburden public health and school nurses. It was decided that the executive secretary of the tuberculosis association, the public health nursing supervisor from the local health department, and the school health educator from the state department of health would formulate plans to establish the new program.

Development of a spirit of cooperation within the community was, the committee decided, the key to the success of the survey. If this spirit were developed, there would be no problem in obtaining community volunteers to assist in the program. If the entire program were worked out in advance and the volunteer group asked to perform specific tasks, difficulties in completing the survey could be reduced. Assistance from many groups in the community was needed, but also vital to the program were obtaining the services of volunteer nurses to assist in the tuberculin testing, obtaining the help of parents to assist with health records, and asking public health nurses to volunteer to work in the evenings so that parents of children with positive reactions could come to the health department for follow-up work at a time convenient to them.

The plan of operation was divided into two separate programs—obtaining community support, and training volunteer help and public health and school nurses to carry out the basic elements of tuberculin testing of the school children and to follow up all positive reactors.

The plan was presented in detail at a meetng composed of the public health staff, all school nurses, the tuberculosis association staff, board of health members, and the press. It was accepted with an enthusiasm that was to accompany all activities of the program in the following two months.

With the community's support, the survey was successfully completed and the following facts were revealed:

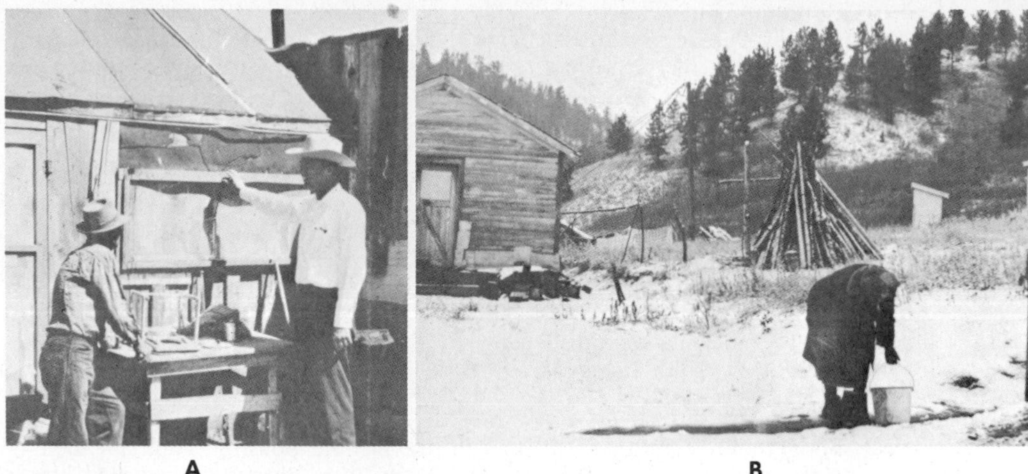

Figure 4–3 *A,* Health educator visits an Indian home to discuss need for new screening with the owner. *B,* Riser pipe keeps water for this Navajo home from freezing in the snow. New privies are a safe distance from the house. (From Kane, R. L.: Community medicine on the Navajo reservation. HSMHA Health Reports, *86*(8):737, August, 1971.)

1. The positive reactor rate for the school-age population was 4 per cent, which is about normal for this part of the country.
2. In a tuberculin testing and follow-up program, the professional nursing staff in the health department is necessary only in the areas of health education, in-service training, planning, and follow-up service.

A MODEL FOR COMMUNITY ACTION

With impetus from a graduate class in mass communications at the University of Denver, the Colorado Department of Health sponsored a mass media venereal disease education campaign in the five-county Denver metropolitan area. The campaign ran for six weeks, with radio and television stations airing a minimum of 12 spot announcements daily. The United Way Department of Community Services provided its telephone number to be used in all spot announcements and on 13 different posters specifically developed for the Denver campaign. Major results of the campaign were as follows. A venereal disease clinic was opened at Colorado General Hospital, which is connected with the University of Colorado Medical School. A total of 1632 patients were seen at local clinics, and 436 were found to be infected. The United Way received 2733 telephone calls, and 255 pharmacies (73 per cent) in the five-county area displayed posters, as did many junior and senior high schools. The State's public health clinics extended their pre-campaign by 18 hours weekly, to the present 60 hours per week. To date, 10 regional laboratories have been officially approved by the Colorado Department of Health for gonorrhea screening activities. Additionally, four universities in the state are cross-crediting a graduate course in venereal disease education for teachers, counselors, school nurses, and others desiring graduate credit. Over 1000 teachers have been trained. The course has been approved by the Colorado Commission of Higher Education.

3. A skin-testing program can be very successful when volunteers are used for interpreting the program to the public, for record work, and for actual skin-testing procedures (only volunteers who are nurses can perform skin tests).
4. It is possible to organize on a community-wide basis a tuberculin testing program that is efficient in terms of service, time, and cost.
5. The survey provided access to new cases and suspects not known before.
6. So far, the results are as follows: new cases diagnosed, one; new suspects, pending diagnosis, 25; other conditions found, seven.[22]

The fourth program illustrates how regular evaluation can lead to action for furnishing a more comprehensive community health service. The Oberlin Plan for Community Health Services was formulated by the Oberlin Health Commission in Oberlin, Ohio, in order to coordinate the services of an increasing number of public and volunteer health agencies, and to meet the needs of the growing numbers of senior citizens. After four years, the achievements of the Oberlin Plan were as follows.

1. Coordination of all health agencies.
2. Medical aid to any needy citizen who does not qualify for service through any other existing agency.
3. Health education that is coordinated with public health, school and voluntary health agency efforts.
4. A Senior Citizens Program that includes physical therapy, occupational therapy and diversional therapy.[23]

A unique approach to help teachers get involved in community health education was presented as an inservice program for elementary teachers in one of this school district's attendance areas. This included a 90-minute, 17-mile, guided "Rubber-neck" bus tour of Community Health Agencies. It was a tour filled with study packets, resource material, guitar music, peanuts, popcorn, and lively commentary. Several months prior to the tour, the need for improvement in these areas was brought to the attention of the school district superintendent and the four directors of School District 4J by the head nurse of the School District Department. A plan for inservice programs was approved and dates for the sessions reserved on the annual calendar. A committee was formed in each of the four high school attendance areas. The committee in this instance was composed of the area director, the high school nurse who served as chairman, a high school health educator, a junior high health educator, and three elementary teachers, representing primary and intermediate levels. This committee represented the high school, two junior high schools, and eight elementary schools in one attendance area.

The purpose of the inservice program was to acquaint teachers with the community's many varied health resources. The goals were: (1) to encourage the teachers to explore and utilize these community health resources in the classroom presentation, (2) to relate the use of these agencies to the lives of their students, (3) to guide students out into the community to enhance their knowledge of health resources, and (4) to help students see health resources in a relevant light. Stress was placed upon the World Health Organization definition of health for every individual: "Health is the state of maximum physical, mental and social well-being; not merely the absence of disease or infirmity.[24]

CITIZENS' LEAGUE AGAINST POLLUTION

Many political scientists argue that one of the ways to deal with pollution lies in regional governments designed to solve environmental abuses on a broad, systematic basis. The U.S. has an impressive model. The seven Minnesota counties that include Minneapolis, St. Paul and their bustling suburbs have recently discarded the old Balkanization of power for something new; the Twin Cities Metropolitan Council, which controls key planning for the region's 2,000,000 people while coexisting with 321 political units.

Separated by the Mississippi River, Minneapolis and St. Paul had long neglected their common problems as the nation's fifteenth largest urban area. On occasion, they joined to fight mosquitoes, build an airport and support big-league athletic teams. But the cities could not agree—among themselves or with their suburban neighbors—on any common solutions for some of the region's more pressing ailments.

Great factories sent pollutants into the good Minnesota air, sub-divisions sprawled over the pleasant landscape, delays mounted at the airport, and traffic began to choke the highways. Most shocking of all, the water table was polluted by thousands of leaky backyard cesspools. Even this problem, which posed an imminent threat to health, seemed beyond resolution. For four straight biennial sessions, the state legislature tried to form a huge metropolitan sewer district. But suburbanites felt city dwellers were going to take advantage of them—and vice versa—so the bill failed to pass.

Finally, concerned residents organized a 3600-member Citizens' League, which helped to devise a regional planning body that both cities and suburbs would trust. With leadership by the League the state legislature passed an act setting up the Metropolitan Council to provide for "the orderly physical, social and economic growth of the area."

Under legislation, the council controls only regional matters like pollution, sewage, highway routes and preservation of open space, leaving to each locality full sovereignty over police, schools, zoning and taxation. The 14 council members are appointed by the Governor from newly created districts of roughly equal population, and their chairman is selected at large. Thus the group avoids being influenced by myopic municipalities. The council is also financially independent. It funds itself mainly through a 70¢ levy on every $1000 of taxable valuation—a property surtax that brings in about $1,000,000 a year. Its staff of 50 experts includes city planners, sanitary engineers and political scientists. It has power to match its vision. Even small local projects concerning bus routes and landfill must correlate with the council's regional plan or be suspended.

If there is a flaw in the council, it is that members are not elected by the public. Yet the group's initial accomplishments suggest that other medium-sized metropolitan areas in the U.S. might do well to emulate the Twin Cities' plan. The council has already vetoed a site for a major new airport, on the ground that it would have brought too much noise and blight to nearby residential areas. On the positive side, the council is developing a mass-transit plan and has mapped out a gigantic sewer district that will unite 34 existing systems running through 121 towns and 300 governmental units.[25]

VICTORY IN THE EVERGLADES

The concrete had already been poured for the first runway of a mammoth jetport that would doom this fabled wilderness 8 miles north of Everglades National Park, Florida, but then an enlightened citizenry began to fight.

Basically, the Floridians won their fight by means and agencies available to all citizens. First, they called upon scientists expert in certain aspects of the local ecology, including the personnel of the U.S. Geological Survey and the U.S. Fish and Wildlife Service. Then citizens' committees were set up to keep the government—both local and federal—informed of their findings. These findings were widely publicized through organizations already set up to disseminate information—the Izaak Walton League, the Florida Audubon Society, and the Florida Federation of Garden Clubs, as well as churches and the press. High school and college students distributed fliers and knocked on doors. Possibly the most important lesson that could be learned from the Floridians is that many of the people who helped to stop the jetport are precisely the ones who, had they not received accurate information, would have supported it. As one scientist put it succinctly: "Man is an intelligent animal—if you show him that he is destroying his environment, he will not persist."

A NUTRITION EDUCATION PROGRAM FOR MIGRANT FARMWORKERS

The Migrant Nutrition Education Project located in the lower Rio Grande Valley, Hidalgo County, Texas, was responsible for surveying the nutritional status of children of Mexican-American migrant farm workers and improving the nutritional status of the target population through nutrition education and increased enrollment in food assistance programs. Preliminary surveys showed vitamin A deficiency in approximately one-third to one-half of the children in the target population. Vitamin D deficiency and anemia were also present. The survey of dietary patterns showed that consumption of fruits, vegetables, and milk products was low, and that snacking was common. Bilingual Mexican-American mothers from the target population were hired and trained as nutrition aides.

Since the most prevalent nutritional problem in the target population was vitamin A deficiency, food sources of vitamin A were emphasized in a variety of ways. The aides selected two styles of dresses (their uniforms) in dark green to represent vitamin A foods. In addition, the uniforms gave the project identity, so that target families could easily recognize aides from the project in different migrant areas. The supervisors and aides wore similar uniforms, which seemed to increase the team spirit. The uniform helped families recognize aides and supervisors ("the ladies in green") in neighborhoods where they weren't already known personally and may have increased the aides' authority in neighborhoods where they lived or were already known as friends.[26]

HOPE IS THE BEST MEDICINE

The U.S.S. HOPE, a 15,000-ton World War II hospital ship, sailed to some of the world's poverty regions with a cargo of about 150 American doctors, dentists, and nurses. Some of these medics were dispersed into the city and countryside to train local people; the rest treated the sick in the ship's model hospital. The ship was retired in 1974.

As a privately financed project (annual budget is $6.7 million, with 70 per cent coming from individuals and 30 per cent from corporations), HOPE went only where it was invited and usually stayed no more than nine or 10 months. It visited fifteen countries on four continents, trained 7000 persons in medicine, dentistry, and nursing, and compiled a list of achievements that ranged from organizing the first nursing school in northern Peru to fabricating the first set of false teeth in Guinea.

Hope public health teams worked closely, with their counterparts, tackling the broader health problems of the country. The philosophy of the approach was summarized by Dr. Walsh: "We don't give the local people charity. We demand work from them. If they've got a worm problem, we don't hand out worm medicine. First they must learn to build latrines and wash their hands. Then we give them worm medicine."

The public health teams sometimes encountered unusual cultural techniques. In one Latin American country, a Hope team went to a small community to immunize all of the villagers. Despite advance arrangements, the people were reluctant to have injections, and very few appeared. When the local police captain heard about the situation, he called his policemen together, presented each one of them with an extra pistol, and suggested that perhaps they could encourage the villagers to report to the Hope truck for injections. The Hope team, not knowing until later the motivating factor, was very favorably impressed with the sudden enthusiasm on the part of the entire populace of the area to get immunized, making the visit the most statistically successful of the entire Hope immunization campaign.

With the growing awareness that America too has poverty pockets, some of the project's workers began to feel that HOPE—like charity—should begin at home. Explains HOPE's founder-director, Dr. William Walsh: "Our country is already approaching something of a crisis in medical care. We have only about half the doctors and medical technicians we need and two-thirds of the nurses. And as you can imagine, it's even worse in poor areas. Therefore, about a year ago, we decided that in addition to our work overseas, we would also try to get something going here in the United States. After looking all around the country, we decided to start in Laredo."

HOPE couldn't have found a better spot to launch its first domestic program. Laredo is a dusty Texas border town of some 78,000 people, a town that in all its sun-baked history has managed to pick up few distinctions, except that it is now the poorest city in the nation. About 85 per cent of the population are Mexican-Americans, many of whom scratch out an existence as field hands. There is much illness, few doctors, and only one 250-bed hospital to serve them and anyone else within a 150-mile radius.

Moreover, with this underexposure to modern medicine, superstition still flourishes. It is not at all uncommon for an appendicitis patient to attempt the home-cure of wrapping his belly with spiced banana leaves, or for a mother to refuse to let a doctor see her newborn baby for fear that he might look upon the child with a *mal de ojo* (evil eye). "So much of this superstition and the sickness that comes with it." concludes José Gonzalez, administrator of the county's public health program, "can be wiped out if only we can educate the people. But we just don't have the medical personnel to do it. That's where HOPE comes in."

Shortly after the eight-member HOPE staff arrived, they began seeking out candidates for their "health assistant" trainee program—a program that in four months intends to make nurses' aides and public health workers out of undereducated housewives and field hands.

Once the health assistants completed their training, they could immediately fill the vacant slots in the public health program and at the local hospital. Yet their education does not stop there. HOPE's staff has begun to map out an inservice training program which will provide ongoing education for the new health assistants, as well as for many other nurses' aides and public health workers.

HOPE has already started similar projects throughout the country. And if HOPE is successful, perhaps other programs, both public and private, will follow suit. "This is just the beginning," says Dr. Leo Cigarroa, Laredo surgeon and co-chairman of HOPE's Laredo project. "If we prove here that housewives and field hands can be made into competent health workers, there's no reason why it can't be done elsewhere."

Meanwhile, the eyes of Texas, and much of the nation, are upon them. They are beginning to see that the ready solution to poor quality medicine in poor areas may not be a lot of doctors and a lot of money, but a classroom full of interested citizens and a little bit of HOPE.*

---

*For further information write Project Hope, 2233 Wisconsin Ave., N.W., Washington, D.C., 20007. "The Spirit of American Medicine," a new health ship, was launched on July 4, 1976.

SOLVING PROBLEMS IN OTHER COUNTRIES

Community Participation in India

In India, the State Irrigation Department, which supplies water for fields through tube-wells, started in the early 1950's to construct overhead tanks and, in some villages, to lay water mains and pipes and to provide water to the communities through public stand posts. This plan, however, failed totally, primarily because (a) the communities were not involved in either the planning or implementation of the project; (b) no arrangements were made to dispose of the waste water; (c) no arrangements were made for regular supply of water and the maintenance of the project; and (d) the people for whom the plan was designed did not own it and therefore considered it a scheme of the government.

In order to determine the reasons for the lack of community support, a survey was taken to find out why the villagers were opposed to the water project. It may be of interest to examine some of their views:

—Water is a free gift from nature; we should not have to pay for it.
—Well water is cool and refreshing and generally superior to tap water.
—Many people using tap water are in hospitals.
—Drawing well water is good exercise for ladies and reduces gossip.
—Sweet memories are associated with the use of wells.
—Well water is always available.

To win the people over to the project, a waterworks executive committee was formed, made up of seven members, i.e., one from each village involved. An educational program was developed with the help of a health educator and a senior sanitarian to counter the negative views expressed by the people. Various approaches were used in educating the people, but the most practical and effective one proved to be participation in the "evening sittings." These are informal spontaneous meetings that take place almost daily in all the villages, at which people gather during leisure hours in small groups to talk about various matters of mutual interest. The sittings are generally held just outside the house of a community leader or at a place where it is convenient for the villagers to sit. The Banki water project finally succeeded, demonstrating that it is possible, through patient health education efforts, to overcome the initial resistance of the population and to achieve community involvement and support—to the point where the people assumed full responsibility for the maintenance of the project.[27]

Selling Vasectomies in India

India's vasectomy program is part of the extensive family planning activities being undertaken by the Indian government. The United States, through the Agency for International Development, has been a major donor in helping the Indian government achieve its goals in this vital area. At two month-long vasectomy festivals in Kerala, India, more than 80,000 people underwent sterilization. This was acclaimed by many as a major success in the concerted family planning compaign in India. (See Fig. 4–4.)

The vasectomy operation for men was chosen as the family planning method to be popularized at the camps because it is the easiest, surest, most permanent method, is less expensive, requires less time, and is best suited to existing conditions of Kerala. There were arrangements at the camp for recanalization operations for all registered cases, medical checkups for the family members of all who were adopting sterilizations in the camp, baby shows, cultural programs, and a family planning exhibition. A sterility clinic provided service to infertile couples through detailed tests, medication, and advice.

Fifty booths with operation tables and accessories were set up. Arrangements were also made for reception, registration, information, and pre- and postoperative waiting rooms. About 100 doctors with supporting paramedical staff and the required number of staff of other categories were stationed at the camp. With the help of the government of India, the Kerala state government, and CARE through AID, a number of incentives were made available to acceptors and promoters at the camp. Each person who was sterilized received 100 rupees (about $12) in cash and goods,—about one month's income for the average Indian.[28]

Public Health in China

The Chinese have managed to improve their system of medical care and enhance the health of their population by making medical changes an integral part of a change in their society as a whole. Discipline and political theory are large elements in Peking's

A
B
C
D
TWO OR THREE Children
THE BEST REMEDY IS
STERILISATION

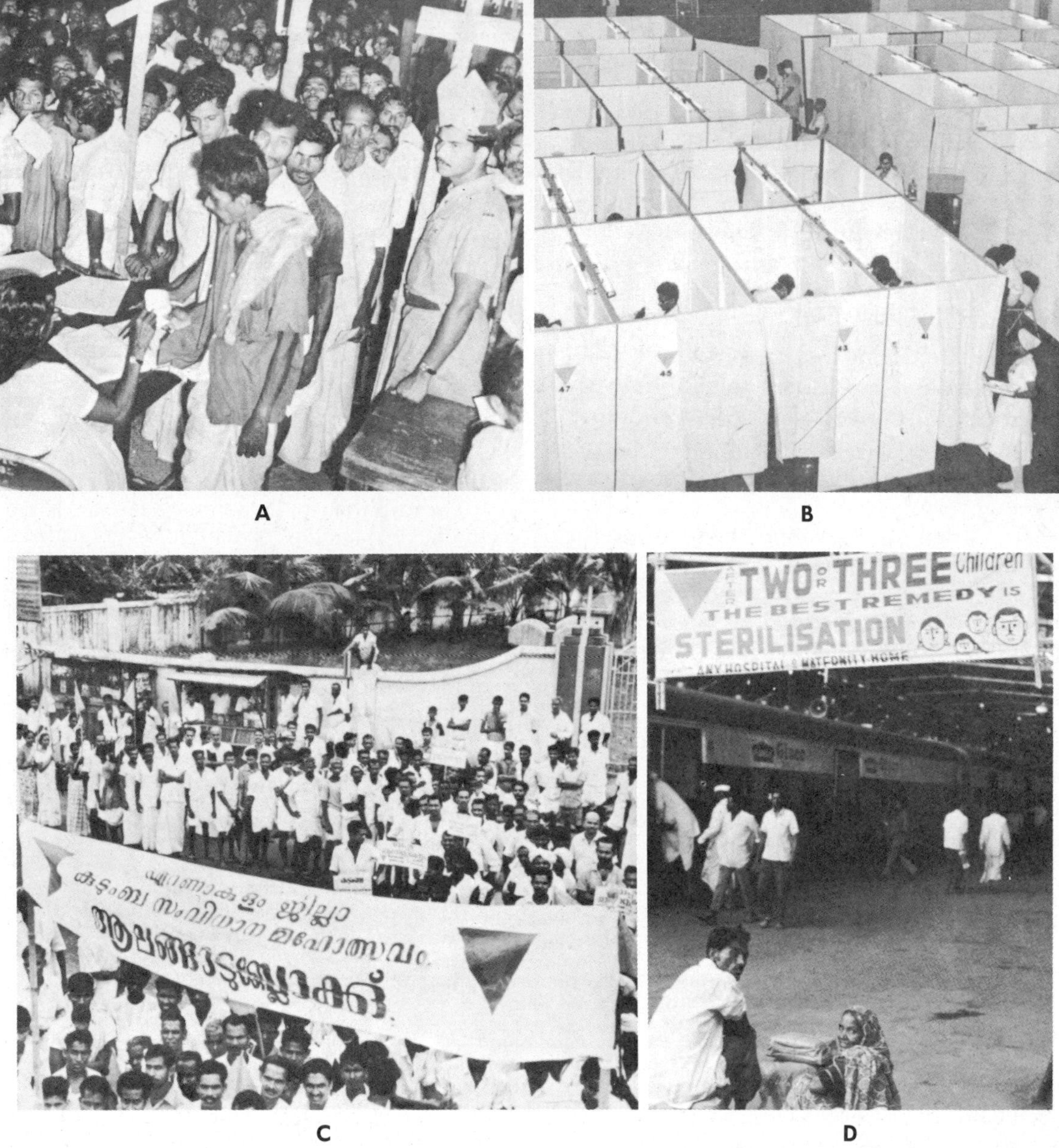

Figure 4–4 *A,* A large crowd of acceptors patiently await their turn to register for the vasectomy operation. *B,* Though the operation usually took less than 15 minutes, the 50 cubicles in the "operating theater" (the Town Hall) were kept busy most of the time. By the end of three weeks the figure on the illuminated scoreboard for completed vasectomies had climbed to 38,000 but people continued to pour into the festival and by the end of the month the number had jumped to almost 64,000. Folk dancers, lights and music helped to maintain a festival atmosphere. *C,* The banner proclaims the name of the festival and the area this group of men come from: "Ernakulam District, Family Planning Festival, Alangad Block." The long line of men waiting for vasectomies was a common sight at the festival. *D,* A Family Planning sign at a Bombay railway station encourages sterilization after a couple have had two or three children; a clinic at the station can perform vasectomies on the spot. (From Palmer, J.: Selling vasectomies in India. War on Hunger (a reprint from AID), January, 1972, pp. 6–9.)

medical policies. Dispensing health care throughout the country took on new momentum when the Cultural Revolution began in 1966. One-third of the country's medical personnel were sent to rural areas where 85 per cent of the population lives.

Four basic principles permeate medicine and public health in the People's Republic of China, guiding the organization and delivery of health services as well as the behavior of practitioners and citizens. Service to the people, prevention as a primary task, cooperation between western medicine and traditional medicine, and participation of the masses in public health work are the ingredients in health care service delivery. The system relies on prevention, rapid expansion of health facilities, and cooperative financing between the state and local governments, extensive use of traditional medicine and ancillary personnel to deliver medical and health care, and citizen participation in health affairs. (See Fig. 4–5.) It has brought to reality a health care system that is indigenous, innovative, and effective in providing care to 800 million people.

Virginia Li Wang has described China's philosophy toward health and health education as follows:

> Health education is recognized as a long-term process and one which must be self-motivating and continuous in order to be effective. As a method of education, the principles are to inform, to motivate, and to involve by doing and by participating in decision making. Health education may relate to environmental sanitation, family planning, or community affairs. In educating the public, first the problem is thoroughly discussed, then consensus is taken before mapping out a course of action. It is felt that once people participate in the decision-making process, they are likely to take a personal interest on their own

有利于抓革命 促生产 促工作 促战备
好好学习
天天向上
有利于培养无产阶级革命事业接班人
有利于支援世界革命
有利于认真学习毛主席著作
有利于巩固无产阶级专政
有利于备战 备荒 为人民
为革命搞好计划生育

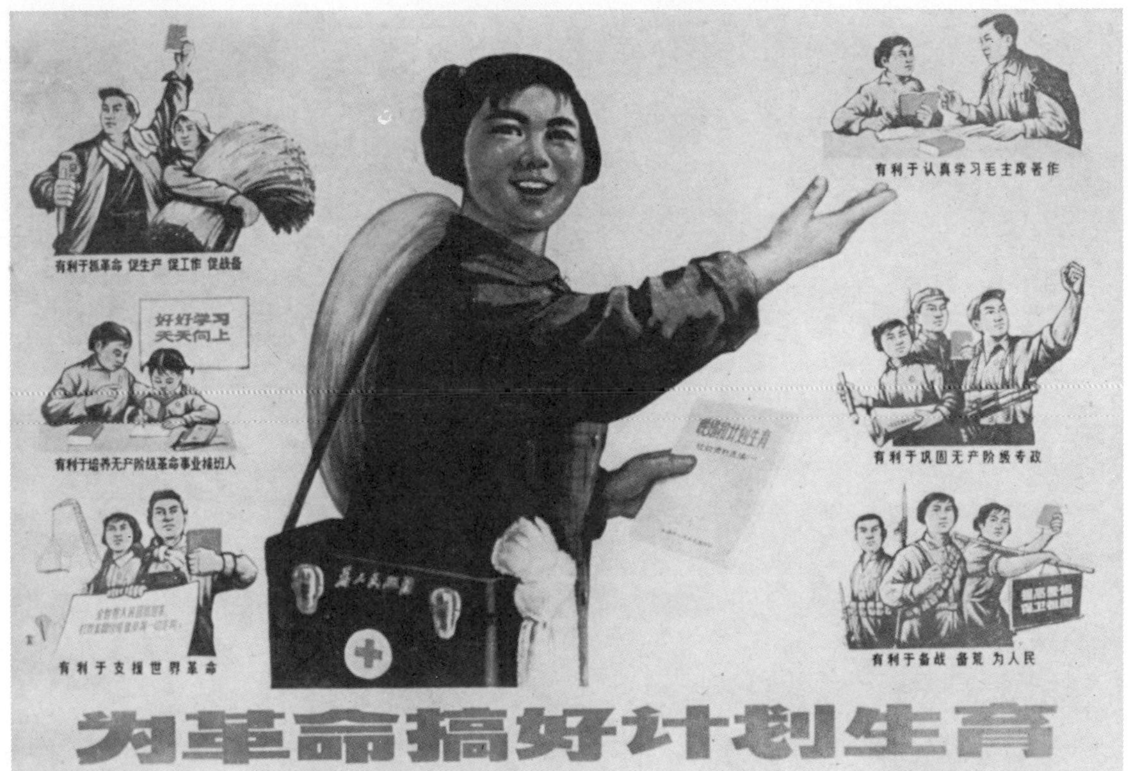

Figure 4–5 Birth control poster shows a woman "barefoot doctor," her medical kit slung over her shoulder, holding a book titled *Late Marriage and Plan for Birth Control.* She points to the first of six vignettes; the captions, somewhat abbreviated, read "To study and apply Chairman Mao's Thought," "To consolidate the dictatorship of the proletariat," "To prepare against war or national disaster and for the people," "To support world revolution," "To raise successors to the revolution" and "To grasp revolution, promote production and prepare against war." The title of the poster is "Plan for Good Birth Control for Revolution"; the five characters on the lid of the medical kit repeat a slogan enunciated at every level of Chinese health care: "Wei ren min fu wu," or "Serve the people." (From The Delivery of Medical Care in China, by R. Sidel and V. W. Sidel. Copyright © 1974 by Scientific American, Inc. All rights reserved.) (Scientific American, Vol. 230, #4, April 1974, p. 20)

behalf as well as that of the community, since health has personal and communal dimensions.

In disease prevention the Chinese believe it is understanding and not fear which education must provoke. When people are fearful of disease, one manner in handling it may be by avoiding contact with health workers or by ignoring its existence. Through education, informed citizens become motivated to improve their health and learn to decide on a course of action among certain alternatives. Making services available and accessible is not the whole answer; people must make use of the services and be motivated to take action in health maintenance and in disease prevention.

The public health department promotes hygiene, physical education, and exercise (Fig. 4–6), food and nutrition, pest control and environmental sanitation, and maternal and child health, and gives leadership to hospital services, manpower, and other resource allocations, and the patriotic health movement.* During the early years, emphases of the patriotic health movement were heavily concentrated in the areas of personal hygiene, sanitation and control of epidemic diseases, and immunization. In recent years, much of its propaganda has been related to acceptance of the combination of traditional and western medicine, cooperative medicine and the barefoot doctor, and family planning.

*The patriotic movement is a continuous series of health campaigns initiated by the public health department and organized with the help of the people in the community. It is patriotic since it promotes socialist construction.

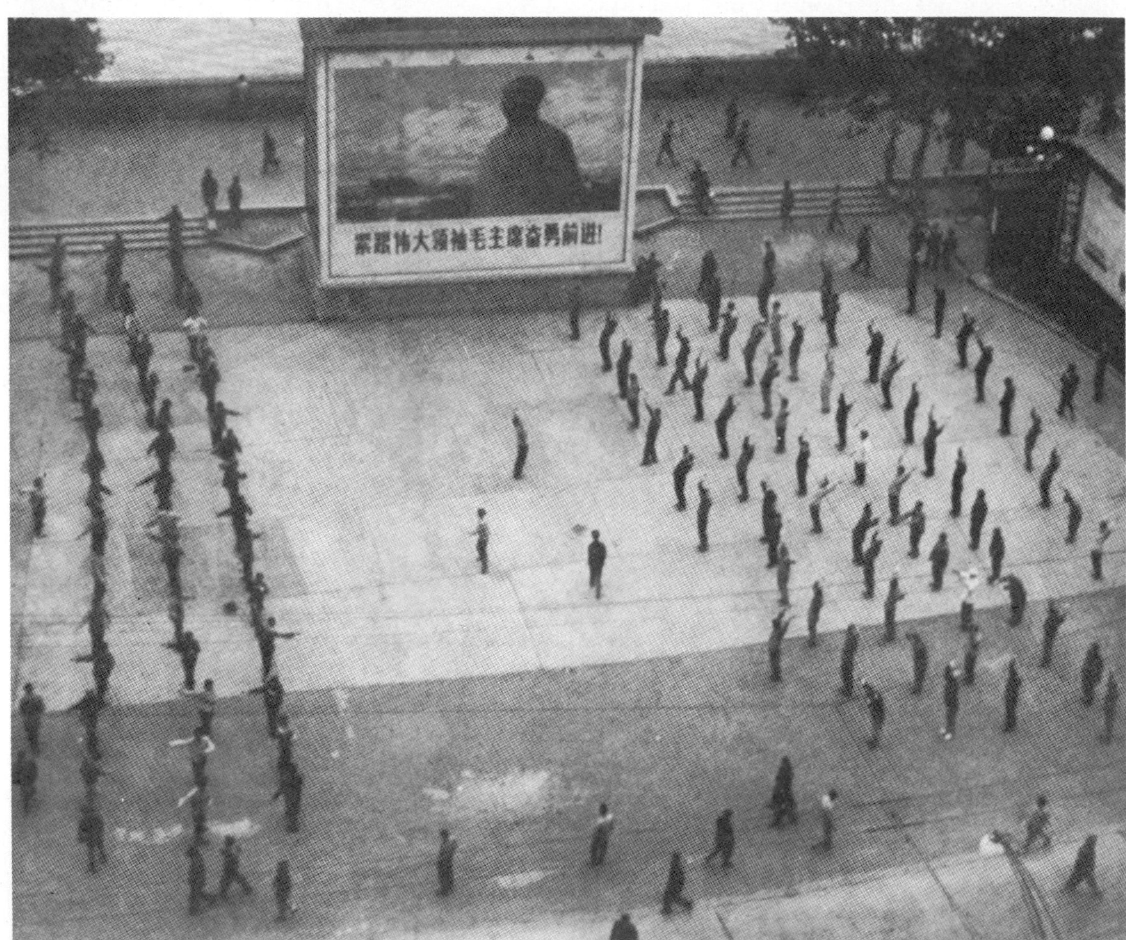

Figure 4–6 Calisthenics groups exercise in a riverside park in the city of Shanghai. One group *(right)* is exercising in Western style and the other is following traditional Chinese routines. Exercise is accepted by traditional Chinese medicine as something more than simple body building. Along with certain respiratory practices it is used as part of both physiological and psychological therapy. (From The Delivery of Medical Care in China, by R. Sidel and V. W. Sidel.)

The extraordinary success in fusing health education into all forms of activities and service delivery is observable. All political subdivisions and administrative units from street level and commune up have a committee appointed for public health. Community leaders and cadres† share the responsibility to inform and motivate, as well as involve all available resources for delivering better health care. They work closely with the public health department, receiving from it guidance and health propaganda materials. The public health department is joined by the hospital and the People's Liberation Army in providing in-service training for health workers and others engaging in prevention and health care.[29]

QUESTIONS FOR DISCUSSION

1. List and briefly discuss six steps that interested groups and individuals may use as a guide to help them improve the health of their community.
2. List the steps you would take in promoting a community fluoridation program.
3. How would you go about *discovering* and *solving* major health problems in your community?
4. How can we evaluate the effectiveness of a community health program?
5. List five reasons that some community health programs are delayed.
6. In your opinion, what are the five major community health problems in your community? State? Why?
7. Give three different examples showing how community health programs failed in your community because of lack of effective communication.
8. Name three important functions that public interest groups can fulfill.
9. Briefly discuss two successful and effective community health programs in your community. What methods were used in obtaining greater active citizen participation?
10. Briefly discuss the purpose of a community health service center.
11. Briefly discuss the philosophy, objectives, approaches, and projects of The National Commission On Community Health Services.
12. Research projects have demonstrated the effectiveness of community opposition to a public health measure despite the endorsement of professional public health and medical associations. List ten results of these studies.
13. Check your community to investigate whether they have had an evaluation study of health needs in the community. If so, how did they get organized? Obtain a copy of the results of the survey and make comments and implications of the study.
14. Describe and evaluate the public health program for the minority groups in your community.
15. What evaluative techniques does the comprehensive health planning organization in your community use? State?
16. Make a study of the duties of the various types of employees of a local health department.
17. What tests are available to help evaluate individuals' attitudes toward health and public health?
18. What statistics are used in public health research?

QUESTIONS FOR REVIEW

1. Who is most responsible for the effectiveness of a community health program?
2. List seven ways in which knowledge of a community's health problems and resources can be gained.
3. What is an ideal instrument for achieving the goal of mobilizing all the forces in a community willing to work for better health services?
4. What is the first task of the above instrument?
5. What is the name of the organization that can take care of most community health surveys?
6. What kind of a laboratory is set up for concentrated research study in a single community? How is it helpful for community health?
7. Give three reasons why a health survey is necessary.
8. List six factors that should be included in a community self-study.
9. What are the two kinds of community service?
10. What are the two factors that seemed to be important in establishing a person's attitude toward personal health, according to the study by Koos?
11. What is one of the most effective approaches to opening new educational channels in a community?
12. What three kinds of support are necessary for the acceptance of health programs and the adoption of health policies?
13. In order for the formulation of goals to be effective, what three steps must be considered?

---

†The word cadre applies to anyone in a responsible position in any organization of government, party, military, industrial, or cultural life. The term also implies loyalty to the Communist Party.

14. Why might an expert who tries to locate and define a specific problem have less influence on the public than an agitator or demogogue?
15. List three general factors that can delay health programs.

REFERENCES

1. Patterson, R. S., and Roberts, B. J.: *Community Health Education in Action.* St. Louis, C. V. Mosby, 1951.
2. National Health Council: *Aids to Community Health Planning Kit.* New York, National Health Council, 1954.
3. American Medical Association: *The Key to Community Health.* Chicago, American Medical Association, 1954.
4. Koos, E. L.: *The Health of Regionville.* New York, Columbia University Press, 1954.
5. Spence, J. C., et al.: *A Thousand Families in Newcastle-upon-Tyne.* London, Oxford University Press, 1954.
6. Leighton, A.: *My Name is Legion.* New York, Basic Books, 1959. See also Hughes, C., et al.: *Cove and Woodlot.* New York, Basic Books, 1960.
7. Strole, L., et al.: *Mental Health in the Metropolis.* New York, McGraw-Hill, 1962.
8. Suchman, E. A.: *Sociology and the Field of Public Health,* New York, Russell Sage Foundation, 1963.
9. Anderson, O. W., et al.: Symposium on community self-surveys in health. Amer. J. Publ. Health, *45*:273, 1955.
10. American Public Health Association: *Guide to the Community Health Study.* 2nd ed. New York, 1961.
11. Kane, W. C.:Coordinating a community study of environmental health. Publ. Health Rep., *79*:539, 1964.
12. U.S. Public Health Service: *Environmental Health Planning Guide.* Washington, D.C., Public Health Service Publication No. 823, 1962.
13. Pyatt, E. E., and Rogers, P. P.: On estimating benefit cost ratios for water supply investments. Amer. J. Publ. Health, *52*:1729, 1962.
14. Wilner, D. M., et al.: *Housing Environment and Family Life.* Baltimore, Johns Hopkins Press, 1962.
15. Warren, D. I., and Warren, R. B.: Six kinds of neighborhoods. Psychology Today, June, 1975, pp. 72–76.
16. Kariel, P. E.: The dynamics of behavior in relation to health. Nursing Outlook, *10*:402, 1962.
17. Freeman, R. B.: *Community Health Nursing Practice.* Philadelphia, W. B. Saunders Co., 1970, pp. 109–117.
18. Wickenden, E.: How to Influence Public Policy: A Short Manual on Social Action. American Association of Social Workers, 1954, pp. 3, 4, 6.
19. American Medical Association: *The Community Health Council.* Chicago, American Medical Association, 1949, pp. 14, 15.
20. Brembeck, W. L., and Howell, W. S.: *Persuasion, a Means of Social Control.* Englewood Cliffs, N.J., Prentice-Hall, 1963.
21. McDonald, W. J.: Community planning for accident coverage. Publ. Health Rep., *76*:1010, 1963.
22. Vandervoort, E. D.: We couldn't do it alone. Natl. Teachers' Assoc. Bull., p. 12, February, 1964.
23. Siddall, A. C.: The Oberlin plan for community health services. Amer. J. Publ. Health, *54*:1317, 1964.
24. Journal of School Health, *40*:414, 1970.
25. Government, Minnesota model. Time, September, 19, 1969, p. 64.
26. Larson, B., et al.: A potpourri of nutrition education methods. J. Nutr. Ed., *6*(1):21, January–March, 1974.
27. Misra, K. K.: Safe water in rural areas. An experiment in promoting community participation in India. Int. J. Health Ed., *18*(1):53, 1975.
28. Palmer, J.: Selling vasectomies in India. War on Hunger, AID, January, 1972, pp. 8, 9.
29. Wang, V. L.: Health education and planning in The People's Republic of China. Int. J. Health Ed., supplement to Vol. 17, No. 2, April–June, 1974, pp. 1–3.

SUGGESTED READING

Anderson, C. L.: *Community Health.* St. Louis, C. V. Mosby Co., 1973.

Benson, E. R., and McDevitt, J. Q.: *Community Health and Nursing Practice.* Englewood Cliffs, N.J., Prentice-Hall, 1976.

Berelson, B. (ed.): *Population Policy in Developed Countries.* New York, McGraw-Hill, 1975.

Bergsma, D., et al. (eds.): *Ethical, Social and Legal Dimensions of Screening for Human Genetic Disease.* New York, Stratton Intercontinental Medical Book Corp., 1974.

Berne, E.: *Structure and Dynamics of Organizations and Groups.* New York, Ballantine Books, 1975.

Bete, C. L.: *About Alcohol,* 1973.

Blum, H. L.: *Planning for Health; Development and Application of Social Change Theory.* New York, Behavioral Publications, 1974.

Burgess, A. W., and Lazare, A.: *Community Mental Health.* Englewood Cliffs, N.J., Prentice-Hall, 1976.

Burton, L. E., and Smith, H. H.: *Public Health and Community Medicine.* 2nd ed. Baltimore, Williams & Wilkins, 1975.

Cohn, V.: Sister Kenny: *The Woman Who Challenged the Doctors.* Minneapolis, University of Minnesota Press, 1976.

Corey, L., et al.: *Medicine in a Changing Society.* St. Louis, C. V. Mosby Co., 1972.

Corrigan, E. M.: *Problem Drinkers Seeking Treatment.* Rutgers Center of Alcohol Studies, Community Council of Greater New York, 1974.

Danish, S. J., and Hauer, A. L.: *Helping Skills: A Basic Training Program.* New York, Behavioral Publications, 1973.

Douglas-Wilson, I., and McLachan, G. (eds.): *Health Service Prospects—An International Survey.* London, Lancet, 1974.

Elling, R. H., and Martin, R. F.: *Health and Health Care for the Urban Poor: A Study of Hartford's North End.* Connecticut Health Services Research Series No. 5. North Haven, Conn., Connecticut Hospital Research and Education Foundation, 1974.

Grant, M.: *Handbook of Community Health.* Philadelphia, Lea & Febiger, 1975.

Greenblatt, B.: *Family Planning Goals and Social Work*

Roles. New York, Planned Parenthood Federation of America, 1972.

Hardy, R. E., and Cull, J. G.: *Severe Disabilities: Social and Rehabiltation Approaches.* Springfield, Ill., Charles C Thomas, 1974.

Hofmann, F. G., and Hofmann, A. D.: *A Handbook on Drug and Alcohol Abuse: The Biomedical Aspects.* New York, Oxford University Press, 1975.

Illich, I.: *Medical Nemesis.* New York, Pantheon, 1976.

Jacobs, A., and Spradlin, W. W.: *The Group as Agent of Change.* New York, Behavioral Publications, 1974.

Johnson, B.: *Marijuana Users and Drug Subcultures.* New York, Wiley, 1973.

Leininger, M., and Buck, G.: *Health Care Issues.* (Health Care Dimensions, Fall, 1974.) Philadelphia, F. A. Davis, 1974.

Manisoff, M. T., et al.: *Advancing the Quality of Health Care: Key Issues and Fundamental Principles.* New York, Planned Parenthood Federation of America, 1972.

McMahon, J. H.: *Social Policy – Improving the Human Condition.* New York, Public Affairs Committee, 1973.

Meyer, R.E.: *Guide to Drug Rehabilitation: A Public Health Approach.* Boston, Beacon Press, 1972.

Montoye, H. J.: *Physical Activity and Health: An Epidemiologic Study of an Entire Community.* Englewood Cliffs, N.J., Prentice-Hall, 1975.

Mushkin, S. J. (ed.): *Consumer Incentives for Health Care.* New York, Prodist (for Milbank Memorial Fund), 1974.

Neleigh, J. R., et al.: *Training Nonprofessional Community Project Leaders.* New York, Behavioral Publications, 1971.

Pitcairn, D. M., and Flahault, D. (eds.): *The Medical Assistant: An Intermediate Level of Health Care Personnel.* Conference, Bethesda, Md., June 1973. World Health Organization, Public Health Papers No. 60. Geneva, 1974.

Planned Parenthood Federation of America: *Guide to Public Affairs.* New York, 1971.

Porkert, M.: *The Theoretical Foundations of Chinese Medicine: Systems of Correspondence.* Cambridge, Mass., MIT Press, 1974.

Rehr, H. (Ed.): *Medicine and Social Work: An Exploration in Interprofessionalism.* Colloquium, April, 1973 New York, Prodist (for Doris Siegel Memorial Fund of Mount Sinai Medical Center), 1974.

Reinhardt, A. M., and Quinn, M. D.: *Family-Centered Community Nursing: A Sociocultural Framework.* St. Louis, C.V. Mosby Co., 1973.

Safar, P. (ed.): *Public Health Aspects of Critical Care Medicine and Anesthesiology.* Philadelphia, F.A. Davis, 1975.

Schindler, E., et al.: *Team Training for Community Change.* Berkeley, University of California Extension, 1973.

Secretary of Health, Education and Welfare: *Second Special Report to the U.S. Congress on Alcohol and Health.* Washington, D.C., U.S. Government Printing Office, 1974.

Strickland, S. P.: *U.S. Health Care: What's Wrong and What's Right.* New York, Universe Books, 1972.

Stycos, J. M., et al.: *Clinics, Contraception, and Communication: Evaluation Studies of Family Planning Programs in Four Latin American Countries.* New York, Appleton-Century-Crofts, 1974.

Waitzkin, H., and Waterman, B.: *The Exploitation of Illness in Capitalistic Society.* Indianapolis, Bobbs-Merrill, 1974.

CHAPTER 5

COMMUNITY HEALTH EDUCATION

Health education has been defined as "the sum of experiences which favorably influence habits, attitudes, and knowledge relating to individual, community, and racial health."[1] In order to provide people in the community with such experiences, it is necessary to make them aware of individual and community health needs and problems, to secure the facts, to disseminate the information, and to motivate them to act. As the above definition points out, any education program must consider the habits, attitudes, and knowledge of the people. In our modern society, the senses of the average citizen are constantly bombarded by publicity, propaganda, advertising, promotional and educational forces. Some of them are subtle; others are not. The community health educator must recognize this competition and must devise and employ techniques that will obtain a fair share of public attention.

EDUCATING THE PUBLIC

Attitudes

It is clear that mass communications media can be of great use in the decision making that must accompany economic and social development. But their usefulness does not lie in frontal attacks on strongly held attitudes or long-valued customs. For example, as advertisers have discovered, once people have decided that a toothbrush is a good thing, then it is relatively easy to convince them that *this* or *that kind* of toothbrush is a good thing. If a new agriculture or health practice can be presented as merely *one instance* of an old honored custom, then it is likely to be accepted. If it can be presented as merely a tiny change in an old honored custom, then it is more likely to be accepted than if it is shown as a frontal attack on an old custom. Strongly held positions are in the domain of personal influence and group norms. If changes are made in stoutly defended customs and beliefs, interpersonal communication is usually required, and group change is usually involved. In such major decisions, therefore, mass media can help only indirectly. They can feed information into the channels of interpersonal influence. They can confer status and enforce norms. They can broaden the policy dialogue. They can help form tastes. When there are no strong attitudes, or when the only change desired is a slight canalization of an existing attitude, they can be directly effective. But for the most part, in the area of entrenched belief and behavior, they can only help.[2]

The attitudes one takes toward health practices suspected of being harmful relate closely to one's own health behavior. In persons who have a habit that might be harmful to good health, there is evidence that twice as many are unwilling to acknowledge its potential harm as compared with an equal number of persons who do not have that habit. Among those who have the habit, the higher the individual's educational level, the less likely the person will be to accept evidence that the habit is harmful. Among nonpracticers, however, the reverse is true—that is, the higher the individual educational level, the more likely sound evidence on health associations will be accepted. Let us use an illustration. If you advise a group composed of 50 smokers and 50 nonsmokers that smoking is harmful, statistics show that twice as many smokers as nonsmokers would reject your report. Of the smokers, the higher the individual educational level, the less likely your evidence will be accepted. Among nonsmokers, the higher the individual educational level, the more likely the evidence will be accepted. Thus, it is postulated that the unbiased nonpracticer of a habit intellectually accepts what he concludes to be solid evidence, while the practicer uses his good intellect to rationalize the same evidence as circumstantial.

Values, attitudes and personality exert an important influence upon how a man perceives, interprets, and responds to illness. Social group membership and individual personality affect a person's perception of pain, his decisions to seek medical care, and his behavior as a patient. His acceptance of medical services and of new ideas and techniques requires more than merely making these available to him—that is, more than changing his physical environment. It may be more important to change his psychosocial environment. Man gains everyday perceptions, interpretations, and behavior through an acquired sensitivity to values and attitudes that are approved of in his group and culture. Today, man is the agent of his own diseases; his state of health is determined more by what he does to himself than by what some outside germ or infectious agent does to him. The medical cause of lung cancer may be a chemical substance in cigarettes, but the psychosocial cause is a behavior—smoking. Cholesterol, heart disease, and overeating can be similarly explained.

The incidence of accidents is related to a wide range of personality factors and to a person's safety practices and attitudes in relationship to risk taking and exposure to hazards. A person may consider risk a challenge to test his skill or to toy with fate—is he vulnerable or not? Reactions are likely to be governed strongly by role expectation, judgment on degree of danger, previous experience, and presence of restraining forces. Demographical variables, including age, sex, ethnic background, religion, political party, socioeconomic class, occupation, educational status, family membership, and marital status, influence attitudes not by membership in these groups *per se*, but by the effect of such membership upon exposure to and patterns of perceiving, interpreting and reacting to health hazards.

Principles Governing Individual Behavior

Today, much emphasis is given to educating the public in the prevention of chronic diseases. Prevention is largely a matter of the initiation of voluntary behavior involving basic changes in health habits and individual responsibility for early detection, combined with medical and welfare cooperation in long-term treatment and rehabilitation programs. Furthermore, the initial emphasis of the public health movement on the building and provision of health facilities and services has been followed by obtaining public utilization of such services—again a matter of individual participation. It is quite apparent that public health has now entered an era of educating the individual citizen to his responsibility and necessarily voluntary cooperation in advancing the general health of the community. Such education requires an understanding of the principles governing individual behavior.

Behavior change in health is most important, since any risk-reduction program is dependent upon changes in personal behavior. Research conducted by Hochbaum and Rosenstock[3] has resulted in the formulation of several principles for accomplishing changes in health-related behavior. These principles can be summarized briefly as follows:

1. *Perception of the threat.* A person must become aware that a threat to health exists.
2. *Belief in the importance of the threat.* The person must believe that the threat is important to him, not that it applies just to other people.
3. *Reduction of the threat.* Some means of action must be available by which the person can reduce the threat. A direct tangible action, such as getting a shot, is more easily accomplished than a less tangible long-term action, such as changing the composition of the diet.
4. *Reinforcement.* This is not one of the Hochbaum-Rosenstock principles; however, continuing reinforcement of the new behavior pattern is important. Rewards for the new behavior should be sought so that the individual gains more satisfaction from the new behavior than he did from the old behavior.

Suchman identifies three important processes that seem to intervene between availability of facts and behavioral response: perception, interpretation, and salience.[4] People observe selectively—that is, from the myriad messages that constantly bombard their sensory receptors, only those for which they already have an initial "set" are perceived. Perhaps the greatest number of health messages never reach the attention threshold of the individual. The interpretation or "meaning" of any given fact that the individual perceives is determined to a large degree by his previous experiences and his current needs. Thus, subjectivity rather than objectivity will characterize the reaction of most individuals to facts about disease. Finally, health knowledge is not the same as health action. To affect behavior, the health information must have salience for the individual in terms of the rewards to be obtained from acting on the basis of the facts. For many, if not most, individuals, especially those with limited social horizons and immediate social or economic needs, the rewards for initiating new or modified preventive health behavior are too remote to carry much weight. The negative consequences of not acting or acting in opposition to the desired response are not obvious enough or dire enough to arouse within the individual the energy required to produce a desired response, such as taking part in a public health program.

These basic principles were found to control the health behavior of a cross-section of low-income mixed racial groups surveyed in Washington, D.C.:[5]

> .... health is not of primary importance to these families. There are too many matters in their everyday lives which would appear to have greater significance.
>
> ... the concept of the ways and means by which health may be maintained as viewed by these families does not include certain measures which are of primary importance, such as immunizations, early diagnosis and prompt treatment.... The concern here, it is seen, is with matters of the moment and not with those which are more remote, and for conditions which are certainly neither pressing nor evident.
>
> ... knowledge concerning a health procedure or verbal acceptance of its importance does not necessarily beget action on the part of these families in obtaining it. As a corollary, lack of knowledge about a procedure does not result in lack of action.

The foregoing analysis is obviously oversimplified and is intended only to highlight the importance of social and psychological factors in the operation of public health programs. We may characterize the difficulty of the problem for public health in terms of two major axes: the degree of meaning the desired health action has for the individual—that is, his recognition of disease as a personal threat—and the degree of effort required in terms of personal decision-making and activity to initiate the desired action. As shown in Figure 5–1, we may hypothesize that the difficulty of securing individual participation in a public health program will increase as one moves from Cell A to Cell D.

Thus, it would be least difficult to induce the individual to participate in a measles vaccination program during the height of a threatened epidemic if convenient and free inoculation stations were provided; it would be most difficult to obtain his cooperation in such a program when only in-

DEGREE OF EFFORT REQUIRED	DEGREE OF RECOGNITION OF THREAT: High	Low
Low	A	C
High	B	D

Figure 5–1 The difficulty of obtaining individual participation in a public health program (see text)

convenient and costly sources of inoculation were available and no immediate threat to the individual from the disease existed. This general combination of personal threat and effort required has been found by a number of studies to underlie the success or failure of many public health programs.

Decision to Participate

In an analysis of public participation in a poliomyelitis vaccination campaign, Rosenstock attributes the individual's decision to participate to two broad classes of factors: personal readiness factors, consisting of perceived susceptibility and seriousness (comparable to recognition of threat); and situational factors, among which he stresses convenience (comparable to effort). In addition, Rosenstock discusses the role of social pressure, which we will analyze later as an external force influencing the perception of threat or effort required.[6]

In another study of an Asian influenza vaccination program, Rosenstock and his colleagues concluded that the failure of individuals to be vaccinated, despite the possibility of a community-wide epidemic, stemmed from "a belief on the part of a great majority of respondents that neither they nor their families were susceptible to Asian influenza, and a belief that Asian influenza was not much more serious, if more serious at all, than usual respiratory illness."[7] This finding again accentuates the importance of personal threat in determining the salience of a health act for the individual.

In an evaluation of research in the field of population control, Berelson stresses the overwhelming importance of such down-to-earth considerations as "not too much bother" and "effectiveness." He predicts that very little progress will be made in instituting birth control measures in a society unless the means for such control are so simplified that they require a minimum of individual initiative and result in a minimum of failure. He points out that even though the individual may have highly favorable attitudes and some positive motivation toward family planning, he or she will not undertake the disciplined behavior associated with such population control measures as abstinence or withdrawal, rhythm, contraceptives, or pills.[8] This is an example of a type of public health program to which public response is most difficult to obtain, because it involves the factors in Cell D of Figure 5–1: high individual behavior (effort) for a continuous period and minimum motivation.

Other studies that support the hypothesis were conducted by Metzner and Gurin in relation to public participation in a mass chest x-ray survey for tuberculosis detection in New York, and by Johnson and associates in regard to public response to a poliomyelitis vaccination campaign in Florida. The New York study is particularly pertinent to the discussion, because it illustrates the influence of factors to be found in Cell C of Figure 5–1. The failure of the program to attain its goal of 80 per cent saturation of the population was attributed to the low salience of tuberculosis to the individual, while the degree of success attained was almost completely attributable to the "immediacy and convenience" of participation.[9]

Social Pressure

The Florida study points up the results of interpersonal influences on individual behavior. Such influences relate to the "social pressure" variable previously mentioned in Rosenstock's study of vaccination campaign. Both studies found that participation was closely related to the perception of the individual that his peers were participating and *that he himself was expected to join them.* As reported in the Florida study:

> Belief that one's friends had taken the new vaccine had a particularly strong association with the respondent's own vaccine status. These informal interpersonal factors, membership in social organizations, social class, and education were the variables found by this survey to be the most powerful predictors of vaccine acceptance and rejection.[10]

The Florida study formulates the proposition on the importance of personal influences quite clearly:

> The respondent's perceived friends are reference group. The actions he believes they took become one basis for deciding what is "the way my kind of people are supposed to act." Thus,

persons who believed their friends took the oral vaccine also believed that their friends would approve and praise them for taking the vaccine, too. Similarly, where the persons important to the respondent were believed to have refused the vaccine, the respondent had the psychological experience group support for his nonacceptance.[11]

The implications of this study for public health programs are obvious. These programs need to develop approaches to the public that touch directly on their customary patterns of behavior, and they need to make the health action "acceptable, desirable, and appropriate." The resistant groups of the population at present do not seem to find any worthwhile benefit in many of the current health programs. They simply do not see these health programs as rewarding or meeting any of their real needs. The presentation of the health program must stress some reward for the individual besides the prevention of a disease about which he feels no great concern. Perhaps the most promising redefinition of public health education is not in terms of teaching "good" personal health behavior, but rather in teaching how people *should* behave in response to the public health programs. This idea is emphasized in the final recommendation for the conduct of public health programs in the Florida study:

> The data of this study do not indicate the necessity of factual discussion of the dangers of polio or the merits of vaccine. All that appears necessary is for people to feel they have a group of friends and to believe that most or all of these friends will be taking or have taken vaccine. Fostering this collective perception should greatly increase vaccine acceptance.[12]

This approach to public health programs takes into account the low salience of purely health appeals for the public and stresses instead an appeal for a kind of social conformity, which requires greater motivation to resist than to accept. The concept offers an interesting possibility for public health practice based on a sociological rather than a psychological approach. Hochbaum's statement in regard to participation in a tuberculosis screening program further supports the validity of group appeal:

> Even when this state of (psychological) readiness is absent or of very low intensity, people were found to come for x-rays *in response to external influences alone.* These may be influences exerted by other individuals or groups. In other words, people may come for x-rays not for any health-relevant reasons, but to please other people, to be accepted by their groups, and the like.[13]

The importance of circumventing motivational appeals keyed to the threat of disease, when the perception of such a treat cannot be made real to the person, is noted by Metzner and Gurin in their final conclusions:

> Much in our society depends on building into it automatic, unavoidable acts which are not directly motivated toward the goals they achieve nor represent conscious decisions to be good or safe . . . and what success we have had in vaccination lies more in making it a part of the relationship with a pediatrician or the school system than in increasing appreciation of and desire for immunity.[14]

The major contribution sociology can offer to public health practice, then, is the development and testing of methods and techniques that make the desired health behavior part of the prevailing value system and pattern of social behavior of the individual, based not on appeals to his health, but rather on the appropriateness of the behavior itself. Thus, mothers may be influenced to take their children to health stations for polio shots not so much to protect the child from disease as because it is "what every good mother is expected to do" and "what other mothers like me are doing." This suggestion is supported by the findings of the Washington, D.C., study of the health behavior of low-income families.

> . . . it may not be necessary for people to be informed provided they can be motivated by other means. The mothers who took their children to be vaccinated, although ignorant about the disease, may have been motivated by the thought that this is what is expected of good mothers.[15]

The mother's definition of such action as appropriate to her role as a mother rather than simply advantageous to the health of the child was also found to be highly significant by Clausen and associates in their study of participation in the poliomyelitis vaccine trials.[16, 17] Another very important consideration is the general example set by parents regarding health care, which will influence their children's behavior patterns and attitudes. The children, in turn, will transmit these attitudes to their children.

Perception and Small Group Dynamics. Two basic theoretical concepts—perception and small group dynamics—have changed our work in health education. These concepts are influencing our present activities in administration, research, and our daily work. Once the significance of perception was appreciated by psychologists, sociologists, and anthropologists, they began to develop methods for understanding and applying the concept in investigating the nature of the learner. One of the most pertinent contributions, as far as educators are concerned, has come from an enlarged concept of the meaning of perception. Today, the literature is rich in reports from continuing research, and new textbooks in education psychology are often built around new principles in perception, self-motivation through involvement, and value systems. The resulting knowledge supplied from the field of the social sciences has helped us undertake what is now one of the first steps in any community health program—*diagnosis of the cultural and educational status of the community.*

The second revolutionary group of theories responsible for our new approach to public education comes from studies of small groups in action. From these studies we are learning to understand what directs the behavior of adults; that is, how basic motivations are aroused, how leadership is demonstrated, and how commitments to action are formed. Of the many advances in all social sciences, it is to these two facets—the meaning of *perception,* and *small group process*—that we are most deeply indebted.[18]

Communicating Health Information

To change behavior, we must first determine the frames of reference held by the target group. The information that we select to make people dissatisfied with their present behavior must be reasonably compatible with their psychological set—attitudes, values, and perceptions. We must make them aware of how this dissatisfaction can be resolved. Rosenstock gives the following suggestions on selecting appropriate health information material:

1. Every attempt should be made to gather good information on the kinds of relevant beliefs initially held by members of the audience. Such data serve as the basis for setting educational objectives. Frequently, different educational campaigns will be required for different groups in the same population.

2. Careful estimates should be made of the psychological distance between current beliefs of the audience and those that reflect sound medical knowledge. If the distance is great, the educational program may have to be divided into a series of related successive steps. We know that communications are most effective in changing the opinions of people when the messages are not excessively dissimilar from the initial opinions. In certain cases, then, belief changes may have to be accomplished slowly, one small change at a time. This approach is similar to, perhaps identical with the often-mentioned "soft-sell."

3. The greater the prestige of the educator or communicator, the more influential the communication. Prestige, of course, is defined by the opinions of the audience and not by the opinions of the profession.[19]

PERSUASION AND ATTITUDE CHANGE

Shock Technique

A shock, wisely administered, can shake individuals out of attitudes of indifference and result in their active concentration on a community problem. On occasion, such action seems necessary. When used, this rather blunt technique should be fully justified by the urgency of the problem and the presentation carefully evaluated for the accuracy of its message. The person using the shock technique is invariably engaging in a frontal assault on individual security, comfort, and complacency, or on that which custom has been established as desirable and respectable. The initial reaction to such a shock may well be fear or antagonism.

In health education, fear is a two-edged sword that, wrongly used, can backfire. Fear that produces mild anxiety that is readily relieved by appropriate action can be a useful motivation. Fear that generates great apprehension but offers no relief through constructive action may be destructive. People affected by great apprehension may find relief by avoiding the problem and rejecting further educational efforts. Health educators drawn largely from the middle socioeconomic classes find it hard to deal with members of the lower classes. There are language difficulties and differing goals and values. Those we call hard to reach may be so only because our techniques are imperfect. We need to find methods and materials keyed to their values rather than our own.[20] The persuader who uses shock as a technique must be prepared to proceed to grounds so vital that they automatically defer negative response and obtain concession that the shock was justified. Winans reports a vivid example of the shock technique.

> Dr. Wiley tells a story of a member of a certain Middle West legislature who sought an appropriation of $100,000 for the protection of public health; but could secure only $5000. One morning he put upon the desk of each legislator before the opening of the session, a fable which ran something like this: A sick mother with a baby is told by a physician that she has tuberculosis and that she should seek a higher altitude. Lack of means prevents her going. She applies to the government and is told that not a dollar is available to save the mother and her child from death. At the same time a farmer observes that one of his hogs has cholera symptoms. He sends a telegram, collect, to the government. An inspector comes next day, treats the hog with serum and cures it. Moral: Be a hog! The $100,000 appropriation was promptly granted. The legislators saw from this vivid presentation of the case that what they had variously called economy, common-sense, business is business, etc., was really putting the hog above the child.[21]

Many studies have been conducted in an effort to explain why groups accept or reject a certain health measure or program. There is no simple answer or solution: a person's behavior involves personal, social, and emotional factors, as well as the time, place, and situation.

Throughout history, however, certain documents, literature, and books have effectively aroused the populace, and they have stimulated creative thinking, research, legislation, and change. Dr. René Dubos points out that:

> . . . the general public has long been aware of the fact that some factors of the modern environment are creating disease problems which become manifest chiefly during adulthood and later years of life. However, this awareness is derived chiefly from statistical evidence, and consequently it is not sufficient to motivate social action. Whether we like it or not, emotional upheavals are still the most effective stimuli for mobilizing public opinion and for generating effective legislation. The hasty legislative action which followed the accidents associated with the use of thalidomide provides convincing even though disturbing evidence that emotional appeal has far more power than deliberate approach based on knowledge and common sense when it comes to moving the wheels of Government and Congress. In view of this fact, the tremendous popular impact of writing such as the articles by Rachel Carson in the *New Yorker* and of her book, *Silent Spring*, cannot help being of importance for organizations concerned with medicine and public health.[22]

Word Manipulations

"He who wants to persuade," said Joseph Conrad, "should put his trust not in the right argument, but in the right word. . . . Give me the right word and the right accent and I will move the world." And Joseph Conrad was right, indeed, for the right manipulation of the words has been moving people since the beginning of human speech. Miller tells this interesting story:

> Clarence Darrow, the famous criminal lawyer, once told me of his early boyhood in Ohio and how he "read law" under a country attorney with a local reputation for unusual success in swaying juries. "Once," said Darrow, "he was trying a libel suit. He was attorney for the plaintiff. The defendant was a newspaper editor. Libel suits are hard to win and yet my friend won his suit.
>
> "Congratulating him later on the favorable verdict the jury had rendered, I said to him, 'Sir, if you don't mind my raising the point, I was puzzled by your pronunciation of the word "libelous." You kept pronouncing it throughout the trial as though it were spelled "libeelious." You know, of course, that that is not how it is pronounced.'
>
> "Certainly I know,' was his answer. 'And also I knew what I was doing when I pronounced it "libeelious," You see, "libelous" correctly pronounced has a dry, technical, colorless sound, but when pronounced "libeelious" it sounds frightfully evil and wicked. I know the men on that jury. I have grown up with some of them. I know how they feel about evil, wicked things and I knew just what response that evil-sounding word would evoke. Well it worked all right. We won.'"[23]

Words that have been used in the heat and fire of daily crises take on "loaded" meanings; they elicit yes or no responses from us. Compare such words as mother, home, hearth, heaven, godly, decent, and

American with rascal, devilish, communist, tyranny, dictator, conniving, liar, and decadent. Such words, when fitted into our system of stereotypes, carry effective motivating power and can move or change the world. The listener must be alert to the types of word manipulations used on him and should be able to assess their justification. The persuader must, within ethical limits, decide what trigger words are needed to release the response he desires from his audience.

Persuasion in Verbal Communications

To a certain extent, attention determines what stimulations the organism will react to. Because this is true, a speaker can expect an audience to respond to his verbal message if he succeeds in focusing their attention on it, but to respond to something else if attention shifts. For example, suppose a speaker is trying to persuade a listener to give money to a cancer research fund, and that he is able to control the listener's attention as he chooses. If we limit, for the sake of illustration, the listener's perceptual field to a few stimuli, we may then graphically depict the role of attention in securing response. The speaker must succeed in keeping attention sharply focused on himself and the idea of giving to the cancer fund. Under these conditions (inasmuch as action is always a response to a stimulus, and the indicated stimulus is the only effective one operating), there is a strong likelihood that the desired action will take place—that the listener will reach into his pocket for money. Thus, although attention is not a cause of action in itself, it helps to determine action by determining which potential stimuli in a perceptual field a person will respond to.[24]

Semantic Differential for Health

Observation of behavior over long periods of time can reveal perceptions, attitudes, and beliefs. Longer periods of time are not always available, so research into rapid methods of determining perceptions and values is being carried out. Patrick, Johnson, and Jenkins developed a technique for measuring beliefs about diseases which they call the Semantic Differential for Health.[25] In applying this instrument, they discovered that diseases are perceived in systematically different ways (as shown on page 102).

Cognitive Dissonance

Although man is generally consistent in his actions, sometimes he feels an inconsistency between what he knows and the action he takes. This leads to rather unexpected communication behavior in order to reduce the discomfort. This process is referred to as *cognitive dissonance.* For example, many people believe that one should brush one's teeth three times a day, after every meal. However, many, or perhaps most, people who believe this do not actually brush their teeth so often. Thus, dissonance exists between this belief and their behavior. We would expect that such people would be readily influenced by a communication stating that it is actually harmful to brush one's teeth too often, or by a communication stating that a certain brand of toothpaste is so good that its use required only one brushing day. Either of these communications, if accepted and believed, reduces the existing dissonance. On the other hand, if an attempt were made to persuade such a person that one should really brush his teeth five times a day, we would expect the communication to be resisted—the per-

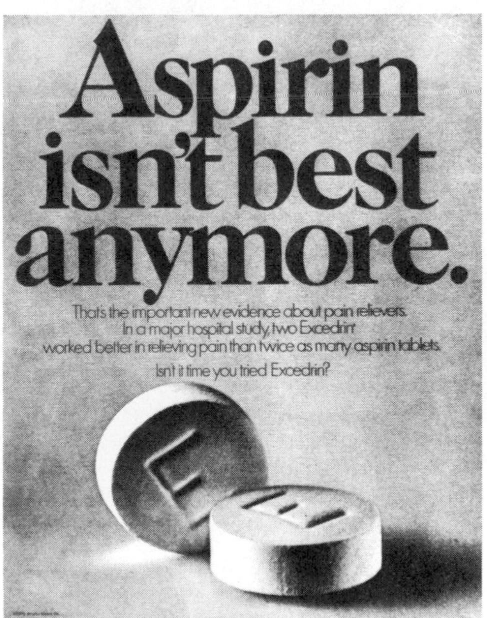

Figure 5–2 Honest and accurate or misleading and deceptive? (Reprinted by permission from Time, the Weekly Newsmagazine; copyright Time Inc., 1970, and the Bristol-Myers Co.)

son would not be influenced. Clearly, if the person accepted this communication, it would merely increase the dissonance between his belief and his behavior.[26, 27]

Methods of Evaluating the Results of Persuasion

A persuader must develop reliable methods of evaluating the results of his persuasion if he is to assess and improve his ability to move men. Some methods that may be used in evaluating face-to-face persuasion follow, with emphasis on methods useful in class-room training.

The Linear Scale. The linear scale may be used when it is desirable to show the movement of attitude change more precisely than does the simple ballot.

Speaker's Name ______________________ Date ____________
Speaker's Purpose ______________________________________

MY ATTITUDE TOWARD THE SPEAKER'S PURPOSE

Before the speech is given, indicate by a circle (O) the position on the scale below that represents your present attitude toward the speaker's purpose. *After* the speech is concluded, again indicate your attitude toward the speaker's purpose by placing a cross (X) on that position on the scale.

0	1	2	3	4	5	6	7	8	9	10
Extremely Favorable					Neutral					Extremely Unfavorable

This ballot is easy to construct and affords opportunity for a type of check on persuasiveness. Like all such scales, it should be administered in such a way as to gain thoughtful evaluations.[28]

The Shift-of-Opinion Ballot. The late Professor H. S. Woodward of Western Reserve University developed the shift-of-opinion ballot. This is another method of measuring the shift of attitudes. It has been used extensively in evaluating collegiate debates. A standard example of the ballot is

Scales of the Semantic Differential for Health (used to measure beliefs about cancer, poliomyelitis, tuberculosis, and mental illness)

A. Many people get it | Some people get it | A few people get it | Almost nobody gets it

|__|__|__|__|__|__|__|__|__|__|__|

B. This is usually a disease affecting:
babies | children | teenagers | young adults | middle; added people | very old people

|__|__|__|__|__|__|__|__|__|__|__|

C. Is extremely painful | Causes much pain | Causes some pain | Causes little pain but is uncomfortable | Causes very little discomfort

|__|__|__|__|__|__|__|__|__|__|__|

D. People recover fully | People recover but are weaker | People have permanent minor body damage | People have obvious permanent disability

|__|__|__|__|__|__|__|__|__|__|__|

E. The chance *you* have of getting it:
Big chance | Some chance | Little chance | No chance

|__|__|__|__|__|__|__|__|__|__|__|

F. Usually causes death | Often causes death | Sometimes causes death | Rarely causes death

|__|__|__|__|__|__|__|__|__|__|__|

G. Clean | Sort of clean | Sort of dirty | Dirty

|__|__|__|__|__|__|__|__|__|__|__|

Scales of the Semantic Differential for Health (used to measure beliefs about cancer, poliomyelitis, tuberculosis, and mental illness) *Continued.*

H. Nothing can prevent it — Hard to prevent — Can be prevented with a little effort — Easily prevented

I. A fast-moving disease — A slow-moving disease

J. A "powerful" disease — A "mild" disease

K. A mystery — Something is known about it — Well understood

L. I think about it *often* — I think about it sometimes — I think about it occasionally — I *never* think about it

M. Attacks mostly good people — Attacks mostly bad people

N. To keep from getting it, I'd give: a day's pay — a week's pay — a month's pay — a year's pay

O. Often talked about — Sometimes talked about — Almost never talked about

P. Cause for pride — Acceptable — Embarrassing — Occasionally talked about — Disgraceful

given below. By comparing the pre- and post-speech checks, the shift of attitude can be determined. Information can also be obtained regarding the person checking the ballot.

TO THE AUDIENCE

The debaters would appreciate your interest and help if you will, both *before* and *after* the debate, indicate on this sheet your personal opinion on the idea proposed for debate.

Please return your ballot to an usher at the close of the debate. This ballot is filed by a man_________, woman_________, student_________, faculty member_________, lay citizen_________.

BEFORE THE DEBATE

_______I believe in the affirmative of the resolution to be debated.
_______I am undecided.
_______I believe in the negative of the resolution to be debated.

AFTER THE DEBATE

I have heard the entire discussion, and now
_______I believe more strongly in the affirmative of the resolution than I did.
_______I believe in the affirmative of the resolution.
_______I am undecided.
_______I believe in the negative of the resolution.
_______I believe more strongly in the negative of the resolution than I did.

The Rating Scale. When a series of proposals is presented, as in a symposium, the rating scale may be used to gain audience reaction to the proposals. It can be given before and after the speech (or speeches) to indicate shifts of opinion. A sample, used for a discussion on "fluoridation" is given below.

Question: What about fluoridation? Below are five possible solutions to this problem. Place a 1 before the solution you believe best, a 2 before the second best, etc.
_______1. The city council should approve and adopt fluoridation plans and procedures for the city water supply.
_______2. The city council should act on the fluoridation issue only after a vote has been taken by persons in the community.
_______3. The city council should not be involved in this issue.
_______4. The public should not be involved in this issue.
_______5. Fluoridation is neither democratic nor prudent under any circumstances.

The Critic Judge's Ballot for Debate. The effectiveness of the various elements of a debate in creating attitude change may be evaluated by the use of the following ballot. It provides a useful breakdown of the important parts of this form of persuasion (as shown on the following page).

Shifting opinions of those opposed is a key problem of persuasion, and many critics of propaganda say that it frequently not only does not achieve its purpose but may reinforce established contrary ideas. Several experimental studies and evidence in politics, social organization, and consumer selling refute this stand.

Persuasive techniques that utilize an appeal to more than one sense appear to be most successful. Movies are often more effective teaching devices than film strips or unaided lecture presentations. Television is a more effective communication medium than radio, and audience participation programs are usually more effective in establishing an idea than the audience lecture or a radio broadcast. The best educational approach lies in effective use of combined presentations that take advantage of the full receptive power of the audience.

Conclusions

We can draw a few tentative conclusions from studies in persuasion. These are contained in the following outline:

A. Concerning content analysis studies in persuasion.
1. The content analysis methods currently employed are capable of rather precise description and quantification of persuasion materials.
2. Content analysis can reveal significant writer or speaker bias.
3. Thematic analysis is useful in locating the basic arguments of a persuader and in determining the degree of his reliance on each.
4. Both qualitative and quantitative analyses are helpful in increasing understanding of a unit of persuasion; statistical measures and consistency are to be considered as supplementary sources of information.

B. Concerning audience analysis studies in persuasion.
1. Extensive interviewing has established great differences in listener preference in radio programs; these are correlated with education and age.

BALLOT FOR JUDGING DEBATES

I. Quality of the Debating

Indicate the relative skill of each debater in each of the six phases of debating by placing numbers selected from the following scale (1, 2, 3, 4, 5, 6, 7) in the appropriate column. 1 is poor; 4 is average; 7 is superior.

	Affirmative 1	Affirmative 2	Negative 1	Negative 2
1. Analysis—plan of case	( )	( )	( )	( )
2. Knowledge, evidence	( )	( )	( )	( )
3. Reasoning, inferences	( )	( )	( )	( )
4. Adapting to opposing case	( )	( )	( )	( )
5. Skill in rebuttal	( )	( )	( )	( )
6. Speaking skill	( )	( )	( )	( )
Totals				

II. Ranks of Debaters

Please rank the debaters in order of their excellence.

First ____________________

Second ____________________

Third ____________________

Fourth ____________________

III. Decision

I believe the better debating was done by the ____________________ team.

(Signed) ____________________

2. A majority of American listeners are satisfied with radio; the discontented minority, however, is largely made up of highly educated people.
3. Tastes of people tend to determine what they hear and read rather than mass communication media causing a change in the tastes of the people.

C. Concerning media comparison studies in persuasion.

1. Direct speech seems to be more persuasive than radio speech or printed materials.
2. The motion picture audience appears to be more suggestible than newspaper or radio audiences.
3. Learning by radio lecture seems to be approximately as efficient as learning by classroom lecture.

D. Concerning studies in methods of persuasion.

1. Listeners prefer a variety of brief motive and logical appeals intermixed to either extended logical or extended emotional appeals.
2. Apparently material conflicting with one's frame of reference tends to be forgotten.
3. Repetition is a strong means of emphasis. Factors of vocal and physical variety are also helpful.
4. Both the beginning and ending of a speech are relatively well remembered; which one has the advantage is in dispute.
5. Specific training in methods of problem solving, argumentation, and debate can increase critical thinking ability of a group.
6. Recognizing propaganda methods does not render the person being persuaded immune to influence from that unit of propaganda.
7. Logical-factual persuasion seems to change attitudes about as effectively as does more colorful and emotional appeals.
8. Attitude changes from persuasion tend to regress more than do those resulting from discussion.
9. Conversational radio delivery seems to be as effective persuasively as dynamic delivery.
10. The status accorded the speaker by the audience is an important determinant of his persuasive effectiveness.
11. Effective persuasion must be "set"

within the experience of the person to be persuaded and use his language.

12. Threats are, generally, ineffective persuasion.
13. Demands of propaganda must not be excessive as judged by reasonable expectations of probable outcomes. Conversely, attitude changes from persuasion are usually modification, seldom conversion.
14. Debate tends to strengthen previous convictions, whereas discussion apparently more often ameliorates them.

E. Concerning case studies in persuasion.

1. Feelings of guilt can be used by the persuader to motivate action. Interviewers in the Merton study found that bond purchase frequently relieved disagreeable tensions.
2. Personal influences rather than issues seem to change votes.
3. Audience response recorders fail when the audience becomes interested in the message and forgets the push button.
4. Film strips are about as effective teaching devices as are sound motion pictures.
5. Dramatic and commentator radio programs are about equally well-liked and equally effective in changing attitudes.
6. Intellectual abilities are closely related to knowledge and opinion.
7. The average number of years of school completed is an accurate index to the intelligence of an *adult* audience.
8. Presenting both sides is effective with highly educated and/or initially opposed auditors.
9. Presenting only one side is effective with the less educated and/or initially favorable auditors.
10. Audience participation techniques help the persuader most with the less educated, less able, and unmotivated audience.[28]

Motivation

In order to motivate people to use their health knowledge, they must be confronted by a basic human emotional urge to take action. The urge may be based on personal emotion such as fear, jealousy, ambition, pride, or any combination of these. However, the health educator desires to motivate people intrinsically, advancing such factors as normal growth, disease prevention, prolonging of life, social and emotional well-being of individuals.

The motives that are likely to be involved in public acceptance to preventive health programs include:

1. Desire to conform to group pattern.
2. Desire to seek relief from fear of disease.
3. Acceptance of screening as a convenient, quick, inexpensive, and usually painless method of examination.
4. Curiosity.
5. Hypochondriasis.
6. Desire for maintenance of optimum health as a factor in job security.
7. Compulsion of a legal, economic, or social nature.
8. Various personal motives.

Motives causing rejection of preventive health programs include:

1. Fear of a particular disease and its accompanying physical effects, as in cancer.
2. Fear of the economic consequences of discovering that one has tuberculosis (e.g., loss of job, cost of care, inability to continue supporting one's family).
3. Fear of social stigma still attached to certain diseases, such as epilepsy and syphilis.
4. Religious or cultist beliefs.
5. Traditions of medical practice (i.e., attachment to personal relationship with a family physician, as against the impersonality of a mass screening procedure, for example, in which examination may be by unknown physicians and technicians).
6. Misinformation or lack of information.
7. Lack of confidence in the effectiveness of a particular procedure.
8. Inconvenience as to time and place at which a preventive service is offered.
9. Indifference (which may often be a cloak for unstated fears with respect either to a particular procedure, to the disease or diseases to which it relates).
10. Cost of the procedure (for the individual).
11. Emphasis of a particular preventive procedure on common aspects of chronic illness rather than on specific disease entities.
12. Cultural and social patterns of ethnic and other subgroups in the population.

A person's motives are linked with and strongly influenced by the groups to which he belongs. An individual can and does belong to a long list of "publics" simultaneously. A person's overlapping membership in many "publics" lends stability to the powerful force of public opinion. Citizens are continually forming, disbanding, and reforming "publics" holding specific views toward specific issues. Community health educators realize the importance of these groups and communicate with the individuals in them. Appeals must be significant and relevant to a particular group interest in a particular situation. The roles people play and the value and attitudes they build around them are largely determined by the group to which they belong. A person's group relationships provide the setting for most of the health education he receives and transmits.

Research in Motivation. Health behavior or practice usually follows a characteristic pattern in each group or individual, and is reflected in his other actions as a way of life, involving attitudes, values, culture, and knowledge. Although a great deal of work remains to be done before we fully understand how best to promote every health program, a research study of the variables related to effective advertising of seat belts as a safety device reflects the complexity of the problem.[29]

The study notes that many experts believe that the automobile seat belt is the most effective single device available for reducing the number of deaths and the severity of injuries resulting from automobile accidents. It is estimated that the use of seat belts would reduce the chance of death or serious injury in automobile accidents by at least one-third. In view of these estimates, it is most disheartening to discover that only about 30 per cent or fewer of the passengers riding in vehicles with seat belts actually use them.

This extremely low level of public acceptance of seat belts has been interpreted in several ways. The explanations have elements in common but contain important distinctions:

1. *Ignorance.* "There has not been enough advertising of seat belts and the benefits they offer." The simplest explanation, this view assumes, is that the low level of use is due merely to lack of information. It states the problem as one of a product obscurity rather than consumer resistance. However, studies indicate that despite group discount and major promotional efforts, including posters, movies, brochures, and newspapers, effected by the manufacturers and distributors to promote seat belts to their own workers, only 3 to 5 per cent of employees have them installed.

2. *Misinformation.* "People are misinformed about seat belts, and additional advertising and promotion must be designed specifically to combat erroneous opinions." To remedy this situation requires also that additional advertising and promotion be directed specifically at predetermined areas of misinformation. Studies also indicate that many persons are receptive to appeals against seat belts because of misinformation. If a person reads the caption "Do seat belts cause abdominal injuries?" the negative link is established, and his reasonable doubts are selectively and distortively reinforced. He may remember what he has read as "seat belts cause abdominal injuries."

3. *Psychological factors.* "Generalized and perhaps unconscious psychological reactions toward seat belts are the principal cause of consumer resistance. The consumer resists the light of psychodynamic concepts of association and anxiety defense."

This explanation of the problem offers the most promising basis for an effective action program. No real evidence has been offered as to the exact nature of psychological resistance factors, but several plausible, though speculative, hypotheses have been advanced.[29]

Representative examples of hypotheses concerning psychological resistance factors are given in the following paragraphs:

1. The seat belt may act as an anxiety producing symbol. The primary purpose of seat belts is the prevention of death or serious injury resulting from automobile accidents, and this is clearly not a pleasant association. Few persons are willing to accept the responsibility of being involved in a serious accident. However, purchasing seat belts is at least tacit recognition of this possibility, and the mere presence of the seat belts in the car serves as a daily reminder. Thus, it has been suggested that seat belts are not accepted because of their unpleasant associations.

2. Use of the seat belt is seen as implying lack of masculinity. This hypothesis indicates that selling seat belts to men is comparable to getting them to wear galoshes on a rainy day. Either is felt to represent a more feminine concern for safety and is indicative of excessive timidity and precaution. For many men, the automobile represents their only chance for reckless bravado and daring; such being the case, they are not apt to install a safety belt.

3. Seat belts may bring about reactions involving resistance to restraint and restriction. It is likely that many persons object to the general idea of restraint and restriction that the use of seat belts involves. Informal observation reveals this objection to be particularly prevalent among women. Perhaps it is associated with a reversal in sex role identification and the resultant strong need for independence and freedom. A highly speculative interpretation is that the seat belt involves association with sexual assault.[29]

More superfluous but frequent objections include the untidy appearance that seat belts give to the car, the concern that individuals voice over wrinkled dresses or suits, the time required to buckle and unbuckle them, and irritation at having lights and buzzers command us! These objections indicate the type of psychological factors that may constitute a basis for consumer resistance. Two related problems occur in effectively combating psychological resistance. The first is determining, by empirical means if possible, exactly what psychological factors are responsible, since present information in this area is admittedly speculative. The second is devising advertising and promotional material that will effectively overcome resistance.

Accepting psychological factors as the most likely explanation of consumer resistance to the purchase and use of seat belts, the research study developed two promotional campaigns to check effect on public attitudes. The first approach involved the identification of seat belts with a professional racing driver, basing the identification on the racing driver's frequent and, we suspect, well-known use of seat belts and consequently the credibility of his endorsement. However, to achieve closer consumer identification, a pointed effort was also made to stress the driver's use of the belt both on and off the job.

This particular approach was selected for several reasons. As previously discussed, it is plausible that men (at least some) regard the use of seat belts as antithetical to a strong masculine role, and further, this reaction may be heightened by the function their driving serves in expressing such "masculine" traits as recklessness. Also, by omission and contrary slant, this approach minimizes association with accidents, death, and injury. The seat belt information that is stressed includes comfort, relaxation, and staying behind the wheel and in charge, the latter having an obvious literal meaning, but also perhaps, an effective figurative implication heightening the masculine tone of the material.

The second campaign used a "scare approach" and relied heavily on anxiety for its desired effect, by stressing the possibility of personal involvement in an accident, and that seat belts constitute the best device for preventing serious injury and death. In both cases, a specific approach is achieved primarily through the illustrations and captions. For the sake of experimental equivalence, both approaches are essentially the same in terms of information content, and such basic perceptual qualities as color and pattern.

Results of the experiment showed that the professional driver approach induced a statistically significant greater number of persons in the test groups to purchase seat belts than did the scare approach. The professional driver approach induced 6 per cent sales, and the scare approach induced 3.4 per cent sales. In addition, audience survey evidence and the evaluation of promotional arguments tend to support the position that the professional driver approach was significantly more effective than the varied but more intensive anxiety approach. It is interesting to note that seat belts are now standard equipment on new cars. People still resist using them, though, so programs to encourage them to "buckle up" are still necessary.

An individual confronted with many images and preformed values and attitudes can justify a number of similar rationalizations (Table 5–1). He may respond to promotion with thoughts about the *subject* rather than a definite attitude toward the *product.* This research study on seat belts offers many constructive suggestions in the use of health communication and motivation:

1. Advertisement of health and safety products should not emphasize the functional role but should emphasize comfort, skill, masculinity, beauty, etc. Some consideration might also be given to stylizing products for their attractive and socially appealing appearance. The general concept of credibility of claims associated with use of the product involves several related factors and is determined by a host of communication variables. We must appeal to the social needs and habits of the various groups in terms of their ideals such as: the heavyweight champion, professional golfer, actress, doctor, and other credible groups.

2. The nature of an advertisement should be dictated by the nature of the response it is intended to elicit and the opportunities for making such a response. If we have to wait any undue length of time to receive immunization or to have seat belts installed, if costs are excessive, or if the availability of the product is limited, the rewarding aspect and motivation diminish.

3. Pleasant, repetitive, simple material will be most readily retained.[29]

TABLE 5–1 Rationalizations Behind Health Behavior

FOR SMOKING	AGAINST SEAT BELTS
Reasonable doubt	Reasonable doubt
No immediate danger; cancer will happen to the other fellow	No immediate danger; accidents will happen to the other fellow
Other causes of lung cancer	Not 100 per cent effective; knows of someone who wore seat belt and was killed
Grandma smoked and lived to be 105	
I can stop anytime	I am a good driver
Many people smoke	Many people don't have belts
Will die someday, anyhow	Will die someday, anyhow
Nervous	Too bothersome, uncomfortable
It's my right!	Don't like machine giving me orders (i.e., buzzers and lights as warnings to put seat belts on)
If I stop, I'll get fat and die from heart disease	

Those of us in public health must seriously evaluate the nature of the public's resistance to community health programs before we can devise more effective ones. Future research must be directed toward discovering approaches that will most effectively lead to positive community health practices and attitudes. This means making use of new principles from advertising, consumer research, and marketing, and cooperating with experts in these fields to promote and protect individual health.

Motivation for Family Planning. The education and communication programs carried on by the Chinese in behalf of "Planned Childbirth" have five distinctive characteristics:

1. They aim at educating the younger generation.
2. They emphasize the personal benefits and responsibilities of reduced childbearing, and attack or ignore Malthusian theories of overpopulation.
3. They use a great variety of techniques, including printed material, posters, films, exhibitions, meetings, and individual follow-up.
4. They combine medical, social, employment, party, and rationing approaches on a broad and coordinated level.
5. They employ social pressure to encourage conformity with national policy.

The Chinese model is the most rational and extensive experiment in family planning of any developing country. It is a system in which grassroots workers and cadres are informed of family planning, contraceptive devices and services are easily available and accessible to all who want them, and social norms are mobilized to create social pressure and social support for small families.

MASS COMMUNICATIONS

In order to disseminate information to increase the knowledge of others or to change their concepts, personal discussions, carried out in terms familiar to the listener and related to his personality and circumstances, are required. For example, a poster stating "Protect . . . get your DPT" may not convey the message as well as "Be wise . . . Immunize." The word *immunize* relates a common experience to most people; few people, however, are familiar with the term DPT (multiple antigen—diphtheria, pertussis, and tetanus). Health education programs depend upon effective communication. Although communication appears to be a simple process, research has successfully isolated and identified the following variables: exposure and access to the message, the media of communication used, the content of the message, the receiver's predisposition to the message, and relationships within groups receiving the message.

Health educators must be able to classify community groups and organizations in order to plan an effective, well-balanced communications program. Although the public is continually growing, moving, and changing, the following groups should be considered before launching a community health education program: teachers and students—all levels; government officials and agencies—local, state and federal; women's groups; service clubs; business and professional groups; industrial groups; church groups; and veterans.

Once identification of the selected groups making up the community has been accomplished, health educators must compare the objectives of their program with the characteristics and interests of each group in order to select the most effective approach to public favor. Understandably, certain groups are better targets than others in any given program. Names and meeting places of various groups may often be supplied by the local chamber of commerce or local health department.

The 7 C's of communication, as advanced by Cutlip and Center, are: *credibility*—competent source; *context*—provides a link with reality and participation; *content*—realistic meaning; *clarity*—simple, clear message; *continuity* and *consistency*—repetition with variation; *channels*—established channels of communication should be used; and *capability*—requires little effort on part of the recipients.

Expansion of topics within the 7 C's of communication results in the following principles, which may help promote better communications for better health:

1. Timing—people must be ready and receptive for a health message.
2. There must be mutual cooperation, understanding, and empathy between members of the communications media and medical communications.
3. The audience's average age, its economic and social status, and the number of people in the audience must be determined.
4. What are the objectives of the information—does it do what it is supposed to do?
5. Pretesting and careful evaluation of materials can save money.
6. Developing several types of pamphlets or materials for multiple or target groups is very effective.
7. A pamphlet must be clear, accurate, attractive, sincere, cohesive, and unified.
8. People who read pamphlets and retain information also use other informational sources much more frequently and readily than the group as a whole.
9. Prompt and accurate information serves the advantage of all health agencies.
10. Health information must be presented to newspaper readers in language they can understand and in a way that enables them to identify with the information. Communicate so that the reader can identify himself with the problem and react.
11. In relating health messages to the readers of a particular magazine, health communicators should study the magazine, the editorial objectives and content, style, range and depth of coverage, the advertisements, and the illustrations, all of which indicate the type of reader the magazine reaches, as well as his interests.
12. In a sound, preventive health program for the family, information has to be repeated.
13. In matters of *personal* health, we may expect too much from mass communication media. They help create a climate of acceptance, but in such a personal matter as health, person-to-person communication is necessary.
14. The use of mass media methods together with face-to-face methods is better than the use of either one alone.
15. Social factors affecting health compel interagency communication.
16. The provision of a central source of authentic information about the many aspects of health organizations, and services, is necessary.
17. The effect of any particular communication depends largely on the prior feelings and attitudes that the parties concerned have toward one another.
18. The effect of any particular communication depends on the pre-existing expectations and motives of the communicating persons.
19. The behavior of the communicant in any communication process is motivated.
20. Communication is likely to be more effective if we perceive the person communicating as one who can be trusted, who is an expert, or who commands prestige.
21. The use of repetition by different mass media, especially repetition with variations, helps to bring about change.
22. A strong threat may be less effective than a mild threat in inducing a desired opinion change.
23. The greater the conflict between what a man thinks and what he has been led to say, the more likely his opinions will change in the direction of what he says—the "saying is believing" phenomenon.
24. The more extreme the opinion change the communicator seeks, the more actual change he is likely to receive.

Promotion Techniques

Although health educators have developed many superior and effective promotion techniques, it is very difficult for them to compete with large businesses in advertising for public attention. The apparent lack of success of health educators in teaching basic

The mother got over her rubella in three days. Unfortunately, her unborn child didn't.

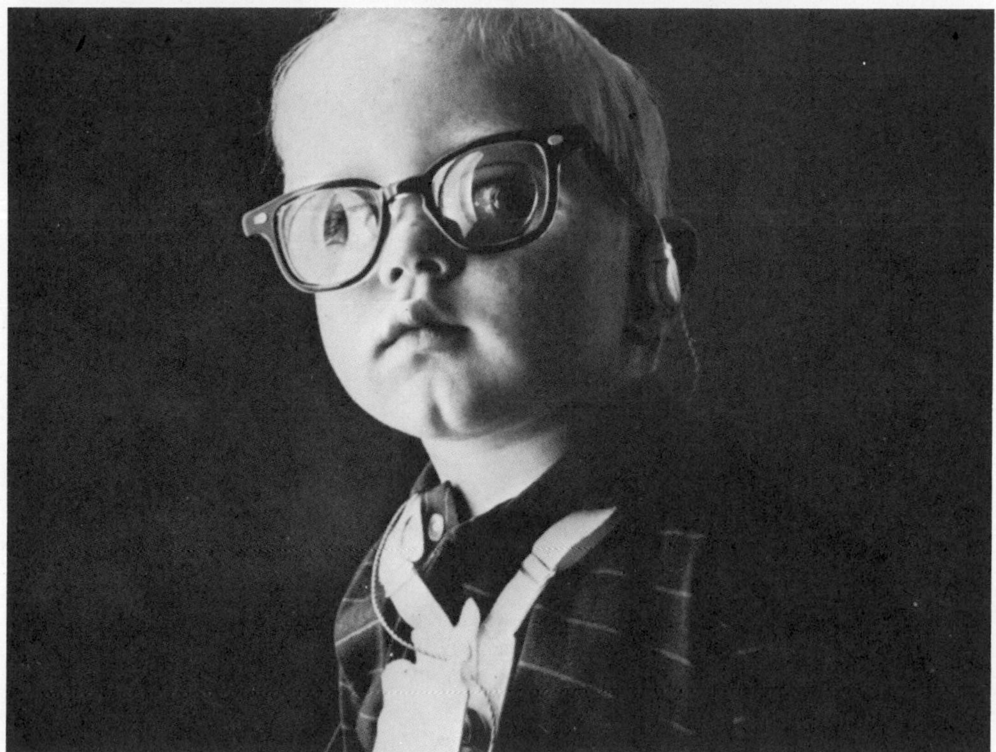

To pregnant mothers, rubella (German measles) means a few days in bed, a sore throat, a runny nose, temperature, and a rash.

But if they're in their first month when they catch it, there's a 40% chance that to their unborn babies it can mean deafness, or a heart condition, or brain damage, or cataracts which cause at least partial blindness.

Only last year, an immunization against rubella became available. But when a pregnant mother gets immunized, the prevention may be as harmful to her baby as the disease.

So if unborn babies are going to be protected, it will have to be by inoculating the kids who infect the mothers who in turn infect the fetuses. And it will have to be done now.

You see, rubella epidemics break out every six to nine years. The last outbreak was in 1964. Which means the next one is due any day now.

In the last epidemic, 20,000 babies were deprived of a normal childhood—and 30,000 more deprived of any childhood at all—because no immunization existed.

It would be unforgivable if the same thing happened again because an immunization existed and nobody used it.

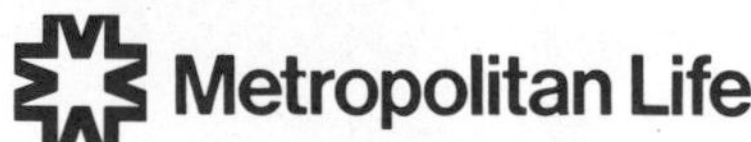

We sell life insurance.
But our business is life.

For a free booklet about immunization, write One Madison Avenue, N.Y., N.Y. 10010.

Figure 5–3

health facts; product discrimination in the purchase of foods, drugs, and cosmetics; and recognition of false health facts may be due to a number of factors:

. . . first, the American public is an overstimulated population, what with newspapers, magazines, radio and television programs, billboards and even space on buses and trains devoted to advertising intended to influence people to buy something. The advertising industry works harder and harder trying to think up new gimmicks to induce the public to purchase all types of goods. For a health educator to get in a few licks

Inoculate them Protect her

Rubella* means German measles.
Although it is a minor ailment for
children, rubella can be destructive
if contracted by a pregnant woman.
It can cause cerebral palsy and
other birth defects. Now, children
can be vaccinated for rubella.
Through your support in the past,
we were able to help in developing
this new vaccine that will remove
one of the causes of cerebral palsy.
There are many more causes to
be uncovered and conquered.
We still need your support.
Give to
United Cerebral Palsy.

*Every child aged one to eleven
should have a rubella vaccination.

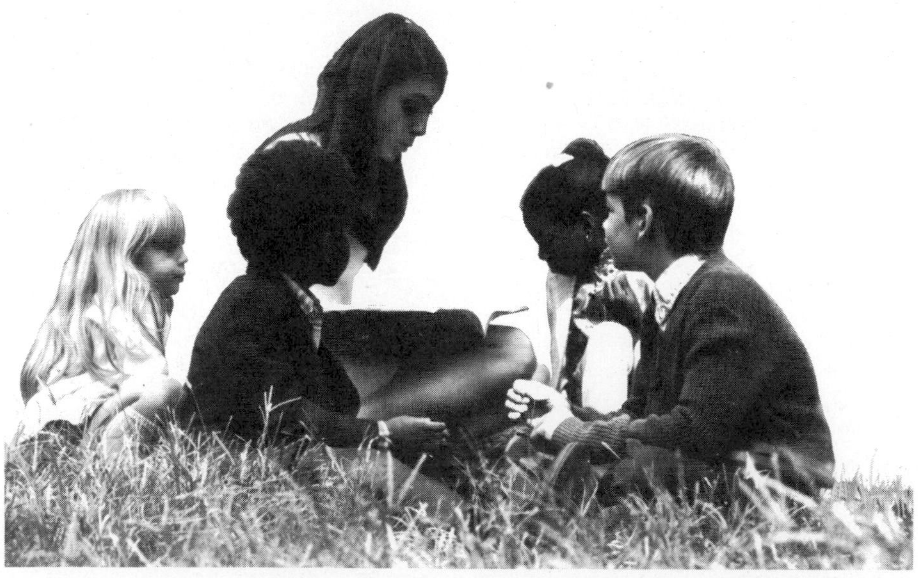

Figure 5–4 (Courtesy of the United Cerebral Palsy Associations, Inc., New York.)

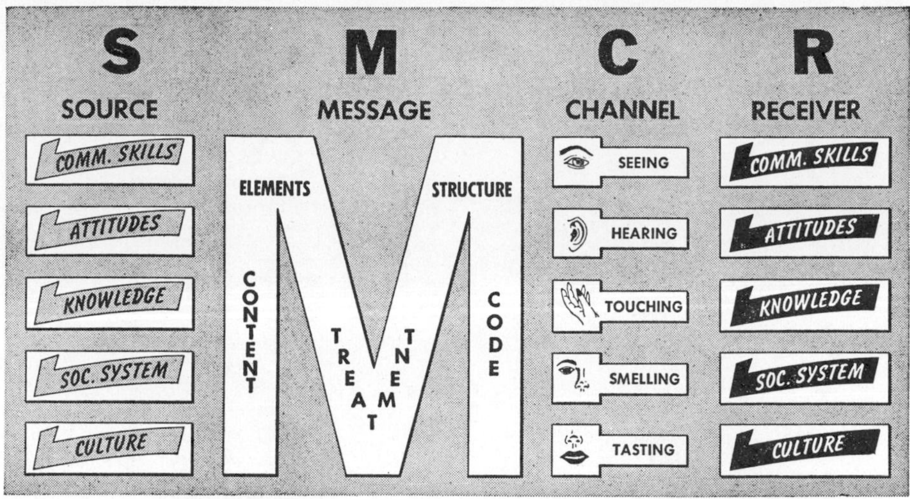

Figure 5–5 A model of the ingredients of communication. (From Berlo, D. K.: *The Process of Communication.* New York, Holt, Rinehart & Winston, 1960.)

on health factors over this threshold of overstimulation will take a real jolt.* Second, the quality and effectiveness of public health "advertising" is amateurish compared to that of the Madison Avenue professionals. Professional advertising is expensive, and few, if any, health departments could justify the expenditure of public funds in such an effort. The rationale of advertising is that if through this medium one can bring about the sale of larger volumes of merchandise, the saving consequent upon greater production volume more than pays for the advertising. It is unlikely that any such saving could be brought about in the field of public health. In fact, it might even produce further increase in expenditure of public funds. Third, there are ethical considerations which prevent health departments from using material in an advertising way, particularly case records which though quite forceful are nevertheless confidential. Even where names are changed to protect the innocent, in a small community individuals and families are easily recognized.[30]

There is no doubt, however, that health educators can learn a great deal about health promotion from techniques used by major industries (Fig. 5–6). For example, the athlete, movie star, and cowboy have been used very successfully in promoting cigarette and alcohol sales. Manufacturers have offered manliness and athletic prowess to men, love and popularity to women, and socialibility to everyone who will buy and use their products. A number of sports celebrities lend their names to testimonials on the implied, if not stated worth, of products as necessary to good health, social status, or personal success. Slogans, such as "kick the habit, it's a matter of life or breath" and "you only go around once" have had tremendous positive appeal, when associated with a national image in sports or other entertainment areas. Special target groups are essential in this type of advertising. For instance, an executive of one major cigarette company commented, "Students are tremendously loyal. If you catch them, they'll stick with you like glue because your brand reminds them of happy college days."[31] Complex political, economic, and social implications make it difficult to improve on the situation, but many countries are now disseminating cancer education materials on tobacco as a possible agent in causing cancer in an effort to help combat the increase in lung cancer (Fig. 5–7).

Industries spend a great deal of money each year on research in relation to advertising. Health educators can learn to effectively apply techniques gained from this information in their campaigns by a study of health product advertising. For example, a toothbrush company with increasing sales learned these valuable lessons:

1. Good distribution can be achieved without high cost. The technique used in this case was

*See the film, *Too Tough to Care* (1964) (18 min.), for light-hearted satire that de-glamorizes cigarette advertising and exposes attempts to manipulate teenagers. Produced for the Marin County (California) Medical Society and the California Medical Society (for grades 7 through 12 and adult groups).

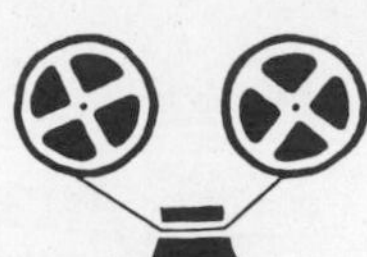

WORDS AND MUSIC. One association gets a popular disc jockey from a local radio station to donate his services. He plays music and chats with those stopping by the X-ray bus, stationed in a high-incidence area. His "show" is recorded on the spot and broadcast later over the radio station.

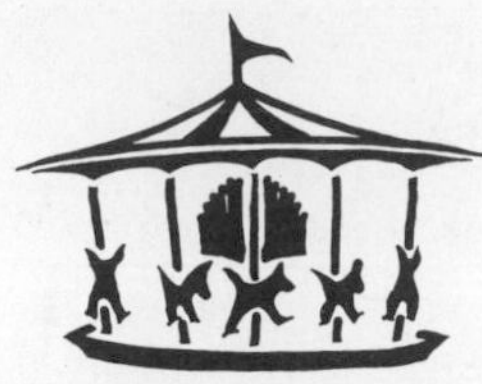

OUTDOOR ENTERTAINMENT. "Your portrait while you wait—for a chest X-ray!" That was the offbeat come-on of a city association, whose volunteer artist did the sketches right on the sidewalk. Another association gave kids a whirl on a merry-go-round while parents were X-rayed.

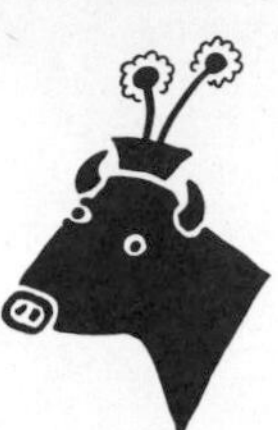

BEEFING UP THE CAMPAIGN. Draw numbers and you'll draw a crowd. Gifts donated by dealers and organizations have included practically anything you can think of and a few you never would. In one midwestern town, the livestock association offered a free beef cow. In another place, the millinery institute dangled a free hat as the reward. In an eastern city, enterprising committee members collected 100 merchandise donations from neighborhood shops. With all that going on, who needs TV quiz programs?

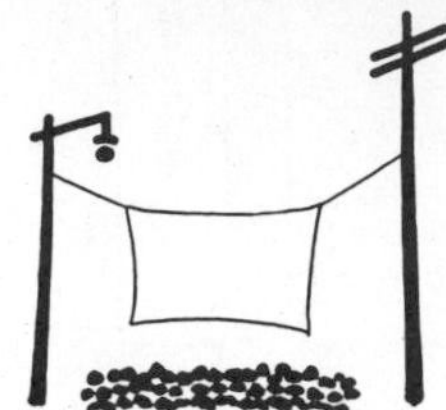

INSTANT FILM FESTIVAL. A bedsheet suspended above the street, a movie projector mounted on the TB association's station wagon—and all was set for an outdoor movie extravaganza. Its purpose was to herald the appearance of the health department X-ray bus on the following night in a high-prevalence urban area. The show was free, and included several entertainment films plus one on TB. Police and civil defense helped with arrangements. P.S.—The yield of active new cases from the subsequent survey proved particularly high.

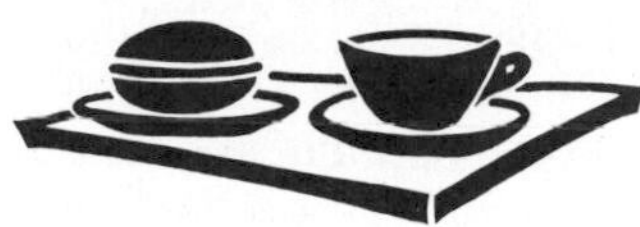

FREELOADING HAS SURE-FIRE APPEAL. In cities, skid row denizens have been offered free eats ranging from a meal ticket to a free carton of milk. In one big city survey, a national hamburger chain gave the skid rowers free hamburgers and coffee.

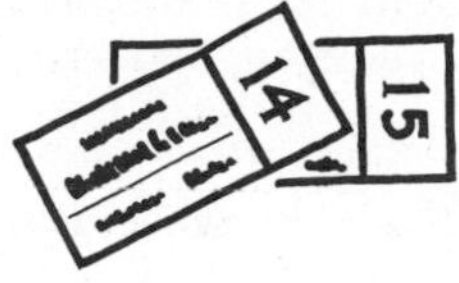

COMPETING FOR ANNIE OAKLEYS. A nice package deal was offered by one TB association: Take part in the X-ray survey and earn the chance to participate in drawing for a couple of big league ball game passes. The drawing for the lucky number was performed by a local diamond star.

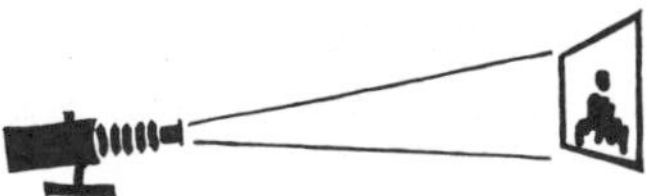

EASTERN ACCENT. In a western city, the Chinese section, considered a high TB incidence area, is surveyed yearly. "Miss Chinatown" makes personal appearances, and liberal use is made of bilingual tapes, news stories in the four local papers —and even Chinese movie house showing of lantern slides!

LIGHTS, SIRENS, ACTION! Lights flashed, bells clanged, sirens whooped as the fire department in one town sent its star engine down through the high-incidence area to tootle up the X-ray survey. Another stunt used in this town: a dancing girl in red leotards parading with a sign.

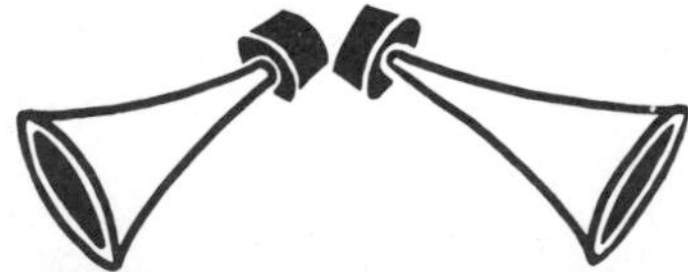

VOCALIZING THE MESSAGE. P.A. loudspeakers are a standard device—one of the best—for reminding people to get their X-rays. In one city, members of a special community group taped announcements to be broadcast from the mobile unit speaker to encourage participation in a high-incidence section. People and recorded music popular in the community were chosen for the broadcasts. In another town, the TB association recruited students from a broadcasting school to man the sound truck.

BIG STAMPEDE. If trading stamps stimulate business, why wouldn't the same thing happen at the X-ray unit? So reasoned members of a Rotary Club sponsoring an X-ray survey with the TB association. The club got a trading stamp company to donate 75,000 stamps for this purpose but wanted to give older people, considered a high-incidence group, extra incentive. Local merchants donated more stamps so that a double quantity could be offered to every person over 65 who came to get his X-ray. Successful? Very.

Figure 5–6 X-ray promotion techniques. These techniques have been used to induce people to come in for their x-rays—especially in high incidence areas. (From NTA *Bulletin*, February, 1964.)

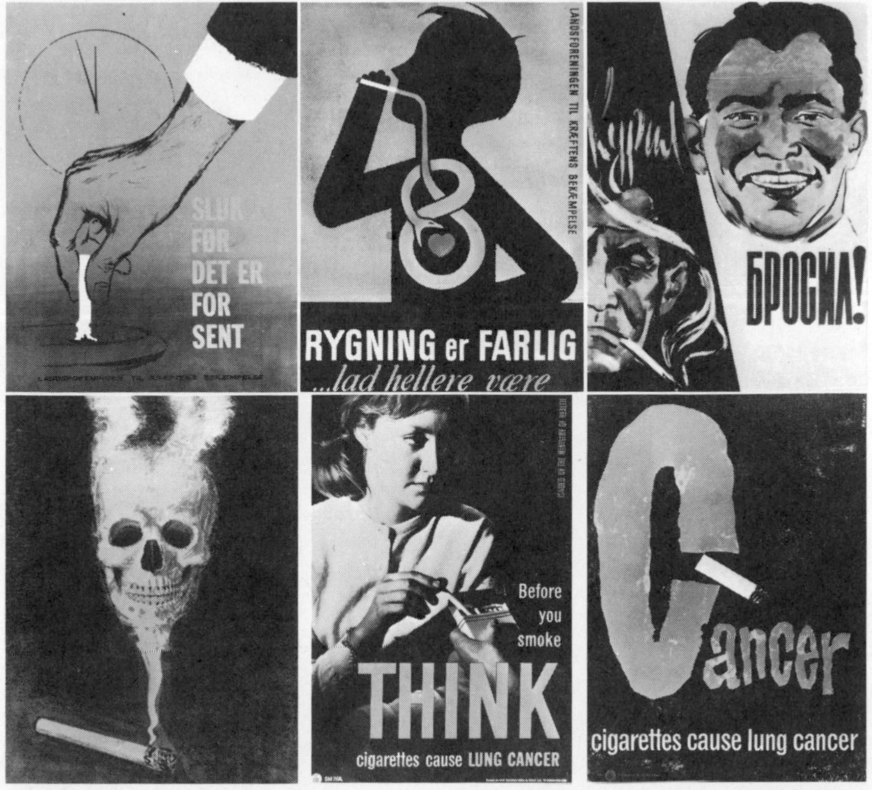

Figure 5–7 Cancer education posters from European countries warn smokers that tobacco may cause lung cancer. (From Brecher, R., et al: *The Consumers Union Report on Smoking and the Public Interest.* Mt. Vernon, N.Y., Consumers Union of U.S., Inc., 1963.)

simply seeking sales for a good product through dental prescription.

2. Ethical groups (dentists, in this case) are not as opposed to consumer advertising as often supposed. They object mainly to misleading and fraudulent claims but will strongly support an educational sales approach for a superior product if it places them and their profession in a good light.

3. A low-pressure approach in both trade and consumer advertising can accomplish your objective even in a highly competitive field.

Current promotion plans of the company call for adherence to the policies that have served so well in the past. This includes effective soft-sell, relying on advice of the dentist as the final authority, avoiding exaggerated or otherwise questionable statements, and a strong program of dental contact through attendance at more than 70 dental conventions annually.

Likewise, a major drug company realized the necessity of cooperating with and seeking advice from physicians in promoting a new vaccine (Fig. 5–8).

Mass Media Impact

The television and radio industries, no small part of the national economy, dwell a great deal on, and gain much of their profit from, medical problems. Medical dramas and soap operas abound. Almost all commerical announcements in the evening concern products that promise to cure constipation, headache, nervousness, sleeplessness or sleepiness, arthritis, anemia, stomach gas, odors, dandruff, hemorrhoids, and almost any other condition short of cancer and heart failure. The food industry plays the role of surrogate physician, advertising breakfast cereals as though they were tonics, vitamins, or restoratives. Each week, Dr. Joe Gannon or Dr. Marcus Welby performs a miracle. This leads to the expectation of mirthis is a reproduction of a message that will

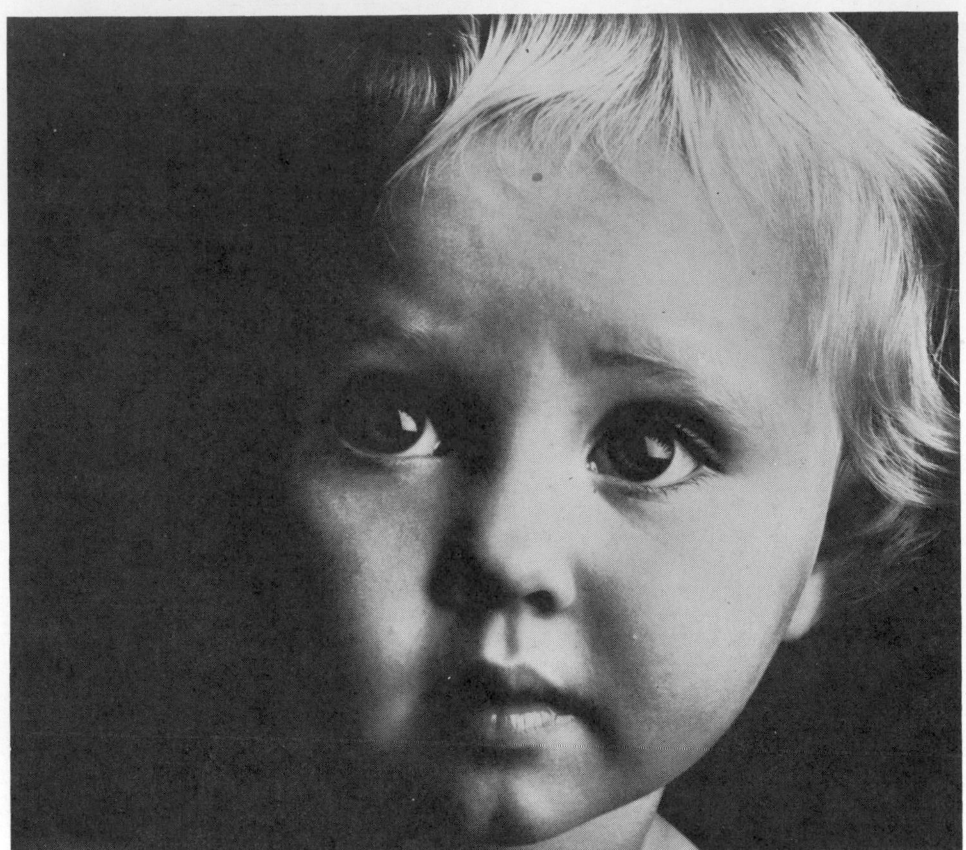

Measles only gave her spots...will your child be as lucky?

For most children measles is certainly distressing and inconvenient. But for some, it can be serious and even tragic. In fact, one child in every six who gets measles develops a secondary bacterial infection such as pneumonia or ear infection. (Most infections, of course, respond to your doctor's care.)

In about one case in 1,000 measles causes inflammation of the brain—encephalitis—an infection for which there is no specific treatment. In some of these children encephalitis causes only temporary changes; in others there is permanent damage such as mental retardation. And, some do not survive.

In 1962, for example, 408 children in the United States died from measles. (Since the conquest of polio, measles causes more deaths than any other common disease of childhood.)

Even when measles is apparently mild, it may accentuate certain problems such as bed-wetting, thumb-sucking, poor school work or tantrums.

If your child hasn't had measles why take any chances? Measles is now preventable, along with other serious and common childhood diseases, through vaccination. Don't wait for your child to catch measles... 9 out of 10 unprotected children will. Call your doctor now about vaccination against measles.

The American Medical Association, the American Academy of Pediatrics, the American Academy of General Practice, the American Osteopathic Association, and the U.S. Public Health Service urge all parents to consult their physicians about measles vaccination for their children.

MERCK SHARP & DOHME
Division of Merck & Co., INC., West Point, Pa.

Figure 5–8 *See opposite page for legend.*

acles by many—the belief that if you go to the right doctor, you'll be cured. Others believe that because they have read the latest magazines and viewed certain special television shows, they are well informed and there is no need to go to a physician. Many have also come to the conclusion that *everything* we eat may be carcinogenic; so why pay attention to any "new and startling" revelations.

Many persons feel we are living in a time of instant gratification. There is an impatience with inconvenience and a demand for magic shortcuts. This irrational trust can turn, if unfulfilled, into an irrational misappear in women's magazines

Doctor,

The advertisement reproduced on the left hand page will soon appear in popular women's magazines like McCall's and Good Housekeeping. It tells parents about the risks of measles and about the availability of measles vaccines.

Before it appears, however, we thought you would want to see the ad. It urges the reader to consult you, the family doctor, for more information about measles and for vaccination against this common, but potentially dangerous, childhood disease.

In addition to providing you with a preview of the advertisement, we want to take this opportunity to tell you why Merck Sharp & Dohme decided to run the ad in the popular press.

First, while several vaccines are available and more than six million children have been vaccinated, it is estimated that more than 22 million children remain unprotected.

Second, the measles program—like the polio program—has been slowed by the public's lethargy toward immunization.

You will recall that it was not until you, your medical societies, public officials, and the public press got behind the polio program that it began to achieve its goals.

Third, before we decided to go to the public about measles immunization, we consulted the U.S. Public Health Service and the major medical societies. All groups consulted strongly endorsed this action.

Last, about the advertisement itself: In field testing the reactions of mothers to health advertising, we have found that only a forceful, objective, no-punches-pulled message would motivate the reader to take the time and effort to consult you about immunization. Our studies also found that only 20% of the mothers interviewed were aware of the potential dangers of "natural" measles.

Unfortunately, not all parents will read the reproduced message. We, therefore, join the A.M.A. in urging you to take the initiative by talking with parents about measles and the availability of measles vaccines. Office posters, with the message seen on the left hand page, are available from your MERCK SHARP & DOHME representative.

MSD | MERCK SHARP & DOHME
Division of Merck & Co., INC., West Point, Pa.
where today's theory is tomorrow's therapy

Figure 5–8 *(Continued)* An example of advertising in which a major drug company cooperates with and seeks the advice of physicians in the promotion of a new vaccine. (Courtesy of Merck, Sharp & Dohme, West Point, Pa.)

trust. Perhaps we must come to the naturalness of disease, the inevitable limitations of medicine, and the real certainty that life itself is a fatal disease. If people are educated to believe that they are fundamentally ill and fragile, perpetually in need of support by health care professionals, and always dependent on an imagined discipline of "preventive" medicine, there will be no limit to the number of health services and facilities required to meet this impossible demand. Conversely, when physicians are on strike, as they were in California because of the malpractice insurance controversy, it was revealed that individuals took better care of themselves and utilized family support systems. The next major advance will come from self-imposed changes in the life styles of all individuals.

Mass Communications in Health in Other Countries

Asia. Linwood Hodgdon, a social anthropologist who has worked for some years with problems of social and economic devel-

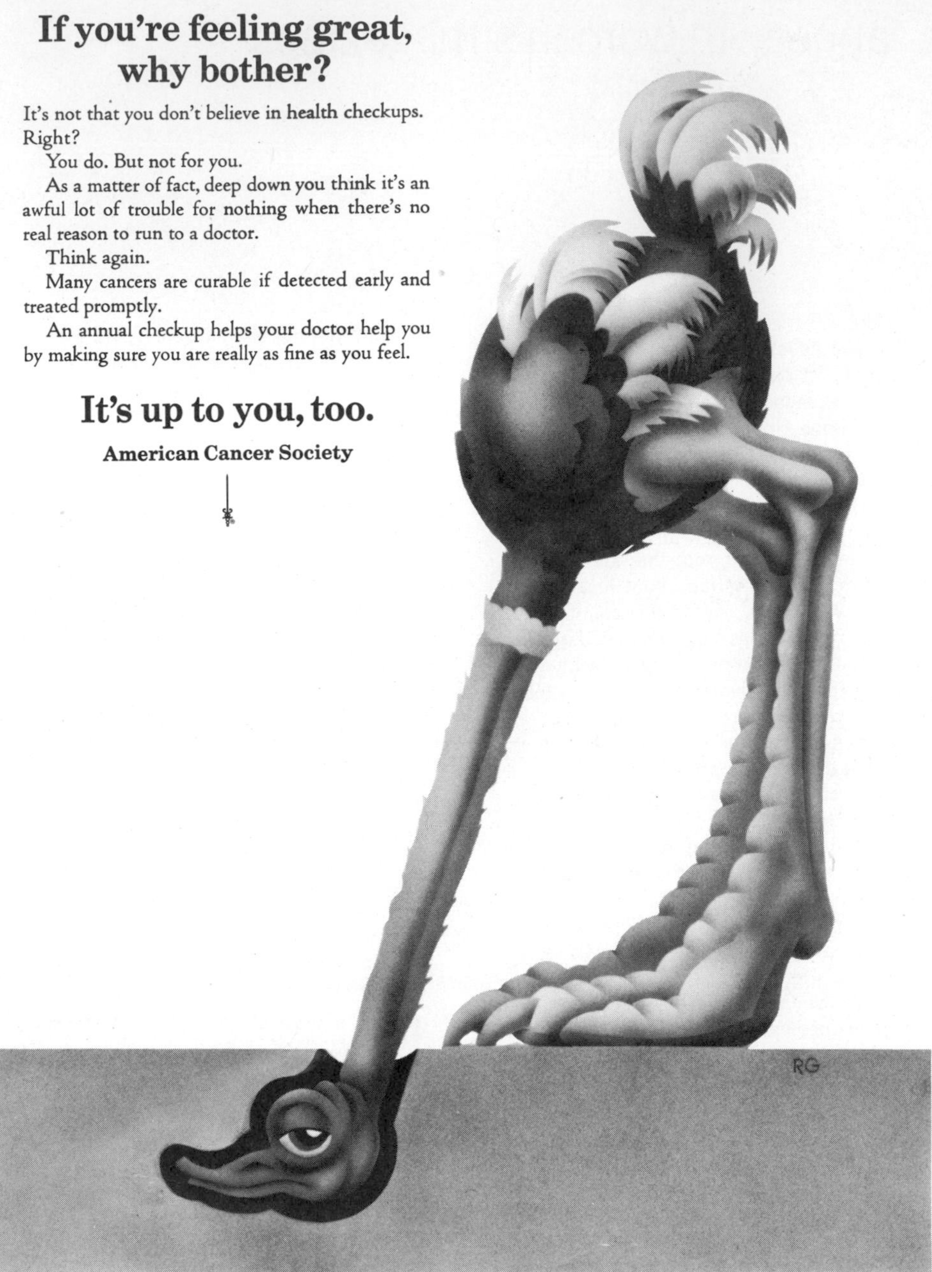

Figure 5–9 (From Cancer News, Volume 23, Winter, 1969/70. Copyright, American Cancer Society, Inc., 1969.)

opment in Asia, had this to say about health improvement programs:

> The further we progress with programs of public health education, the more our educational efforts will have to be concerned with the individual, and with the sociological and psychological factors which influence his behavior.
>
> In the initial stages of a malaria control program we are not directly concerned with either cultural values or individual attitudes and beliefs. Our efforts are concerned with doing things *to* people or *for* people, rather than *with* people. However, when we are interested in promoting a family planning program, or in changing the dietary habits of a group of people, we impinge directly upon the realm of individual attitudes, values, and beliefs. We must strive to help the people make a fundamental change in their personal behavior. In these instances we will find that

progress can be made only as we understand and work through these values and attitudes. We will also discover that public health programs cannot be legislated into existence, but rather the focus must be upon the educational process.[32]

In health campaigns, as long as we are concerned with doing something to or for people, the task is not too difficult, and an information campaign, although useful, is not crucial. But as soon as it becomes necessary for the villager to make a decision and change his behavior, then effective information is crucial. At this stage, as health development officers have discovered, if we expect our campaign to succeed and our information to be effective, then (1) we must base the whole campaign on an understanding of the life, beliefs, and attitudes of the villagers, and the social factors that help to determine how they live; (2) we must expect to provide face-to-face communication with field workers or other individuals who understand the village and villagers as well as the dynamics of social change, and use the mass media to support and extend the work of this field staff; and (3) we must use a combination of communication channels, employing each in such a way and at such a time as to contribute most to the total usefulness of the informaiton.

India. A report of the General Health Education Bureau of India indicates how that organization goes about applying information to the speeding up of community development in health practices. In the first place, there is an active field staff of public health workers, with traveling doctors and health clinics spaced over the country. To these people, the Bureau and the state offices furnish a stream of materials, in the planning and selection of which the field workers presumably have a voice. The Bureau uses all mass communication media to reach the public health workers, the health educators, and the general public. It maintains a film library on health subjects, previews new films to advise other users, and helps the Information Ministry in the production of films on health problems. It also stocks filmstrips. It arranges radio talks and publishes the scripts in a monthly journal, *Swasth Hind.* The Bureau is beginning to experiment with India's one television station. It publishes pamphlets carefully pretested with a target audience, issues press releases, takes advertisements, and publishes posters. It has participated in a number of health exhibits. Now it plans a new nontechnical health journal in a vernacular language for people with minimum education. In a typical campaign, such as the one aimed at smallpox vaccinations, it produces brochures and pamphlets for popular use; posters on the need for vaccination for six different target groups; handbills, bus panels, and chalk boards, explaining about vaccination; feature articles and press conferences for newspapers; "talking points" and technical background material for the field staff; a special number of the journal; and radio features, advertisements, and a group of slogans for campaign use.[33]

To the extent that facilities and personnel are available, a public health campaign in almost any developing country wil resemble this program. That is, it will be a wide-range effort utilizing mass media in support of an intensive interpersonal campaign. In dealing with rural and often illiterate people, health information planners have found film and radio especially effective in support of public health workers. Examples of each of these follow.

Philippines. The government of the Philippines has been operating 22 mobile film vans, built on trucks, and carrying their own power generators, projection screens, loudspeakers, microphones, exhibits, pamphlets, and other supplies. These vans go from community to community, showing films on health and sanitation, better agricultural practices, government organization, civic responsibility, and so on. After the film has been shown, the microphones and loudspeakers of the vans are often used in a discussion of the problems introduced by the film. People throng to see the films. Audiences range from 500 to 3000. In the course of a year, millions of people are reached.

South Korea. In South Korea, in an area where electricity and radio receivers were scarce, ingenious use was made of a limited number of inexpensive battery-powered radios. Twenty such receivers were obtained, and a 50-watt transmitter was built for a few hundred dollars. A program was designed to disseminate some needed information about tuberculosis, typhoid fever, and intestinal parasites in areas where these were the principal health problems. This information was featured in a three hour program, which also included a considerable amount of entertainment—a singing contest, local bands, a man-on-the-street interview, and so on. The program was broadcast three times a day. After each broadcast, volunteers moved the receiving sets to another community. Thus, in three days, the broadcast on the 20 sets was heard in 180 different locations. The broadcast was a huge popular success, and it taught the information it was intended to teach. A sample of viewers was pretested and post-tested. After the broadcast, the number of people who believed that tuberculosis was hereditary was reduced by 50 per cent, almost everyone had learned how encephalitis is transmitted, and 50 per cent more people knew the source of typhoid fever.

Information can also be effectively transmitted verbally (parables and storytelling), pictorially (painting, carving, drawing), and dramatically (games and plays).

China. Wang describes the health education approach in China as follows:

> Since the educational principles of informing, motivating and involving by doing have been successfully and broadly applied in the development of political, economic and social organizations, and in the transformation of the society, they are now being applied in health matters involving the individual and the community.
>
> The total absence of commercial advertising in the streets, shops, newspapers and magazines is immediately noticeable to the visitor. In its place are slogans such as "combining theory with practice"; "in order to be a teacher, one must first be a student of the people"; and Mao's thoughts and teaching and Party ideology. They are usually painted in bright red and bear the closest resemblance to commercial advertisements in other societies. Instead of selling a product, they sell an ideology. On the other hand, the visitor is just as much impressed by the use of the loudspeaker, which is the principal means of mass communication in China.
>
> Group interaction is extensively used to create social norms and instill new values. Having people study with and talk to each other is an important and successful means of solving social problems and bringing about social change.
>
> Criticism and self-criticism, a technique employed by the Party and universally adopted as a method in educating the cadres and the people through group interaction, is a forceful form of persuasion when issues and conflicts are brought to the open. The participants, after soul-searching self-examination helped by others, usually reach the decision of commitment or compliance.
>
> Wide use is also made of propaganda teams for health promotion and disease prevention. These teams consist of artists, writers, film makers, and youth and community members, who help launch the health education campaigns to educate the citizenry. There are also prevention teams who spread the messages on prevention from neighborhood to neighborhood and check on the spread of diseases.
>
> As a monolithic society, China has chosen propaganda to spread an ideology and to reinforce the goals and aspirations of the state. Health messages receive unilateral support at every level and from every organization. Health care is a shared responsibility of citizens and health workers.
>
> People of socialist China are health conscious. Old and young alike are found in the park at the break of day doing calisthenics and exercises. In cities martial music is played through the loudspeakers several times a day. At the sound of music people stop what they are normally doing and leave the shops or offices, go out to the street and start exercising. They are vigilant in keeping the homes and streets clean and free of mosquitoes, flies and rats. At the earliest sign of illness, people go to the clinics and health stations for care. The new mass culture has changed the value of the once "sick men of Asia". They want to be healthy not only for themselves, but for the sake of the state and for the productivity of their work team.[34]

TOOLS OF COMMUNICATION

The most economical and effective avenue of contact with the general public is through mass media—newspapers, pamphlets, radio, television, and magazines. The health educator must understand how, when and where to utilize the media in community health programs.

There has been much resistance among newspaper and broadcasting officials to other than news-type mention of certain health problems. This attitude has gradually been replaced by one of cautious support of health education efforts and programs. In spite of this resistance to carrying public health and personal health communications in this programming, the mass media remain our best means of dispensing information.

Newspaper

The newspaper is perhaps the most universally available printed medium for use in a community health program. As an important social agency, the local paper ranks high

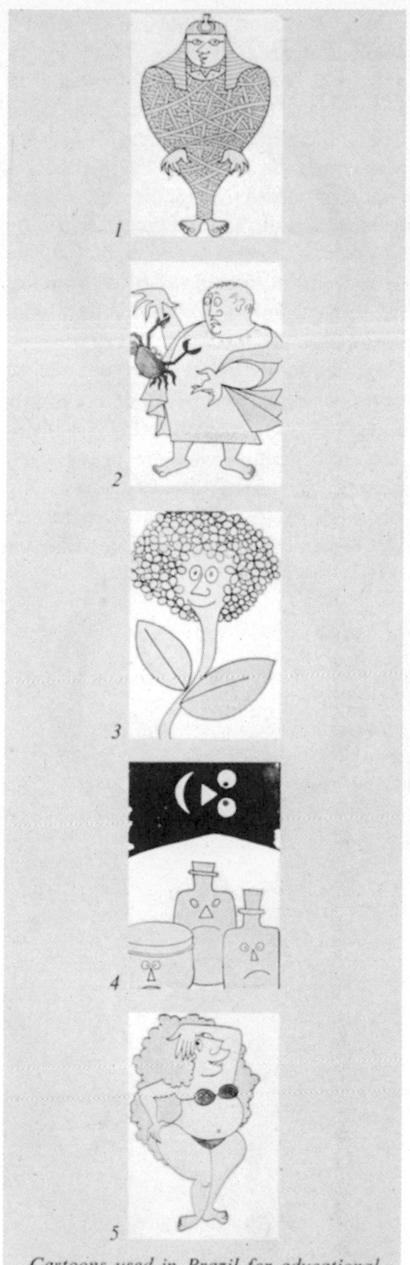

Cartoons used in Brazil for educational purposes.

1. There was cancer in ancient Egypt as the examination of mummified bodies has shown.

2. Karkinos or cancer in Greek means crab. Annoyed at being associated with the disease, a crab nips Hippocrates.

3. Ipoxia flowers, though sweet, do not cure cancer.

4. Don't take drugs without consulting a doctor.

5. Too much sunshine can cause cancer.

Figure 5–10 (From Wakefield, J.: Learning to save lives. World Health, February–March, 1970, p. 34.)

as an effective ally of health groups. If health activities are to receive the desired space in the press, health officials must gain and retain the respect of both news and editorial staffs.

Advantages of the newspaper include the intimacy and confidence of local publics, large community circulation; possibility of descriptive pictures, favorable medium for a cumulative publicity build-up or promotional campaign; foundation for promoting television and radio programs, and the leisure and convenience with which a newspaper can be read and digested. On the other hand, the newspaper has certain limitations. Perhaps the major limitation is the fact that most people read only a portion of the daily newspaper, and that portion may have little to do with community problems. It is interesting to note, however, that one survey revealed that 66 per cent of the persons polled wanted additional coverage of public health, medicine, and other scientific information.[35] It is questionable, though, whether or not the facts and information in a newspaper lead to changes in attitude and behavior. For example, many physicians have among their patients obese women who read every column and article on reducing but continue to gain weight.

A few suggestions for health committees to keep in mind when preparing an article for the press are:

1. Write simply and use words that can be understood by the least educated reader.
2. Keep the story interesting, brief, and concise.
3. Present the *facts*—who, what, where, when, why and how.
4. Write sympathetically, especially about false notions that may be present in the community.
5. Use a positive approach and try to avoid controversial material.
6. Write about recent local events that occur near home.
7. Do not overlook the possibility of using local group and organization publications as vehicles for messages to special audiences.
8. Keep in mind the various community groups that will read the article. (There must be reader interest.)
9. Convey the message intended.
10. Give the main points and the reason the item is important in the first paragraph.
11. Write a story with a real reason for being written. (It must be of public interest.)
12. Submit the original draft to several interested persons and groups for suggestions.

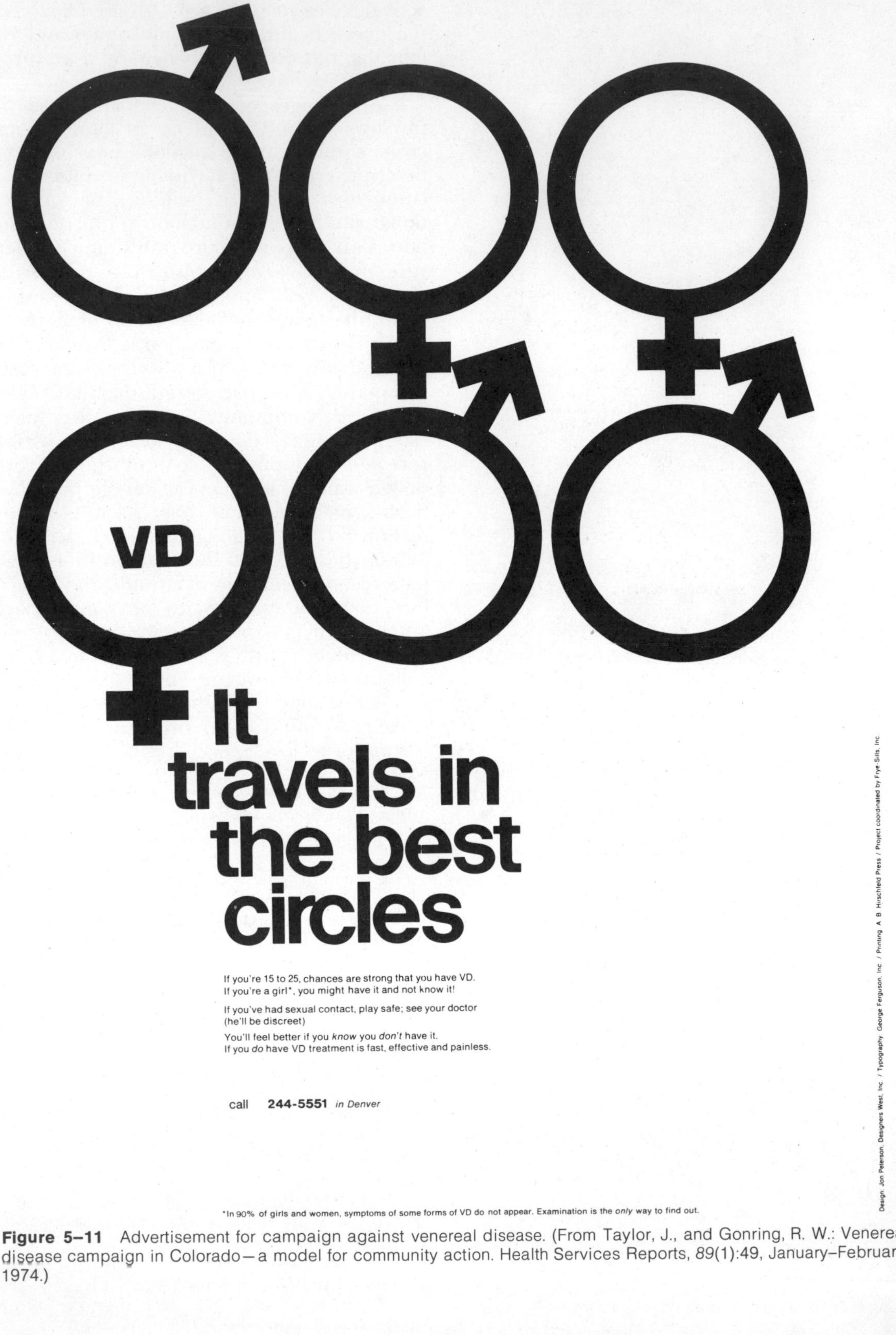

VD

It travels in the best circles

If you're 15 to 25, chances are strong that you have VD.
If you're a girl*, you might have it and not know it!

If you've had sexual contact, play safe; see your doctor (he'll be discreet)

You'll feel better if you *know* you *don't* have it.
If you *do* have VD treatment is fast, effective and painless.

call **244-5551** *in Denver*

Design: Jon Peterson, Designers West, Inc / Typography: George Ferguson, Inc / Printing: A B Hirschfeld Press / Project coordinated by Frye-Sills, Inc

*In 90% of girls and women, symptoms of some forms of VD do not appear. Examination is the *only* way to find out.

Figure 5–11 Advertisement for campaign against venereal disease. (From Taylor, J., and Gonring, R. W.: Venereal disease campaign in Colorado—a model for community action. Health Services Reports, *89*(1):49, January–February, 1974.)

13. Type the final copy neatly and recheck for errors in spelling, content, and meaning.

14. Place routine material in the editor's hands at least 24 hours prior to the day of publication.

15. Write articles that emphasize the problems, programs, and organizations, not individuals.

16. Be impartial in distributing newsworthy stories.

17. Consider inviting reports and editors to witness certain programs or incidents occasionally.

18. Seize the opportunity for follow-up with other articles, if practical.

To make writing more readable, there are three general rules to follow:

1. The more words there are in a sentence, the harder it is to read and understand that sentence.

2. The more parts there are in a word, the harder it is to read and understand that word.

3. The more personal references there are in a passage, the easier it is to read and understand that passage. (Personal references include pronouns, names, and words that refer to people, like *boy, friend, sister.)*

Although the press is an excellent medium, it cannot be used to the exclusion of all other media. Dissemination of information involves launching an attack via all channels of communication.

Radio

Radio has become part of our daily lives and exerts a strong influence on the public. One major advantage of the radio is the flexibility of the medium. For example, the ubiquitous radio may be present in two or three rooms of a home, the garage, and the automobile. The advent of the transistor, the pocket radio, and increasing number of FM stations has made the radio more popular than ever. Other advantages include low cost of operation, ease of shifting from one station to another, large number of programs, possibility of selecting specific audiences, current news, and music. There is no need for visual attention, and the spoken word can be more compelling, more personal, friendlier, and timelier than other media. However, ease of turning the dial may often be a disadvantage to educators.

Most radio and television stations allot a certain amount of air time for nonprofit programs of an educational nature, among which are included public health programs and commentaries. Short spot announcements or 15- to 30-minute programs can be very effective. Quiz programs, panel discussions, or brain storming may warrant different approaches.

Television

Television has impact and realism, is welcome in the home, and is readily available as an informational medium for the community health worker. The number of medical television programs has markedly increased. Such programs as *Marcus Welby, M.D.,* and *Medical Center* have enjoyed good ratings, as well as imparting accurate information. Television's first series about health, "Feeling Good," was initiated in 1974 at a cost of 7 million dollars. The potential of this medium is so great that we have already witnessed its impact on presidential elections, criminal investigations, diplomatic and foreign policies and relations, education, and medical research and surgery. We're on the threshold of a new era in medical and psychiatric consultation. Through closed-circuit TV, specialist and patient may be brought together in seconds. The time saved in emergency situations alone can mean the difference between life and death. For example: A man recently suffered what appeared to be a heart attack. In less than a minute, a cardiac specialist at Massachusetts General Hospital was studying the patient's electrocardiogram over the system, confirming the diagnosis and advising on treatment. Shock therapy suggested over the system brought a Bedford patient out of deep depression. A Massachusetts General Hospital therapist started a Bedford patient on the road to recovery from loss of speech, and MGH speech specialists are using the system to teach special techniques to nurses at Bedford. A stubborn depressive case at Bedford was helped when an MGH psychiatrist, after an interview on the system, ascertained that the man's depression was linked to his relationship with his wife. He suggested therapy for the couple, and it is already beginning to work. The day will come when anyone can obtain instant expert emergency treatment over interactive TV channels between his own tele-

Anatomy of a TV commercial

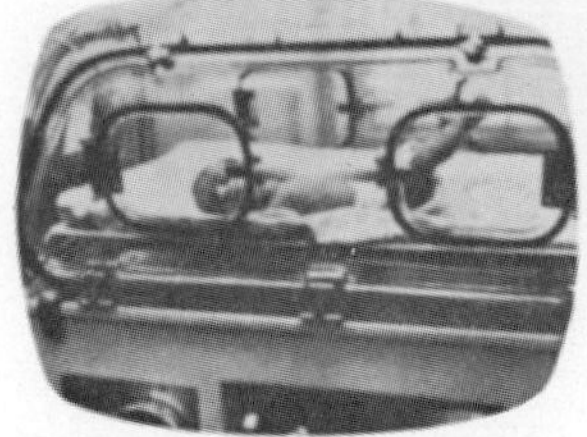

Commentator VO:

This is what can happen if you smoke when you're pregnant. You may deprive your baby of oxygen. You may poison it's bloodstream with nicotine.

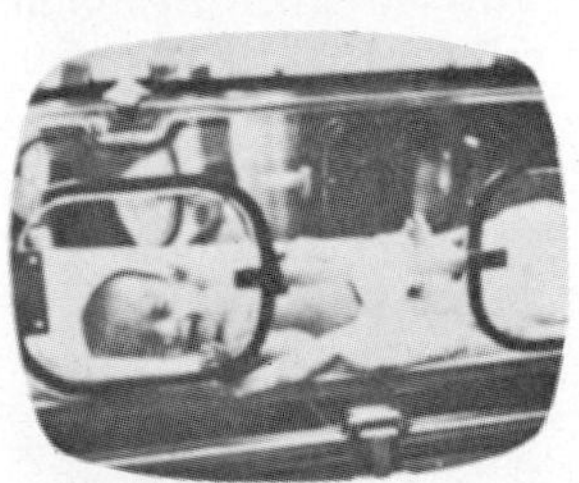

Smoking can make your baby premature. And not just small but undernourished with thin arms and wasted flesh. It can make him vulnerable to illness for months. It may even threaten his life.

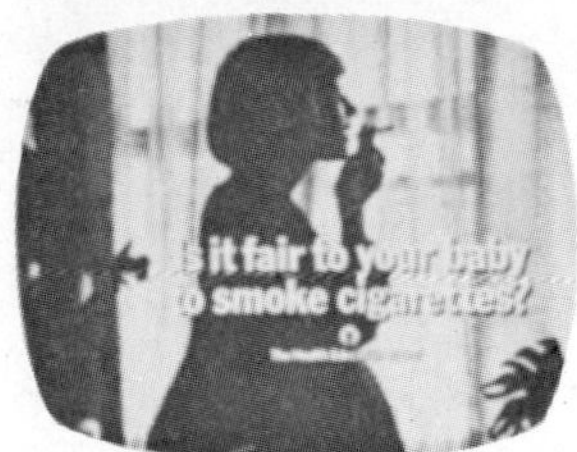

Is it fair to your baby to smoke cigarettes?

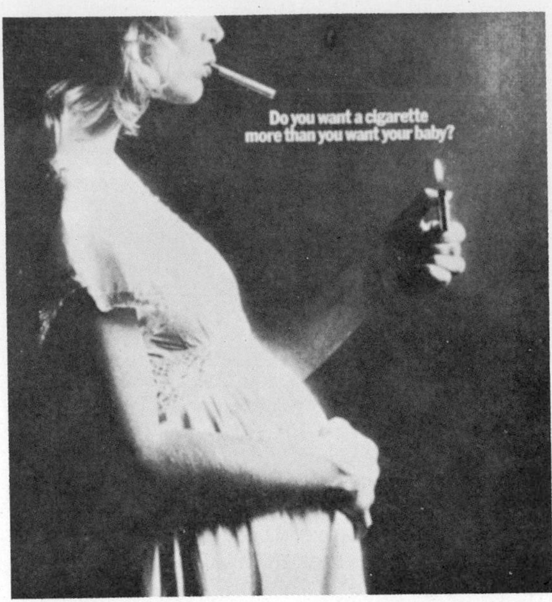

Figure 5–12 Campaign against smoking in pregnancy, sponsored by the Health Education Council, 78 New Oxford St., London, England. (From Health Education Journal, *34*(1):13–14, 1975.)

vision set at home and a nearby hospital or doctor's office.

Commercial stations throughout the nation donate thousands of hours of free public service time to educational organizations in the interest of community culture and welfare. Since many public groups are inclined to visualize only their needs and interests in asking for time on commercial stations, it is well for community leaders to understand the considerations of station personnel in granting requests for free broadcasting in terms of value, availability of time, and quality of the public service program. For example, a half-hour television program may cost a great deal of money, and time is at a premium. The public service program must compete with programs scheduled at the same time on other channels. Station personnel want to schedule public service programs that meet high broadcasting standards and attract as wide an audience as possible. Health education possibilities are infinite. For example, a series of programs devoted to explaining and discussing the various health problems within a certain community is certainly an excellent springboard to community health organization and planning.

Baltimore's health information television series, *Your Family Doctor,* which began on December 15, 1948, was the oldest continuously produced medical television series. Health information and education emanated from the family doctor as he dealt with his patients and their diseases. The family doctor is interested not only in promoting individual health, but also in improving the health of the community. In accomplishing these aims, *Your Family Doctor* utilized every available source of medical material and every practical audiovisual technique. In so doing, it enlisted the cooperation of every important health agency in Baltimore, both official and nonofficial. Viewers enjoyed the program.[36]

Your Family Doctor was designed to promote interest in and understanding of personal and community health, and was produced on a surprisingly small budget. Its prime functions were to increase the public's knowledge of the basic practices for keeping well, to encourage consultation with the individual's family doctor when there was any doubt about illness, to present public health problems and their local application to the community, and to inform and familiarize the public with the activities of the local health department. In essence, *Your Family Doctor* skillfully joined education and entertainment in the encouragement of healthful living.

Overall responsibility and supervision of program production rested with the director of the bureau of health information in the city health department. Programs were selected on the basis of timeliness and need by a television committee composed of the commissioner of health, the assistant commissioner of health, key city health department administrators, the script writer, the studio producer-director, and the director of the bureau of health information, who acted as chairman of the committee. Besides the selection of program topics, the committee designated well-known authorities as specialist advisers for each program. The following procedure ensured the authenticity and accuracy of each program:

> A preliminary conference is held to decide on the information to be presented. The method of presentation is discussed and decided on. The conference is attended by the specialist adviser, the scripwriter, the studio producer-director, and the director of the bureau of health information. After the preliminary conference, a script is prepared and submitted to the director of the bureau of health information for his approval. The director of the bureau of health information and the specialist adviser critically examine the script. They check on the accuracy of each statement and for the possible omission of essential facts. Final approval is given, and copies of the script are prepared by the bureau of health information for distribution to the studio and the cast. The participants memorize their lines, in this way avoiding the possibility of misrepresentation.[37]

Health directors who contemplate producing a television series or a single program may obtain information regarding the availability of source materials from the World Health Organization, Division of Public Informationa, Palais des Nations, Geneva, Switzerland; from the Pan American Sanitary Bureau, 1501 New Hampshire Avenue NW, Washington, D.C. or from the Bureau of Health Education, American Medical Association, 535 North Dearborn Street, Chicago, Illinois.

Refer to your county schools office, local health department, and local colleges and universities for many new and interesting TV health films designed for use in the classroom with children in grades K through 12.

PHONE-IN TELEVISION PANEL

Connecticut's "phone-in" sessions were an added half-hour to the "Food for Youth" course. A panel of experts, on live camera, answered questions on nutrition called in by the viewing audience. During the 10-week series, 120 questions were answered. The viewing audience consisted mainly of school-age children, homemakers, school food service personnel, physicians, and other adults, each with different interests, but each searching for accurate information on the food that people eat or should eat daily.

Questions varied from "Why can't I buy Coke instead of milk with my school lunch?" to "Does grapefruit have enzymes that help dissolve body fat?" The course stimulated an overwhelming response, with 1570 Connecticut school food service personnel and interested adults registering in the course. While the "phone-in" series required substantial work, the results in terms of interest generated by the viewing audience were well worth the effort.

The importance of radio and television in a statewide program of public health education in Texas is emphasized in the Texas State Department of Health Biennial Report:

> *Radio and Television:* The extent to which mass media managers of Texas contribute time and space to public service materials escapes the notice of the public generally; however, persons who—in the conduct of their work—must solicit time and space are very much aware of media generosity. For example, each month during this biennial period, this office has written and mailed

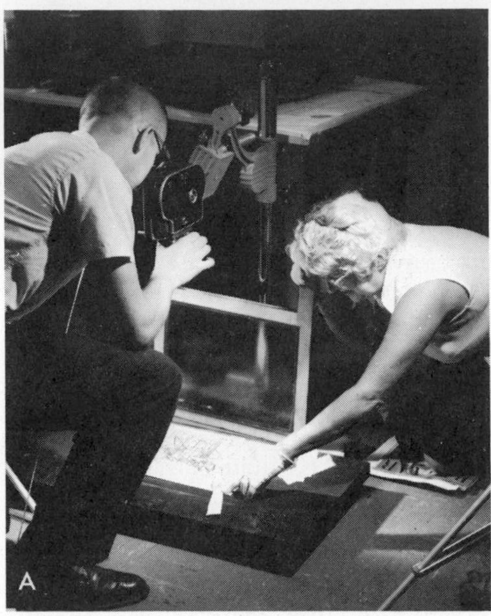

Don't Flip Your Lid

Producing a fast-moving cartoon color film for the Ohio (State) Division of Sanitation was a slow, painstaking process for Creative Services Photographer Dick Kraut and Artist Dorothy Kelley. Here you see them filming the action in the picture at the top. Dorothy moves a cut-out of the arm with the newspaper-wrapped garbage a fraction of an inch, then Dick snaps another picture, photographing the movement frame by frame. This process was repeated 56 times to move the arm a total of five inches.

The flyer (c) accompanied the film when it was distributed to television stations throughout Ohio.

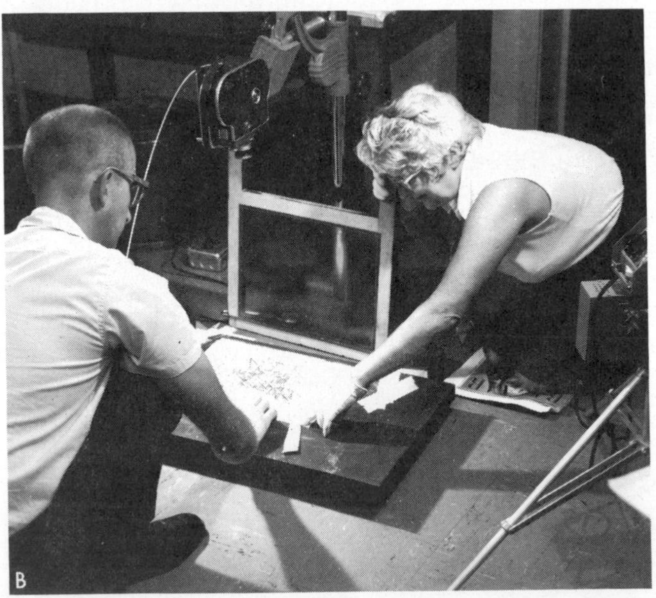

Figure 5–13 (From *Ohio's Health,* State Department of Public Health, Ohio, November–December, 1969.)

To: Public Service Director
of This Television Station

Solid waste storage, disposal, and collection is one of the serious pollution problems facing Ohio today. Many have referred to the problem as "The Third Pollution." Ohioans are required to store approximately 45 million pounds of refuse daily. Most of this is stored in garbage cans. Improper storage results in nuisances involving rodents, flies, odors, etc. Proper storage of garbage will do more to rid communities of rodents than anything else.

"Dont' Flip Your Lid" is the subject of a 20-second, animated 16 mm sound color spot announcement produced by the Ohio Department of Health in cooperation with local health departments. This spot points out the importance of proper storage of garbage and refuse on the premises.

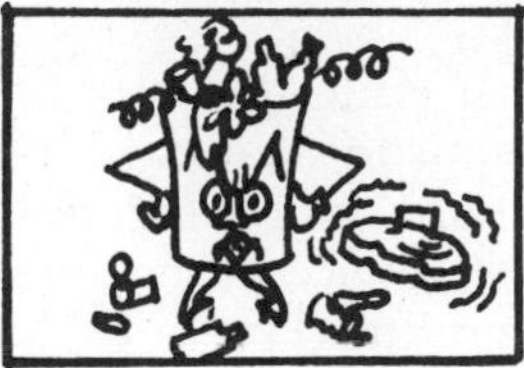

Yes I've flipped my cool and lid...

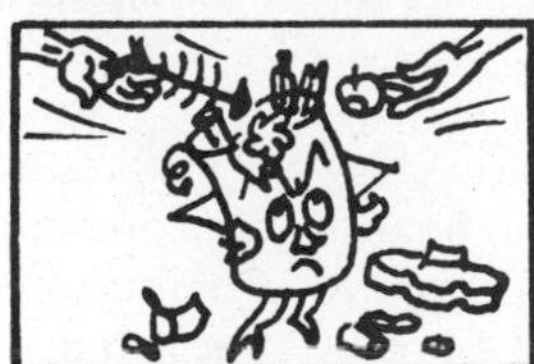

With all this trash there's nothing hid.

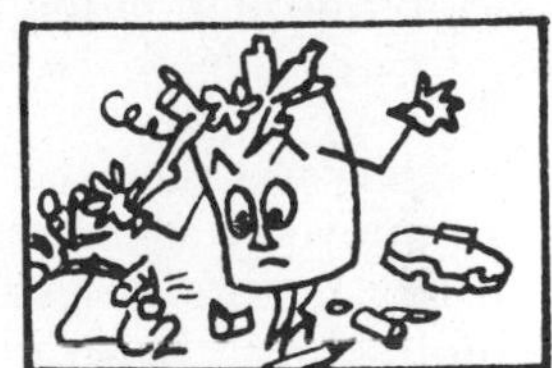

Rats and flies, they dine in style Germs do travel for a mile.

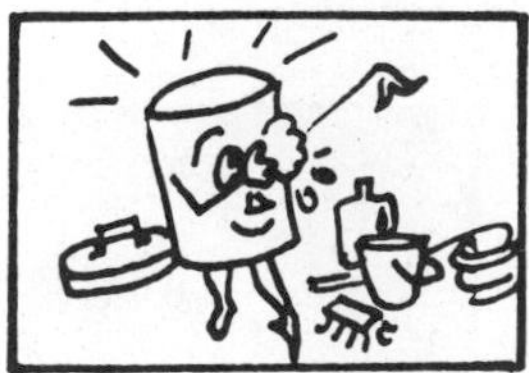

But, if I'm scrubbed and disinfected...

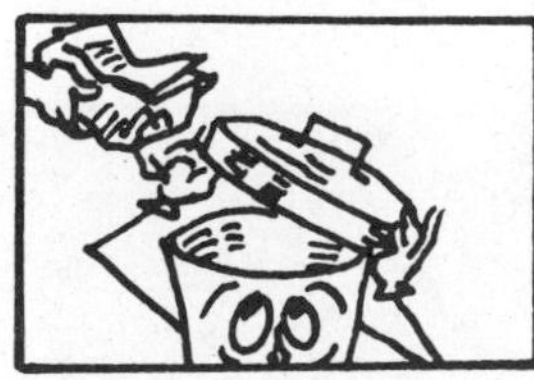

Garbage wrapped, paper protected.

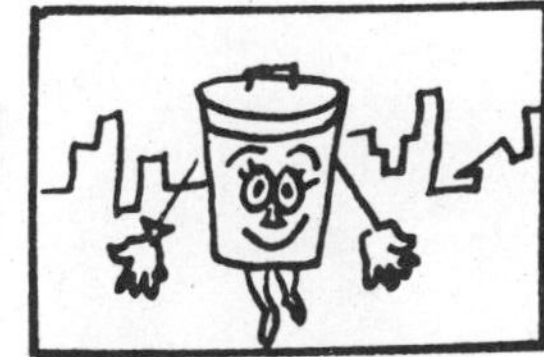

With my lid on always tightly This city'll be healthy, less unsightly.

C

Figure 5–13 *Continued*

to each radio station in Texas a packet of four 30-second radio "spot" announcements on topical health subjects, for a total of 23,520 repetitive messages. Conservately calculating thirty seconds of prime time at seven dollars for the average station, and assuming that each spot was read just once during the month of its intended use, Texas radio stations clearly donated an aggregate of $164,990 toward the Texas public health education movement. In addition to the radio announcements, 936 television slides with written commentaries in three different time lengths were distributed to Texas television stations, with only one known instance of a station refusing to display a slide because of an interest conflict. Radio Station WOAI, a powerful station whose signal is receivable all over the State, made time available each Sunday during the biennium for broadcasting a fifteen-minute health program produced by personnel of this Division. The weekly show was begun in 1937 and has continued without interruption each week since.

The most effective means of reaching Texas' 1,500,000 Spanish speaking citizens with health reminders continues to be a matter of importance to this Division. A dozen or so radio stations which broadcast Spanish-language shows continue to cooperate by airing weekly fifteen-minute music-health message programs produced by this office. Although radio is known to be perhaps the most efficient means of reaching this audience en masse, the necessary personal contact with stations has fallen off because of the press of other obligations.[38]

Because television is becoming more significant and important as a source of health education, a few factors necessary for planning and conducting a program will be discussed. In television, as in all other media of expression, an idea must be present. The main theme may revolve around major community health problems, obstacles, objectives, needs, programs, services, and accomplishments. If these things can be shown as well as explained, the embryo of a television program is present.

The program idea must be tested or refined by asking the following questions:

1. Is the subject of direct interest to my audience?
2. Can the importance of the subject be clearly shown to my audience?
3. Is it timely in terms of current developments, research findings, local problems, or seasons of the year?
4. Does it further community health education programs?

A good educational presentation involves research and careful planning. It is important that participants be given enough time to prepare a program to insure a feeling of security and excellent results.

Any format can be made interesting and meaningful if performers are carefully chosen, the subject is attractive to a wide audience, and audiovisual techniques are employed to provide variety and clear communication.

Pamphlets

Most health educators and health committees are often confronted with the task of preparing an educational pamphlet for distribution to the public. Authorities have recommended certain standards for use as guides in the selection and production of effective educational materials. The following outline is a brief summary of standards that apply to health education materials, and is

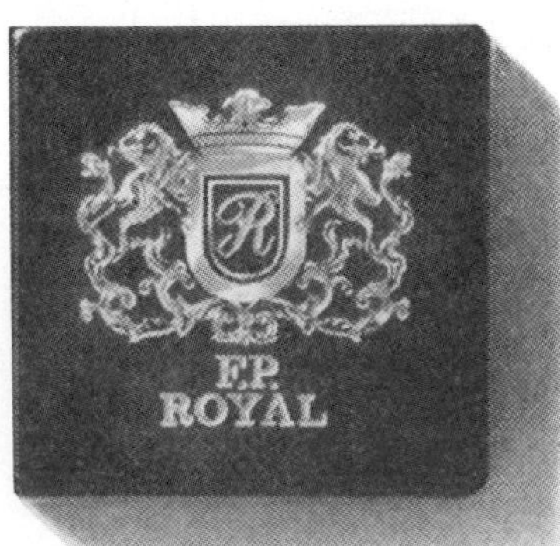

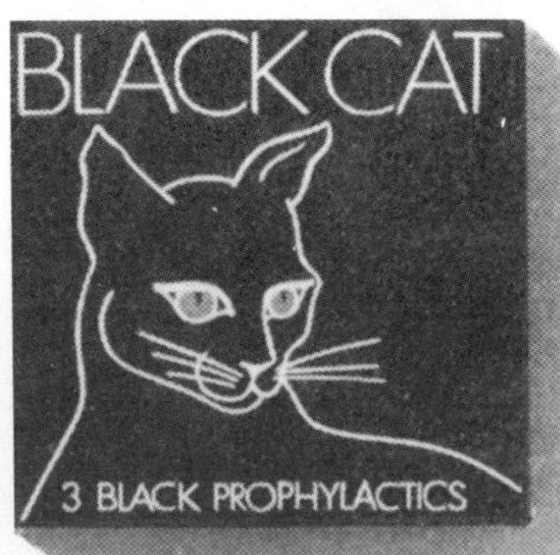

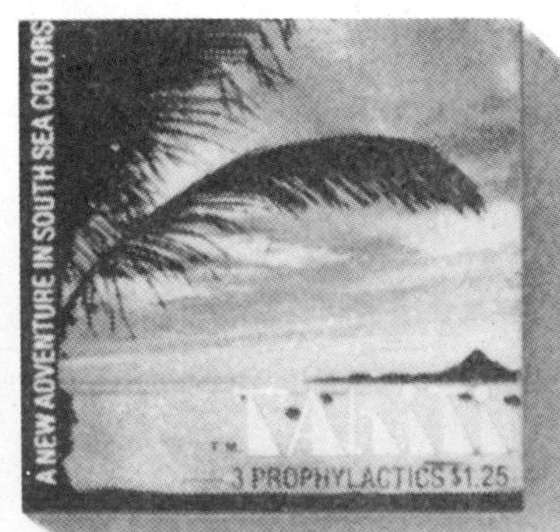

Figure 5–14 Condom packs: "Marketing experience has shown that packaging is as important as the service or the product." (From People, *1*(2):16, January, 1974. International Planned Parenthood Federation, 18-20 Lower Regent St., London, England.)

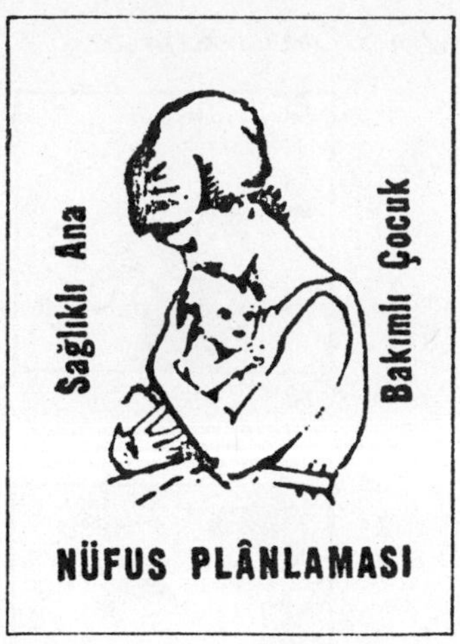

Figure 5–15 Family planning slogans in cigarette packets are Turkey's new technique for combating population growth. (From People, *1*(1):40, October, 1973. International Planned Parenthood Federation, 18-20 Lower Regent St., London, England.)

intended for use by health educators, teachers, health council members, and other persons whose responsibility is to compose health pamphlets for distribution among people in the community:

1. Is it accurate? Is it up-to-date? Are source, author, date noted?
2. Is it impartial? For what kind of readers are you choosing the pamphlet?
3. Is the purpose of the pamphlet to arouse interest, develop attitudes, give information, or stir to action?
4. Is the reader expected to read and keep the pamphlet, or read it and throw it away?
5. Is it attractive in format? Is it easy to read? Is it eye-catching; would illustrations enhance the appeal?
6. Does it cover essential and factual information?
7. Is the material well-written, well-organized, and easy to understand?
8. Will readers remember essential points?
9. Is it personalized?
10. Does it have the positive approach?

"Yo Soy Margarita . . ."

A unique series of colorful brochures have been printed in Spanish and geared to the specific health questions and linguistic nuances of California's rural Spanish-speaking population. The brochures were developed by a Chilean health educator and have been produced by the Farm Workers' Health Service.

The first four leaflets in the series are now in print, and will be distributed to health officers and health education directors in California counties where sizeable Spanish-speaking minorities live or work The titles are:

"I am Margarita, and I would like to explain immunization . . ."

"I am Benjamin, and I would like to explain what every child needs to be happy . . ."

"Protect your children by vaccinating your dog . . ."

"Take care of your child's health . . ."

The series is unusual in a number of ways. It is the first such project to be undertaken by the California State Department of Public Health using Spanish as the original language. Its drawings and much of the content were developed by Mrs. Raquel Carmona, a native of Chile with extensive experience in rural health education in that country. And the subjects chosen were not necessarily those deemed most important by health professionals, but rather those which community health aides in California's farm worker projects decided they had been asked about most frequently or found most difficult to explain.

A good case in point is the pamphlet on rabies vaccination for pets. The Farm Workers' Health Service was surprised to learn that community health aides found this the most puzzling of concepts to convey to their clients, and placed the subject first among their priorities for the series.

"In developing the pamphlets," noted the coordinator of the Farm Workers' Health Service, "we tried to understand and use the values of the people we wanted to reach. That's why we started with Spanish. A lot of Americans might not be in agreement with some of the things we say—for example, the leaflet describing what a child needs to be happy. Each culture has different emphases, but we tried to put across what Spanish-speaking people want, and what will have meaning to them. Many translations, she added, "although very good, still retain the cultural frame of reference of the English-speaking majority. And a lot of times these subtle differences can significantly weaken their impact." (Incidentally, the ingredients the brochure listed as essential to a happy childhood were love, protection, harmony in the home, independence, security, discipline, and understanding. Not vividly controversial.)

Lo que todo niño necesita para ser sano.
Amor
El niño necesita del cariño de sus padres tanto como de la alimentación.
Alimentación
1
2
3
4
Para que pueda desarrollar bien su cuerpecito, necesita comer alimentos de los cuatro grupos, todos los dias.
Inmunización vacunas
Las vacunas protegen al niño contra las enfermedades infecciosas como: polio, sarampión tos ferina, etc.
Prevención de accidentes
La vida del niño debe protegerse de los accidentes en la calle y dentro del hogar.
Higiene
La higiene es un factor muy importante en la salud del niño.
Control médico
Para preservar la salud del niño debe llevarse a control médico periodicamente.

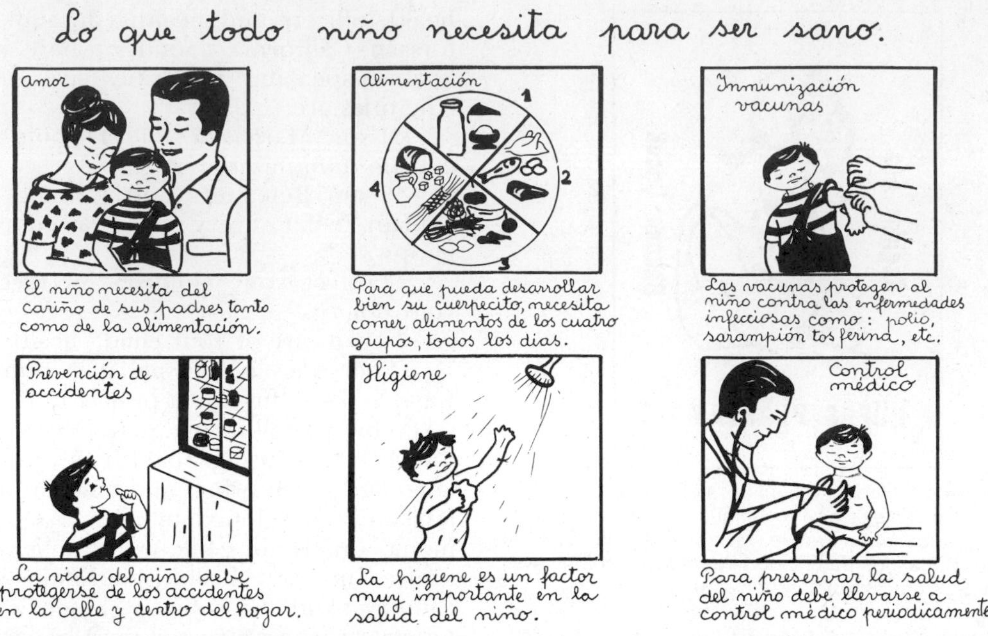

Figure 5–16 (Courtesy of the Farm Workers Health Service, California State Department of Public Health.)

The pamphlets are printed in four colors because color is extremely important to Latin Americans. Moreover, the drawings, the handwritten text, and the approach from a child's point of view all contribute to the booklets' liveliness, vitality, and intimate flavor.

Although they are tailored especially to Mexican culture, the pamphlets, with the help of bilingual staff members of the Farm Workers' Health Service, are also suitable for other Spanish-speaking groups in California, such as the Cubans, the Puerto Ricans, and other Latin Americans. They are, however, aimed primarily at rural dwellers.

Additional brochures are planned in the series, discussing such subjects as dental hygiene, family planning, prenatal care, and healthful living and working conditions in rural areas.

Films

Films are valuable adjuncts to any community health education program. Free 16 mm. films covering all aspects of community health are available from many sources.* The following sources are especially valuable: state and local health departments, county schools office or local college visual-aids departments, state and local voluntary agencies, and the large insurance companies. When a group or agency has embarked upon a definite project with clear-cut objectives for which it needs public understanding, support, or participation, and for which cooperating national or state agencies cannot supply suitable films, the agency may be justified in making its own films.

Nothing destroys the value of a film presentation more quickly than an antiquated film which is patently dated by outmoded wearing apparel, automobiles, buildings, and other scenery, materials, and techniques. To get the most from films, they must be previewed by the educator, introduced to the group, shown, and discussed by the group. Comments and criticisms should be encouraged. Lighting, seating, the condition of the film itself, mechanical smoothness of projection equipment, environment, and room temperature are important factors to consider when presenting a film. Before a film is decided on, the following questions should be raised:

1. Is a film the best medium to accomplish the objectives set for a particular meeting, or would other materials and methods be more suitable?
2. Is a particular film best suited to the pur-

*See appendix for suggested health films.

pose you would like it to serve, e.g., to raise issues as a stimulus to discussion, to present information on a certain subject, or to arouse emotions for action to follow?

3. Has the film been previewed before use?
4. How can you get the most out of it?

After the film has been decided upon, the following questions should be raised:

1. Has the request for the film been confirmed? (Order it at least one month ahead of time.)
2. Have you arranged for an operator who knows how to run the projector efficiently?
3. Is the projector in good working order? Is the sound mechanism working correctly?
4. Is an electric outlet handy? Are there two- or three-pronged adapters? Will an extension cord be needed?
5. Is an extra projection lamp available? Is there an exciter bulb for sound?
6. If the film is to be shown during the day, are there adequate window blinds in the room?
7. Has the screen been set up where it can remain during the whole meeting?
8. Are chairs and tables placed so that they need not be moved for showing?
9. Is the film ready to run when the time comes to use it?
10. Is the film in good condition?
11. Have you run through the entire procedure?

Exhibits and Health Fairs

Combining design, illustration, color, and modern materials with brevity, clarity, and emphasis, the exhibit *can* be a most valuable educational medium. Many exhibits are available on loan from local, state, and federal health agencies. Although there is considerable interest in using exhibits and health fairs to educate the public about health programs and problems, and although many communities have operated successful health fairs, recent studies have indicated that certain types of health fairs may not be worth the time, effort, and money invested in them.

In an effort to evaluate a diabetes fair in Boston, a number of penetrating questions were raised.[39] The major objectives of the fair were to educate and stimulate interest in the public concerning diabetes and its detection, and to stimulate people to go to their family doctors for a urine test and a blood test, if necessary. It is interesting to note that almost half of all persons who attended the

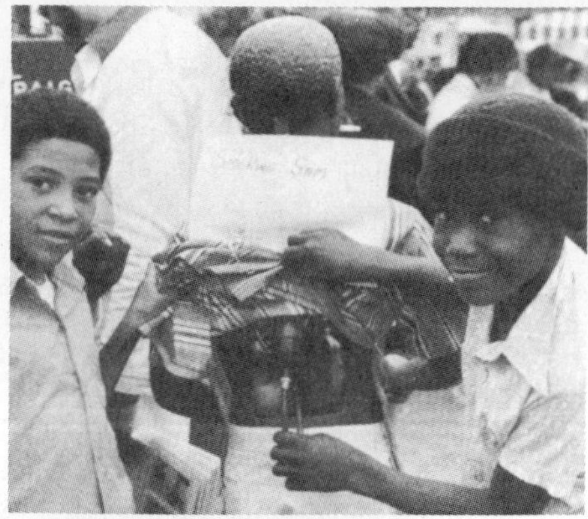

Figure 5–17 "Smoking Sam," an exhibit at a Los Angeles health fair, gives youngsters an inside view of what smoking does to the lung. (From Healthnews, December, 1974, p. 3. California Department of Health, Sacramento, Calif.)

fair credited the newspapers as a chief source of information about the fair, and most of them came to take advantage of the free service. However, an evaluation of 20 exhibits contributed little, if anything, of importance to the education of the viewers. An analysis of some of the individual criteria scores is also illuminating:

Nine of the 20 exhibits were scored 50 per cent or less on item one because the material printed on the exhibits could not be read from the point of observatoin.

Ten of the 20 exhibits were scored 50 per cent or less on item two because the charts, graphs, and other statistical presentations were not readily intelligible.

Eleven of the 20 exhibits were scored 50 per cent or less on item three because the vocabulary and style of writing were not applicable to the majority of the audience.

Thirteen of the 20 exhibits were scored 50 per cent or less on item four because they did not hold the viewer's interest long enough to be read. Obviously, an exhibit cannot be an effective tool unless people look at it long enough to read the message printed on it.[39]

Other difficulties, which all health educators have experienced only too often, included:

1. *Audience.* This consisted mainly of two groups—a larger one composed of older diabetics and members of their families, and a smaller one composed of students. A total of about 150 people were in attendance at the beginning of the talk, but there was much moving in and out throughout the session, causing considerable noise and distraction.

Boston Diabetes Fair
Registration Form (No Signature Required)

Check the appropriate items

1. Age: Under 20 ☐ 20-39 ☐ 40-59 ☐ 60 or over ☐
2. Sex: Male ☐ Female ☐
3. Occupation (please list) ____________
4. Town or City where you live ____________
5. Has diabetes ever been found in any member of your family or in you?
   Yes ☐ No ☐

6(a) Have you ever attended the Boston Diabetes Fair before? Yes ☐ No ☐
(b) If yes, how often? ____________

7. How did you learn about this fair? (Check all those items that apply.)
   Newspaper ☐ Television ☐ From a friend or relative ☐
   Radio ☐ Posters ☐ Other (please specify) ☐
8. What was your chief reason for coming to this fair?

Summary of Evaluation of APHA Exhibits*

Exhibit sponsored by ____________

		Value Not to Exceed	Evaluator's Score
1.	Is it physically possible to read the exhibit from the point of observation?	10	______
2.	Will all graphs, charts, and diagrams be clearly understood by the intended audience? Has the use of statistical presentations been kept to a minimum?	10	______
3.	Is the vocabulary and style of writing used such that the intended audience can comfortably follow and understand the exhibit?	10	______
4.	Does the exhibit sustain interest long enough to read completely?	10	______
5.	Supplementary items (qualified attendant present; visual aid used; visitor-operated devices used and contributing to exhibit; literature supporting the exhibit objectives)	10	______
6(a)	Does the exhibit tie in with the interests of the visitor?	10	______
(b)	Does the exhibit offer the visitor a chance to participate in satisfying a personal purpose?	15	______
7.	Does the exhibit impart the message that it is designed to impart?	25	______
		100 Total	

*Revised October, 1956.

Figure 5–18 Questionnaires used in the evaluation of exhibits at the Boston diabetes fair. (From Young, M. A. C., Kiernan, O., Nangle, G., and Snegireff, L.: Evaluation of a diabetes fair. Amer. J. Publ. Health, *53*:761, 1963.)

2. *Mechanics.*

a. The microphone was out of order during most of the session, and thus it was almost impossible to hear clearly from the rear of the hall where we were sitting. The noise mentioned above added to this auditory difficulty.

b. Since the physician who was answering questions from the audience did not repeat the questions, we heard only his answers, which were not meaningful apart from the questions raised.

c. The film that was to be shown after the talk was not shown because the sound equipment attached to the projector was out of order. Although an effort was made to repair it, after considerable delay the film showing was called off. (By the time the film was about to begin, the majority of the audience had left the hall.)

3. *Content.*

a. The language used by the physician was highly technical much of the time, replete with jargon, initials of various drugs used by diabetic patients, and so on. Our analysis of the responses on the registration form leads us to believe that the material could not have been clearly understood except by those who were directly and intimately involved with diabetes and its treatment.

b. The types of questions raised indicated that those who asked the questions had diagnosed diabetes; in fact, many questions referred to themselves and their condition directly. Therefore, the answers given by the physician were also related to the technical aspects of diabetes and its treatment.[39]

Positive attributes of these talks were the enthusiasm of the physicians, their superlative medical information and knowledge of the subject, and their patience with and understanding of the problems of the participants.

The evaluation committee concluded that the original objectives were not met. The fair did, however, motivate more than 3000 people to have a simple routine urine test made, the results of which were quite "loosely" interpreted, leaving most of those who were screened to form their own opinions of the values and with the procedure and its results. Other suggestions included: make certain that the fair visitors know the significance of the tests before they take them, interpret results properly, making testing arrangements attractive and private, and shorten the time lapse between taking the screening test and the report on results, and follow up. It appears that for a similar sum, a well qualified professional person could be employed to work full time with the cities and towns serviced by the agency, and assist them to organize and operate diabetes detection programs at the local level.

A health fair held in Los Angeles in 1973 turned out to be a great success, as illustrated in Figure 5–19. Teenagers, who paid for entertainment, enthusiastically responded to another interesting and successful health exhibit on venereal diseases set up at a commercial teenage fair in Los Angeles County, California. They took the time to view the exhibit and ask many pertinent questions (Fig. 5–20). A knowledge inventory of 20 questions given to a sample of 1800 exhibit viewers was helpful in gaining an understanding of what teenagers in southern California know about venereal diseases. Forty-two per cent of the participants incorrectly answered questions relating to how syphilis and gonorrhea are acquired, 63 per cent missed questions on symptoms, and 74 per cent missed questions on methods of diagnosis. There was no significant difference between the responses of girls and boys. Ages ranged from 13 to 21, but 71.3 per cent were in the 15- to 19-year-old bracket, the age group in which most of the increase in venereal disease had occurred.[40]

Other Tools of Communication

Culture by Mail. Rheumatic heart disease can be eradicated by adequate control of its precursor, streptococcal infection, through pharyngeal culturing. One method of adequate culturing is the mass mail-in system used in Colorado. Cultures are taken in the physician's office and mailed to central laboratories, where they are processed. Reports of positive cultures are telephoned to the physician, who then institutes adequate therapy and does family contact cultures when indicated. This system requires no equipment or space in the physician's office, and it is readily adaptable to a visiting nurse service, screening programs, and clinics. It is low in cost and offers the advantages of monitoring community prevalence of streptococcal disease. This system has been widely accepted in Colorado by physicians and the public. Data indicate that rheumatic fever has been reduced in areas where culturing is extensive. An essential factor in the rapid growth and acceptance of Colorado's culture program has been the vigorous promotion by the Colorado Heart Association directed toward both physicians and the lay public.

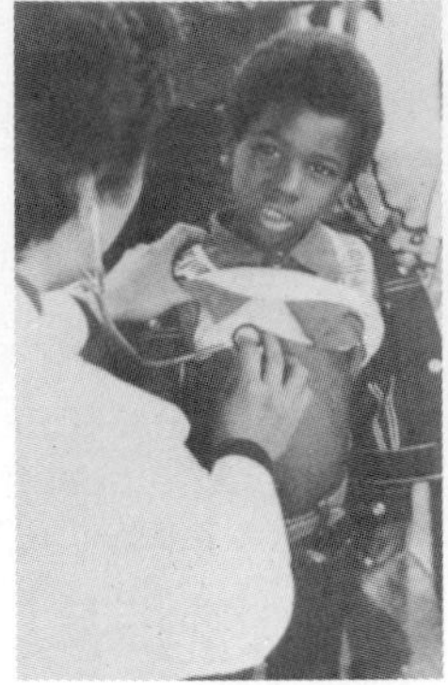

Photos / Ginny Staley

Perhaps the first and most important step in promoting a healthy community is making good preventive health care easily accessible to the people . . . and what better way than to move the clinic out into the street, organize an old-fashioned fair, and invite the public to come. That's exactly what the Central Los Angeles Health Plan did on Saturday, October 16. Between 1,600 and 2,000 people showed up for hot dogs and hematocrits, mariachi music and measles shots, soda pop and sickle cell testing, chest X-rays and rock music. Tiny tots rode merry-go-rounds while their parents learned more about how to protect them from dangerous childhood diseases. Tears that came with life-protecting immunizations were soon erased with snow cones, balloons and cotton candy.

Staying healthy can be fun, when you go to a prepaid health plan fair. During the six hours of festivities the PHP staff gave 500 immunizations, 420 chest X-rays, 800 anemia counts and 150 sickle cell tests. Health education discussions and literature were in abundance and now nearly 2,000 community people know a lot more about prepaid health plans, preventive care and the Central Los Angeles Health Plan.

Prepaid Health Plan Street Fair – A Fun Approach to Community Health

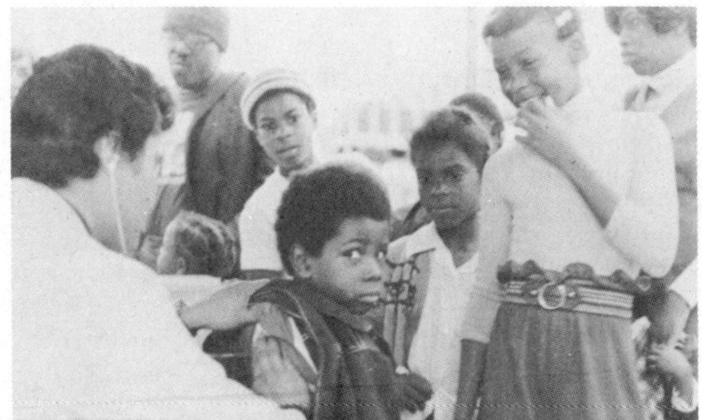

A cold stethoscope doesn't appeal to this young visitor to the PHP Health Fair in Los Angeles. Big sister laughed too soon – she was next in line.

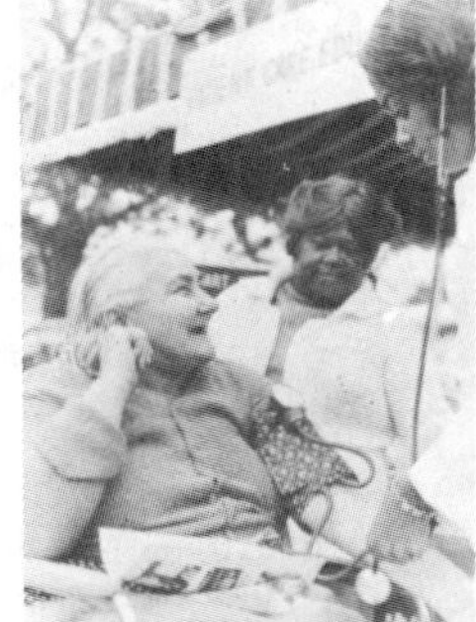

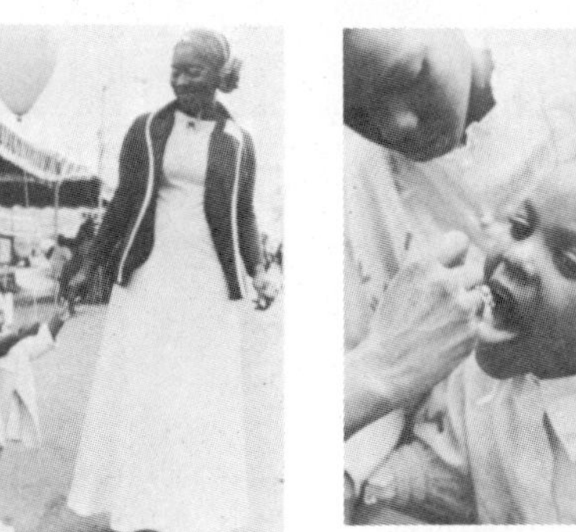

Along with the pleasure of meeting new friends and the satisfaction of getting free medical attention such as the blood pressure test given to a local woman (right), neighborhood residents were also treated to the happy sounds of guitars and Mariachi singers (below) as they strollea from booth to booth down the street.

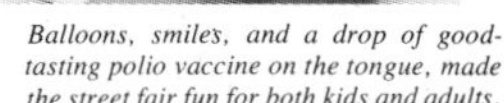

Balloons, smiles, and a drop of good-tasting polio vaccine on the tongue, made the street fair fun for both kids and adults.

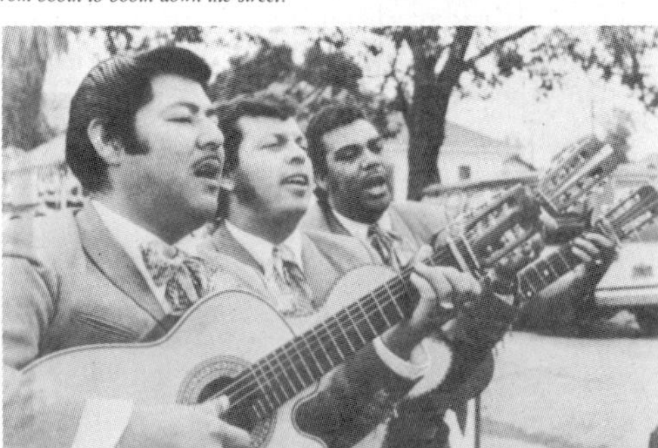

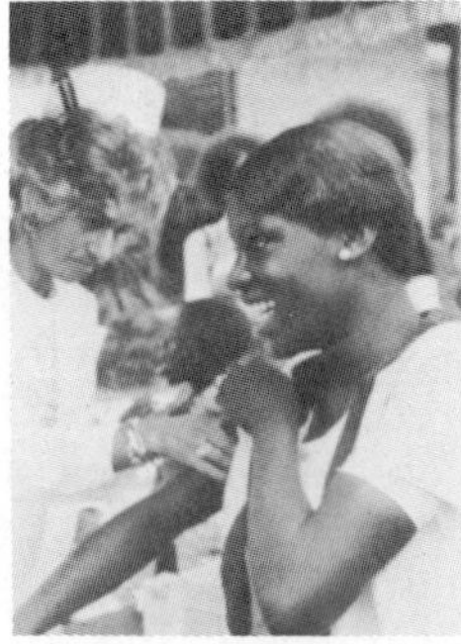

Figure 5–19 A successful health fair held in Los Angeles in October, 1973. (From Healthnews, November, 1973, pp. 7–8. California Department of Health, Sacramento, Calif.)

Questionnaire Used at Exhibit and Percentages of Wrong Answers

How much do you know about venereal diseases?

Statement	% wrong
1. Since syphilis germs can live a long time outside of the body, it is possible to acquire the disease in a variety of ways	42
2. Sores and rashes can always be found on people who have syphilis, therefore people usually know when they are infected	21
3. The symptoms of syphilis will go away even if a person does not have proper medical treatment for the disease	64
4. If a pregnant woman has syphilis, she can transmit the disease to her unborn child if she does not receive treatment soon enough	14
5. Syphilis can be inherited and passed on for generations	41
6. Once a person has syphilis and the disease is cured in the early stage he can never get the disease again	8
7. Some people have syphilis yet may never have any outward signs of the disease	16
8. If syphilis is not found and treated, it may cause blindness, insanity, cripple, or even cause death	9
9. Gonorrhea is often caused by lifting a heavy object (strain)	16
10. If gonorrhea in the female is not found and treated, it may cause sterility (prevent the woman from ever having a baby)	18
11. The symptoms of gonorrhea will go away even though the person is not cured of the disease	62
12. If a person has gonorrhea once and is cured, he will never get it again because he has become immune	15
13. It is possible for a female to have gonorrhea and not know it	19
14. If gonorrhea is not treated, it will turn into syphilis	25
15. Syphilis and gonorrhea are almost always acquired by sexual contact with an infected person	14
16. It is possible for a person to have both syphilis and gonorrhea at the same time	36
17. A blood test can be used to diagnose both gonorrhea and syphilis	74
18. Both syphilis and gonorrhea are frequently acquired by contact with any object an infected person has used such as toilet seats, lipsticks, and towels	42
19. People with syphilis or gonorrhea have a distinctive appearance so that it is possible to tell an infected person just by looking at him	11
20. Both syphilis and gonorrhea can be cured by proper medical treatment	5

Figure 5–20 Questionnaire used at exhibit and percentages of wrong answers. (From Torribio, J. A., and Glass, L. H.: Venereal disease exhibit at teenage fair. Public Health Reports, *80*:4, 1965.)

Tel-Med Tape Library. Tel-Med is a public service of the San Diego (California) Medical Society, in cooperation with other medical and health agencies. The system was developed and pioneered by the San Bernardino County Medical Society. It is a library of over 200 tapes on health and medical information that is available to the general public via telephone. The Tel-Med phones are answered by live operators who also speak Spanish.

The Tel-Med Tape Library is designed to help people remain healthy by giving them preventive health information, by helping them recognize early signs of illness, and by helping them adjust to a serious illness. The tapes are three to seven minutes long, are easy to understand, and have been carefully screened by panels of medical experts. Tel-Med is *not* (and this is important) to be used in an emergency, as a self-diagnosis medium for symptoms of disease, or as a replacement for a family doctor.

The system is a boon to the public and physicians alike. For the public, it offers easy-to-understand messages on health and medicine that the average person may wonder about, but seldom gets to discuss with an expert or is able to read in a booklet or brochure. For the physician, it is a valuable timesaving device; many office hours are saved by having the patient call Tel-Med and get background on his particular problem after diagnosis and during treatment. Or, as a preventive measure, the pediatrician, for example, can advise the parents of his patients to listen to tapes on earache, fever, rheumatic fever, tonsillectomy, and other common childhood diseases.

The system works very simply. The person calls the telephone number and asks for the number of the tape he or she wants to hear. (Brochures listing the tapes are being distributed, or can be obtained from the Medical Society and/or Smoking Research.) The tape discusses the illness or problem, and gives steps to be taken to recognize or prevent it. If callers want the tape repeated or want to hear any other tapes, they simply redial the number and tell the operator.

PROGRAM METHODS AND LEADERSHIP

Program Planning

A good program can be planned by interested group members who consider the needs and interests of all members. Needs and interests may be obtained by various

TABLE 5–2 Community Health Council—Sample Questionnaire

FROM: Program Committee
TO: All Members
SUBJECT: The kind of program you want to have next year. If you would like to help us plan next year's program, please fill out this questionnaire and return it today.

I. *I am most interested in:* — *Specific service, speaker or area.*
- A. Services of voluntary health agencies
- B. Services of local health department
- C. Chronic or communicable disease
- D. School health program
- E. Mental health
- F. Dental health
- G. Drug abuse
- H. Safety education
- I. Environmental sanitation
- J. Maternal and child health
- K. Air pollution—Water pollution
- L. Geriatrics
- M. Suicides
- N. Alcoholism
- O. Women's Health Issues
- P. Health care
- Q. Nutrition
- R. International health
- S. Population issues

II. *Our group needs:*	*Very much*	*Some*	*Not at all*
A. A stronger treasury			
B. More members			
C. More fellowship			
D. More active participation			
E. More significant programs			
F. ________________			

III. The five most important health problems our community faces are:*
1.
2.
3.
4.
5.

* Put a circle around the number of the problem, if any, you think our group can do something about.

methods, including interviews, informal conversations, meeting census, registration cards, suggestion or question boxes, and questionaires. Other considerations in program planning include choosing a topic that is capable of solution and limited in scope. A good program should: (1) start with the interest of members, (2) have a variety of subjects and methods, (3) start and end on time, (4) have a good speaker, film, reading or other needed resource, (5) make provision for fellowship, (6) get members doing things, (7) provide for physical comfort, and (8) add something to each person's life.[41]

Program Methods

A good community health program involves group discussions or an exchange and critical examination of ideas between individuals. Through such participation, the individual adds to his information and has his own contribution evaluated by others. Thus discussion is an important part of the learning process. There are also emotional values that accrue to the individual through his participation in discussion. Discussion, therefore, aids in the personal and social development of individuals. Tensions are relieved

TABLE 5–3 Checklist of Some Program Methods

METHOD	CHIEF CHARACTERISTIC	SPECIAL USEFULNESS	LIMITATIONS
Lecture, film, reading, recitals, etc.	Information giving	Systematic presentation of knowledge	Little opportunity for audience to participate
Forum	Information giving, followed by questions for clarification	Audience can obtain specific information on particular aspects of the subject	Formality; lack of freedom to interchange ideas
Symposium panel or debate	Presentation of different points of view	Issues, approaches, angles spotlighted; analysis stimulated	Personality of speaker may overshadow content; program can be monopolized
Discussion	High degree of group participation	Pooling of ideas, experience and knowledge; arriving at group decisions	Practical with only limited number of people
Project, field trip exhibits, etc.	Investigation of a problem cooperatively	Gives first-hand experience	Requires extra time and energy for planning
Buzz groups	100 per cent participation by large audiences through small clusters of participants	Makes individual discussion, pooling of ideas possible in large groups; develops leadership skill in members	Contributions are not likely to be very deep or well organized.
Group interview	Spontaneous giving of opinions and facts by experts in response to questions	Brings knowledge from a number of sources to bear on one problem	Becomes disorganized without careful planning of material to be covered

through the airing of beliefs and opinions; talking through a problem may have emotional value for all who participate. Suppressed biases and prejudices are brought into the open for examination. Group discussion is a cooperative effort to use facts in the solution of a problem, to test facts proposed in the solution of a problem, to propose alternatives for the solution to a problem, and to present divergent points of view on a problem. Desired outcomes of effective discussion include: (1) increased knowledge or information, (2) increased ability to use knowledge in new situations, (3) increased skill and precision in thinking and in communicating thoughts to others, (4) marked changes in individual interest, (5) more and new rational attitudes, (6) improvement in the social and personal adjustments of individuals, (7) increased awareness and appreciation of the source of materials used in their solution, (8) increased skill in reaching concensus concerning possible action, and (9) directing effective *action* to the attainment of present goals.

The group method is the basic method of democratic socialization, and the framework in which the individual can improve himself as a contributing member of society. The following types of meetings are utilized in group discussions: speaker, symposium, forum, panel, institute, working conference, workshop, group dynamics, role-playing, buzz sessions, and brainstorming. See Table 5–3 for a checklist of program methods.

Leadership in Discussion Groups

Behind every effective discussion group there is usually an able and competent leader. He considers the needs and interests of each member and guides the group toward the achievement of its goals (See Table 5–4). Eventually, the leader becomes a productive group member and actually increases his contribution to the group. He fosters and propels continuous communication between group members in a climate of freedom and mutual respect. Good leaders have many

TABLE 5–4 Group Leader's Outline*

TOPIC: How should children be educated about sex in Midville?
TIME: Sixty-minute panel discussion followed by fifteen minutes of audience participation.

2 min. Preliminary words of welcome to audience by group leader

6 min. I. *The Felt Difficulty*
- A. Statement of problem and why it is important
  - 1. Failure of the home to impart sex education
  - 2. Restrictions placed upon formal education in this regard
  - 3. Increasing incidence of delinquency relating to sex
- B. Introduction of panel members
- C. Definition of terms
  - 1. Sex education
  - 2. What constitutes "children"
- D. Limitation of subject
  - 1. Sex education
  - 2. Of children
  - 3. In Midville

25 min. II. *Analysis of the Problem*
- A. Background
  - 1. Is our problem part of a national one? (scope)
  - 2. When did sex education become a problem here?
- B. How is this problem manifested?
  - 1. Is this problem serious?
  - 2. Who is affected?
- C. Casual factors
  - 1. Why do we have this problem?
    - a. Ignorance of psychological aspects of sex
    - b. Obstacles in the path of dissemination of accurate sex information
      - (1) Social lag
      - (2) Educational lag
  - 2. What are the effects of this problem?
    - a. Promiscuity
    - b. Unwed mothers
    - c. Venereal disease
    - d. Neuroses and mental illness
    - e. Sex crimes and perversion
    - f. Divorce
    - g. Research aimed at solving problem
- D. Goals
  - 1. It is possible to educate children in this regard?
    - a. Children should have sex education commensurate with their mental age
    - b. Information must be scientific and accurate
    - c. The solution should be long range, carefully planned, and efficiently administered

10 min. III. *Finding Possible Solutions*
- 1. In the light of the preceding discussion, what solutions are suggested?
- 2. What solutions have been attempted?

15 min. IV. *Evaluation of Proposed Solutions and Choice of Best Solution*
- A. Will some offered solution meet our present need?
- B. Will it lessen or eliminate the cause of the problem?
- C. Will it work?
- D. Will its advantages outweigh its disadvantages?

V. Applying the Solution [In this discussion presentation there would be no means of evaluating the plan in action inasmuch as it would not have been tried.]

2 min. Concluding summary by chairman

15 min. Forum period

Friends, you have heard our proposed solutions. Have you any questions or can you help us with suggestions?

*(From Wagner, J. A.: *Successful Leadership in Groups and Organizations.* San Francisco, Calif., Howard Chandler, 1959, p. 28.)

qualities in common: (1) they accept all contributions as something to be considered thoughtfully, (2) they are tactful and friendly, (3) they have a good knowledge of the topic being discussed, (4) they have no preconceived notions about where the discussion should go, (5) they take no particular viewpoint in the discussion, (6) they help the group recognize the main issues in the discussion, (7) they see to it that every member of the group gets an opportunity to make a contribution, (8) they prevent the development of bad feelings among members, and (9) they make certain that the group knows what conclusions have been decided.

Good participants prepare for discussion, cooperate with the leader, think before speaking, consider the feelings of others, speak correctly, challenge ideas they cannot accept, and listen.

Group Problem-Solving

What is the actual procedure a group uses for problem solving? Usually it's some variation of the scientific method: gathering the facts, analyzing them, and attempting to come up with solutions. Groups frequently run into difficulty because of role confusion and because the members think they should operate in a democratic fashion. The roles, if they are to function well, should function like this: "the leader is the servant of the group, the group members are the servant of the problem, and the expert is the representative of the problem."

People must be able to express their own ideas freely and to build on each other's ideas, rather than simply defend their own ideas and attack the ideas of other people. Information can be most readily understood and dealt with when the presentation is in visual form, so groups are well advised to use big pads of paper and marking pencils. A good technique is for the leader (after the expert has presented his analysis) to visually divide the statements made into goals and solutions (most group statements fall into one or the other category). Another technique is to separate the good and bad components of each idea. It can often develop that the "one per cent good" component of an idea may contain the nucleus of an original solution to the problem. The leader should also take the responsibility of turning a negative statement or concern into a positive goal, which is of course much easier to deal with. The group must try to generate unusual ideas and desirable goals.

Group Process

The basic assumptions held by most group dynamicists may be summarized by means of the following four propositions:

1. Groups are inevitable and ubiquitous. It is clear to social scientists that conformity is as extreme among such groups of nonconformists as anywhere in society.

2. Groups mobilize powerful forces that produce effects of utmost importance to individuals. A person's very sense of identity is shaped by the groups of significance to him—his family, his church, his profession or occupation. A person's position in a group, moreover, may affect the way others behave toward him and such personal qualities as his level of aspiration and self-esteem. Group membership itself may be a prized possession or an oppressive burden; tragedies of major proportions have resulted from the exclusion of individuals from groups and from enforced membership in groups.

3. Groups may produce both good and bad consequences. The view that groups are completely good and the view that they are completely bad are both based on convincing evidence. The only fault with either is its one-sidedness. An exclusive focus on pathologies or on constructive features leads to a seriously distorted picture of reality.

4. A correct understanding of group dynamics (obtainable from research) permits the possibility that desirable consequences from groups can be deliberately enhanced. Through a knowledge of group dynamics, groups can be made to serve better ends, for knowledge gives power to modify human behavior and social institutions.[42]

Leadership in Community Health Programs

Community organization involves good leadership. Conviction on the part of leaders will cause large groups of people to accept any promulgated idea and will provide a basis for community-wide support and solidarity in relation to the particular program under consideration.

One study indicates that a person may be nominated for leadership in a community if:

1. He belonged to a recognized power clique.
2. He had the will to exercise power and leadership.
3. He had a moderate amount of wealth or property.
4. He had strong relationships with major civic associations.
5. His community residence was satisfactory.
6. He controlled a number of employees.
7. He had control of a corporate enterprise.
8. He was of prime age, or about 50 years old.
9. He was closely allied with major economic or political enterprises.
10. He maintained good press relations.
11. His personal qualities were in conformity to standard community conduct.
12. His social clubs and church affiliations were in conformity with his station in life.
13. He had good interaction with other community leaders.[43]

A man lost in power rating if:

1. He was known to be a follower of another person in such manner or degree that his opinions could not be considered his own.
2. He accepted responsibilities for a community project, and the project failed.
3. He made an unsuccessful bid for public office.
4. His personal qualities were objectionable to top leaders.
5. He was considered a controversial figure by top leaders.
6. He belonged to an ethnic group that did not have the praise of leadership groups.[43]

Although strong leaders are necessary to organize and promote health action groups, other major influencing factors include personal motives such as desire for social prestige, personal gains, or traits of personality. But above and beyond individual concerns, people participate because they feel a sense of loyalty and obligation to the community.

It is interesting and important to note here that there is a lack of consensus among physicians as to their role in community health affairs. Dr. Louis H. Bauer, Past President of the American Medical Association, emphasized the lack of medical leadership in community health affairs:

The medical profession has been so long devoted to its own scientific affairs that until recently it has not been very active in civic affairs. Even now many of the profession pay little attention to what should be an important part of their lives. While physicians must always remain physicians, they are citizens first. One of the reasons why the country has experienced inflation and attempts at socialization and has wandered away from the principles and traditions of true Americanism is that so many citizens, particularly the professional groups, have neglected the duties of citizenship. Physicians ought to interest themselves in the civic affairs of their community. Their failure to do so is one reason why so many other groups have "run off with the ball" in health matters. I have previously stated that physicians should be the leaders in community health councils and activities. We ask our fellow citizens to support us in our activities and problems and yet fail to give the leadership we should. . . .[44]

Physicians, as a group, cannot be classified as community power leaders and policy makers, but like other professional groups, they have recognized delegates who speak for the entire group. Individual practitioners are usually aware of the generalized pattern of community power and authority, even though they may not participate directly in the overall processes of decision making.[43]

SOURCES OF COMMUNITY HEALTH EDUCATION MATERIALS

The best sources of audio-visual aids in health education are the local and state health departments. Other major contributors are the local voluntary health and safety agencies. In order for community health workers to keep well informed and abreast of current local, national, and world health

TABLE 5–5 Suggested List of Periodicals

Name of Periodical	Cost	Where Published
War on Hunger	Free	Department of State, Public Division Agency for International Development Office of Public Affairs Room 4953, State Department Building Washington, D.C., 20523
Morbidity and Mortality: Weekly Report	Free	U.S. Department of Health Education and Welfare Public Health Service Communicable Disease Center Atlanta, Georgia 30337
Public Health Reports	$12.20/year (6 issues)	Superintendent of Documents U.S. Government Printing Office Washington, D.C. 20402
Sex Information and Education Counsel of the United States (Plus other materials and films available from SIECUS: Suite 922 122 East 42nd Street	$9.00/year (bimonthly)	Behavioral Publications 72 Fifth Ave. New York, New York 10011
The Nation's Health (monthly newsletter)	$3.00/year for APHA members; $5.00/year for nonmembers	American Public Health Association 1015 18th St., N.W. Washington, D.C. 20036
Human Organization	$7.00 for students $14.00 for others	Journal of Society for Applied Anthropology 1703 New Hampshire Ave., N.W. Washington, D.C. 20009
American Lung Association Bulletin	Free (10 times/year)	American Lung Association 1240 Broadway New York, New York 10019
Archives of Environmental Health	$25.00/year (monthly)	American Medical Association 535 North Dearborn St. Chicago, Illinois 60610

affairs, they may subscribe to the list of suggested periodicals in Table 5–5.

Pamphlets

Sources of health education materials are infinite: the local health department and the local voluntary health and safety agencies will have most of the current materials available free of charge. However, they may not have the materials from the following agencies available for distribution, since there is usually a small cost involved:*†

*For a more complete list of national sources of health education materials, see How to find what health education materials you're looking for, Amer. J. Publ. Health, *46*:1460, 1956. For a selected list of public health periodicals published in various countries, see Rosen, G.: *A History of Public Health.* New York, MD Publishers, 1958, p. 516.

†Dagger indicates that the agency also supplies films.

Department of Health, Education, and Welfare
United States Public Health Service
Washington, D.C. 20402

National Institutes of Health (publications list)
Bethesda, Maryland

†American Dental Association
222 East Superior St.
Chicago, Illinois 60611

†American Medical Association
535 North Dearborn St.
Chicago, Illinois 60610

National Health Council
1740 Broadway
New York, New York, 10019

†National Safety Council
429 N. Michigan Ave.
Chicago, Illinois

TABLE 5–5 Suggested List of Periodicals *(Continued)*

NAME OF PERIODICAL	COST	WHERE PUBLISHED
The Journal of School Health	$20.00 includes membership (monthly)	American School Health Association Kent, Ohio 44240
American Journal of Public Health	$30.00/year (monthly)	1015 Eighteenth St. N.W. Washington, D.C. 20036
Health Education Report	$12.00/year (6 issues)	Box 728 Ojai, California 03023
The Journal of Social Issues	$9.00/year (quarterly)	Box 1248 Ann Arbor, Michigan 48206
Health Education	$15.00/year (6 issues)	American Alliance for Health, Physical Education and Recreation 1201 16th St., N.W. Washington, D.C. 20036
Family Planning Population Reporter	$18.00/year (monthly)	Alan Guttmacher Institute Planned Parenthood Federation of America 1666 K St., N.W. Washington, D.C. 20006
World Health	$5.00/year (monthly)	World Health Organization (WHO) Ave. Appia 1211 Geneva 27, Switzerland
People	$6.00/year (monthly)	International Planned Parenthood Federation 18–20 Lower Regent St. London, SWIY 4PW England
The Victor-Bostrom Fund Report	Free (4 times/year)	1835 K St., N.W. Washington, D.C. 20006
International Journal of Health Education and Health Education Monographs	$14.50/year (6 issues)	Charles Slack 6900 Grove Rd. Thorofare, New Jersey 08086
Journal of Community Health	$15.00/year (quarterly)	Behavioral Publications 72 5th Ave. New York, New York 10011

Public Affairs Pamphlets
381 Park Ave. South
New York, New York, 10016

American School Health Association
Kent, Ohio 44240

SIECUS (Sex Information and Education Council of the United States)
1855 Broadway
New York, New York 10023

American College Health Association
2807 Central St.
Evanston, Illinois 60201

†American Alliance for Health, Physical Education, and Recreation (AAHPER)
1201 16 St., N.W.
Washington, D.C. 20036

World Health Organization (WHO)
Palais des Nations
Geneva, Switzerland

Mental Health Materials Center
419 Park Ave. South
New York, New York 10016

Spanish Language Health Communication Teaching Aids: a list of printed materials and their sources (free)
Health Services Administration
5600 Fishers Lane
Rockville, Maryland 20852

Spenco Medical Corp
P.O. Box 8113
Waco, Texas 76710
(Charts, take-apart models on health science and family planning)

Films

The best sources of community health education films are the local and state health departments. Individuals may write to these departments for a list of available films. Other major contributors include local schools and voluntary health and safety agencies. A catalogue of many health films that can be borrowed without charge is available from the Pan American Health Organization, 525 23rd St., N.W., Washington, D.C. 20037. See Appendix for list of suggested health films.

For further information, write for:
Guide to Audiovisual Aids for Spanish-Speaking Americans (free)
Health Services Administration
5600 Fishers Lane
Rockville, Maryland 20852

Health Library Catalogue
American Education Films 132 Lasky Drive
Beverly Hills, California 90212

QUESTIONS FOR DISCUSSION

1. In what ways can we motivate people to participate in a community health program?
2. Give three different examples showing how effective communication aided and supported successful community health programs in your community.
3. What community groups are we most concerned with in our health programs?
4. What is the nature and function of a community health council?
5. What are the major qualifications of a superior community health leader?
6. Briefly discuss the major tools of communication available to health educators in disseminating information to the public.
7. Prepare a brief health article for the press.
8. Prepare an educational pamphlet relating to a major health issue for distribution to the public.
9. List five major sources of health education materials in your community.
10. Name five periodicals dealing with community health.
11. "Although health educators have developed many superior and effective promotion techniques, it is very difficult for them to compete with large business." Discuss this sentence.
12. "The fear technique in health education can never be useful in motivating the public." Discuss this comment.
13. List and discuss three methods of evaluating the results of persuasion.
14. List 10 general conclusions we can draw from studies in persuasion.
15. Hypothetically, how can we analyze the difficulty of obtaining individual participation in a public health program?
16. "Motivation in health behavior should be intrinsic, not extrinsic." Briefly comment.
17. Briefly explain how perception and small group dynamics have changed our work in health education.
18. What is meant by "cognitive dissonance"?
19. What type of health advertisement do you feel is most effective? Explain.
20. Briefly discuss motivational research in relation to seat belts.
21. Briefly discuss motivational research in relation to posters.
22. Briefly discuss motivational research in relation to corporation images.
23. "Emotional upheavals are the most effective stimuli for mobilizing public opinion and for generating effective legislation in public

health." Discuss this statement and site examples.

24. Should the professional training of a school health educator include courses in community health? Public health? What are some of the courses offered by schools in your area? What courses would you add to these?
25. What kinds of mass media programs are being conducted in other countries? Site examples.
26. List 10 general rules or principles that promote better communications for better health.
27. What major factors must be considered in preparing a health exhibit?
28. What major factors must be considered in preparing a health fair?
29. What professional organizations are helping to promote community health?
30. Some communities employ a Director for Comprehensive Health Planning. What are his duties?

QUESTIONS FOR REVIEW

1. What are three processes that seem to stand between the availability of facts and a person's behavioral response, according to Suchman?
2. Briefly summarize Hochbaum's and Rosenstock's principles for accomplishing changes in health-related behavior.
3. What is another important principle that should be added to those of Hochbaum and Rosenstock?
4. The general combination of what two factors has been found by studies to cause the success or failure of many public health programs?
5. To what two broad classes of factors did Rosenstock attribute an individual's decision to participate in health programs, in his analysis of a poliomyelitis vaccine campaign?
6. What are three methods of persuasion for health education?
7. List four methods of evaluating the results of persuasion.
8. What are eight motives that are likely to make the public accept preventive health programs?
9. List three fears that could cause the rejection of health programs.
10. What are the three general categories of reasons for the low level of public acceptance of seat belts?
11. Which advertising campaign worked better for the use of seat belts—the professional driver approach or the scare approach?
12. What are the seven C's of communication described by Cutlip and Center?
13. List three reasons why health educators have a hard time competing with the rest of the advertising industry?
14. What is the most economical and effective avenue of contact with the general public?
15. List the chief characteristic, special usefulness, and major limitation of a group interview.
16. What are the best sources of audiovisual aids and films in health education?

REFERENCES

1. *Fourth Yearbook of the Department of the Superintendent of the National Education Association.* Washington, D.C., 1926.
2. Schramm, W.: *Mass Media and National Development, The Role of Information in the Developing Countries.* Stanford, Calif., Stanford University Press, and the United Nations Educational, Scientific and Cultural Organization, 1964.
3. Hochbaum, G. M.: *Basic Concepts of Health Science.* Belmont, Calif., Wadsworth, 1970, pp. 55–58.
4. Suchman, E. A.: *Sociology and the field of Public Health.* Philadelphia, W. F. Fell Co., Russell Sage Foundation, 1963, pp. 86–94.
5. Cornely, P. B., and Bigman, S. K.: *Cultural Considerations in Changing Health Attitudes.* Howard University, Washington, D.C., 1961, pp. 168–169.
6. Rosenstock, I. M., et al.: Why people fail to seek poliomyelitis vaccination. Publ. Health Rep., *74*:98, 1959.
7. Rosenstock, I. M., et al.: *The Impact of Asian Influenza on Community Life.* Washington, D.C., United States Public Health Service, Publication No. 766, Government Printing Office, 1960, p. 75.
8. Berelson, B.: Communication, communication research, and family planning. In the *Emerging Techniques in Population Research.* New York, Proceedings of the 39th Conference on the Milbank Memorial Fund, 1963.
9. Metzner, C. A., and Gurin, G.: *Personal Response and Social Organization in a Health Campaign.* Ann Arbor, University of Michigan, Bureau of Public Health Economics, Research Series No. 9, 1960.
10. Johnson, A. L., et al.: *Epidemiology of Polio Vaccine Acceptance.* Florida State Board of Health, Monograph No. 3, 1962, p. 98.
11. Ibid., p. 42.
12. Ibid., pp. 90–91.
13. Hochbaum, G. M.: *Public Participation in Medical Screening Programs.* United States Public Health Service, Publication No. 572, 1958, p. 1.
14. Metzner, C. A., and Gurin, G.: *Personal Response and Social Organization in a Health Campaign.* Ann Arbor, University of Michigan, Bureau of Public Health Economics, Research Series No. 9, 1960, p. 33.
15. Cornely, P. B., and Bigman, S. K.: *Cultural Considerations in Changing Health Attitudes.* Washington, D.C., Howard University, 1961, p. 169.
16. Clausen, J. A., Seidenfeld, M. A., and Deasy, L. C.: Parent attitudes toward participation of their children in polio vaccine trials. Amer. J. Publ. Health, *44*:1526, 1954.
17. Suchman, E. A.: *Sociology and the Field of Public Health.* Philadelphia, W. F. Fell Co., Russell Sage Foundation, 1963, pp. 86–94
18. Nyswander, D. B.: Modern trends emphasize the individual. California's Health, *22*:74, 1964.

19. Rosenstock, I. M.: *Keys to People: a Report to the Fifty-First Annual Meeting of the Wisconsin Anti-tuberculosis Association.* Milwaukee, Wisc., April, 24, 1959.
20. Hein, F. V.: Bridging the gap between medical discovery and public utilization of that discovery. From *Proceedings of the Health Education Seminar for Extension Specialists.* Chicago, American Medical Association, 1964.
21. Winans, J. A.: *Public Speaking.* New York, Appleton-Century-Crofts, 1917, pp. 209–210.
22. Dubos, R.: The conflict between progress and safety. Arch. Environ. Health, 6:449, 1963.
23. Miller, C. R.: *The Process of Persuasion.* New York, Crown Publishers, 1946, pp. 119–120.
24. Minnick, W. C.: *The Art of Persuasion.* Boston, Houghton Mifflin, 1957, pp. 38–41.
25. Jenkins, C. D.: The semantic differential for health. Int. J. Health Educ., *10*:135, 1967.
26. Schramm, W. (ed.): *The Science of Human Communication.* New York, Basic Books, 1963, pp. 17–27.
27. Festinger, C.: *The Theory of Cognitive Dissonance.* New York, Basic Books, 1963.
28. Brembeck, W. L., and Howell, W. S.: *Persuasion, a Means of Social Control.* Englewood Cliffs, N.J., Prentice-Hall, 1963.
29. Blomgren, G. W., and Scheuneman, T. W.: *Psychological Resistance to Seat Belts.* Research Project RR–115, The Traffic Institute, Evanston, Northwestern University, 1961.
30. Roney, J. G., Jr.: *Public Health for Reluctant Communities.* River Edge, N.J., River Edge Printing Company, 1962, p. 41.
31. Brecher, R., Brecher, E., Herzog, A., Goodman, W., and Walker, G.: *The Consumers Union Report on Smoking and the Public Interest.* Mt. Vernon, N.Y., Consumers Union of U.S., Inc., 1963, p. 165.
32. Hodgdon, L. L.: Psychological and sociological factors in rural change. Paper presented to the 16th general aseembly of the World Medical Association. Bombay, India, November 13, 1962.
33. Schramm, W.: *Mass Media and National Development: the Role of Information in the Developing Countries.* Stanford, Calif., Stanford University Press, and the United Nations Educational, Scientific and Cultural Organization, 1964, pp. 154–158.
34. Wang, V. L.: Health education and family planning in the People's Republic of China. Int. J. Health Ed., Supplement to Vol. 17, No. 2, April–June, 1974, pp. 11, 12.
35. Krieghbaum, H.: *Readers Crave News of Health, Science.* Published and edited by H. Krieghbaum, 1958.
36. Gordon, J.: Health education via television. Publ. Health Rep., *68*:818, 1953.
37. Health television in twelfth year. Publ. Health Rep., *75*:494, 1960.
38. *Texas State Department of Health, Biennial Report, September 1, 1960–August 31, 1962,* p. 16.
39. Young, M. A. C., et al.: Evaluation of a diabetes fair. Am. J. Publ. Health, *53*:761, 1963.
40. Torribio, J. A., and Glass, L. H.: Venereal disease exhibit at teenage fair. Publ. Health Rep., *80*:5, 1965.
41. Knowles, M. S.: Your program planning tool kit, the leader's digest. Adult Leadership, *1*:64, 1952.
42. Cartwright, D., and Zander, A.: *Group Dynamics: Research and Theory.* New York, Harper & Row, 1968.
43. Hunter, F., et al.: *Community Organization: Action and Reaction.* Chapel Hill, University of North Carolina Press, 1956.
44. Bauer, L. H.: The president's page. JAMA, *151*:390, 1953.

SUGGESTED READING

American School Health Association: *Guidelines for the School Nurse in the School Health Program,* 1974.

American School Health Association: *Teaching About Drugs: A Curriculum Guide, K–12* (1975).

Barrett, M.: *Health Education Guide: A Design for Teaching. A Program Continuum for Health Instruction.* 2nd ed. Philadelphia, Lea & Febiger, 1974.

Beisser, A. R., and Green, R.: *Mental Health Consultation and Education.* Palo Alto, Calif., National Press Books, 1972.

Bowers, J. Z., and Purcell, E. F.: *Schools of Public Health: Present and Future.* Josiah Macy, Jr., Foundation, 1974.

Brown, L. R.: *In the Human Interest.* New York, W. W. Norton & Co., 1974.

Chenault, J.: *Human Services Education and Practice: An Organic Model.* New York, Behavioral Publications, 1975.

Chiappa, J., and Gelolo, M.: *A Shortcut to Venereal Disease Education.* Saluda, N.C., Family Life Publications, 1973.

DeCarlo, J. E., and Madon, C. A.: *Innovations in Education in the Seventies: Selected Readings.* New York, Behavioral Publications, 1973.

Drugs are Dangerous; Dangerous to Your Health. Two films available from Public Relations Department, Oxford Films, Los Angeles, California.

Eisner, V., and Callan, L. B., *Dimensions of School Health.* Springfield, Ill., Charles C Thomas, 1974.

Hubbard, C. W.: *Family Planning Education: Parenthood and Social Disease Control.* St. Louis, C. V. Mosby Co., 1973.

Moustakas, C.: *Teaching As Learning.* New York, Ballantine Books, 1975.

Nemir, A., and Schaller, W. E.: *The School Health Program.* Philadelphia, W. B. Saunders Co., 1975.

Nutrition Education Center: *Teach Nutrition with Bulletin Boards.* Montclair State College, Montclair, N.J., 1974.

Oberteuffer, D., et al.: *School Health Education.* 5th ed. New York, Harper & Row, 1972.

Packard, R. C.: *The Hidden Hinge.* New York, Ballantine Books, 1975.

Pavy, R. N., and Metcalfe, J. V.: *The Teacher's and Doctor's Guide to a Practical Approach to Learning Problems.* Springfield, Ill., Charles C Thomas, 1974.

Payne, J. S., et al.: *Education and Rehabilitation Techniques.* New York, Behavioral Publications, 1974.

Rogers, E. M.: *Communication Strategies for Family Planning.* New York, The Free Press, 1973.

Superintendent of Documents: *Continuing Education in Mental Health.* Washington, D.C., U.S. Government Printing Office, 1974.

Uslander, A., et al.: *Their Universe—The Story of a Unique Sex Education for Kids.* New York, Delacorte Press, 1973.

Vacher, C. D., and Stratas, N. E.: *Consultation-Education: Development and Evaluation.* New York, Behavioral Publications, 1975.

Wechsler, H., et al. (eds.): *Social Work Research in Human Services.* New York, Behavioral Publications, 1975.

World Health Organization: *Development of Educational Programmes for the Health Professions.* Public Health Paper No. 52. Geneva, Switzerland, 1973.

CHAPTER 6

Organization and Administration of Official and Voluntary Health Agencies

The constitution, as originally adopted in 1788, made no direct reference to public health. Public health had not become as significant a national need as other more pressing problems, and thus public health became a responsibility of the individual states. Fear of importation of disease prompted state legislatures to draft and adopt minimum health codes and to establish state health departments. These state laws were soon expanded to provide for local ordinances pertaining to community health and sanitation, and this precipitated the birth of county and city health departments.

Public health workers have witnessed rapidly growing, complex health organizations striving to keep pace with rapidly growing, complex societies. Public financial support has been growing steadily with increased understanding of how public health services actually save the taxpayers' money as well as their lives. Unfortunately, many areas still lack the services of a health department. Since public health can move no faster than the public allows, education has always been basic to all public health work. Although the health departments have responsibility for enforcement of a great many laws and regulations, compulsion has never been their most important method of protecting the health of the public. The ultimate responsibility for community health, therefore, rests with the interested people of the community.

LOCAL HEALTH DEPARTMENT ORGANIZATION

Health departments continue to emphasize their two major objectives—preventing disease and prolonging life. The organization of local health departments varies in complexity and in number of staff. Figure 6–1 shows a typical state health department.

The staff, in general, consists of well-trained professional persons. The health officer and his physicians usually hold M.D. degrees plus Masters of Public Health (M.P.H.) and/or Doctors of Public Health (Dr.P.H.). There are also many executive officers who are trained in business administration and have no M.D. degree. Special academic preparation is also required of the public health nurse, public health laboratory technician, dentists, sanitarian, industrial hygienist, statistician, chemist, health educator, social worker, and many others. For recommended qualifications for public health personnel, write to American Public Health Association, 1015 18th St. NW, Washington, D.C. 20036. The following professional schools of public health offer various degrees in the field (as of this printing):

University of California
School of Public Health
Earl Warren Hall
Berkeley, California 94720

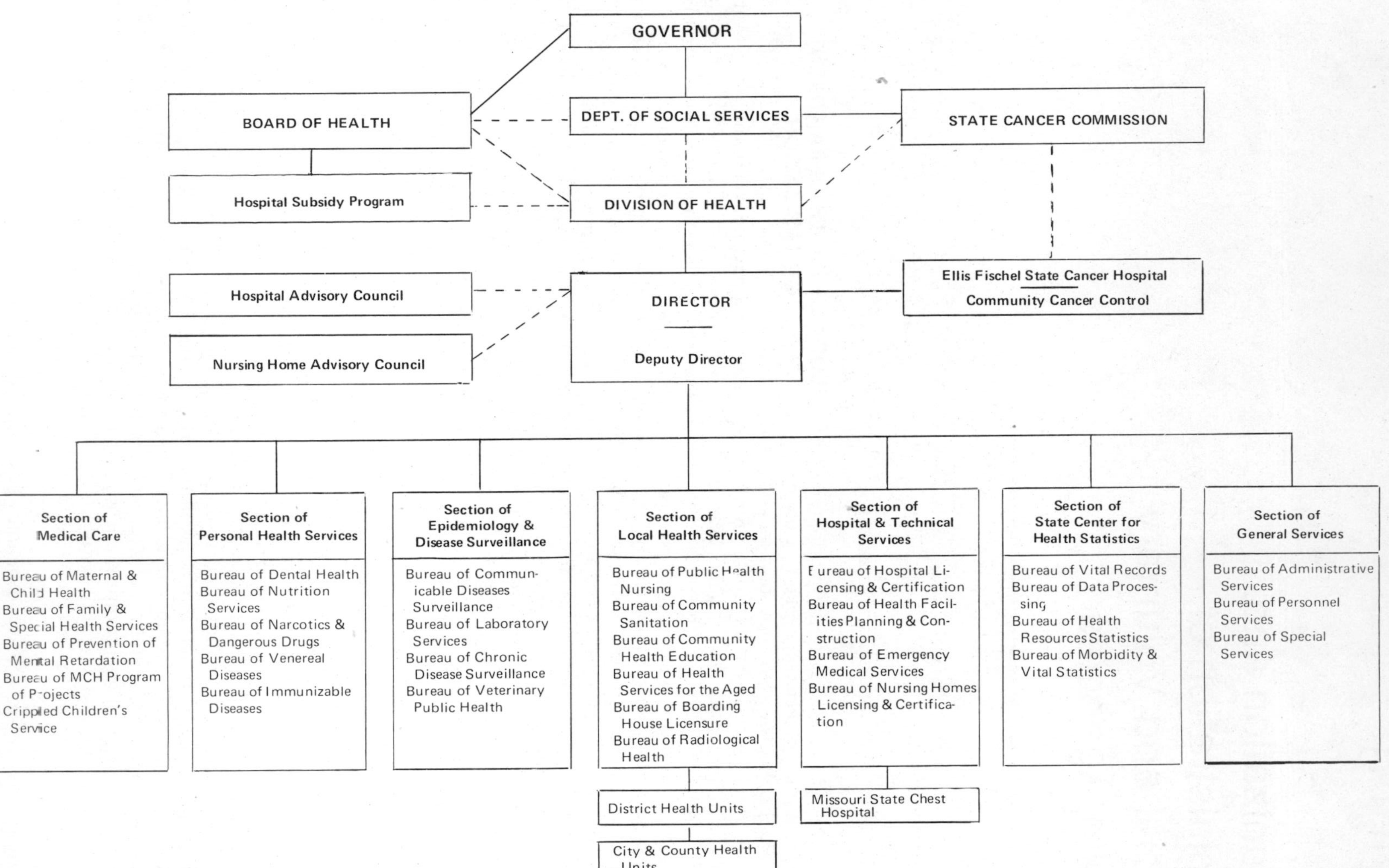

Figure 6–1 Organization of state health department of Missouri.

University of California at Los Angeles School of Public Health
Los Angeles, California 90024

Columbia University
School of Public Health
600 West 168th Street
New York, New York 10032

Harvard University
School of Public Health
55 Shattuck Street
Boston, Massachusetts 02115

University of Hawaii
School of Public Health
1860 East West Road
Honolulu, Hawaii 96822

University of Illinois at the Medical Center
School of Public Health
P.O. Box 6998
Chicago, Illinois 60680

Johns Hopkins University
School of Hygiene and Public Health
615 North Wolfe Street
Baltimore, Maryland 21205

Loma Linda University
School of Public Health
Loma Linda, California 92354

University of Michigan
School of Public Health
Ann Arbor, Michigan 48104

University of Minnesota
School of Public Health
1325 Mayo Memorial Building
Minneapolis, Minnesota 55455

University of North Carolina
School of Public Health
Chapel Hill, North Carolina 27514

University of Oklahoma
College of Health
Health Sciences Center
P.O. Box 26901
Oklahoma City, Oklahoma 73190

University of Pittsburgh
Graduate School of Public Health
Pittsburgh, Pennsylvania 15213

University of Puerto Rico
School of Public Health
Medical Sciences Campus
GPO Box 5067
San Juan, Puerto Rico 00905
(Teaching in Spanish)

University of Texas at Houston
School of Public Health
P.O. Box 21086
Houston, Texas 77025

Tulane University
School of Public Health and Tropical Medicine
1430 Tulane Avenue
New Orleans, Louisiana 70112

University of Washington
School of Public Health and
Community Medicine
F 356d Health Sciences Building
Mail Drop SC-30
Seattle, Washington 98195.

Yale University
Department of Epidemiology and Public Health
School of Medicine
60 College Street
New Haven, Connecticut 06510

California State University at Northridge
Department of Health Science
Northridge, California 91324

Hunter College
Community Health Education Program
Institute for Health Sciences
105 East 106th Street
New York, New York 10029

University of Massachusetts
Department of Public Health
Amherst, Massachusetts 01022

University of Missouri
Division of Community Health Education
M-504 Medical Sciences Building
Columbia, Missouri 65201

New York University
School of Education
Division of Physical Education,
Health and Recreation
Washington Square
New York, New York 10003

San Jose State University
125 S. Seventh Street
San Jose, California 95114

University of Tennessee
College of Education
Knoxville, Tennessee 37916

GENERAL PURPOSE OF AN OFFICIAL HEALTH AGENCY

The Arden House Task Force described the three major areas of responsibility of health agencies as: (1) promotion of personal and community health; (2) maintenance of a healthful environment; and (3) an aggressive attack on disease and disability

Dr. Hugh Leavell, venerable and prestigious public health leader, discussed the basic ingredients necessary for an effective public health program as follows:

The dignity and importance of putting public health into practice;

The need for the kind of team-work that is built on respect for the essential contribution of other professions, and on understanding of their professional strivings;

The real value of group discussion and decision, recognizing that times come when the leader must decide;

The concept of comprehensive health care as a unifying idea to coordinate the work of many and sometimes divergent forces;

The importance of the social sciences in helping the practitioner do a more efficient job, in systematizing knowledge of the community, and in providing research tools and concepts which can add new knowledge;

Health education as the channel which brings to the people the fruits of the laboratory;

Mental health as a key to improved interpersonal relationships and as a support to the weak—and to the strong in their weak moments;

Community diagnosis to discover what our community patient needs, what he wants, and how he may be reached;

International health not only as a fascinating career but also as a bridge for two-way traffic to bring nations together;

The inescapable responsibility of the health officer to view his community as patient, and to be impatient with any who persistently refuse to play their proper roles in the total community health enterprise.[1]

A detailed description of services that should be provided by local health departments has been published as an official statement of the American Public Health Association (APHA)* and a similar statement has been published concerning state health department services.†

The official health agency should furnish primary leadership toward assuring that all community health needs are met. This may be accomplished either through direct provision of services, or indirectly through other official and voluntary agencies and the private sector. The usual pattern is a combination of the two approaches. The components are: promotion of physical and mental health and prevention of disease if possible; if not, then halting the progress of illness, prevention or treatment of the complications or sequelae; and rehabilitation. This is achieved through analysis and improvement of (1) the systems which provide for the delivery of personal and environmental health services; (2) the quality of health services which these systems provide; and (3) the adequacy of resources in these systems for giving quality health services to the entire community.

*The Local Health Department—Services and Responsibilities. Amer. J. Publ. Health, *54*:131, 1964.

†The State Public Health Agency. Amer. J. Publ. Health, *55*:2011, 1965.

General Responsibilities of the Director of an Official Health Agency

The director must increasingly have interest in and concern for all aspects of the community that may affect health in the broadest sense. He should, therefore, participate and provide leadership in such important activities as those listed below, together with representatives of other official and voluntary agencies, appropriate health related interests, and professional groups.

1. Continuous study of the health status of the community as indicated by morbidity and mortality reports of important physical and mental health conditions, medical care and hospital statistics, environmental health data, special health survey data, and all relevant demographic information;

2. Assessment of the community's heatlh resources, including official, voluntary, and private facilities, services, and manpower;

3. Development of clear, measurable objectives of the total health program and of specific program components, and comprehensive health planning on state, regional, and local levels to provide for the most effective use of resources to meet community needs in relation to these goals;

4. Coordination of services and programs in

order to create and maintain the most productive relationships among all suppliers and recipients of service;

5. Encouragement of professional education and community action to provide needed additional or expanded resources. Such activities should involve not only educational institutions and the suppliers of health services, but also the power structure of the community as well as consumers of service;

6. Evaluation of the effectiveness of community health programs by study and interpretation of such aspects as mortality and morbidity trends, the communicable disease control program with special attention to levels of immunity in the population, progress in case finding and disposition of cases so discovered, progress in delivery of personal health services and availability of personal health care, hospital utilization, and environmental control programs;

7. Encouragement of education and research to provide competent manpower, and to develop new knowledge about health problems and how to deal with them. This may be carried out directly by health agencies or in conjunction with universities or research institutions.

8. Promotion of high standards of organization and administration of all personal health service programs in the community.[2]

MISSION OF THE HEALTH DEPARTMENT

The mission of the Health Department is to promote and protect the public health by supplementing the coordinated efforts of all those contributing to personal and community health. This is made possible by appropriations of county funds by the Board of Supervisors, State Health Department subsidy, and allocations of Public Health service funds.

Specifically, the objectives of the department are: first, to gather and disseminate information for the maintenance and improvement of the health of the county's populace; second, to assist in the provision of preventive health services and the control of communicable diseases, by laboratory services for physicians, and by participating in counseling services for parents and others when indicated, regarding medical, emotional, and social problems; third, to maintain and raise standards of environmental sanitation; fourth, to augment or support treatment and rehabilitation services where needs are not otherwise met and health department resources permit.[3]

Health planning goals include high-quality comprehensive health care for all; efficient, effective, and equitable use of facilities, manpower, and other health resources; life-enhancing interactions between man and his environment; a citizenry that carries out healthful living practices; and implementation of planning by constructive action. The ultimate goal is optimum health and well-being for all persons.

RECENT CHANGES IN HEALTH DEPARTMENT ORGANIZATION

Some of the major shifts and changes in direction in health department organization and programs in recent years include the following:

1. Business administrator sharing key responsibilities with health officer (personnel, legal action, budget, complex paper work).
2. Program emphasis from communicable disease control and sanitation to mental health.
3. Integration of health department, social services, and mental health to form Human Resources Agency.
4. Employment of more women in environmental health division.
5. Assignment of health educators in larger departments to specific programs (air, water, mental health, alcohol).
6. Expansion of programs to meet changing needs, including geriatrics, counseling to child-abusing parents, methadone programs, counseling for alcoholics, and "rap" sessions for all ages.

SERVICES OF THE LOCAL HEALTH DEPARTMENTS

The activities of a local health department are varied and interrelated, but they still include the following seven broad categories that are essential: health education, sanitation, disease control, maternal and child health, vital statistics, laboratory facilities, and mental health.

Mental Health Centers

Community mental health centers operate on the belief that the community is responsible for the promotion of mental health and the prevention of mental illness. Many health departments now have an entire facility devoted to mental health activities. Mental health centers vary dramatically in terms of personnel and services. Larger departments may have a combination of persons with different professional backgrounds related to mental health. This multidisciplinary professional staff may include mental health physicians (psychiatrists or other M.D.'s), clinical psychologists, psychiatric social workers, psychiatric nurses, and other specialists to deal with special problems (for example, drug abuse, child abuse, or alcoholism) or to provide rehabilitative services in such areas as occupational therapy or vocational adjustment. Other mental health personnel may include psychiatric technicians, health educators, indigenous nonprofessional mental health community workers, and program clerks.

Centers may provide, either directly or through contract, basic treatment services, including 24-hour care (inpatient services), outpatient services, emergency services, and a program of partial hospitalization (day, evening, night, or weekend care and treatment) for patients able to spend part of their hospitalization periods at home. Many centers have a community services program, which includes consultation, education, and community organization services. Other special programs are developed in response to community needs as a part of the planning process, and implemented as funding may be available, according to established priorities. As programming becomes more decentralized and more responsive to the communities served, there is less uniformity in the internal organizational structure and staffing patterns within individual centers.

Basic services available to many community members include assistance in dealing with problems related to temporary life crisis situations (on a 24-hour basis), prolonged emotional problems, and alcohol or other drug abuse. Some centers also have suicide and crisis telephone services, methadone clinics, play-therapy sessions, individual, family, and group psychotherapy, emergency "mobile" clinics, "rap" sessions, programs for the aged, and occupational and recreational therapy. Short term counseling, treatment, and referral assistance is available in most mental health centers. In the last few years, mental health programs and services have expanded at a rapid rate, in an effort to meet the increasing needs of a drug-oriented, mobile, "stressful" society.

Health Education

The local health department's long-range objectives through education include:

1. A community that accepts responsibility for its health
2. A community informed of its health status, i.e.,
   a. Morbidity and mortality
   b. Individual measures for the prevention and control of health problems
   c. Availability of community facilities and services for the prevention and control of health problems
   d. The program and services of the health department
3. A community participating in coordinated planning and programming for:
   a. Appraisal of community facilities and services
   b. Utilization of existing community facilities and services
   c. Provision of additional needed community facilities and services.
4. A community composed of individuals motivated to observe the personal practices conducive to physical, mental and emotional health.

The health education division is the focal point of the wide variety of educational programs carried out by the health department in an effort to accomplish the educational objectives. The division assists in the educational work of the department; provides educational materials; disseminates reliable health information to the public through newspaper, radio and television; advises on the use of educational methods pertinent to public health programs; and assists in community health education programs sponsored by the department or other community agency. Educational materials not available from other sources are prepared or assembled in the health education workshop. These include films, slides, exhibits, pamphlets, posters and other teaching aids for use in conjunction with the education programs carried out in schools, homes, industries, communites and professional groups.

Health education is stressed by each member of a local health department in an effort to prevent disease. For example, the sanitation division of most local health departments conducts training classes regarding the proper handling of food. Upon completion of this course by restaurant employers and employees, each class member receives a card that recognizes his training.

HEALTH SERVICES AVAILABLE AT ONE LOCAL HEALTH CENTER

Services	*Description*
Advice on health problems	A public health nurse (on call), to answer health questions
Childbirth and baby care classes	For teenage mothers 12–19 years
Child health conferences	Immunizations, examinations, and medical advice for children 6 weeks to 5 years
Dental clinic	Emergency and consultation service only for children 3–18 years
Screening for diabetes, glaucoma; Pap test	Over age 30, or over 21 with a history of diabetes in family, or referral by a private M.D.
Family planning clinic	Education and birth control methods for women
Immunization clinic	Immunization for adults and children over 2 years (parents must accompany child); Diphtheria-pertussis-tetanus, polio, measles, rubella (under 12 years), smallpox, tuberculin skin test
Validations ($1.00 or more)	For international travel
Mental health	Psychiatric counseling, alcoholic clinic, suicide prevention clinic; methadone clinic
Minifilm chest x-ray	Open to anyone 15 years or older
Mistogen	Test to obtain sputum sample, private M.D. referral only
Mother baby care classes	Special classes for expectant parents
Pregnancy testing and counseling	Pregnancy testing arranged for anyone, with special counseling available for unwanted or teenage pregnancy
Sickle cell anemia screening	Open to anyone
Youth clinic	Young people
VD clinic	Open to anyone
Geriatrics center	Problems associated with aging

Recording of Vital Statistics

Two major services, vital registration and statistical tabulation and analysis, are performed by local health departments. All births and deaths occurring in the health department jurisdiction are registered and routed to the county recorder and state health department. The statistics division also receives records and tabulates reports of communicable diseases. From records of such vital events, analyses are made of trends and changes in the overall public health situation. With this information, the health department is able to measure progress and to plan its work efficiently and realistically. Although all states have adopted regulations relating to the immediate reporting of certain communicable diseases to the health department, it is quite evident that this is not the case in most situations; therefore, local and state statistics are only as reliable as the reporting person or agency. The statistics division also records health department activities, issues certified copies of births and deaths, and keeps private physicians and the public informed of changes in the health status.

Disease Control

Immunization, sanitation, and *health education* are key words in disease control. Immunizations against diphtheria tetanus, pertussis, measles, German measles, mumps, poliomyelitis, and smallpox are given to preschool and school-age children who have not been immunized by their family physician. These immunizations are recorded in the student's cumulative health record.

Sanitarians work for the suppression of disease transmission by controlling potential sources of disease through the regular supervision of food establishments, water and milk supplies, sewage disposal systems, and insect and vector control.

The health department provides both treatment and education in its venereal disease clinic. Visits include those people who have been referred to the clinic by their family physicians and others who come voluntarily for diagnosis or treatment. Contacts of venereal disease patients are investigated to prevent further spread of the disease. Premarital and prenatal examinations are also available.

Community protection against tuberculosis is accomplished by case finding, referral to diagnostic and treatment services, and nursing supervision of cases and contacts. Records of all known cases of tuberculosis within the county are recorded and filed in the Tuberculosis Case Registry, which is the key to the control program. The registry is used by private physicians, the lung association, local sanitarians, and public health nurses to coordinate case findings, treatment, and home care of patients.

The eradication of disease and the prevention of illness require continual surveillance. The program is facilitated by the cooperation of private physicians, medical and health agencies, and laymen who are informed and interested.

The program for the diagnosis, control, and prevention of communicable diseases is supported by: (1) epidemiological investigations, surveillance, and consultation to the private physician, (2) services of the public health laboratory for identification of communicable disease by morphological, biochemical, cultures, and serological techniques, (3) services of environmental health, (4) control over public milk supply, with inspection and control of milk, dairy products, milk handlers, and processing plants, (5) home visiting and individual consultation by public health nurses, (6) morbidity reporting and statistical analysis, (7) regular publication to physicians, (8) alerting physicians and individuals concerning unusual outbreaks of serious disease, (9) providing appropriate information to the general public, (10) immunization against preventable diseases, (11) immunizations for foreign travel, (12) provision of international certificate of vaccination booklets for persons traveling to foreign countries, (13) smallpox vaccinations, and (14) yellow fever immunization.

The chronic disease control program provides multiphasic screening services, including special projects for diabetes, cancer, glaucoma, chest diseases, and cardiovascular diseases. The program works in conjunction with mental health programs, and assists in the development of neighborhood health clinics.

PUBLIC HEALTH NURSING

The field of public health deals with three major factors: population, environment, and agents of disease. Change produced by this interaction gives rise to social uncertainty, uncontrolled environment, multiple health needs, shifts in public behavior and values, and continual change in priorities for service. Therefore, the expert community health nurse needs to develop a high degree of ability (1) to make individualized, practical, independent, judgments that are firmly rooted in relevant theories and concepts, (2) to integrate her perceptions of health needs with those of the family and of the community in determining alternate courses of action, (3) to consider the community the primary focus in working with the many direct contacts and complex interrelationships of communities, families, and public health and other community workers, (4) to apply knowledge in effecting meaningful communication and in motivating families and communities to utilize protective health practices and services, and (5) to evaluate and utilize herself and the contributions of other health workers in effecting community health.

The philosophy of community health nursing is that of service to the total family. The goal is to help the family to help themselves in solving their own problems, with respect for the individuals' right to make the final decision. Contact is mainly in the home, where family interaction can be more easily assessed.

Organization and Administration

The purpose of community health nursing is to further community health through the selective application of nursing and public health measures with the framework of the total community health effort. In the local health system, community health nurses may be expected to function in many difficult organizations and structures. The Division of Community Health Nursing Practice of the American Nurses' Association endorses the following definitions:

> Community health nursing practice is a field of nursing practice for which there exists a body of knowledge and related skills which is applied in meeting the health needs of communities and of individuals and families in their normal environments such as the home, the school, and the place of work. It is an area of practice which lies primarily outside the therapeutic institution.

A statement developed by the Canadian Public Health Association defines the philosophy of public health nursing in the following terms:

> Public health nursing is professional nursing that focuses its attention, through organized community effort, on serving people in their usual environments of home, school, and work. As one part of the community's total arrangement for health promotion, public health nursing is concerned with well people and with the sick and disabled. It strives to prevent disease or to retard its progress; to reduce the ill effects of unavoidable disease; to provide skilled nursing care for the non-hospitalized sick and handicapped; to support those facing crisis situations; and the community as a whole for the development and practice of habits conducive to health.

Thus community health nursing may be said to represent elements of both nursing and public health practice.

A community health nurse may function in many areas, some of which are listed here:

A. Official agencies (tax-supported)
   1. Public health (state, county, city)
   2. Veterans' hospitals
   3. Schools—active role in child health, as well as being counselor and educator
   4. Social work or welfare agencies

B. Non-official agencies
   1. Visiting Nurse Associations (liaison nurse in hospitals to analyze for home care)
   2. Industry—preventive aspects as well as treatment
   3. Mental health centers
   4. Suicide prevention
   5. Alcoholic rehabilitation
   6. Drug abuse centers
   7. Speech centers
   8. Consultants to nursing homes
   9. Adoption agencies
   10. Children's centers
   11. Hearing clinics

C. In doctors' offices as an extended care person

The activities of the public health nurse include educational and demonstrational work in the home, the clinic, the school, industry, and community health centers. Emphasis is always placed upon the prevention of disease, the promotion of health, and rehabilitation of patients. A few specific services include the following:

Family Spacing. Counseling in various contraceptive methods and make appropriate referrals.

Prenatal Counseling. Provided to referrals of private physicians and County Hospital clients, on diet, general hygiene, and preparation for the infant. Injections given as ordered.

Postnatal Care. Assistance in interpreting and following the doctor's order in the home.

Premature Infant Care. Before a premature infant goes home from the hospital, the nurse visits the home to counsel the mother and to determine whether the environment is safe.

Infant and Preschool. Follow up on phenylketonuria-positive infants until negative test results are obtained or condition is under treatment. Continued follow up if disease is identified.

Counseling. Physical appraisal, diet and immunizations counseling, anticipatory guidance in growth and development, and advice on accident prevention are provided to those born at County Hospital and to those referred by a private doctor.

Preparation for School. Vision testing, hearing testing when indicated, preschool physical, and anticipatory guidance; prevention of child abuse.

Crippled Children Services. Interpreting the meaning of condition to child and family; interpreting the importance of care as necessary.

Child Development Clinic. Diagnosis, recommendations and follow-up by multidisciplinary specialists when mental retardation or other mental health problems are suspected.

Schools. Vision, hearing, and dental screening, referral for care when conditions are identified, physical examinations and immunizations when they cannot be provided by a private physician.

Communicable Disease. Instructions given to the family on adequate isolation, immunization, how to obtain necessary laboratory specimens. Taking epidemiological histories in order to complete follow-up.

Venereal Disease. Urging prenatal patients to have adequate follow-up care when indicated by previous blood test. Interviewing teenagers at the request of private physicians.

Tuberculosis. Giving injections when ordered by private physician. Making a plan for tuberculosis skin testing, x-rays of contacts, sputum and gastric specimens from the patient. For case finding purposes, referring clients to the proper resource when indicated.

Home Health Agency. Bedside nursing for the sick at home by Registered Nurses and Home Health Aides.

ENVIRONMENTAL HEALTH

This division is responsible for the elimination or reduction of hazards in the environment by applying principles of education and law enforcement combined with practical and technical measures.

Sanitation Bureaus

1. Bureau of General Environmental Sanitation is responsible for the supervision of the following environmental factors: housing, solid waste disposal, liquid waste disposal (industrial and sewage), water pollution control, swimming pools, water supplies, insect and rodent vector control, recreational sanitation, food, food service worker training, and general sanitation of environment. Periodic supervision and consultation to operators of food establishments require a great amount of the sanitarian's time. Guidance and education of the operators have replaced reprisals and legal action in the vast majority of instances.

2. Bureau of Milk and Dairy Services has the responsibility to insure that milk and dairy products are safe and free from milkborne disease through routine surveillance of establishments to observe that they have clean and healthy environment where milk is produced and handled, clean and healthy milking animals, clean and healthy personnel in milk plants and dairies, and clean and sterile milk handling equipment and procedures.

3. Bureau of Sanitary Engineering is responsible for surveillance of domestic water systems for the purpose of issuing permits to purvey water and of water pollution control plants to assure protection of the environment. Consults and assists with review of subdivision sewage disposal and domestic water systems and related engineering aspects.

4. Bureau of Housing is responsible for the assurance that housing for all citizens provides a safe and healthful environment; routinely conducts maintenance, sanitation, ventilation, and use and occupancy inspections of motels, hotels, apartments, mobile home parks, resorts, and organized camps.

5. Bureau of Vector Control is responsible for the suppression of insects and animals which adversely affect public health. It does this by environmental conservation measures, appropriate chemical and biological control, consultation, and dissemination of information.

6. Bureau of Industrial Hygiene or Occupational Health routinely inspects the working environment and investigates occupational disease reports to observe the presence of occupational health hazards; consults and advises industry as to the prevention and control of industrial hygiene hazards.

7. Bureau of Animal Control is responsible for control of diseases transmitted from animals to man. The program includes the isolation of known or suspected rabid dogs, control of stray animals, investigation of animal bite cases, and isolation of known or suspected rabid animals.

General Responsibilities of the Sanitarian

The sanitarian enforces laws and regulations providing for the protection of public health. In this connection, he investigates sanitary conditions in food processing and serving establishments, water systems, sewage and garbage disposal systems, inhabited structures such as hotels and apartments, industrial plants, laundries, beauty shops, and even pet shops, kennels, and stables.

Public health sanitarians aim to provide long-range protection from all known environmental health hazards. They also protect individuals from the day-to-day possibility of encountering food poisoning in an ill-kept restaurant, or of contracting diseases from water or milk. This is one of the most essential of all jobs, although it is seldom publicized, for it provides all citizens with better living conditions than were available to even the richest and most powerful members of earlier societies.

Public health sanitarians are responsible for the maintenance of acceptable standards of sanitary conditons for entire communities. They may also be called sanitary inspectors, public health inspectors, or food and environmental health inspectors.

While education and persuasion are

usually effective in ensuring that health standards are maintained, there are individuals who persist in violating sanitation laws. Elaborate, time consuming, and often ineffective measures must be resorted to while a clear hazard to the public's health may continue unabated. Certain counties issue citations when (1) there is a condition of immediate hazard to the public health, (2) reasonable persuasive methods have been exhausted, or (3) there is a well-documented case with prior notification given.

Duties

The major part of a sanitarian's time is spent in investigations. He makes routine inspections of establishments open to the public to ensure that they maintain required standards, and he investigates complaints regarding either public places or private dwellings. About one-quarter of his work is concerned with food control. He inspects food processing and serving establishments, such as bakeries, slaughter houses, restaurants, retail and wholesale food markets, and all food-carrying vehicles.

Sources of Information

Your Career in Public Health
State of California
Department of Public Health
Sacramento, California

National Association of Sanitarians
1550 Lincoln Street
Denver, Colorado 80203

International Association of Milk, Food,
and Environmental Sanitarians
Blue Ridge Road, P.O. Box 437
Shelbyville, Indiana 46176

*Related Occupational Guides**

Biological Scientist, Health Physicist, Medical Technologist-Bioanalyst, Plant Scientist, Plant Pathologist, Plant Quarantine Inspector, County Agriculture Inspector, Public Health Nurse.

*Write to your state health department or comprehensive health planning office for your county for copies.

LABORATORY SERVICES

The facilities of the public health laboratory (see Fig. 6–2) are used by private physicians and health department personnel to assist them in diagnosing, treating, and controlling communicable diseases.

Professional services include the following:

1. Microbiology laboratory for microbiological examinations for the detection and identification of infectious and communicable microbial agents, parasites, and rabies.
2. Serology laboratory for qualitative and quantitative serological tests for syphilis, diagnostic agglutination tests, and routine hematology and urinalysis procedures on county preemployment physical examinations.
3. Tuberculosis and mycology laboratory for diagnostic and determinative mycology and mycobacteriology and for testing tubercle bacilli for susceptibility to various drugs.
4. Sanitation laboratory for routine analysis of milk, water, and sewage and for bacteriological examination of utensils used in restaurants.
5. Veterinary services in accordance with funds and personnel available.
6. Information services to inform students, community leaders, physicians, nurses, sanitarians, laboratory technologists, and allied medical personnel of laboratory objectives, functions, services, and so on.
7. Training (a period of instruction to selected college graduates for certification as a Public Health Microbiologist).

CRIPPLED CHILDREN SERVICES

The Crippled Children Services Programs are state-wide programs administered by the State Department of Public Health in most states. These programs, established by state law for the purpose of providing corrective treatment to children with certain types of physically handicapping conditions, are organized and financed by cooperative effort of the federal and state health and welfare agencies. The Crippled Children Services Program provides a wide range of medical services, including expert diagnosis, medical and surgical treatment, hospital care, physical and occupational therapy, and the necessary appliances and special materials. For the purpose of the program, a physically handicapped child is defined as a person under the age of 21 with certain physical defects resulting from congenital anomalies,

The Quintessence of Quality is the Skill of People

The quality of diagnostic laboratory services available from the Berkeley laboratories of the state Department of Health directly reflects the quality of the many dedicated researchers and technicians who contribute to the health and welfare of the individual Californian.

Many of the procedures by which infectious disease agents, adulterants of food and drugs and specific pollutants of air and water are identified can be carried out in local laboratories. However, certain techniques are so complex and require such specialized equipment that they must be performed by the highly trained staff of the Berkeley laboratories.

These laboratories provide reference and analytical services to other laboratories throughout the state. They influence, in a supportive as well as a regulatory manner, the compliance of all laboratories with standards which assure delivery of reliable health-related testing services to Californians.

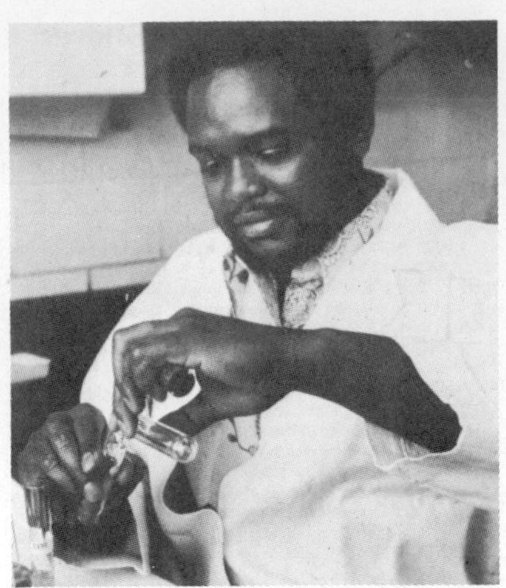

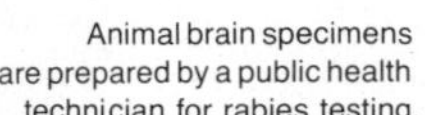

Animal brain specimens are prepared by a public health technician for rabies testing.

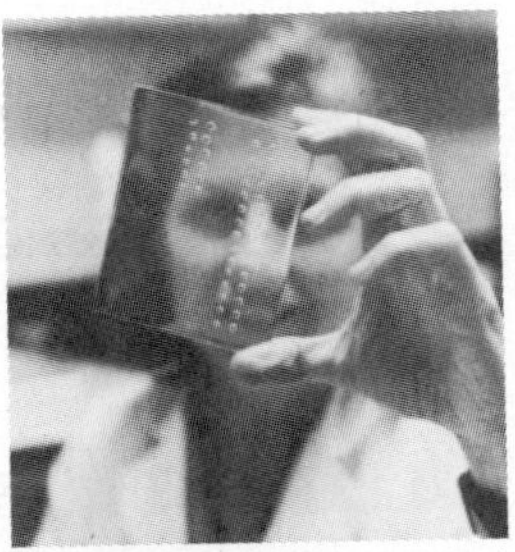

In the virus lab human serum samples are tested for hepatitis.

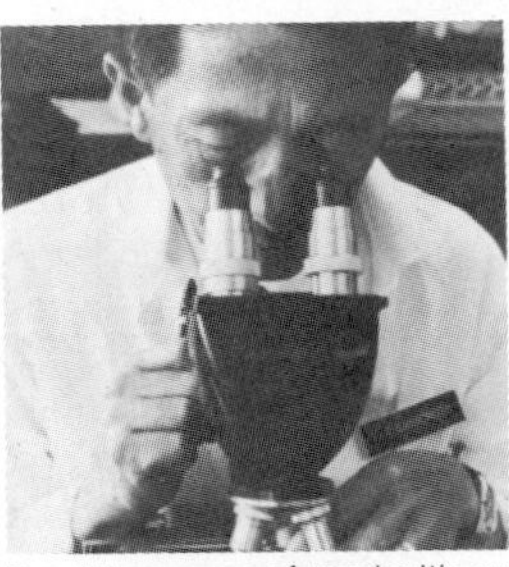

Possible causes of meningitis are investigated by examination.

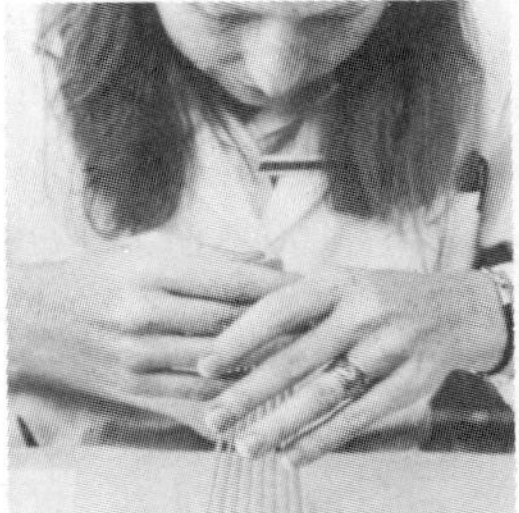

Microbiologist in the virus lab performs rubella tests on a baby's blood.

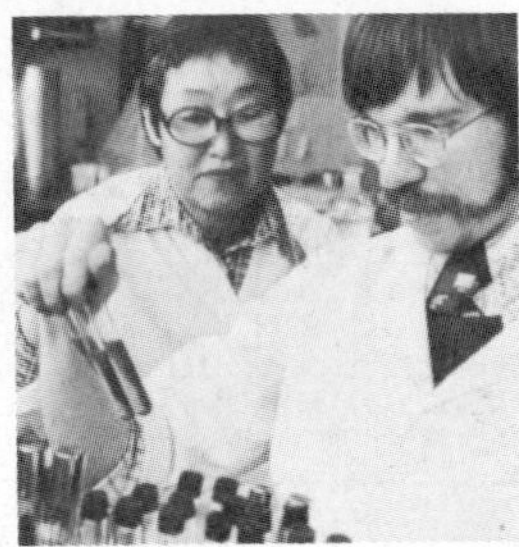

In the microlab bacterial cultures are read for identification.

Figure 6–2 State laboratory services available in California. (From Healthnews, August, 1973, p. 5. California Department of Health, Sacramento, Calif.)

or acquired through disease, accident, or faulty development.* At the state level, the Crippled Children Services Program is generally administered by the State Department of Public Health through its Bureau of Crippled Children Services. The program is administered locally by county health departments or county welfare departments. The medical aspects of each child's condition and the financial status of his family are factors in determining whether a child is eligible for care under the program. Certain exceptions are provided in cerebral palsy for the purpose of efficient administration.

In general, the program provides treatment services for the child whose physical defects are disabling and can be either corrected or arrested. The following categories of conditions are eligible for care:

1. Defects of an orthopedic nature due to infection, injury, or congenital malformation. Examples include clubfoot, poliomyelitic paralysis, or cerebral palsy.
2. Defects requiring plastic reconstruction. Examples include cleft palate and lip, contractures, or disfigurement due to burns.
3. Defects requiring orthodontic reconstruction. These include dental-facial deformities accompanying cleft palate.
4. Eye conditions leading to a loss of vision, such as cataract or strabismus, not ordinary refractive errors.
5. Ear conditions leading to a loss of hearing—chronic otitis media, chronic blockage of eustachian tubes, or congenital deafness.
6. Rheumatic or congenital heart disease.
7. Other disabling or disfiguring deformities, such as extrophy of the bladder or severe hemangiomas.
8. Brain damage.

The Crippled Children Services Program is financed by tax funds from county, state, and federal sources, and by repayments from families who can afford to pay a portion of the cost.

*Epilepsy and cerebral palsy programs are an integral part of the total program in many states.

PUBLIC HEALTH SOCIAL WORK

Help is given to patients through clinics and conferences, enabling them to deal more adequately with psychosocial and socioeconomic problems, upon referral by physician. Individuals with health and social problems are guided to appropriate community services. Liaison social work is conducted between the health department and other social agencies whose clients are also health department patients.

Consultation

The social worker provides consultation to staff, individuals, and groups on the biological, psychological and sociological aspects of human behavior. The goals are more effective handling of pathological situations.

The community organization method is employed by the public health social worker in the exploration, expansion, and creation of services to meet health needs. Services are needed when potentially hazardous situations exist and pose threats to significant numbers of people.

PUBLIC HEALTH SOCIAL WORK[4]

Social workers are becoming increasingly important as members of health departments. The South Carolina State Health Department describes its program as follows: *Function:* To identify and modify social, psychological, and environmental factors which contribute to health problems of individuals and families or influence their maximum use of health and medical services provided by the Agency.

Significant Activities: The total number of social workers employed by the Agency is 41:

Master's degree – 32
Baccalaureate degree – 9

The social worker functions as a member of a multidiscipline health team in program planning and implementation. Social work services are provided to individuals and families through clinic and hospital structures, home visits, interagency conferences and referrals, and participation in related community activities, i.e., advisory groups, planning councils, and various committees.

A major effort is being made to develop an effective recording and reporting system of social work activities.

The following activities were reported:

Direct services cases	11,931	Assessment and diagnostic interviews	11,342
Home visits	1,582	Referrals to community resources	2,375
Consultations	1,842		
In-service training	356		

COORDINATION CENTER FOR THE RETARDED AND HANDICAPPED

Many health departments are establishing coordinating centers for the retarded and handicapped. Such centers develop communication between individuals and agencies. Maximum service with a minimum of time and expense can be provided by avoiding duplication and gaps in services.

Information is given to groups, professionals and families regarding aids and facilities. Guidance and support are provided to families. Community education through groups is provided by literature, films, and speakers. Those concerned are alerted to new courses, legislation, services, facilities, and materials. Communities are aided in assessing needs, determining priorities, and developing new services for employment, diagnosis, recreation, and supervised care.

NUTRITION SERVICES

Nutrition services are promoted by the entire staff through consultation to agency personnel and to personnel of other health and welfare agencies, medical and dietetic nutritional consultation, and studies to determine needs and resources. The staff tries to improve food habits by demonstrating educational methods to teachers, nurses, and welfare workers. It also provides leadership in the development of community nutrition programs. Some larger departments have nutritionists on their staff.

THE PRIVATE PHYSICIAN AND COMMUNITY HEALTH

Private physicians are urged to promote community health. They can do this in the following ways:

1. Promptly reporting births, fetal deaths, and other deaths.
2. Promptly reporting communicable and other diseases, reporting first by telephone, with confirmation later in writing for the following conditions: botulism, diarrhea of the newborn, diphtheria, dysentery, food poisoning, meningitis, poliomyelitis, paratyphoid, plaque, psittacosis, rabies (human or animal), smallpox, typhoid, and thyphus.
3. Reporting diarrheal and streptococcal infections, including scarlet fever, in food service and dairy workers. This should be done immediately by telephone. Morbidity Report Cards and a list of reportable diseases and conditions may be secured from the nearest health center of a county health department.
4. Promptly reporting tuberculosis: report all positive results of chest x-rays; submit information regarding contacts. Refer for follow-up when necessary.
5. Reporting venereal disease patients who have lasped from treatment. Training epidemiologists from the local health department are available to assist the doctor in follow-up and in bringing to treatment the source and spread of these infections.
6. Promptly reporting by telephone all cases of communicable disease in the homes of persons employed as food handlers or school teachers.
7. Explaining to underprivileged communicable disease patients the service of the health department in such cases, if laboratory examinations, medicine, or diagnostic services are available without charge.
8. Verifying that patients have been immunized against diphtheria, tetanus, pertussis, poliomyelitis, and smallpox.
9. Prompt administration of diphtheria antitoxin if indicated, rather than waiting for the laboratory report.
10. Promptly reporting all persons bitten by animals or a species subject to rabies.
11. Relaying information relating to occupational health hazards which will contribute to the prevention and control of occupational diseases.
12. Cooperating with public health officials in all measures to promote community health.

Cooperation

The professional cooperation of the physician is indispensable in the implementing of community public health programs. The accuracy of local morbidity reports and the appraisal of health needs within a community depend on the prompt and accurate flow of disease reports, especially communicable disease reports, received from private physicians.

If requested to do so, a representative from the Department of Health will meet with any local medical society to explain reporting procedures as well as laboratory, consultative, and other departmental services offered to private physicians.

Many local departments prepare a publication which appears monthly, discussing the current communicable disease situation throughout the county. The physician or interested person is invited to ask the department to place his name and address on the mailing list.

PROBLEMS CONFRONTING LOCAL HEALTH DEPARTMENTS

There are many problems confronting local health departments. A few include a scarcity of qualified personnel; opposition by certain groups; inadequate salaries, facilities, and buildings; overlapping of services in the city and county; administrative line relationship between city council or county board of supervisors and the health officer; continual complex and confusing reorganization; quickly changing health legislation; and in many instances, health workers are "afraid of stepping on someone's toes!" There seems to be a dichotomy between being a public servant and at the same time trying to promote community health by enforcing state and local laws.

The gravity of the situation caused by personnel shortages was emphasized by the Health Commissioner of Toledo, Ohio:

> It is recognized that there is a great need for public tax funds for all municipal services; howev-

er, and we quote from a report of the Toledo District Board of Health of several years ago '. . . this department would fail in its obligations to the citizens of this community if it did not point out that in certain areas there is no longer the question of whether a city *can afford to do* a program, but whether it *can afford not to*. . . .' It is increasingly clear to the Board of Health and other official and non-official agencies that the basic needs in the areas of public health nursing and environmental health cannot continue to be met with the number of field nurses and sanitarians presently employed.

Most official agencies find it quite difficult to obtain adequate funds necessary for the "ideal" staff.[5]

The Committee on Professional Education of the American Public Health Association has developed educational qualifications for most positions found in a local and state health department. The statement includes the general scope of position, functions, education, background and desirable competencies, graduate education, personal qualities, length of preparation, and schools for graduate education.*

Under the impact of expanding community problems, such as water and air pollution, family planning, drug abuse, malnutritions, poverty, and chronic illness, increased attention is being given to program evaluation and reorganization of services. Facilities are needed that are adaptable to new patterns of service. Health department workers must actively participate and demonstrate leadership in the community health councils. In this way all health agencies and interested persons can define health problems and objectives and cooperate more effectively in an effort to solve community health problems. Community health workers must constantly review and evaluate the changing problems and needs in a rapidly changing society.

Many people in our communities are poorly informed about public health agencies and activities. For example, in one study the respondents discussed the health department as a dispenser of medical care or a garbage and refuse collection agency, and the public had inadequate knowledge of where to obtain health services. Public ignorance about community services was not limited to knowledge of the health department.[6]

*If interested in one or more specific positions, write to: American Public Health Association, 1015 18th St. NW, Washington, D.C. 20036.

Although public health agencies have the responsibility of preventing disease and promoting health through community action, the citizens must also share *their* responsibilities to seek this objective. These responsibilities include:

1. Understanding the problems, policies, and functions of the department.
2. Formulating opinions based on fact and logic.
3. Making sure of proper citizen representation.
4. Protecting the health of oneself and one's family through individual means.

Unfortunately, members of the healing professions, through indifference or ignorance, often aid and abet the noncompetitive, low-quality selection of employees in government health service positions. In some cases, government jobs have been regarded as havens for relatives. Such attitudes hold down salaries, minimize competition for government jobs, and hinder recruitment of competent personnel. Prevalence of resistance to correction of these problems was noted by Blum and Leonard:

> At the same time that such democratically undesirable situations exist, many health departments make every attempt to offer a superior quality of service, particularly in medical care. In spite of inadequate salaries, unusually competent but not competitively oriented persons have often been attracted to agencies with dedicated purposes. The resolve to fulfill the agency's obligations in the best possible manner has in some cases been extended and has set higher-quality standards for the whole community, even though at significant cost to government in the process. A good many examples, such as the specialist standards required in the Crippled Children's Services program in California, are available for scrutiny. Much bitterness has resulted among many practitioners as a result of government's insistence on standards of performance higher than those met routinely in the private cared-for segment of the community. Since human lives justify concern, the only argument that can be advanced against government's providing excellent care is that of "wasting" money on people who are not at the moment the most financially successful members of society.[7]

THE HEALTH DEPARTMENT AND THE SCHOOL HEALTH PROGRAM

The primary responsibility for the health of children rests with the parents or guardians, who are obligated to provide adequate medical and dental care, and such home conditions as are conducive to good health. As the children mature, however, they should assume more responsibility for their individual health. The local board of education and the local health department coordinate and cooperate to give aid and seek correction of physical and emotional problems through family physicians and other appropriate agencies. The health department contributes to the school health program by periodically appraising the health of school children, providing health education services, and supervising the sanitary facilities of the school.

Many schools cooperate with members of the health department in an effort to appraise the health of certain students who have been referred by the teacher. Screening in the school health program is a preliminary examination by fairly simple and routine procedures for the purpose of identifying those children in need of further examination or diagnosis by qualified specialists. In this way, many disorders can be prevented and many defects corrected. Screening tests most commonly performed by teachers and nurses include growth and development measurements and vision and hearing testing. The school physician, who may or may not be a member of the health department, gives periodic health appraisals to students who have been referred by the teacher or nurse, new students, prekindergarten children and those who will engage in competitive athletics. Immunizations are also provided for those students who desire them, if they have obtained parental permission for this service. Observations, deviations, and corrections are carefully noted on the student's cumulative health record. Consultation, referral to the family physician or specialist, and follow-up are necessary adjuncts to the program. Health department officials suggest that regular medical supervision by the family's own physician is preferred.

Other public health services to schools provide for consultation to school administrators, parents and students; health information and conferences with teachers in the areas of dental health, smoking, drug abuse, etc.; and communicable disease control by immunizations, tuberculin testing, surveillance, and inspection.

Recent studies indicate that the routine and periodic physical examination of school children seems to be of limited value in revealing previously undisclosed important health problems.[8 9] These studies question the accepted value of periodic school health examination, absence surveillance, and health-room nursing care. If these established procedures do indeed have low value in school health programs, a difficult question is raised: what activities of physicians and nurses in schools can best maintain and improve the health of the nation's youth? This question is at present unanswered. It may well be that the time and effort now spent by high school physicians and nurses on low-yield activities dealing with physical health problems should be redirected toward identifying and managing the social and emotional health problems of adolescent pupils.

The need to begin health education at an early age is significant now because many of the problems that concern us are problems children and adolescents are facing and with which they must learn to cope. Today's school-age children and youth are directly affected by and involved in a number of major health problems and hazards, and the need for adequate instruction in the schools has never been more urgent.

The following four cases illustrate how the health department and the schools are inextricably linked in their efforts to prevent disease. Cooperation is essential to protect the health of school children and adults.

STAPHYLOCOCCAL INFECTIONS IN IOWA WRESTLERS

Eight cases of significant skin infections requiring medical treatment were reported among high school wrestlers at five high schools in Des Moines, Iowa . . .. When compared to previous experience, based on the memories of the coaches and the school nurses, this was a marked increase. Only one case could be recalled during the previous wrestling season and one case about four years previously.

The infections in all but one of the wrestlers were probably contracted at one high school. Five cases were associated with abrasions produced by the mats and two to scratches. The source of one infection is not known. Cultures were taken in three of these eight cases and *Staphylococcus aureus* coagulase positive (nontypable phage type) was found to be the offending agent. Clinically, the other cases were compatible with staphylococcal infections. A culture survey of the wrestling mats

OPERATION BRUSH-IN—FACT SHEET FOR TEACHERS

What Is It? Operation "Brush-In" is a voluntary program to reduce tooth decay in school age children in Santa Clara County, California.

Additional Facts: Santa Clara County does not have the benefit of a fluoridated water supply, which has proven to be the cheapest and most effective means of preventing dental decay. Thus other methods of preventing tooth decay should be used. One such method is applying stannous fluoride directly to the teeth. This procedure normally is performed by a dentist in his office.

Operation "Brush-In" is a procedure much like the one performed in the dentist's office—except the student is given a tooth brush and proper brushing instructions and does the work himself!

Each student applies fluoride protection to his teeth by using a special paste. The paste incorporates 9 per cent stannous fluoride with zirconium silicate. Zirconium silicate is an effective cleaning and polishing material which removes dental plaque, allowing the stannous fluoride to react with the tooth structure.

Stannous fluoride applied directly to the teeth reacts with the surface enamel to form various compounds. These substances become part of the enamel surface structure and make it less soluble in mouth acids which are produced by the bacteria present in the mouths of most people. These bacteria thrive on sugar-rich diets. The fermentation process which the bacteria initiate releases acids which dissolve or decalcify tooth enamel, causing a cavity.

This self-application of stannous fluoride has been thoroughly tested by Indiana University and by the U.S. Navy, resulting in as much as 90 per cent reduction in dental decay.

Operation "Brush-In" is a preventive action. Other preventive activities are also needed to maintain good dental health, such as a well-balanced diet, mouth protectors for contact sports, and regular visits to the dentist.

at the five schools revealed a high concentration of potentially pathogenic staphylococci on the mats of the one implicated high school and of one additional school. The strains isolated from the mats at the implicated high school were nontypable staphylococci. The mats at the other three schools showed negative cultures or very few pathogenic staphylococci.

The following case history suggests that active infections were probably important in transmitting the disease.... One high school wrestler developed a mat burn on his hand, which subsequently became infected. The infection was accompanied by lymphangitis, regional adenopathy, and fever, requiring antibiotic therapy. Following the wrestling season, he had difficulty with several boils on his legs. Early in the wrestling season, he developed several abscesses in his left axilla, which spread down the left side of his chest. He did not seek treatment for these and did not curtail his wrestling activities. The lesions persisted for about two to three weeks before gradually clearing.[10]

CONJUNCTIVITIS IN OKLAHOMA

Within one week, 41 of the 350 boarding students at Sequoyah Vocational School reported to the school clinic with eye complaints. All reported symptoms of eye irritation but denied photophobia or purulent discharge. Four patients gave a history of recent sore throats but all denied fever or other systemic symptoms. One patient was observed to have cervical lymphadenopathy. Ophthalmological examination of the patients revealed minimal bulbar conjunctival erythema. There was a lower tarsal follicular reaction, most marked in the lower conjunctival cul-de-sac, as well as a few follicles on the upper tarsus and occasionally on the bulbar conjunctiva. Slit lamp examination of the upper limbus and cornea was normal in all cases. The clinical history and ophthalmological examination suggested the diagnosis of viral conjunctivitis.

...The entire student body was examined with the aid of a magnifying loupe for acute follicular conjunctivitis. Eighty-four (27 per cent) of 311 students examined were found positive. In addition, three students demonstrated healed trachoma, and one boy was found with early active trachoma and started on therapy.

The attack rate (36.8 per cent) for female students was significantly higher than that for male students (16.2 per cent). Interestingly, the use of eye make-up among female students was widespread, and several supervisors noted that it was common for several girls to share the same eye make-up on any one day. The attack rate for those using eye make-up was significantly higher than for those not using eye make-up.

Extensive laboratory studies have not revealed an etiologic agent. Bacteriologic and virologic examinations were unrevealing, although cytologic examination of the conjunctival cells was consistent with viral conjunctivitis. There was no serologic evidence of recent adenovirus infection.[11]

DIPHTHERIA IN OKLAHOMA

An epidemic of diphtheria, with 13 clinical cases, including two deaths, occurred in Adair County, Oklahoma, between late October and early December. An additional 12 carriers were discovered in the course of investigation.

The epidemic was discovered when two brothers were hospitalized in Arkansas with membranous pharyngitis in early December. Diphtheria was suspected clinically, and confirmed by culture. Then, it was learned that an older sister had experienced a sore throat in early November. She was treated with penicillin; the pharyngitis appeared to be improved. Three days later, however, she developed cardiac failure. She died 13 days after the onset of her illness. An autopsy was not performed. Diphtheria was not suspected.

A physician remembered a 13 year old girl he had treated with penicillin for a severe sore throat in late October. Cultures, taken prior to antibiotic, were interpreted as having normal flora; cultures were not taken specially for diphtheria. Despite antibiotic therapy for six days, she developed nasal regurgitation, and cardiac arrhythmia. She died 11 days after onset of the symptoms.

These two dead girls had attended the same school, where a DPT immunization drive had been held during the fall. A 90 per cent response of school age children resulted; the two girls were among the 10 per cent not receiving vaccine.

After the first case was recognized, a nurse went to the home to immunize the remaining family members.

Intensive investigations by health department authorities subsequently revealed nine additional cases, all but two of whom could be traced to direct or indirect contact with recognized cases. Notably, six of the 13 cases occurred in a family of 13 children. Of the 13 cases, 11 had not received primary immunization; two were inadequately immunized (no booster dose within the past four years).

Oklahoma Public Health officials took cultures from all students at the two schools and all known contacts. Of 12 carriers detected, most were siblings or close contacts of the known cases.

A county-wide immunization program was held when the epidemic was recognized. Approximately 7000 of the county's 13,000 residents responded.[12]

STAPHYLOCOCCAL FOOD POISONING IN FLORIDA

On November 21, an explosive outbreak of food poisoning occurred at four adjacent schools in a Florida city. Before the investigation was concluded, 898 cases of illness, with varying degrees of abdominal cramps, diarrhea, dizziness, nausea, and vomiting were noted. The total enrollment of the four schools was 2500, giving an attack rate of 35.9 per cent. The first case occurred about one hour after food ingestion, while the median onset of illness was five hours after ingestion in 28 cases chosen for study. One child was hospitalized but was discharged in three hours.

The investigation revealed that the food for the four schools was prepared in the kitchen in one school and then distributed to the three adjoining schools for serving. The attack rates were similar in all the schools, suggesting contamination in the central kitchen. The central kitchen employed 18 persons. These were all examined, and the chief cook was found to have a chronic-appearing paronychia on one finger. A culture was made, and the laboratory reported growth of coagulase-positive staphylococci.

The meal had consisted of baked turkey, dressing, string beans, cherry sauce, cake with candied fruit and raisins, mashed potatoes, and giblet gravy. The turkeys had been prepared in stages and, during their preparation, were left at room temperature for varying lengths of time. A few of the turkeys were heated before serving, but most of them were served cold with piping hot gravy poured over the turkey. The chief cook made the giblet gravy and helped in the preparation of the turkey. Samples of the giblet gravy, potatoes, and dressing were not available for laboratory study, and the remaining food showed no positive findings. A review of the food ingested by those who became ill revealed that all had eaten the turkey over which the gravy had been poured.

It appears likely that the outbreak was caused by staphylococcal enterotoxin contamination of the turkeys or giblet gravy by a cook with a staphylococcal paronychia.[13]

The school health program helps prevent communicable disease, helps find and correct physical and emotional problems, helps prepare for emergency or disaster situations, helps lay the foundation for sound health knowledge, attitudes, and habits, and helps promote the physical, social, and emotional well-being of the students. Emphasis

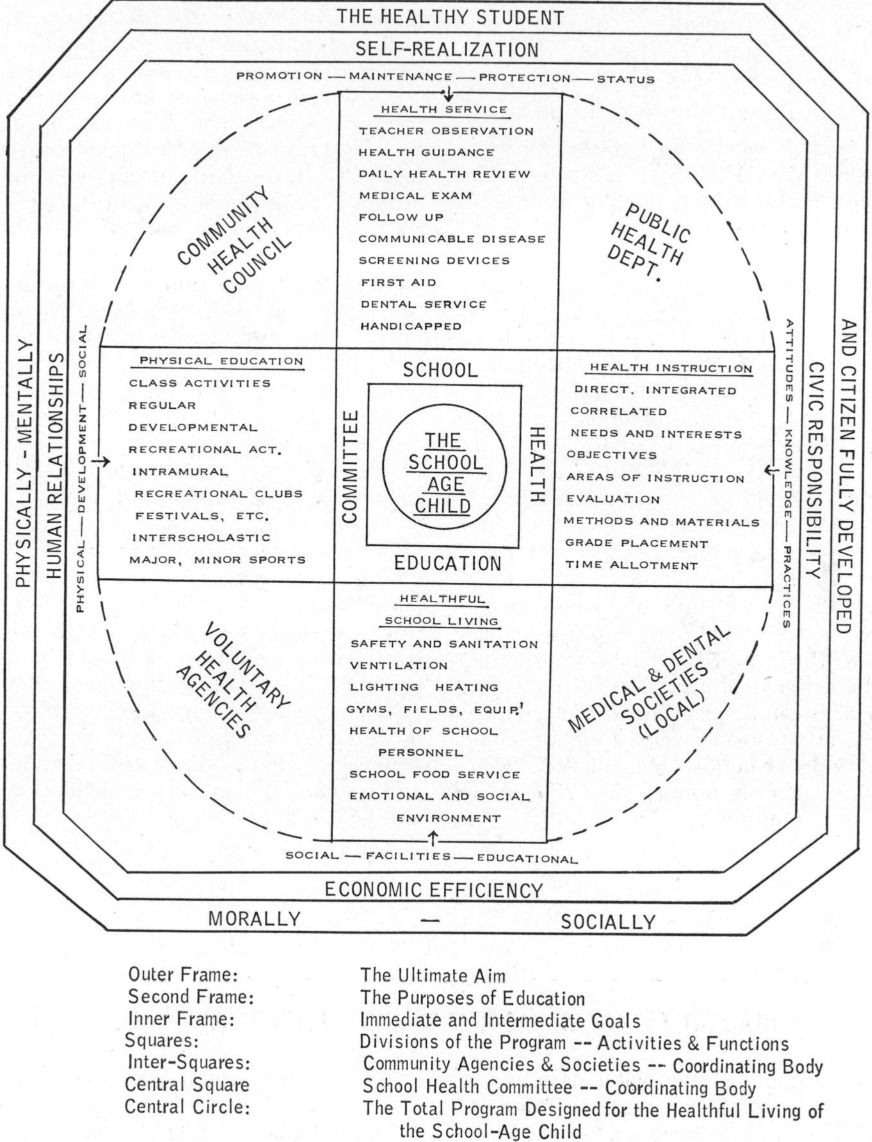

Outer Frame:	The Ultimate Aim
Second Frame:	The Purposes of Education
Inner Frame:	Immediate and Intermediate Goals
Squares:	Divisions of the Program -- Activities & Functions
Inter-Squares:	Community Agencies & Societies -- Coordinating Body
Central Square	School Health Committee -- Coordinating Body
Central Circle:	The Total Program Designed for the Healthful Living of the School-Age Child

Figure 6–3 (From Sparks, L. J.: *The School Health Program.* Unpublished syllabus, Willamette University, 1939.)

must be placed upon community coordination and cooperation, as indicated by Figure 6–3.

THE SCHOOL HEALTH EDUCATION STUDY: A FOUNDATION FOR COMMUNITY HEALTH EDUCATION

By far the most comprehensive, creative, and sophisticated project in health education curriculum planning and development, utilizing the conceptual approach, is the School Health Education Study. Financial support was first underwritten by the Samuel Bronfman Foundation of New York City, and later by the 3M Company of St. Paul, Minnesota. The Study produced its publication, *Health Education: A Conceptual Approach to Curriculum Design,* along with two sets of teaching-learning guides and several series of related transparencies. The Study's curriculum materials provide a complete set of guides for educators to utilize in initiating new or revising present health instruction programs in grades kindergarten through twelve. School personnel have available a conceptual model stemming from the definition of health and depicting its dimensions. The model demonstrates also a supporting hierarchy of concepts which provides an excellent framework for health education. The framework is adaptable and flexible enough to allow the incorporation of new knowledge as it is derived from research findings and the use of individual patterns of curriculum development and organization.

How can a program of school health education contribute to the health education of the community? First of all, some obvious but fundamental assumptions must be made: (1) that learning begins in infancy and should be continuous throughout a lifetime; (2) that community health education is only one stage in the continuum of the life-long learning process; (3) that much of what an individual knows, thinks, and does about health in his adult life stems from habits formed in the early and impressionable years; (4) that the educational setting of the school provides an environment in which certain skills and practices can be learned most efficiently and effectively; and (5) that over 50 million children, each of whom spends an estimated 2000 days in school, usually six hours a day, represent the future adult community.

The possession of knowledge and facts is not sufficient to cope with the complexity of the many health problems in today's society. For it is the ability to apply the behavioral skills of the process to the knowledge that leads to an intelligent and self-directed population and realization toward a productive and constructive way of life.

Traditional and artificial barriers among schools, colleges, and communities for health education responsibilities must be eliminated. Schools and colleges, through the virtue of a conducive environment and climate for learning, can build a solid foundation for continuing education for health in the community setting. Health needs, interests, and responsibilities change throughout one's lifetime. Old and emerging health problems and radical changes in our way of life await all of us. The rapidity and acceleration of medical advances and new knowledge will require continuing efforts to bridge the gap between knowledge and application.

The conceptual approach to health education offers potential for imposing order on an endlessly variable environment; it holds promise for patterning of facts into a statement of relationships to which new truths can be added and by which those no longer valid can be discarded. It provides for the development of cognitive, affective, and action-oriented skills through its focus on behavior and it offers a theoretical curriculum framework that is translated into an operational and functional plan for the facilitation of teaching and learning.[14]

MAJORITY OF MAJOR U.S. CITIES FLUORIDATED

A listing of the status of fluoridation in the U.S. cities with populations over 250,000 shows an overwhelming majority are fluoridated.

Old-timers who have enjoyed the benefits of fluoridation for over 20 years are Baltimore, the District of Columbia, Indianapolis, Milwaukee, San Francisco, Pittsburgh, Nashville, Louisville, Tulsa, Miami, St. Paul, Norfolk, Rochester, New York, and Richmond.

Philadelphia, Denver, and Oklahoma City implemented fluoridation 20 years ago.

In addition to these areas, Chicago, Cleveland, St. Louis, Buffalo, Minneapolis, and Toledo have fluoridated their water supplies for over 15 years.

From a total of 57 cities with over 250,000 in population, 40 are fluoridated and 17 are fluoride-deficient. The biggest unfluoridated cities are Los Angeles and Boston. New Orleans and Jersey City have approved fluoridation, but the measure has not yet been implemented.

Houston and San Jose are partially fluoridated; El Paso and Jacksonville are fluoridated naturally, at a level adequate to protect against tooth decay.

Cincinnati has been ordered to fluoridate in compliance with Ohio's state law. However, the city is in the process of contesting the order.

Fluoridation was implemented briefly, but then discontinued in San Diego and Kansas City, Missouri, after losing referendums.[15]

A CONCEPTUAL APPROACH TO HEALTH EDUCATION

Three Key Concepts: Processes Affecting Health Behavior and Serving as the Unifying Threads of the Curriculum.

GROWING AND DEVELOPING: A dynamic life process by which the individual is in some way like all other individuals, in some ways like some other individuals, and in some ways like no other individual.

INTERACTING: An ongoing process in which the individual is affected by and in turn affects certain biological, social, psychological, economic, cultural, and physical forces in the environment.

DECISION MAKING: A process unique to man of consciously deciding to take or not take an action, or of choosing one alternative rather than another.

Ten concepts of the School Health Education Study which serve as the major organizing elements of the curriculum reflecting the scope of health education in the curriculum:

1. GROWTH AND DEVELOPMENT INFLUENCES AND IS INFLUENCED BY THE STRUCTURE AND FUNCTIONING OF THE INDIVIDUAL.

Growth and development is a stage in the process of growing and developing. In this concept the individual is viewed as a complex interacting and decision-making organism with certain hereditary potentials. Body functions, environmental conditions, the use of certain substances, and other factors may promote or hinder growth and development at any given point on the continuum of growing and developing.

2. GROWING AND DEVELOPING FOLLOWS A PREDICTABLE SEQUENCE, YET IS UNIQUE FOR EACH INDIVIDUAL.

Growing and developing is a dynamic process. There is a predictable sequence to the process, yet each person grows and develops in a unique way influenced by heredity, environment, and personal behavior. An individual may be ahead of, the same as, or behind others of the same age and sex in regard to social, emotional, and physical maturity. Also, unique variations exist between the sexes of the same age.

3. PROTECTION AND PROMOTION OF HEALTH IS AN INDIVIDUAL, COMMUNITY, AND INTERNATIONAL RESPONSIBILITY.

The individual, through independent and cooperative action, has a basic responsibility for safeguarding, maintaining, and enhancing health. In some instances, raising the health status of people or solving specific health problems can be done best by organized community efforts. Community as perceived in the context of this concept includes the family, neighborhood, villages, towns, metropolitan areas, states, regions, nations, and our expanding universe. The community as well as health knows no boundaries.

4. THE POTENTIAL FOR HAZARDS AND ACCIDENTS EXISTS, WHATEVER THE ENVIRONMENT.

Many sources of danger are present in the environment, some of which may produce injury, illness, disability, or death. Sensory, motor, emotional, and a complexity of other factors are involved in reducing and modifying hazards. The conceptual understanding in this instance is that of learning to enjoy life to the fullest with its adventurous pursuits, but respecting the potential for hazards and accidents through adequate planning, preparation, and foresight.

5. THERE ARE RECIPROCAL RELATIONSHIPS INVOLVING MAN, DISEASE, AND ENVIRONMENT.

The dynamic interplay of the individual, disease, and environment results in varying degrees of health. In this relationship, conditions may be produced in man which range from death to high-level wellness. These varying levels of wellness may be the result of transactions involving biological and physical aspects of man's environment. In an effort to achieve high-level wellness the individual may adapt to, or modify the environment. Man, in essence, is not apart from environment.

6. THE FAMILY SERVES TO PERPETUATE MAN AND TO FULFILL CERTAIN HEALTH NEEDS.

The family is a social group in which members interact with one another and relate most intimately to each other. As a social unit the family grows and develops in its own unique way. Through its structure it provides for the expression and exploration of a range of emotions, communicates the meaning of family, satisfies certain health needs, offers an opportunity for the expression of human sexuality, and serves in the transmission of culture and the perpetuation of man.

7. PERSONAL HEALTH PRACTICES ARE AFFECTED BY A COMPLEXITY OF FORCES, OFTEN CONFLICTING.

The choices an individual makes regarding sleep, relaxation, activity, care of teeth, and other facets of personal health are influenced by many factors. As an individual grows and develops personal goals, social pressures, value structures, ethnic and religious beliefs, and past experiences create perplexing alternatives regarding health practices. Deliberate and informed decisions affect the level of well-being.

8. UTILIZATION OF HEALTH INFORMATION, PRODUCTS, AND SERVICES IS GUIDED BY VALUES AND PERCEPTIONS.

Health status, knowledge, background experiences, feelings, health expectations, and related personal and interpersonal factors influence the utilization of health information, products, and services. In addition, one's value system—those tangibles and intangibles which an individual considers to be important and desirable in life—will guide in decision making and help direct actions.

9. USE OF SUBSTANCES THAT MODIFY MOOD AND BEHAVIOR ARISES FROM A VARIETY OF MOTIVATIONS.

The mood and behavior of an individual may be modified if alcohol, amphetamines, tranquilizers, coffee and similar beverages, hallucinogens, and other substances are used. This modification may be beneficial or harmful in some direct or indirect way. Social reasons, personal needs, psychological motives, and other pressures and circumstances underlie the use of such substances.

10. FOOD SELECTION AND EATING PATTERNS ARE DETERMINED BY PHYSICAL, SOCIAL, MENTAL, ECONOMIC AND CULTURAL FACTORS.

Food is basic to life. Selection of foods and eating patterns help determine nutritional status which, in turn, influences growth and development and well-being. In addition to serving physiological needs, food selection and patterns of eating affect and are affected by social and psychological forces in daily life. Such factors as economics, availability, group pressures, body size, food preferences, ethnic background, and mass media also affect nutritional behavior.[16]

*Framework For Health Instruction**

For many years, representatives from the fields of education and health have recommended the development of a framework that would provide a structure for the development of a planned sequential health education curriculum and yet be flexible enough to meet local needs and to provide for the changing health problems facing children and youth. A Framework for Health Instruction in California Public Schools, Kindergarten Through Grade Twelve, has been developed to meet these requirements. It is intended as a foundation for local curriculum development upon which a comprehensive program of health instruction may be built.

Questions commonly asked by groups working on the development of a health education curriculum include the following: What should be emphasized when health-related information is so abundant today? How can attitudes and behavior be the focus rather than the provision of health knowledge? What are the objectives students are expected to attain? To help answer such questions, the concept-oriented approach to curriculum development has been utilized in this publication, and emphasis is placed upon behavioral objectives. Concepts provide a needed framework for knowledge and for thinking—both essential aspects of health instruction. The behavioral objectives listed for each grade-level concept provide specific illustrations of ways in which learners may demonstrate competencies.

*California State Department of Education: *Framework for Health Instruction in California Public Schools, Kindergarten Through Grade Twelve* Sacramento, Calif., Office of State Printing, 1970.

THE STATE HEALTH DEPARTMENT

A state health department is organized on basically the same pattern as a local health department. The responsibilities of the state health department are contained in concise sections of the health and safety codes of the states. From these stem a myriad of laws, rules, and regulations which mold the activities, functions, responsibilities, programs, and projects of the department.

In brief, the state health department is generally responsible for: examination into the causes of communicable disease in man and domestic animals; investigation of the sources of morbidity and mortality; investigation of the effects of localities, employments, conditions and circumstances on public health; licensing of hospitals and nursing homes; detection and prevention of adulteration of food and drugs; examination for and the prevention of pollution of public water and ice supplies; and preparation and distribution, at cost, of antitoxins, vaccines, and other approved biologic products for the control or prevention of communicable diseases. The department may advise all local health authorities, and when, in its judgment, the public health is menaced, it controls and regulates their action.

The department encourages and stimulates local health departments to meet the public health needs of the areas that they serve. Direct public health service to the people of the state is provided by local public health departments; the state department provides only direct service that cannot be provided locally. The state department strives to help maintain superior local health services by providing:

1. Leadership in assisting communities without full time health departments to recognize their public health needs
2. Financial aid in the establishment and strengthening of local health services, including the provision of staff and other resources

3. Provision of educational opportunities for staffs of local health departments
4. Establishment of standards of service and personnel
5. Coordination of the total public health program within the state and of local, state and federal programs.

The California State Health Department, for example, is guided in its activities by the 10 members of the State Board of Public Health, of which the director acts as executive officer in addition to his duties as administrative head of the Department. Members are appointed by the governor for four-year terms, so staggered that there are always some experienced members to give continuity to policy. The Board functions as a policy-making, regulatory, judicial, and licensing body.

Goals

The following represents a statement of the goals of the California State Department of Health:

1. Identify health needs and develop programs to meet them, giving consideration to relative priorities and effectiveness.
2. Promote an environment that will contribute to human health and well-being.
3. Assure the availability of comprehensive health services for all Californians, utilizing both public and private health resources.
4. Assure that quality standards for health programs and services are established and maintained.
5. Assist in coordinating the activities of health agencies—state and local, public and private—along with medical schools, hospitals, and private practitioners, in providing health services.
6. Promote the development of new knowledge concerning the causes and cures of illness and the means of delivering health services to the public.
7. Help all the state's citizens to understand the essentials of positive personal health and the effective use of available health services.
8. Provide maximum protection of the general public health environment.

FINANCIAL SUPPORT OF LOCAL AND STATE HEALTH SERVICES

The financing of local health services has always been a critical matter in developing community health programs. With the increasing competition for tax funds, and with the uncertainties of the future role of federal grants-in-aid, financing is currently more critical than in the past. It is important that both citizens and public officials learn more about the intricacies of the local tax situation in relation to public health.

The provision of community health services in the United States today is a cooperative project, with responsibility shared by federal, state, and local units of government. As a result of these combined efforts, 90 per cent of the country's total population now resides in areas that have some form of organized health services. However, there is a lag between the development of new public health practices and their application in state and local health departments. This situation is partially caused by lack of funds necessary to establish new programs.

The national government is concerned with the public's health because disease moves freely and frequently from one state to another, and the strength of the nation is dependent upon the health and productive capacity of its people. The federal government contributes to public health in the form of assistance to states. In general, federal grants make up the highest proportion of total expenditures in states with small total population, and in those states with low per capita income. Even with extensive aid from federal sources, however, low income states still devote a larger share of their own resources to health than do the wealthier states. Generally, the federal government gives the most assistance to those states that frequently have the greatest health problems, have the least financial resources, and are putting forth the greatest effort in public health in relation to their own financial capacity.[17] Two constituents of the United States Department of Health, Education, and Welfare make grants-in-aid to the states for health purposes. These are the Public Health Service and the Children's Bureau of the Social Security Administration.

The public health movement gathered momentum through stimulation from various public and private sources. The American Red Cross and private foundations such as the Rockefeller Foundation, the Commonwealth Fund, and the Kellogg Foundation were very active in the development of community health services. By 1919 all states had a governmental branch exclusively concerned with health, and some local health

programs and services

From July 1, 1973 to June 30, 1974, public health programs and services in Arizona's state and county health departments cost a total of $42,985,808.

The state share of this cost was $28,679,500. This comes to slightly more than 3 percent of total cost of state government—$876,251,716.

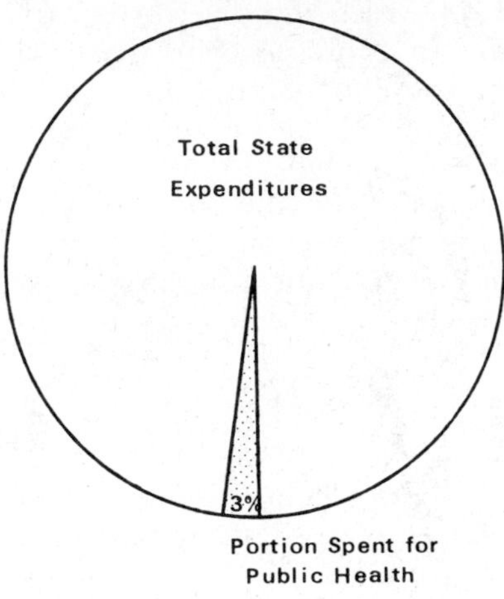

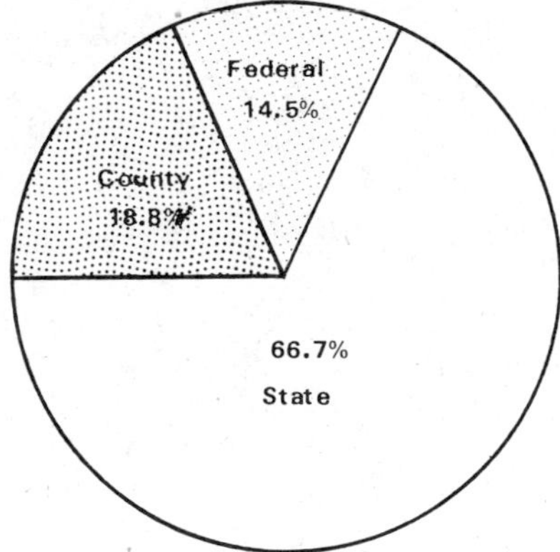

The three levels of government shared the cost of public health programs and services as follows:

County	$ 8,061,408
State	28,679,500
Federal	6,244,900
TOTAL	$ 42,985,808

Figure 6–4 Distribution of funds for public health programs and services in Arizona. (From *The First Year, Annual Report of the Arizona Department of Health Services,* 1973–74, pp. 17–18.)

departments had been established. At the federal level, in 1912, the Public Health and Marine Hospital Service was reorganized by act of Congress into the U.S. Public Health Service.

Federal health grants to states were first instituted in 1918 when funds were appropriated to the Public Health Service for venereal disease control services (Chamberlain-Kahn Act). Grants-in-aid for the protection of the health of mothers and children were initially provided through the Children's Bureau in the Sheppard-Towner Act of 1921. The provisions of this act expired in 1925.

The Narcotics Control Act authorized construction of hospitals for case and treatment of drug abusers in 1929.

The Social Security Act of 1935 promoted the expansion of public health programs throughout the nation. Under this Act, general health grants, which support basic state and local public health services, and special grants for maternal and child health and crippled children services were inaugurated. Since that time, grants

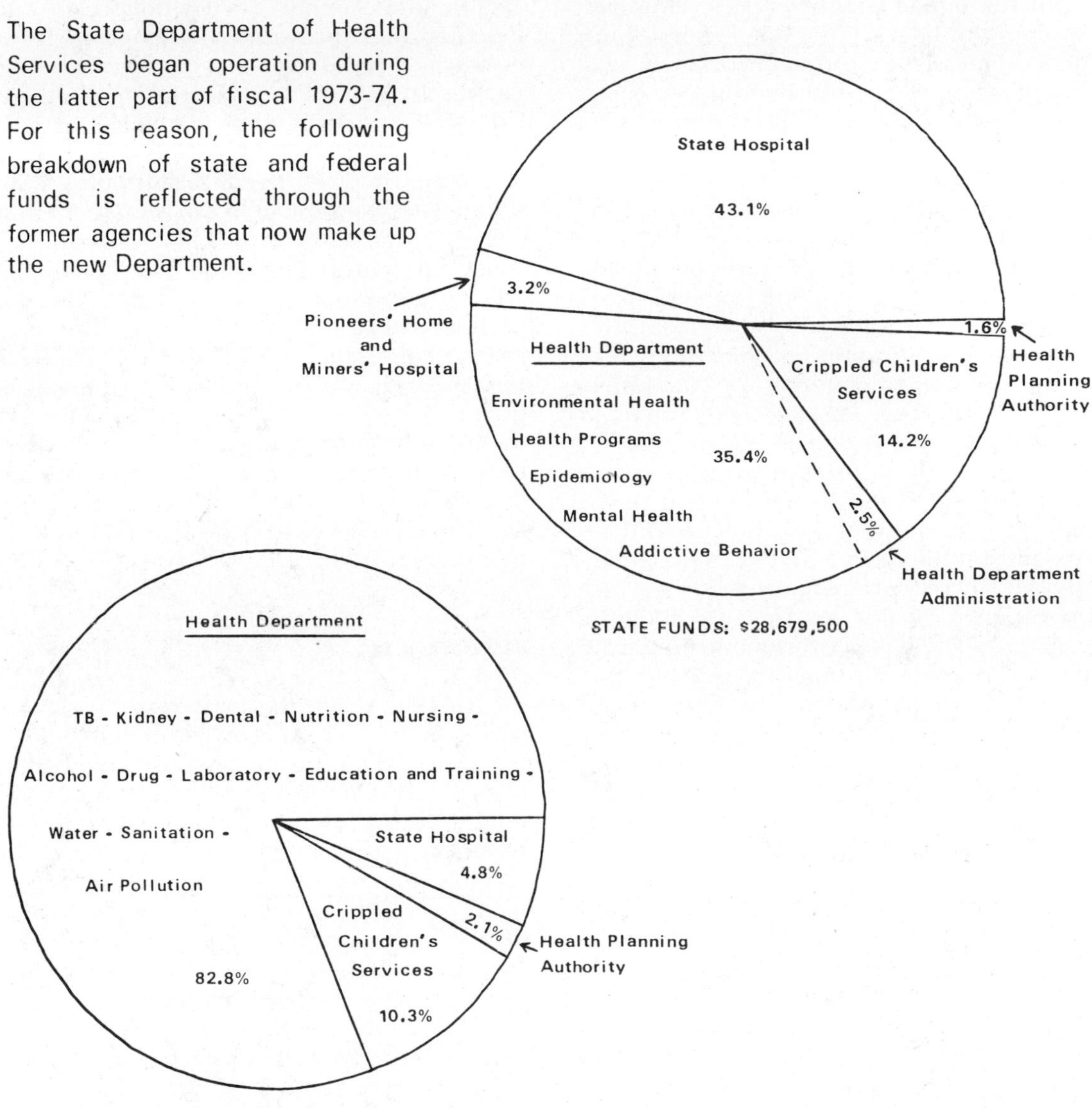

Figure 6–4 *(Continued)*

have been extended to cover a much larger range of activities, including hospital construction. Congress passed the Hospital Survey and Construction (Hill-Burton) Act in 1946. Since then it has been amended to permit federal assistance in the construction of health centers, nursing homes, and many other types of health facilities. Federal contributions are matched by from one-third to two-thirds of state and local funds.

Local health departments are usually supported by a tax levy on the assessed valuation of taxable property, personal income, sales tax, business and industry taxes, and other sources. However, it is a very difficult problem to provide adequate public health services in those rural areas that are so sparsely populated that they cannot support independent local health departments. In an effort to solve this problem, many state health departments furnish special services in such areas. California has enacted legislation with provisions for a county with a population of less than 40,000 to enter into a contract with the State Department of Public Health for public health services. However, the county board of supervisors must request the contract and appropriate at least the minimum acceptable amount per capita for their total population. This contract plan stimulates local interest and responsibility and fosters autonomy.

State funds are allocated to assist local health departments for a wide variety of public health purposes. In addition to subsidizing local health departments, states make grants for mosquito abatement, for construction of hospital and health centers, for care of crippled children, for community mental health programs, and for support of tuberculosis sanitoriums.

Many new health services and programs must be provided to care for current public health problems. Local governments and citizens must understand and support financially the increased costs necessary to provide superior health services. In addition, the state and federal government must continue to provide stronger leadership and greater financial support to encourage and assist in the development and improvement of local services.

Legislation

The 1965–66 session of the 89th Congress was responsible for some of the far-reaching federal health legislation ever passed. The Social Security Act was amended to provide funds for health care of the elderly (Medicare) and of the medically indigent (Medicaid). The Heart Disease, Cancer, and Stroke Amendments, authorizing regional medical programs to combat the three "killer" diseases, emphasized the concept of regionalization and gave a boost to professional programs in continuing education. The Comprehensive Health Planning and Public Health Services Act of 1966 created the Partnership for Health program to promote the most efficient use of our health resources and the ready availability of health services to all who need them. It called for planning councils and required that they have consumer as well as provider representation. The Narcotic Addict Rehabilitation Act of 1966 offered treatment and rehabilitation services in lieu of prosecution or sentencing to addicts who have been convicted of federal crimes.

In 1967 the Child Health Act broadened the base of the earlier Maternal and Child Health and Mental Retardation Acts, and together they provided the impetus for a network of projects and programs across the nation. In 1968 the Health Manpower Act extended and expanded a number of laws already in effect.

With the growth of health programs, stimulated by these federal acts, there was a greater demand for health care personnel. Emerging patterns included health maintenance organizations, comprehensive neighborhood health services, home care programs, emergency health services, National Health Service Corps, and peer review programs. The government has encouraged these programs to help eliminate inequities in the delivery of health care. The programs are intended to help fill the gaps in the existing framework and to provide basic elements in a reorganized structure.

Federal Grants

In 1935, Congress passed the Social Security Act, which authorizes under Title V the appropriation each year of certain sums of money to be used in helping states to extend and improve their maternal and child health, crippled children's, and child welfare services. No part of any of these grants is paid to children or their parents. These grants are used by states to extend and strengthen their services. Some child welfare services grants pay the cost for foster care of children.

All three types of grants are available to official state agencies. Typically, maternal and child health grants go to state departments of health, crippled children's grants to state crippled children's agencies, and child welfare services grants to state public welfare agencies. Every state, the District of Columbia, Guam, Puerto Rico, and the Virgin Islands have such agencies and all, with one exception, receive grants for the three programs. Arizona does not apply for grants for its crippled children's services.

Federal grants help to get new services started, to reach more children, and to improve through the application of new knowledge and findings from research and the training of workers the quality of care children receive. The grants are not intended to meet all costs of health and welfare services for children in any state. To be eligible for a federal grant, a state must show that it is spending state and local money on these programs and must develop a plan for the allotment of funds to the state. Over the years, federal funds have proved to be magnets, as well as helpers, attracting more and more state and local effort in behalf of children.

Every state agency entitled to share in the annual grants to states develops a state plan for the best use for this money. Characteristically, state agencies work out their plans in consultation with Children's Bureau specialists. Each state plan must carry out the intent of the law. But the intent of the law can be broadly interpreted, and the needs of children are many, giving state agencies much latitude to develop their programs within the limits of the funds available and their special needs.

Most services provided by state and local agencies for mothers and children are health promotion services. States use grants to help pay the cost of maternity clinics, where women are given advice by doctors, nurses, nutritionists, and medical social workers. Grants also help to pay for pediatric clinics, visits of public health nurses to homes before and after babies are born, clinics where mothers can obtain health supervision and competent advice on the health care of their babies and preschool children, school health programs that detect youngsters who need medical or dental treatment and help them get it, topical fluoride applications, and immunizations against contagious diseases. Most states conduct special clinics where diagnostic evaluation, counseling, and follow-up services are provided for mentally retarded children.

One of the most recent developments in the expression of the Bureau's concern for children has been its new emphasis on programs for mentally retarded children. In 1971, over 60,000 mentally retarded children and their families were receiving services from projects initiated through the federal-state partnership. About three-fourths of these children were less than nine years old, and more than half of them had other handicaps in addition to mental retardation.

The keystone to further progress in maternal and child health programs lies in the broader distribution of services to groups of mothers and children who are inadequately reached. These services are still lacking or inadequate for some socially and economically deprived groups in cities.[18]

DEPARTMENT OF HEALTH, EDUCATION AND WELFARE

The Department of Health, Education and Welfare (HEW) was established in 1953 for the purpose of organizing the various health and welfare agencies of the government under one administrative unit, thus promoting better cooperation and efficiency in serving the needs of the people. Today, this department employs over 100,000 persons, has a budget of over 100 billion dollars, and is a huge and expanding force in today's society. This department consists of four major branches: Public Health Service, Social and Rehabilitation Services, Social Security Administration, and the Office of Education. HEW is responsible for two institutions of higher learning—Gallaudet College and Howard University, both in Washington, D.C.—scores of hospitals and clinics, the American Printing House for the Blind, and dozens of research laboratories.

HEW scientists tell people what drinks, drugs, foods and cosmetics are unsafe. HEW's National Clearinghouse for Smoking and Health bombards the media with anti-cigarette advertisements and literature. Except for Social Security, the large bulk of departmental spending is in grants to states, localities, universities, school systems, hospitals, laboratories and foundations. Nearly every American is affected by HEW. Ninety per cent of the outlays are made through state and local governments and nonprofit agencies, including universities. HEW finances day care for infants, hot lunches for toddlers, counseling for troubled teenagers, the Pill for impoverished housewives, and welfare for the aged. In one corner or another of the nation, at any hour of the day, HEW-financed research delves into national and personal problems—suicides, drug addiction, headaches, delinquency, child abuse, and "hard-core" poverty.

Social historians suggest the following reasons for the rapid growth of HEW:

1. Educational outlays began multiplying after Russia's early successes in space convinced many Americans that deficiencies in American schools were responsible—and that the shortcom-

ings could be cured only by vast infusions of federal aid to schools and institutions of higher learning.

2. Social problems such as urban decay, racial conflict, and youth unrest forced their way close to the top of national concerns. These problems, for the most part, came within the range of HEW's responsibilities when calls arose for government action.

3. The war on poverty, among other things, gave the poor a voice as well as legal weapons for making their wants known to politicians and bureaucrats. This accelerated the push toward Medicare, Medicaid, bigger welfare payments with fewer restrictions, and special aid to students and schools in poverty areas.

4. Dramatic gains in medicine since World War II produced widespread expectation of longer and healthier lives for all—and widespread demands for massive, government-backed programs of research to perform more "miracles."

To its admirers, HEW today is seen by many as having solid achievements to its credit. Three of its scientists have won Nobel prizes. In recent years, HEW has conducted or subsidized research that brought big advances in cancer treatment, the first vaccine against rubella (German measles) and the first laboratory synthesis of a gene, the unit of heredity.

The critics of HEW, however, claim that the agency has grown into a bureaucratic, uncoordinated, ungovernable jungle that is often confused, wasteful and ineffective. They maintain that guidelines and regulations developed for states are too rigorous and inflexible, that regional offices are concerned with misinterpreting and misconstruing information and directives, and that there is too much bureaucratic red tape for many who apply for financial grants. They object to overlapping, duplicated, splintered programs. For example, Medicare is in one agency and Medicaid in another. Both are outside HEW's major health agencies. Also, five programs offer public library grants, seven offer medical-library grants, and vocational-education grants can be obtained in 15 ways. The critics call HEW a house divided by professional pride and jealousies. They point out that funds have been wasted on projects that were poorly designed, produced no useful information, and were not evaluated and followed up. On the other hand, news of many successful projects was not relayed to the public.

The federal government provides states with funds and minimal guidelines, but the individual states can operate any type of program they choose. The result is a mixture of diverse programs, variation in benefits, and an inadequate response to the needs of the people. The current administration is modernizing its procedures and lines of authority and is probing the effectiveness of HEW programs. The emphasis is on the total complex of "people" problems. Future actions must reflect a better integration of our capabilities in order to deal effectively across the entire spectrum of human needs. For example, look at a low-income family in any of our inner cities and you find, first of all, a lack of money to pay for necessities. Often there is little schooling; the head of the family is likely to be functionally illiterate and lacking in working skills. There may be a history in one or more family members of alcoholism or physical handicap or emotional illness. The social programs established to deal with these problems haven't done as much as they should, because they haven't been adequately coordinated. Each particular part of the social-services bureaucracy treats one aspect of the family's problems. To overcome this, 19 states have consolidated their state agencies dealing with the problems of people into single departments of human resources or social services. Mutually reinforcing health and welfare programs are being brought together under a single unit.

UNITED STATES PUBLIC HEALTH SERVICE

The United States Public Health Service was established by a congressional act in 1798 sponsored by Alexander Hamilton, then Secretary of the Treasury. It is the oldest of the organizations that make up the Department of Health, Education and Welfare and is the principal health agency of the federal government. Through the Service, the federal government works with others to discover and apply knowledge that will help conquer disease and improve health. Public Health Service programs are conducted in close partnership with other agencies of the Department,* with the states and territories, and with many voluntary organizations, professional groups, institutes, and international agencies. The Public Health Service has consolidated into six major agencies:

—*National Institutes of Health,* for the research mission (see Fig. 6–6);

*Department of Health, Education and Welfare

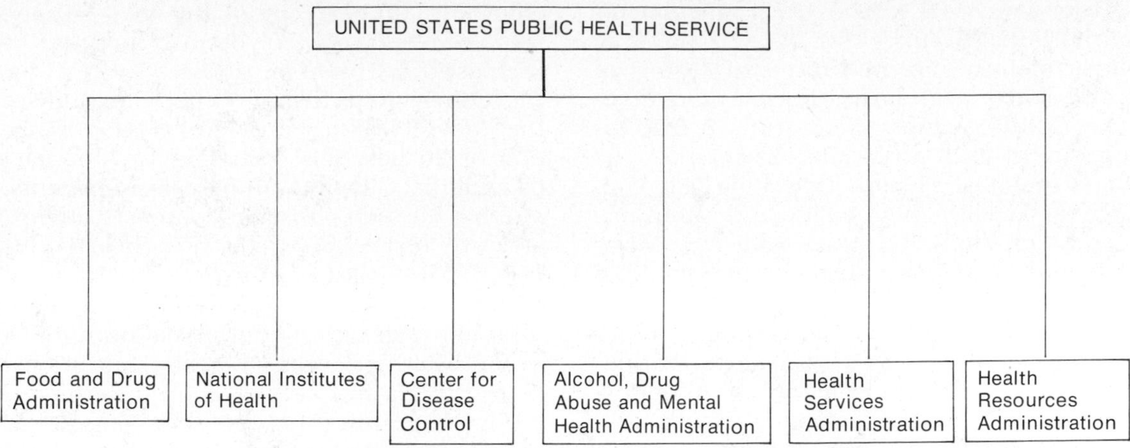

Figure 6–5 Divisions of the United States Public Health Service.

—*Food and Drug Administration,* for the regulatory functions related to consumer protection;
—*Health Services Administration,* for responsibilities related to the delivery of health care and the quality of care;
—*Center for Disease Control,* for the preventive medicine and public health responsibilities;
—*Health Resources Administration,* to help develop health service resources and improve the use of those resources;
—*Alcohol, Drug Abuse and Mental Health Administration,* to deal with the socio-medical problems of alcohol abuse, drug abuse, and mental illness.

The ultimate purpose of this new structure is to provide better health services for the American people. Concurrent with the restructuring of its health component, the Department is working to improve the availability and quality of health care and to combat a number of specific health problems; as discussed in the following paragraphs.

Health Care Review. Acting on au-

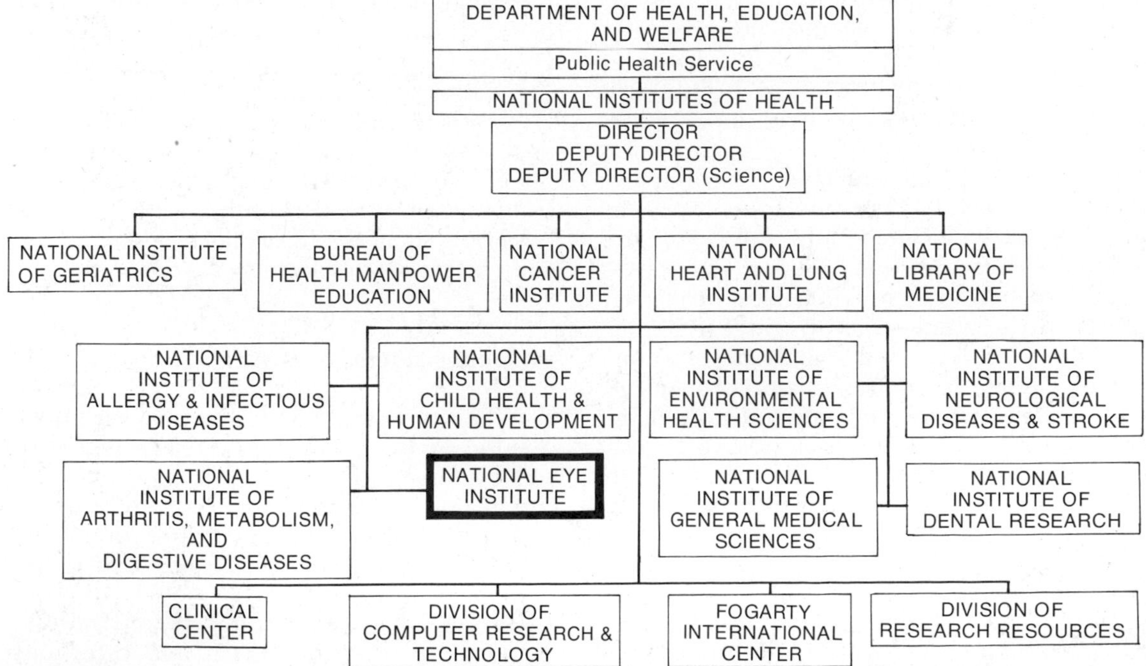

Figure 6–6 Organization of the National Institutes of Health. (Adapted from Amer. J. Ophthalmol., December, 1972, p. 1014.)

thority contained in the 1972 amendments to the Social Security Act (P.L. 92–603) the department began the process of setting up Professional Standards Review Organizations (PSRO's) across the country. A PSRO is a group of local physicians chartered by the Department of Health, Education and Welfare to review the quality and appropriateness of medical care provided to Medicare and Medicaid patients by hospitals and other institutions in the group's area.

Lead-Based Paint Poisoning Prevention. Special grants were given to 42 cities for the establishment of lead paint poisoning detection, treatment, and prevention programs. These programs sought to screen 200,000 children, especially those under 6 years of age.

High Blood Pressure. In a long-range educational effort that may provide a prototype for developing other health education programs, the federal government has joined with the health professions, pharmaceutical and communications industries, and a range of private and voluntary groups in a nationwide campaign to make the general public and medical professions more aware of the importance of diagnosing and controlling high blood pressure.

Venereal Disease Plan. The Center for Disease Control augmented its nationwide attack on the venereal diseases by launching a Venereal Disease Communications Plan. The Plan is designed to create awareness of the venereal diseases, change attitudes and behavior, increase self-referrals for diagnosis and treatment, and encourage health care providers to conduct screening and contact-tracing programs.

National Blood Policy. The Department produced and put into effect a plan to upgrade the efficiency and safety of the blood collection and distribution system. Of the 8.8 million units of whole blood collected yearly in the United States, roughly 25 per cent becomes outdated and is never transfused. Disease is another major problem in the present system. Several studies indicate that there are 17,000 cases of overt post-transfusion hepatitis each year, resulting in about 850 deaths. A major feature of the Department of Health, Education and Welfare plan is the elimination of commercial blood-banking in favor of an all-voluntary donor system. Available data indicate that while commercial blood organizations provide only 15 per cent of the total supply, they are responsible for up to 45 per cent of the post-transfusion hepatitis.

Other Activities. Other activities of the Public Health Service are: (1) the operation of 26 hospitals, including two for narcotic addicts, two for tuberculosis patients, one for Hansen's Disease (leprosy) patients, and two for neuropsychiatric problems, (2) research in health conducted at the National Institutes of Health at Bethesda, Maryland, (3) training grants to educational institutions in the health sciences, (4) fellowship grants, (5) assisting states in their public health education programs, (6) supervisory control and licensure of the manufacturers of biological products used in the prevention and treatment of disease, (7) the publication of vital statistics pertinent to the public health programs, and (8) supervision of St. Elizabeth's Hospital for the treatment of mentally ill beneficiaries of federal employees.

Responsibilities of the Public Health Service also involve safeguarding the health of inmates of federal prisons, personnel of Coast Guard stations, residents of Indian reservations, users of and visitors to the national parks and monuments, projects of the Bureau of Reclamation, and the extensive recreational areas in the national forests. Other important environmental Public Health Service research centers include the Industrial Hygiene Laboratory in Atlanta, Georgia, the Environmental Health Center in Cincinnati, Ohio, and the Communicable Disease Center in Atlanta, Georgia.

The United States Public Health Service is administered by the Surgeon General, who is appointed by the President of the United States. The Surgeon General also plans and conducts an annual conference of state and territorial health officers and other special committees and conferences as needed.[19]

National Institutes of Health

This principal research arm of the Public Health Service is primarily concerned with the extension of basic knowledge regarding the health problems of man and how to cope with them. The institutes include the Office of the Director, Bureau of Health Manpower, National Cancer Institute, National Geriatrics Institute, National Heart and Lung Institute, National Institute of Allergy and Infectious

Diseases; National Institute of Arthritis and Metabolic Diseases, National Eye Institute, National Institute of Child Health and Human Development, National Institute of Dental Research, National Institute of General Medical Sciences, National Institute of Neurological Diseases and Stroke, National Library of Medicine, and the Fogarty International Center. A clinical center provides patient facilities and makes possible clinical investigations for the institutes.

The institutes conduct both laboratory and clinical research to discover better methods of preventing, diagnosing, and treating and curing serious diseases. Emphasis is placed today on research relating to the chronic diseases, since these have become increasingly significant; the incidence of infectious diseases is declining in comparison with that of the past. Much of the research is conducted outside the institutes in nonfederal institutions such as medical schools, universities, hospitals, and other research agencies.

The National Library of Medicine houses the greatest collection of medical literature in the world. The collection is in excess of a million items. The library was developed to aid in the advancement of medical and related health sciences. Books, periodicals, and other materials are organized, catalogued, indexed, and made available to help disseminate and exchange scientific information in medicine and public health. Bibliographical guides to medical literature are published, and reference and research assistance is provided by the library staff.

The main function of the Bureau of Health Manpower is to develop and coordinate programs designed to provide a larger quantity of better qualified and more effectively utilized personnel for the nation's health services.

Food and Drug Administration: Authority and Activities

The authority of the Food and Drug Administration (FDA) is limited to the scope of laws passed by Congress and assigned to the agency for enforcement. Principal responsibility is enforcement of the Federal Food, Drug, and Cosmetic Act, enacted to insure wholesome foods, safe and effective drugs and medical devices, harmless cosmetics, and truthful labeling of such products. Other laws administered by the FDA include:

1. *Radiation Control for Health and Safety Act*—protects the public from unnecessary exposure to radiation from medical x-ray and electronic products such as color televisions and microwave ovens.
2. *Public Health Service Act*—regulates the quality of biologic drugs and the sanitary practices of interstate carriers; provides for a sanitation program designed to minimize public health problems associated with the production, processing, and distribution of products prepared by the food service, milk, and shellfish industries.
3. *Fair Packaging and Labeling Act*—requires truthful and accurate packaging and labeling; FDA authority in this area is limited to foods, drugs, cosmetics, and therapeutic devices.
4. *Tea Importation Act*—designed to insure quality of imported tea.
5. *Import Milk Act*—requires certification that imported milk products meet United States requirements.
6. *Caustic Poison Act*—requires that such substances be specially labeled.

Health Services Administration

The Health Services Administration (HSA) agency of the United States Department of Health, Education, and Welfare was established in 1973. Part of the Public Health Service, HSA seeks to improve the delivery of health services available to the people of the United States through various grant-in-aid and other financial assistance programs, through contracts for state and local health care providers, and by integrating service delivery programs. The agency also provides direct health care through its personnel and facilities to certain segments of the population. In addition it is responsible for assuring the quality and containing the costs of health care provided through the public financing programs.

The Health Services Administration carries out its duties through the Office of the Administrator and four bureaus and services:

1. The *Indian Health Service* provides direct comprehensive health care for American Indians, Eskimos, and Aleuts through a system of over 450 hospitals, centers, stations, and satellite field clinics, and in addition acts as their principal federal advocate in the health field. The Service also assists them to strengthen their capacities and manage their own individual and institutional health affairs.

2. The *Federal Health Programs Service,* through hospitals and outpatient clinics located mostly in port cities, offers care to merchant seamen, coastguardsmen, and federal employees with work-related injuries and illnesses. A division of the Service is also responsible for coordinating emergency health services nationally during major disasters.

3. The *Bureau of Community Health Services* encompasses maternal and child health, health maintenance organizations, family planning, neighborhood and family health centers, and migrant health grant programs which seek to meet the health care needs of communities across the nation. The Bureau's National Health Service Corps provides for health manpower in critical shortage areas and for new mechanisms for health care delivery at the community level.

4. The *Bureau of Quality Assurance* ensures that Medicare, Medicaid, and other federal health care programs provide services that are consistent with recognized professional standards. It also works toward limiting costs of health care services while assuring optimum quality.

Center for Disease Control

The Center for Disease Control (CDC) is responsible for the national attack on communicable and vector-borne diseases, and also certain other preventable but noninfectious conditions. CDC cooperates with state and local health departments to reduce the toll of illness and death from these conditions by providing them, on request, with specialized services that can be furnished best and most economically by a central agency. These services include the national surveillance of disease incidence and trends, epidemic aid, investigations of disease vectors and environmental health problems, laboratory reference diagnostic services for unusual problems, production of biological reagents that are unavailable commercially, and licensure of clinical laboratories engaged in interstate commerce. Laboratory services are supported by applied research to develop improved diagnostic and control methods and to establish national standards for performance of diagnostic procedures.

Much of CDC's technical and training assistance to health departments is delivered by personnel assigned directly to them or to the Department of Health, Education and Welfare regional offices. Among other services, CDC provides assistance and guidance to health departments that receive federal grants for control activities related to venereal disease, tuberculosis, childhood diseases preventable by immunization, lead paint poisoning, and urban rat problems. The CDC administers the foreign quarantine program, the national clearinghouse for smoking and health, and, in conjunction with the Department of Labor, certain occupational safety and health activities.

Other federal agencies, as well as volunteer health agencies, hospitals, and industries, often request and receive CDC's specialized services when they are confronted with problems that fall within the Center's range of competence. Because diseases can spread rapidly all over the globe as millions of people jet annually to faraway places, CDC functions as part of the international network for surveillance of diseases. Its objective is to locate, contain, and control outbreaks before they can spread to other countries. Many of CDC's medical and scientific personnel serve on various expert committees for the World Health Organization (WHO). Fifteen of CDC's laboratories have been designated by the World Health Organization as national, regional, or international reference centers in an international network of more than one hundred laboratories that collaborate on important disease problems.

Health Resources Administration

The Health Resources Administration (HRA), an agency of the United States Department of Health, Education and Welfare, was established in 1973. Part of the Public Health Service, the Health Resources Administration has the task of health planning, manpower training, and research and evaluation of health resources and resource needs. The agency combines manpower, research, planning, and statistical elements brought together from agencies of the old Health Services and Mental Health Administration and the National Institutes of Health. The HRA consists of three bureaus and a national center with varying but nonetheless interlocking responsibilities. The *Bureau of Health Services Research and Evaluation* has overall responsibility for development of health services research strategy within the Department of Health, Education and Welfare. The *Bureau of Health Manpower* focuses on production, distribution, and rationalization of human and physical resources in the health services field. The *National Center for Health Statistics* collects, analyzes, and disseminates data on vital events and health, including the physical, mental, and physiological characteristics of the population. The *Bureau of Health Planning and Resource Development* is responsible for developing health services plans for areas with populations of between 500,00 and 3 million persons. The mission of the *Health Resources Administration* is to help develop the nation's health care resources and to improve the use of those resources. The Administration is made up of three major bureaus: Health Statistics; Health Services Research and Evaluation; and Health Resources Development.

Alcohol, Drug Abuse and Mental Health Administration

The Alcohol, Drug Abuse and Mental Health Administration (A.D.A.M.H.A.), an agency of the United States Department of Health, Education and Welfare, was established in 1973. Part of the Public Health Service, A.D.A.M.H.A. administers three coequal institutes: a National Institute of Drug Abuse, a National Institute on Alcohol Abuse and Alcoholism, and the National Institute of Mental Health.

The *National Institute of Drug Abuse* is responsible for the administration of a program aimed at preventing and reducing drug abuse in the United States. Activities include the awarding of grants and contracts to states, localities, and institutions for research, treatment, and rehabilitation; and training and education programs. The newly created Institute reports an emphasis on international drug abuse issues (including collaborative research projects with several foreign countries and joint work with NATO nations and Mexico); and activity aimed at the drug abuse problems of children and youth, including exploring alternatives to drug use.

The *National Institute on Alcohol Abuse and Alcoholism* is the primary focal point for federal activities in the area of alcoholism. It is responsible for formulating and recommending national policies and goals regarding the prevention, control, and treatment of alcohol abuse and alcoholism, and for developing and conducting programs and activities aimed at these goals. Its most immediate goal is to assist in making the best treatment and rehabilitation services available at the community level. A longer range goal is to develop effective methods for preventing alcoholism and problem drinking. The Institute is fostering, developing, conducting, and supporting broad programs of research, training, and development of community services and public education.

The *National Institute of Mental Health,* established in 1946, has the mission of developing knowledge, manpower, and services to treat and rehabilitate the mentally ill and to promote the mental health of all Americans. Its programs, covering a whole range of problems relating to mental health, are carried out in partnership with the states, communities, professions, and thousands of concerned citizens. A dramatic drop in the public mental hospital population has been brought about through new approaches to care and through new treatment techniques, including the use of recently developed drugs and community-based outpatient facilities. Progress in mental health research, training, education, demonstration projects, and community services have contributed to the century's greatest reforms in the treatment and prevention of mental illness.

THE CHILDREN'S BUREAU

This Bureau was established in 1912 as a branch of the Labor Department, but it is now a division of the Social and Rehabilitation Service of the Department of Health, Education, and Welfare. Some of the activities of the Bureau include: (1) allocation of grants to the states for the promotion of maternal and child health, (2) allocation of grants to the states for crippled children and child welfare services, (3) allocation of research grants, (4) distribution of educational material relating to maternal and child health, (5) promotion of the White House conferences on children and youth (held at 10-year intervals since 1908), (6) conducting surveys and studies relating to child health problems, (7) allocating financial aid for specialized training projects, (8) cooperating and working with official and nonofficial organizations and institutions, and (9) serving as a center for the development of standards of care and protection for children in the United States.

Two of the major programs of the Children's Bureau are Maternal and Child

Health Services and Crippled Children Services. Appropriations are made to every state and territory to improve the health of children by giving care to the mother during pregnancy and birth and by supervising the health of the child during his growth and development. Funds provide for: (1) maternity clinics, in-patient hospital care for delivery in select cases, and dental treatment of expectant mothers, (2) well-child conferences, sometimes known as well-baby clinics, (3) school health services, consisting of physician examinations, checks for vision, hearing, and dental defects, and administering immunizations, (4) family planning, in which oral contraceptives and intrauterine devices are the most common methods selected, (5) mental retardation clinics and the prevention of increased retardation through early case-finding, (6) homemakers' services, foster home care, and day-care centers for children of employed mothers, (7) aid to unwed mothers, (8) case-finding and rehabilitation of children with defects (this covers the cost of diagnosis and medical and surgical treatment), and (9) educational programs in such things as family life and the hazards of smoking.

Some of the research studies funded by the Children's Bureau include juvenile delinquency, child care arrangements of working mothers, an analysis of infant and perinatal mortality, family planning, mental retardation, development of prostheses for children, nutritional status of preschool children, protective services for neglected, abused, and delinquent children, day and foster care services, adoption services, services to unmarried parents, and manpower utilization and training.

OTHER FEDERAL AGENCIES ENGAGED IN HEALTH WORK

Since public health involves disease prevention and prolonging life, and since health is defined as the social, mental, emotional, and physical well-being of individuals, it is not surprising that many agencies of the federal government are involved in some aspect of health. For example, the United States Office of Education, which is a branch of the Department of Health, Education, and Welfare, promotes health, safety, physical education, and recreation programs and services for the public schools throughout the United States. It also contributes information to the school health service program and the school lunch program. All the divisions of the Department of Health, Education, and Welfare are linked with health in some way. In general, the federal government is most concerned with interstate health protection and prevention of disease from abroad.

Various public health programs and services are offered by all federal departments. For instance, many branches of the Department of Agriculture, which functions to serve the farmer and the agriculture industry, either directly or indirectly contribute greatly to the knowledge of health and the prevention of disease. One branch of this Department, the Agricultural Research Administration, directs and coordinates the physical and biological research programs of the Department. Research is done in the fields of human nutrition, animal diseases, insecticides, control of insects affecting man and animals, antibiotics and serums for the control of animal diseases, and rural family housing programs. All have a direct bearing on health, medical knowledge of disease, and health practices.

A few other federal departments interested in public health include: the Department of Commerce, collecting and publishing basic statistics that are used widely in planning public health programs; the Department of Defense, responsible for medical care programs of military personnel and their dependents; the Department of the Interior, supervising health programs in the territories of the United States (various branches in this Department include the Bureau of Mines, which prevents health hazards and promotes safety, the Fish and Wildlife Service, which promotes programs for the destruction of rodents and elimination of stream pollution, and the National Park Service, which insures recreational sanitation); the Department of Justice, providing medical, psychiatric, dental, and nursing services to inmates of federal penal institutions; the Department of Labor, coordinating enforcement of wages, hours, child labor, and safety and health laws; the Department of State, supervising all international health programs; and the Department of the Treasury, enlisting the Bureau of Narcotics to investigate and detect violations of narcotic and related laws. These are only a few of the many agencies which contribute to the prevention of disease and prolonging of life.

ACTION

ACTION is the federal agency combining the Peace Corps, VISTA, and other voluntary agencies into a single force to deal with poverty-related social and economic problems in the United States and in developing countries.

Peace Corps

The Peace Corps was founded in 1961. Ever since, Peace Corps volunteers have been sharing their skills and training manpower in developing nations around the world. Many believe their success is due largely to their ability to relate to people while working together for a common purpose. In many instances, Peace Corps volunteers are the only Americans living and working as a part of local communities in these countries. They gain credibility and prove effective because they speak the local language, appreciate local customs, and adapt to living and working conditions that are considerably different from those they left at home. Peace Corps volunteers work to create a mutual understanding between Americans and the people they serve. As one volunteer states, "When there is no contact between the cultures, there is no understanding." With over 15 years of American contact via 50,000 Peace Corps volunteers, American understanding of other cultures and their understanding of ours has had a chance to grow.

Host countries value the unique contributions that the volunteers are making through their jobs. They especially appreciate the sensitive manner in which the volunteers pass on the technical skills that enable their people to solve their own problems, and which they in turn can pass along to their fellow countrymen. Medical doctors, nurses, dentists, and other health professionals in underdeveloped countries are encountering diseases that we had considered conquered long ago and fighting heroic battles against one of the world's most tragic enemies, malnutrition.

The Peace Corps has volunteers representing most medical specialties, including physicians, registered nurses, licensed practical nurses, dentists, dental hygienists, nursing instructors, medical technologists, occupational therapists, physical therapists, speech pathologists, x-ray technicians, pharmacists, public health administrators, biostatisticians, sanitarians, health educators, and epidemiologists. There are also volunteers who have no professional medical background but work in many disease eradication and control programs.

VISTA

VISTA volunteers serve on projects throughout the United States where special knowledge of the language and cultural tradition of the people served is needed. They serve recent immigrants and elderly ethnic residents in large cities, American Indians, Mexican Americans, Puerto Ricans, Portuguese Americans, and many other ethnic groups. VISTA volunteers in the health field serve on community-run health clinics in urban ghettos and rural poverty pockets—wherever they can bring better health services to the people. These services include preventive procedures and education as well as diagnosis and treatment. Volunteers include medical doctors, registered nurses, dentists, comprehensive health planners, community health workers, pharmacists, lab technicians, and others in related health fields such as nutrition and education.

WORLD HEALTH ORGANIZATION

The creation of the World Health Organization (WHO) in 1948 was the culmination of a long series of efforts made over the centuries to prevent the spread of disease from one continent to another and to achieve international cooperation for better health throughout the world. The organization occupies the status of a specialized agency in the frame-work of the United Nations. It is not necessary, however, for a country to be a member of the United Nations to be a member of WHO.

The World Health Organization has its headquarters in Geneva, Switzerland. It derives its authority from the 131 member states that have ratified its Constitution since 1948. It puts out a daily epidemiological radio bulletin, and conducts a medical research program, which includes projects in human reproduction, drug evaluation, and

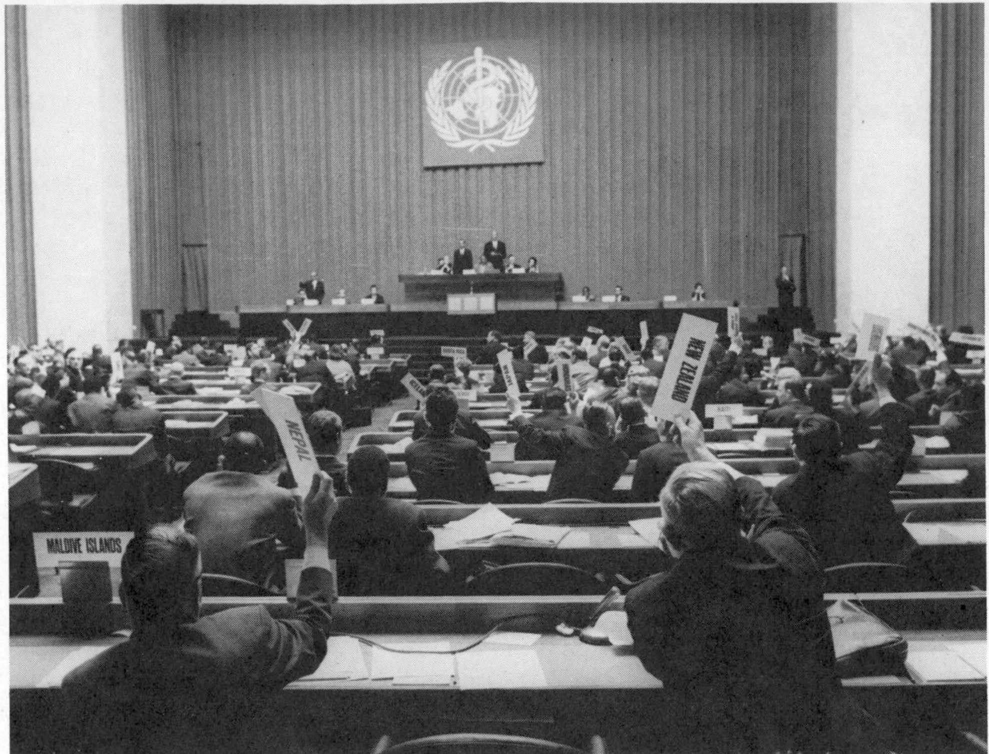

Figure 6–7 (From *WHO—Twenty Years of Work.* World Health Organization.)

environmental pollution. It gives technical assistance to improve sanitary conditions in over 100 countries, warns of outbreaks of epidemic disease, promotes and coordinates research, recommends international standards for drugs and vaccines, and is the world clearing house for medical and scientific information.

Central Technical Services

These form the basis of international health activities, and benefit all countries. Some of these services were taken from earlier international health organizations and have since been developed and extended by WHO. They include epidemiological intelligence and quarantine, international health statistics, standardization of therapeutic substances, atomic energy and health, health laboratory methods, and publication and documentation.

Epidemiological Intelligence and Quarantine. The adoption of the International Sanitary Regulations (1952), which replaced 13 out-of-date conventions, is an important accomplishment of WHO. International Sanitary Regulations apply to land, sea, and air traffic throughout the world. They provide the maximum protection against epidemics with minimum interference in international transport and travel.

The Epidemiological Intelligence Service collects information about the occurrence of disease anywhere in the world, and broadcasts information daily over an international radio network to health authorities, ports, airports, and ships at sea.

International Health Statistics. International health legislation, promulgated by the World Health Assembly, provides for uniform health statistics of diseases and causes of death, thereby making it possible to evaluate health problems more accurately, and therefore to adopt more effective public health measures. The list established by WHO comprises 999 categories of diseases, injuries and causes of death.

Standardization of Therapeutic Substances. Another important work of WHO is to recommend international standards for therapeutic substances. WHO has published the first International Pharmacopoeia that contains recommended specifications for use of drugs in all countries. WHO participates in international efforts for the control of drug addiction, and studies new synthetic drugs suspected of causing addiction.

Atomic Energy and Health. The World Health Organization has been instructed by its member states to study the health problems that arise from the use of atomic energy. Although the peaceful application of atomic energy will improve living conditions, it also threatens the health of workers in atomic establishments and of the general public; the amount of background radiation increases with the development of this source of power. Radioactive wastes, if not carefully disposed of, may pollute the air, soil, and water, and radiation may even have harmful effects on human heredity. In order to provide protection against these dangers, WHO, in cooperation with the atomic energy industry, has been requested to collect information and to advise governments and public health agencies regarding these dangers.

Health Laboratory Methods. WHO helps to establish public health laboratories, promotes simplification and standardization of techniques and diagnostic methods, and coordinates research on various laboratory investigations, including the potential dangers of chemical additives to food.

Publication and Documentation. WHO collects documentation on problems relating to health. It produces a considerable number of technical publications in the fields of health and medicine. A number of films are also available. For further information, write to World Health Organization, c/o American Public Health Association, 1015 18th Street, N.W., Washington, D.C. 20036.

WHO ADDRESSES

Africa P.O. Box 6, Brazzaville, Republic of the Congo

Americas Pan American Sanitary Bureau, 525 23rd Street, N.W., Washington, D.C. 20037, U.S.A.

Eastern Mediterranean P.O. Box 1517, Alexandria, United Arab Republic

Europe 8 Scherfigsvej, Copenhagen Ø, Denmark

South-East Asia World Health House, Indraprastha Estate, Ring Road, New Delhi-1, India

Western Pacific P.O. Box 2932, Manila, Philippines

How WHO Functions

The World Health Assembly is composed of delegates representing WHO member states and is the Organization's supreme governing body. It determines policies, votes on the annual program and budget, reviews the work done, and has the power to adopt regulations on international health questions such as quarantine requirements. Just as in the General Assembly of the United Nations, each member state has one vote. Meetings of the World Health Assembly are annual, lasting generally three weeks, and are attended by observers from many intergovernmental and nongovernmental international bodies concerned with health. The Executive Board of WHO is composed of 24 health specialists who serve on the Board for three years in an individual capacity. Eight of them are replaced every year, and it is the Health Assembly that selects the countries entitled to designate a person to serve on the Board. The Board prepares the work of the Health Assembly, gives effect to the Assembly's decisions, and may authorize emergency aid between meetings of the Assembly. Among other statutory tasks, it decides what nongovernmental organizations of member states may enter into official relations with WHO. It meets at least twice a year. The regional committees consist of representatives of the member states in the various regions. As a rule, their meetings take place once a year, usually in the autumn, when they review the work of their regional office and plan its continuation. Regional plans are amalgamated with plans for work at headquarters, and the resulting draft program goes forward in the first half of the following year to the Executive Board and then to the Health Assembly.

Voluntary Contributions. In 1955, the World Health Assembly established the Malaria Eradication Special Account and called on members and others to contribute so that malaria control could be intensified and the disease eradicated throughout the world. A Voluntary Fund for Health Promotion was created in 1960 to receive contributions to help finance the campaign against smallpox, to intensify medical research, to develop community water supplies, and to accelerate international assistance in the field of health to newly independent and emerging countries. Contributions can be made to this fund also for other specific health purposes. The fund has been used to carry out many health projects which could not be accommodated within the regular budget.

United Nations International Children's Emergency Fund (UNICEF). The General Assembly of the United Nations established UNICEF to meet emergency and long-range needs of children, particularly in underdeveloped countries. Much of its work is related to health.

In many projects, UNICEF and WHO collaborate closely, WHO being responsible for technical planning and advice and UNICEF for supplies. The two organizations cooperate in maternal and child health, in fighting malaria, tuberculosis, leprosy, yaws, and communicable eye diseases, in community water supplies, and in other fields. UNICEF also provides food, medical supplies, vaccination services, and demonstrations on the control of yaws and malaria.

WHO Throughout the World

Doctors, nurses, engineers, administrators, scientists, statisticians, interpreters, translators, secretaries, and others make up the staff of WHO. They are international civil servants recruited from many countries. The Director-General, from whom they take their instructions, is appointed by the World Health Assembly on nomination of the Executive Board. Regional Directors are appointed by the Board in agreement with the competent Regional Committee. Other staff members are appointed by the Director-General.

The Capital of WHO: Geneva

The first World Health Assembly met in 1948 and chose Geneva, Switzerland, as the location of the organization's headquarters. This is where the Director-General and his immediate staff work and where the world services of WHO are concentrated: international quarantine, the classification of diseases and causes of death, biological standardization, etc. Although the executive responsibility for projects of direct assistance to governments is decentralized to the WHO regional offices, technical units at headquarters have central advisory responsibilities. They contribute to WHO's medical research program, serve the WHO expert panels and advise regional offices on planning and methods. WHO headquarters also serves the World Health Assembly and the Executive Board, and fulfills overall administrative functions.

International Health Agencies

In the western hemisphere, the Pan American Sanitary Bureau was founded in 1902. It worked on health problems in both North and South America, particularly malaria and yellow fever eradication. After the organization of WHO, this Bureau became WHO's representing agency for the Americas. In 1960, PASB changed its name to Pan American Health Organization.

The Alliance for Progress, subscribed to by 18 nations in the Americas has the following objectives:

> Greater and more rapid progress in improving nutrition of the neediest groups of the population, taking advantage of all possibilities offered by national effort and international cooperation. Promotion of intensive mother and child welfare programs and of educational programs on overall family guidance methods.[20]

Emphasis is placed on modernizing the living conditions of rural populations, raising agricultural productivity in general, and increasing food production for the benefit of both Latin America and the rest of the world.

The Institute of Nutrition of Central America and Panama (INCAP) has developed and marketed a high-protein vegetable mixture called Incaparina. It has also stimulated studies of the use of indigenous plants as a source of protein, promoted iodinization of salt, and continued investigation of the extent of vitamin A deficiency and nutritional anemias. Basic research is being done on the interrelationship between nutrition and infection, malnutrition and mental and psychomotor development, and the effects of chronic inadequate nutritional intakes on adult work capacity.

The Caribbean Food and Nutrition Institute is under the auspices of local governments, the Pan American Health Organization, and the Food and Agriculture Organization. It is a center for training and research in the areas of food supplies and human nutrition.

There are other international agencies that carry on extensive programs. One is the International Development Agency, which is a part of the United States Government. The function of IDA is to provide military, economic, and technical assistance to nations desiring such aid. The Food and Agricultural Organization, which has its headquarters in Rome, works with the World Health Organization. Its purposes include the expansion of total food production, determination of ways by which the buying power of people in poor areas can be increased, and the improvement of distribution of foods between nations so that farm economics will be stabilized and starvation and surplus will not coexist. The Peace Corps volunteers work with people in underdeveloped countries to improve living conditions and the level of health.

VOLUNTARY HEALTH AGENCIES

Voluntary health agencies are supported by funds from public subscription, such as the Cancer Crusade, sale of Christmas Seals, March of Dimes, Heart Fund, and others. Funds are budgeted according to needs. The first voluntary health agency was the National Tuberculosis Association (now the American Lung Association), which had its beginning in Philadelphia in 1892.

Most of the major voluntary health agencies have a major national administrative office that is responsible for supervising and guiding the activities, functions, responsibilities, programs and projects of its state officers. The state office, in turn, aids the local offices. The local society is usually administered by a salaried executive secretary who efficiently organizes a board of directors that represent the entire county. One major committee of each agency is the health education committee. The function and selection of committee members for a typical local branch of the American Lung Association are shown in Table 6–1.

Services provided by these agencies include education, service, and research. Each agency stresses prevention through health education, and disseminates health information through films, pamphlets, television, radio, exhibits, and other media. The American Lung Association, the American Heart Association, and the American Cancer Society, in particular, have trained, professional, qualified public health educators on their staffs who assist individuals, schools, and community agencies and organizations in understanding and adopting preventive health measures.

Services offered by the voluntary agencies include such activities as first aid, water safety, and prenatal classes, offered by the American Red Cross; bandages, friendly home visits, limited aid to needy patients, and tumor clinics, offered by the American Cancer Society; chest x-rays and counseling to the patient and his family, offered by the American Lung Association; and sheltered workshops, rehabilitation clinics, weight control programs, and nutrition counseling offered by the American Heart Association. In recent years, the heart, cancer, and tuberculosis funds have devoted a major share of their public education programs to warning the public about the health hazards of smoking. It must be pointed out here that volunteer layworkers, physicians, and other professional persons give their time and support to all of these agencies, and many agencies frankly admit that effectiveness would decrease rapidly without volunteers.

The research aspect of the voluntary program is most rewarding and dramatic, as evidenced by the discovery of the Salk poliomyelitis vaccine. Dr. Jonas Salk and others were working under a research grant sponsored by the National Foundation for Poliomyelitis (now called the National Foundation). This agency is now directing its efforts toward viruses, congenital malformations, and arthritis. Thousands of public health research grants are awarded to individuals, schools, colleges, and universities by voluntary agencies each year. The American Heart Association, as well as many other voluntary agencies, also offers undergraduate and graduate scholarships to motivate and encourage students to work in the public

TABLE 6–1 A Health Education Committee for a Local American Lung Association

Functions

1. Assist in planning and implementing a health education program based on needs
2. Support and interpret the health education program to the public
3. Reflect public opinion, bring problems to attention of committee
4. Give skilled advice on health education techniques.

Group composition

It should be:

–representative of groups within the community (the "consumers," the "what-the-people-want" group)

–representative of persons who can give skilled advice on health education techniques (the "producers," the "how-to-do-it" folks).

The chairman of the health education committee could well be a member of the board of directors.

Selection of members

Members could be selected from the following:

Education	Director of health education, state department of education (for state association) School administrator P.T.A. representative Health educator in health department College person interested in health education Adult education or night school teacher Classroom teachers.
Physicians	The health officer A physician interested in health education A physician from the tuberculosis hospital A school physician.
Social and Nursing Service	Public health nurse Representative of welfare department.
Community Relations	Newspaper editor or reporter Representative from radio or TV station Representatives of various religious faiths Representative of service club Representative of Y.M.C.A. or similar organizations.
Business	Representative of labor and management.
Industry	Representative of management
Agriculture	Representative of farm group: Farm Bureau, Grange, Home Extension Service.
Special Groups	Foreign language groups Groups with high tuberculosis prevalence.

health field. Scholarships are available to physicians, nurses, educators, and other interested professional persons. For further information, contact your local voluntary health agency.

Types of Voluntary Agencies

Voluntary health agencies fall into several categories. Most important is a large group of agencies supported by citizen contributions and donations. Hanlon divides these into the following four types, which demonstrate a remarkable degree of specialization:

1. Agencies that are concerned with specific diseases, for example, the American Cancer Society, the American Heart Association, the American Lung Association, the National Foundation (poliomyelitis and birth defects), the American Social Hygiene Association (venereal diseases,

narcotics, and alcoholism), and the American Diabetic Society.

2. Agencies that are concerned with certain organs or structures of the body, for example, the National Society for the Prevention of Blindness, the American Society for the Hard of Hearing, the National Society for Crippled Children, and the American Heart Association.

3. Agencies that are concerned with the health and welfare of special groups in society, for example, the American Child Health Association (now extinct), the Maternity Center Association, and the American Negro Health Association (now the National Health Association).

4. Agencies that are concerned with particular phases of health and welfare, for example, the National Safety Council and the Planned Parenthood Federation of America.

Hanlon goes on to describe the other kinds of voluntary health agencies:

The second large group of voluntary agencies engaged in health work is composed of foundations established and financed by private philanthropy. Prominent among them are the Rockefeller Foundation, the W. K. Kellogg Foundation, the Carnegie Foundation, the Commonwealth Fund, the Johnson Foundation, the Milbank Memorial Fund, the Mott Foundation, the Rosenwald Fund, and the Markle Foundation. Organizations of this type have functioned in a variety of ways, particularly by promoting and subsidizing local health departments, especially those in rural areas, and by supporting basic research as well as public and professional education. The third main group of voluntary health agencies is made up of professional associations such as the American Public Health Association, the American Medical Association, the National League for Nursing, and their state and local affiliates. In addition to providing a meeting ground for professional workers in their respective fields, these associations do much to establish and improve standards and qualifications, encourage research, further health education, and promote programs.

Integrating agencies such as health councils and community chests and councils constitute what may be considered a fourth group. There are now more than 1000 of these multiple interest organizations. They are found on local, state, and national levels; their purpose is the coordination of the activities of the many specialized voluntary agencies. A fifth group of nonofficial agencies that may be considered to have some interest in the public health consists of an increasing number of commercial organizations that have found it worthwhile for one reason or another to participate in the promotion of sanitary and health habits and programs. Predominant among these are several of the large insurance companies that have carried out extensive and effective educational programs and demonstrations. Some activities have also been engaged in by industries concerned with the manufacture and sale of soap, sugar, milk, meat, eating and drinking utensils, and other products. Generally speaking, this latter group must be treated cautiously, since their programs are based primarily on a desire for increased profits and improved public relations.[21]

For a directory of National Voluntary Health Organizations, write Box D, Department of Health, AMA, 535 N. Dearborn Street, Chicago, Illinois.

The Gunn-Platt Report on Voluntary Health Agencies

The Gunn-Platt study listed eight basic functions of voluntary health agencies:

1. *Pioneering.* This involves exploring or surveying for needs not being served and for new methods of dealing with needs already recognized.

2. *Demonstration.* Voluntary health agencies have rendered particularly significant service by carrying out or subsidizing experimental projects designed to demonstrate practical methods for improvement of public health and for the wider application of proved methods by official and other agencies.

3. *Education.* This is probably the single most important function of voluntary health agencies; all other functions have education as their goal.

4. *Supplementation of Official Activities.* With no legislative restrictions to encumber them, the voluntary health agencies have very frequently found themselves in a position to augment the activities of official health departments.

5. *Guarding of Citizen Interest in Health.* Voluntary health agencies, because of their nature, representation, and support, have often found themselves in a position to guard the public interest not only by promoting the official health program but also by defending it against political interference.

6. *Promotion of Health Legislation.* In every state and community there is a constant stream of proposed legislation of concern to the public's health.

7. *Group Planning and Coordination.* These functions have been particular concerns of health councils and social agencies. With the development of many voluntary agencies in a community, there has resulted a great need for action in this field. Related to it is the need for increased coordination between the programs of the voluntary agencies and those of the official agencies in the community.

8. *Development of Well-Rounded Community Health Programs.* This is the total cumulative result

of the successful accomplishment of the foregoing purposes and functions. By protecting and promoting the official health department, by increasing the health consciousness and awareness of the community, and by support with funds and facilities, the voluntary health agency may make the difference between a mediocre community health program and one that is truly superior.[22]

Problems

Voluntary health organizations have given many persons an opportunity to become actively involved in serving members of their community. At the same time, it helps these volunteers to keep active and self-satisfied, and provides them with a feeling of community spirit and cooperation. Many organizations are responsive to the needs of the community, and have devoted members, a great degree of participation, easy access to positions of leadership, and a full voice in policy. Most important to health interests, of course, is that these group efforts lead to promotion of health and prevention of disease. There has been an increasing interest on the part of United Funds in setting up health foundations interested in medical research, service through donations to hospitals or other medical agencies, and community health education.

Voluntary health agencies, however, are not without their problems. Where voluntary agencies coexist with a governmental health department in a community (and this is the situation in almost all communities) frequently there is healthy competition. However,

> . . . there may be lack of cooperation, which is not so healthy. This may result in duplication of official and voluntary agency functions. The voluntary agency, usually being the older organization (particularly in reluctant communities) and made up of volunteers from the community, may look upon the newer health department as the usurper of its functions. The health department on the other hand may look down its organizational nose at the voluntary agency as being "nonprofessional." Such events need not happen. With an enlightened and active group of citizens interested in health and with emancipated health department personnel, they will not happen.[23]

A continuing major problem, however, revolves around fund-raising. Because of the growth of voluntary agencies, the demand for the charity dollar has become extremely competitive. Tax increases and growth in federal appropriations for health research have led many persons to establish impressive theories of organizational good and evil to disqualify the fund raiser without jeopardizing their own standing as philanthropists. In the interest of protecting the public against never-ending campaigns for funds in communities, consolidated fund-raising has been attempted by organizations such as Community Chest and United Fund. Those in favor of this plan argue that the health of a community is essentially a single interest with many different aspects. To promote one aspect of community health at the expense of other essential factors is unscientific, wasteful, and misleading. Furthermore, supporters of a single community charity campaign claim that more money can be raised in a single appeal with less annoyance to the donors. Such claims, though logical, receive considerable single agency opposition, and campaigns are rarely completely successful. Some major agencies continue to reject the United Fund approach in favor of a separate campaign. For example, the members of the American Cancer Society concluded that, although the United Fund idea is a sound method for raising money for strictly local services, it is not suited to mounting and increased national attack against cancer. Points that led to this conclusion include the following:

> 1. The great majority of the Society's units and divisions never participated in united funds. Of the Society's 3000 local units, only 15 per cent at a peak period were member agencies of united funds.
>
> 2. A six-year study comparing the financial growth of 54 units in federation with the units outside of federation showed that, while those conducting independent crusades showed increases of 94 per cent during this period, those in federation showed increases of only 46 per cent.
>
> 3. In situations where units were member agencies of united funds, the Society's nationwide research program plans were being judged by non-medical, non-scientific laymen on local budget committees who were not qualified to recommend the essential funds needed for a nationwide attack against cancer.
>
> 4. United funds have no organizational machinery nationally for evaluating and implementing nationwide programs of organizations like the American Cancer Society.
>
> 5. The Society would have agreed to retain the status quo of 15 per cent of its units in federation and 85 per cent independent. But some local united funds, ill-equipped to meet the budgetary

250 Agencies and Services will share in Your Gift

American Red Cross
Chester-Wallingford Chapter
Southeastern Pennsylvania Chapter
(14 branches)
Central Montgomery County
Chester Pike
Eastern Delaware County
Main Line
Metropolitan
Northeast
Northwest
Old York Road
Swarthmore
Upper Main Line
Wayne
West
Western Delaware County
Wissahickon
American Social Health Association
Arthritis Foundation
Eastern Penna. Chapter
Associated Day Care Service
Big Brother Association
Boy Scouts of America—Chester Co. Council
Boy Scouts of America—Philadelphia Council
Boy Scouts of America—Valley Forge Council
Chestnut Hill Hospital
Child Development Center
Child Guidance and Mental Health Clinics of Delaware County
Child Psychiatry Clinic and Child Study Center of Philadelphia at St. Christopher's Hospital
Children and Family Service—Episcopal Community Services
Children's Aid Society of Montgomery County
Children's Aid Society of Pennsylvania
Children's Heart Hospital of Philadelphia
Children's Service
College Settlement of Philadelphia
Community Health Association
Community Nursing Service, Delaware Co.
Community Services of Pennsylvania
Conshohocken Free Library
Council on Social Work Education
Crime Prevention Association
R. W. Brown Boys' Club
South Philadelphia Boys' Club
West Philadelphia Boys' Club
West Philadelphia Girls' Club
Defender Association of Philadelphia
Delco Child Day Care Association
Diagnostic and Rehabilitation Center/Philadelphia, The
Diversified Community Services

Episcopal Hospital
Family Service of Delaware County
Family Service of the Main Line Neighborhood
Family Service—Mental Health Centers of Chester County
Family Service of Montgomery County
Family Service of Philadelphia
Federation of Jewish Agencies
Association for Jewish Children
Community Medical Home Care Program
Downtown Children's Center
Eagleville Hospital and Rehabilitation Center
Einstein Medical Center
(Northern and Samuel H. Daroff Divisions)
Female Hebrew Benevolent Society
Golden Slipper Club Camp
Home and Hospital for the Jewish Aged
J. W. B. Armed Services & Veterans Committee—USO
Jewish Employment and Vocational Service
Jewish Family Service
Jewish Y's and Centers of Greater Philadelphia
Moss Rehabilitation Hospital
Philadelphia Psychiatric Center
Rebecca Gratz Club
S.G.F. Vacation Camp
Samuel Paley Day Care Service
Vacation Bureau
Fellowship House of Conshohocken
Florence Crittenton Service of Philadelphia
Freedom Valley Girl Scout Council
Friends Neighborhood Guild
George Washington Carver Community Center —Norristown
Germantown Boys' Club
Germantown Dispensary and Hospital
Germantown Settlement
Girl Scouts of Delaware County
Girl Scouts of Philadelphia
Graduate Hospital of the University of Penna.
Greater Phila. Federation of Settlements
Hahnemann Medical College Hospital
Health and Welfare Council
Delaware County District
Montgomery County District
North Central District
Northeast District
Northwest District
Southern District

West District
Community Information and Referral Service
Council on Volunteers
National Social Welfare Assembly
Health and Welfare Council of Chester County
Homemaker Service of Chester County
Homemaker Service of Delaware County
Homemaker Service of the Metropolitan Area
Horizon House
Hospital of the Medical College of Penna.
Hospital of the University of Pennsylvania
Housing Association of Delaware Valley
Inter-Church Child Care Society
International Social Service, American Branch
Jane D. Kent—St. Nicholas Day Care Centre
Jewish Community Center—Norristown
Legal Aid Society of Philadelphia
Lighthouse, The
Lutheran Social Mission Society
Memorial Hospital, Roxborough
Mental Health Assn. of Southeastern Penna.
Mercy-Douglass Hospital
Montgomery County Homemaker—Home Health Aide Service
Montgomery County Mental Health Clinics
Montgomery Hospital
National Committee on Employment of Youth
National Council on Crime and Delinquency, Penna. Council
National Recreation and Park Association
Nationalities Service Center of Philadelphia
Neighborhood League of the Upper Main Line (Public Health Nursing Service)
Nicetown Club for Boys and Girls
North Light Boys' Club
North Penn Visiting Nurse Association
Northeast Boys' Club
Northeastern Hospital of Philadelphia
Pennsylvania Hospital
Pennsylvania Mental Health
Pennsylvania Prison Society
Philadelphia Center for Older People
Philadelphia Child Guidance Clinic
Philadelphia Mouth Hygiene Association
Philadelphia Society to Protect Children
Retired Citizens Community Centers
Riverview Osteopathic Hospital—Norristown
Sacred Heart Hospital—Norristown
St. Christopher's Hospital for Children
St. Luke's and Children's Medical Center

Salvation Army
51 Services in the area include:
Booth Memorial Hospital
Camp Ladore (Fresh Air Camp)
Community Centers (7)
Corps Units (9)
Correctional Service Bureau
Day Camp (Norristown)
Family Service Bureau
Harbor Light Corps
Ivy House (Children's Home)
Men's Social Service Center
Missing Persons Bureau
Mobile Emergency and Disaster Canteens (5)
Music Department
Overnight Lodge (Norristown)
Service Extension to Outlying Areas
Settlement and Day Care Center
Thrift Stores (9)
Women's Emergency Service (Norristown)
Women's Service Bureau for the Armed Forces:
Red Shield Club, Philadelphia
Servicemen's Lounge (International Airport)
Central Volunteer Bureau
Home League Department
League of Mercy
Senior Citizens Program
Valley Forge Military Hospital Program
Senior Adult Activities Center of Montgomery County
Settlement Music School
Shut-In Society, Pennsylvania Branch
Southern Home for Children
Stephen Smith Home for the Aged
Stetson Hospital of Philadelphia
Temple University Hospital
Thomas Jefferson University Hospital
Travelers Aid Society
USO of Philadelphia
United Cerebral Palsy Association of Philadelphia and Vicinity
United Cerebral Palsy of Delaware County
United Communities, Southeast Philadelphia
United Health Services
United Seamen's Service
Urban League of Philadelphia
Visiting Nurse Association of Conshohocken

Visiting Nurse Association of Eastern Montgomery County
Visiting Nurse Association—Norristown
Visiting Nurse Society of Philadelphia
Wharton Centre
Wissahickon Boys' Club
Women's Christian Alliance
Young Men's Christian Association of Germantown
Young Men's Christian Association—Norristown
Young Men's Christian Association of Philadelphia and Vicinity:
Abington Branch
Ambler Branch
Armed Services Branch
Camp Branch
Central Branch
Christian Street Branch
Columbia Community Branch
Community "Y", Eastern Delaware County
Main Line Branch
North Branch
Northeast Family Branch
Parkside Community Branch
Penn Center Academy
Reed House
Roxborough Area
West Branch
York Road Area
Young Women's Christian Association of Central Montgomery County
Young Women's Christian Association of Germantown
Young Women's Christian Association of Philadelphia:
Community "Y", Eastern Delaware County
Cooperative Living Residence
Crozer Residence
Frankford Branch
Kensington Branch
Mid-City Branch
North Central Branch
Northeast Center
Southwest-Belmont Branch
Spring Garden Center
Youth Service

Figure 6–8 (Courtesy of Philadelphia, Pa., United Fund Brochure, 1971.)

requirements of the Society, were exerting undue pressures on the 85 per cent to join.

6. The Society's crusade is completely different from a United Fund drive. The sole purpose of the latter is to raise money. The crusade is both a life-saving education effort and an effort to raise funds. The former is vital to the fight against cancer. Life saving is a responsibility of the individual, who must take the step of seeing his physician for early detection and diagnosis. People must be informed about cancer.

7. The Society's program must be accelerated at a much faster rate than united funds can sustain. The rich promises in research, education, and service need a greater investment of funds than ongoing welfare services that are the touchstone for the determination of united fund goals.

8. In many American communities, units of the American Cancer Society which raise money independently work harmoniously with united funds. Volunteer leaders help raise money for both interests and contribute to both interests. The Society believes firmly that this live-and-let-live behavior pattern is a practice which can be achieved in many more local areas of the country.

The American Heart Association has also expressed its view of these matters:

> The educational value of the independent campaign is largely lost in federated fund raising. Although there are those who say that an educational campaign could be conducted in February apart from any fund-raising effort, neither past experience nor an examination of the practicality of such a plan would indicate that this is so. It is doubtful whether the army of... volunteers... recruited... to conduct the Heart Sunday campaign could have been secured only for the purpose of distributing educational material from house to house. . . . By charting the inquiries received at the national headquarters, it is clear the impact which the campaign has on the public, for it reveals that inquiries reach a peak during and immediately after the campaign, which is far above the number of inquiries at any other time of year. In 1955 it was interesting to note that although the number of inquiries rose following President Eisenhower's heart attack, nevertheless, this rise was not as great as that which takes place each year at campaign time. In other words, we not only know that a great deal of educational material goes to the public during campaign time, but we also are certain that this stimulates their interest in the problems of heart disease. . . . A problem with the scope represented by cardiovascular diseases cannot be budgeted by local committees in individual communities throughout the country. It is self-evident that a group of citizens in any given community could not determine what amount of money the American Heart Association needed from that community in order to carry on its program.

Dr. Robert W. Wilkins, former president of the American Heart Association, says:

> Our chapters participating in united funds were losing organizational vitality, showed a definite lessening of volunteer interest upon which a democratically run organization such as ours is wholly dependent, the program was being curtailed and the amount of money being raised was markedly less than that being raised by our Associations which conducted independent campaigns. These unfavorable results we now believe are inherent in the 'united way' of raising and allocating funds. As we have seen it the 'united way' approaches taxation in its mechanical and, not always subtle, coercive technique of raising and allocating funds. This technique is usually under the control of powerful, locally-oriented citizens, mostly industrialists, who arbitrarily allocate funds raised primarily through payroll check-offs. These citizens are less concerned with, if not totally ignorant of, nationally coordinated programs of medical research. Therefore they tend to favor the local charities over the national health agencies.
>
> The dissension and controversy has cast a shadow over the entire field of philanthropy. The older established agencies with well-developed and effective fund-raising techniques do not wish to give up their stamp sales or their seasonal drives which have become familiar to and accepted by the public. The newer and smaller agencies are more willing to join a united fund-raising effort and to accept their share of the pot. This development has resulted in a schism within the voluntary agency ranks: the independents and the united fund adherents. The battle has been marked by emotional accusations on both sides, resulting in a possible loss of prestige of both. It has been my observation that if agencies can cooperate first in regard to carrying out a community health program in a successful way, then perhaps this may lead to further cooperation in regard to how they may obtain their funds with greater efficiency and with less annoyance to the public.[23]

In addition to stimulating public and government interest in specific health problems, each voluntary agency and each drive offers a person a chance to put his charity dollars where he feels they will do the most good. Furthermore, private health funds do many important things that government agencies are unable to do. They can often move more quickly and take more risks than a government agency can. Thus, they are in a position to pioneer new frontiers of research, to experiment, and to develop new methods.

One problem is that there is sometimes

a tendency for contributions to flow most liberally to diseases that are most readily dramatized—particularly those which affect children. This sometimes results in serious imbalances. For example: alcoholism afflicts 10 times as many Americans as does cerebral palsy, but the United Cerebral Palsy Association generally receives many times as much in public contributions as the National Council on Alcoholism. Also, about 200,000 Americans suffer from muscular dystrophy; more than 9 million have serious mental illnesses—but the Muscular Dystrophy appeal brings in about as much each year as the public contributes to the National Association for Mental Health.

The most striking example of the American public's tendency to keep giving to an organization which has captured its emotional fancy is the Seeing Eye, Inc. It was organized in 1929 to train and provide guide dogs for the blind. Experience soon demonstrated that the vast majority of blind people (particularly the elderly) do not want or are not able to use guide dogs. But the Seeing Eye project had won the public's heart, and contributions continued to mount—even after the agency announced in 1959 that it was discontinuing public solicitations. Result: Seeing Eye, Inc., now has about $19 million saved in banks and securities, and its $2 million annual income from these reserves and from unsolicited contributions and bequests is nearly twice what it is able to spend on guide dogs, even though it searches the country diligently for blind people who want them. Meanwhile, the National Society for Prevention of Blindness, which sponsors glaucoma screening tests and conducts a valuable program of public education on preventing blindness, struggles along on an income of $1.3 million a year.

In any case, most authorities agree that the voluntary agencies will continue to flourish and to offer the public and its governments the kind of creative leadership and vital services that have distinguished these agencies for many years.

Agency Evaluation

Most people get almost daily appeals for funds. And each one raises the question: How do you distinguish between the worthy and the unworthy organizations? It is an important question, because last year Americans gave charities $60 million a day, or a total of nearly $22 billion, establishing an all-time record for generosity.

Even well-known national charities have not been above reproach. The reputation of the Sister Kenny Foundation was ruined when the activities of its dishonest operators were uncovered. They were later convicted of mail fraud and conspiracy. The Disabled American Veterans Organization has been severely criticized for the excessive fund-raising costs of its mailings of unsolicited miniature auto license tags. The National Foundation, known as the March of Dimes (originally the National Foundation for Infantile Paralysis), has been criticized because of excessive costs for fund raising and administration as well as for possible conflict of interest in fund disbursements; also, for six years it did not announce the change of status of its president from volunteer to paid employee. Other well-known national charities have not provided the full financial reports requested by such monitoring agencies as the Council of Better Business Bureaus.

In 1973 investigators for the Senate Subcommittee on Children and Youth, headed by Democratic Senator Walter F. Mondale of Minnesota, came up with substantial evidence that all is not as it should be in the charity field. The committee revealed that only 10 per cent of the $3.1 million collected by the Epilepsy Foundation of America in 1973 went for direct help to epileptics, and only 3 per cent went for research. By its own figures, more than 40 per cent of the money it received went to meet fund-raising costs, a much higher percentage than that reported by such well-known charities as the American Heart Association (15 per cent) and the National Multiple Sclerosis Society (19 per cent).

Most people know of the National Tuberculosis and Respiratory Disease Association (renamed the American Lung Association), a pioneer in the health agency field and famous for its Christmas seals. The Association deserves credit for its role in helping reduce the prevalence and effects of active tuberculosis. In recent years the Association has added other lung diseases such as chronic bronchitis and emphysema to its program. But critics point out that although chronic bronchitis and emphysema are serious and prevalent, they cause significantly fewer deaths than several other diseases fought with inadequate funds. They note, too, that assets of the Association and its chapters now exceed $55 million. Over 90 per cent of these funds, most of which go for operating expenses, are in the hands of local chapters, not all of which, say the critics, are spending their funds to the best advantage.

Organizations of professional fund raisers, such as the American Association of Fund Raising Council and the National Society of Fund Raisers, as well as independent monitoring agencies like the National Information Bureau and the Council of Better Business Bureaus, have established ethical standards by which they judge charitable organizations and fund appeals. The following are standards to which all reputable nonprofit charitable organizations should adhere:

1. Fund-raising and administrative costs should be reasonable. There is no easy agreement on what is reasonable, but reputable professional fund raisers feel that a well-established organization should spend less than 25 per cent of the funds it collects for fund raising. The best-managed agencies spend far less, sometimes only about 10 per cent, and in the case of capital campaigns of leading universities and hospitals, perhaps only 4 or 5 per cent. A new charity with special start-up costs might exceed 25 per cent in its first few years, but then fund-raising costs should begin to come down. If administrative expenses together with fund-raising costs continue to absorb as much as half of every dollar contributed, the organization's efficiency in achieving its presumably worthy purpose should be questioned.

2. Full and truthful financial disclosure should be made on request and should clearly indicate fund-raising and administrative costs. The accounts should be audited annually. Even detailed financial data doesn't necessarily show that a charity is effectively operated.

3. The organization should have an active and responsible governing board whose members serve without pay, meet regularly, and control the administration of the charity and its funds. A letterhead filled with "important" names doesn't necessarily mean much. Although many prominent people serve on charity boards with dedication, others accept board membership indiscriminately and may even be unaware of the true nature of the enterprise to which they are lending their names. Among those formerly listed on the "honorary advisory board" of the American Kidney Fund (not to be confused with the National Kidney Foundation) were four Senators, four Congressmen, former New York City Mayor John V. Lindsay, and entertainer Barbra Streisand. This fund asks for help to "pay for more kidney machines and more treatment for people with kidney failure." However, only five cents of every dollar raised has gone directly to help in this way.

4. The charity should work effectively toward a legitimate goal and should avoid duplication of the work of other reputable organizations.

5. The charity's promotion and fund-raising practices should not be questionable; that is, the charity should *never*:

a. Pay commissions or percentages to fund raisers.
b. Use overstated emotional appeals or exaggerated claims about its purpose or accomplishments.
c. Condone pressure on business clients or associates, customers or employees to make "voluntary" contributions.
d. Mail unordered merchandise with a request for money in return.
e. Raise funds by general telephone solicitation.
f. Use recognition devices such as pins and buttons in public places or canisters passed through captive audiences where nongivers would be conspicuous.
g. Mail solicitations that look like bills. Postal regulations now require that such letters note that the material is a solicitation and that no money is due.

6. The organization should make available to anyone requesting them a budget and an annual report that includes an audit prepared by an independent certified public accountant. Even detailed financial data don't necessarily show that a charity is efficiently run. Twenty-three states, the District of Columbia, and several dozen cities do have laws regulating charities, but most of these are ineffectual, unenforceable, or unenforced.

Money wisely given will not only reach those who need it most but will also discourage incompetent or unethical charities.

Sources of Information

Here are some ways we can learn more about a charity:

1. Write directly to the national office of a charity and ask to see a report that shows (a) what percentage of the funds raised actually goes to beneficiaries of the cause and (b) other data you can use to evaluate the agency. A critic of charity ethics recently requested financial reports from 80 charities that solicit donations in this country to help people abroad. He received financial data from fewer than two-fifths of them; general information, but no financial report, from over two-fifths; and nothing at all from one-

fifth. A charity's response to your inquiry can be a quick clue to its worthiness.

However, keep in mind that financial facts may be obscure or misleading. Even if they're clear, you probably won't be able to tell from the report of a charity whether its efforts duplicate those of other agencies, whether its fund-raising practices are ethical, or how effective it is.

2. Consult the Council of Better Business Bureaus, Solicitations Review Section, 1150 17th Street, N.W., Washington, D.C. 20036. The CBBB collects information on charities soliciting funds nationally and internationally. It does not rate them, but maintains files on more than 5000 agencies and supplies objective information with which you may be able to judge a charitable organization. You can obtain available CBBB reports free through your local Better Business Bureau or the CBBB.

3. Join the National Information Bureau, 305 E. 45th Street, New York, New York 10017. The NIB is a nonprofit independent monitoring organization that reports on about 500 national and international organizations that solicit funds from the public. It provides background information not usually available in the charities' own reports and evaluates them according to its eight basic standards. Reports are available only to NIB members on a confidential basis. The minimum membership costs $15 a year for an individual and $25 for a corporation, and entitles you to NIB reports on any of the organizations it evaluates.

4. Check with your city or state government. About half of the states and a number of cities require some form of registration of licensing of charities that solicit there. In nine states and some cities, charities are further required to file annual financial reports along the lines of nationally recognized uniform accounting standards. Few of these laws set standards, and registration alone does not necessarily deter charity operators from violating the bounds of ethical conduct.

THE AMERICAN MEDICAL ASSOCIATION

Founded in 1847, the American Medical Association has as its primary mission the advancement of the art and science of medicine. It promotes and maintains professional standards through various committees. It supports a Bureau of Health Education, which has many kinds of educational programs. *Family Health* magazine now incorporates *Today's Health,* which was formerly published by the AMA. This monthly magazine is devoted to the latest information on health, nutrition, and preventive medicine, and can

United or Federated Fund Raising

PROPONENTS OF FEDERATED FUND RAISING BELIEVE—	OPPONENTS BELIEVE FEDERATED FUND DRIVES JEOPARDIZE THESE PRINCIPLES—
1. It provides a balanced approach to meeting health and welfare needs.	1. The right of human beings to organize themselves for direct action against social problems.
2. It eliminates duplication of agency services through centralized budget control and cooperative community organization approach to determining needs and rendering services.	2. The right of such social organizations to control their own policies, programs, and budgets.
3. It enables agencies, relieved of time-consuming fund raising responsibilities, to devote more time to program and service.	3. The right of the individual, after private negotiation with his conscience, to give time and money to any cause that pleases him.
4. It eliminates the annoyance and confusion of separate and often-times competing campaigns.	4. The right of the individual to withhold support from any cause in which he lacks personal interest.
5. It reduces the cost of fund raising by consolidating the costs of many appeals in a single operation.	5. The impermissibility of employer interference in the personal affairs of their employees (in this case, their philanthropic affairs).
6. It conserves time by concentrating volunteer participation in a single effort.	6. The ethical outlook that places the needs of the recipient above the convenience of the giver.
7. It provides a method for fair distribution of funds, through annual budget review, to local and national agencies alike.	7. The duty of government to meet, through tax-supported activity, whatever social needs are not met through voluntary activity.[24]
8. It provides a method for dividing most equitably among all communities the support of national agencies whose services benefit the entire community.	
9. It represents a pattern of giving more acceptable to most people.	

be obtained by subscription at $5.97 per year. (Write to Family Health Magazine, 149 Fifth Ave., New York, N.Y. 10010.) The staff also will answer general questions about health and medical problems. Many pamphlets, films, and posters representing many areas of health are available at a small cost from the Association. Another program is devoted to school health. Every two years is a Conference on Physicians and Schools, which concerns itself with school health services. Many local member associations maintain school health committees that work closely with school personnel to plan and promote programs.

Another activity of the AMA is the Institute for Biomedical Research, established in 1965 by the American Medical Association Education and Research Foundation, which also sponsors a medical student loan program and distributes funds to medical schools, hospitals, and universities, In the Institute, "scientists and technicians search for basic information involved in understanding of life and disease: how the normal cell works, how it sends 'signals' to other cells, and how its function is altered by diseases of many kinds." In 1968, the Institute had 30 scientists. Hanlon reports that:

> Research freedom such as that granted at the Institute would hardly be possible under government grants, which support almost all research carried on today in American universities, hospitals, and institutes. The Institute for Biomedical Research is unique in that it is supported entirely by voluntary contributions from private physicians, other interested individuals, and private organizations.[25]

THE AMERICAN PUBLIC HEALTH ASSOCIATION

Each of the medical and paramedical specialties or groups usually has its own professional association which assists in improving and maintaining the standards of their members. APHA, founded in 1872, draws its members from different disciplines, and its purposes are "to identify objectively the health needs of the American people and to formulate a public policy posture with respect to health issues, and to provide for the collective evaluation by health workers of technical and professional matters related to health as a basis for improving the utilization of health knowledge." The promotion of professional education is accomplished by (1) publication of the *American Journal of Public Health,* (2) production of authoritative manuals of procedure in nearly all phases of public health work, (3) establishment of statements of standards for examination of water, food, and housing, (4) accreditation of graduate schools of public health in North America and defining the educational qualifications for various professional categories, and (5) objective testing through their Professional Examination Service, which is available to interested agencies. Most tests are used by merit system and civil service agencies in the selecting of employees. Some tests are used by state examining boards in such fields as medicine, veterinary medicine, and physical therapy.

The Association stimulates research through providing personnel to cooperate in research programs, providing funds, and sponsoring programs. In order to reduce the time lag between the discovery of data and their application, regional institutes are held throughout the country. (This is done cooperatively with other official and nonofficial agencies.) Officers and members of the organization maintain close liaison with official agencies, legislators, and congressional committees. Professional advice and support are available on proposed health legislative matters. Some of the health legislature to be considered includes concentrating federal health responsibilities in a more effective, coordinated organizational structure, through the establishment of a National Department of Health and Welfare; strengthening and carrying out comprehensive health planning for state and local health programs through provision of more adequate federal bloc grant funding to further augment state and local support of their programs; re-establishing the essential health protection element of water pollution control by taking that program from the control of Department of the Interior and returning it to the Department of Health, Education, and Welfare; continuing and extending federal programs for encouragement of health facility planning and construction, with needed state participation; and increasing federal effort in the recruitment and training of health personnel.

THE NATIONAL HEALTH COUNCIL

The coordinating body at the national level is the National Health Council. It provides the structure that welds together all efforts for health at the national level.

The Council has three principal functions: helping member agencies work more effectively together in the common interest; helping to identify, call attention to, and promote solutions of national health problems; and promoting better state and local health services, whether governmental or voluntary. A continuing work of the Council is the promotion of state and local health councils, similar in action to the national council. It is through these councils that groups can work together, identify needs for services, and carry out effective planning.

The functions of the National Health Council include promoting health education, serving as a clearinghouse for public health information, developing new state and local health councils, assisting all such councils, promoting full-time local health departments, offering a consultant service on community health and other services to individuals and groups, and coordinating the activities of the national health agencies. One of the most significant recent contributions is the sponsorship of the Health Career Horizons Project and the distribution of health career publications. The National Health Council is the medium for community organization at the national level. The National Health Council also sponsors the National Health Forum and assists in the important community studies undertaken by the National Commission on Comprehensive Community Health Care, 1740 Broadway, New York, New York 10019.

FEDERATION OF WORLD HEALTH FOUNDATIONS

A newly organized attack on disease and suffering among peoples in developing countries was launched in 1972. The W. K. Kellogg Foundation of Battle Creek, Michigan, financed the initial organization of the Federation of World Health Foundations with a grant of $1.3 million. An agreement with World Health Organization authorities in Geneva makes that organization's professional and technical expert assistance available to the new system. Headquarters of the Federation of World Health Foundations is at 1211 Geneva 27, Switzerland, with a branch office in Los Angeles. The United States Division of the Federation of World Health Foundations has its office in Houston. Through the participation of so many financially strong corporations and corporate foundations, it is evident that this new private organization for medical aid to developing nations will be a strong and active organization that will supplement the efforts of separate governments and of such public organizations as the World Health Organization.

THE PROFESSIONAL ORGANIZATIONS

Many professional agencies are organized on a national, state, or local basis, and furnish a wide variety of information and service. These organizations are financially supported by professional membership fees, donations, professional magazine sales, educational materials, and books. Each of these organizations is usually staffed by specialists in their particular field. They help develop new methods and materials, conduct studies and research, promote professional standards, and publish educational journals and data. A few such professional organizations are:

American Association for Health, Physical Education, and Recreation, a Department of the National Education Association, 1201 16th St., N.W., Washington, D.C.

American Association of School Administrators, a department of the National Education Association.

American Council on Education, 744 Jackson Place, Washington, D.C.

American Dental Association, 222 East Superior St., Chicago, Ill.; National Foundation, 800 Second Ave., New York, N.Y.

American Medical Association, 535 N. Dearborn St., Chicago, Ill.

American Public Health Association, 1015 18th St., N.W., Washington, D.C.

American Social Health Association, 1790 Broadway, New York, N.Y.

Association for Childhood Education, International, 1200 15th St., N.W., Washington, D.C.

National Committee for Mental Hygiene, 1790 Broadway, New York, N.Y.

National Council on Family Relations, 1126 East 59th St., Chicago, Ill.

National Council on Schoolhouse Construction, George Peabody College for Teachers, Nashville, Tenn.

National Education Association, 1201 16th St. N.W., Washington, D.C.

National Health Council, 1790 Broadway, New York, N.Y.

National Safety Council, 429 N. Michigan Ave., Chicago, Ill.

National Society for the Prevention of Blindness, 1790 Broadway, New York, N.Y.
National Society for the Study of Education, 5835 Kimbark Ave., Chicago, Ill.
National Society of State Directors of Health, Physical Education, and Recreation, State Department of Education, Los Angeles, Calif.
American Lung Association, 1790 Broadway, New York, N.Y.
United States Office of Education, Washington, D.C.
SIECUS (Sex Information and Education Council of the United States), 1855 Broadway, New York, N.Y.

QUESTIONS FOR DISCUSSION

1. Define public health.
2. List and briefly discuss the six basic services of a local health department.
3. "Since we have state health departments, it is not necessary to have local health departments." Comment upon this statement.
4. What factors led to the creation of your state health department? Local health department?
5. Briefly discuss the significance of the following acts in relation to public health:
   (a) Sheppard-Towner Act
   (b) Hill-Burton Act
   (c) Social Security Act, Titles V and VI
   (d) Marine Hospital Service Act.
   (e) National Quarantine Act
6. Draw and label the organization and administration of your state health department.
   (a) How is it financed?
   (b) Briefly describe the major services and functions of each of the divisions.
7. Draw and label the organization and administration of the Department of Health, Education, and Welfare.
8. Briefly discuss the services of the World Health Organization.
9. List five major voluntary health agencies in your community. What do these agencies have in common? What services does each agency offer?
10. "We must gear our public health programs and services to the changing community problems." Briefly discuss this statement.
11. "Each member of the health department staff is a health educator." Briefly discuss this statement.
12. How can we attract more and better qualified personnel in public health?
13. Briefly discuss the basis of financial support of local health departments.
14. List the major expenditure for:
    (a) federal health programs
    (b) state health programs
    (c) local health programs
15. Describe the administrative set-up of your local public health department. Describe the activities that they offer to the community.
16. Describe the activities of your State Public Health Department. Distribute samples of the Bulletin used by your State Health Department.
17. List the voluntary and professional health organizations in your community.
18. Discuss with local officials the problems in drug investigation and control.
19. Why is group action necessary to help provide health services in a community?
20. What organizations in your community contribute to environmental health? Public health? Consumer protection?
21. How does WHO help control environmental health in the various countries it serves?
22. What are the requirements for a career in sanitation? Health Education? Dental hygiene? Medicine? Nursing? Dentistry?

QUESTIONS FOR REVIEW

1. What are the two main objectives of a health department?
2. According to the Arden House Task Force, what are the three major areas of responsibility of a health agency?
3. List six broad categories that are essential activities of a local health department.
4. What are the two major services performed by the vital statistics division of a health department?
5. What are the three main aspects of disease control?
6. What are the major factors in the field of public health?
7. Give four examples of a nonofficial health agency in which a community health nurse might function.
8. What are five major jobs related to the preparation for school which the public health nurse performs?
9. What is the major part of a sanitarian's job?
10. What are the goals of a social worker's provision of consultation?
11. How is a physically handicapped child defined by the Crippled Children Services Program?
12. How is the Crippled Children Services Program funded?
13. According to recent studies, of how much value are the routine and periodic physical examinations of schoolchildren in disclosing important health problems not previously known?
14. How does the school health program help children?
15. What are the three key concepts of school health education?

16. Explain why it is said that many health workers are "afraid to step on someone's toes."
17. What are four of the citizens' responsibilities toward the objectives of preventing disease and promoting health?
18. How many years does a term for a member of the State Board of Public Health last and how does a member come into office?
19. Which two constituents of the U.S. Department of Health, Education and Welfare make grants-in-aid to the states for health purposes?
20. How are local health departments usually supported?
21. Which three types of grants are authorized under the Social Security Act passed in 1935?
22. What two things must a state do in order to become eligible for one of the grants listed in the preceding question?
23. What are the four major branches of HEW?
24. What are the major functions of the U.S. Public Health Service?
25. What are the central technical services of the World Health Organization?
26. From where does the World Health Organization derive its authority?
27. What was the first voluntary health agency?
28. What are two of the major problems connected with voluntary agencies.
29. What can a voluntary health agency do that a government agency cannot?
30. What is the main goal of the AMA?
31. What is the name of the organization that coordinates all efforts for health at the national level?
32. How are professional agencies financed?

REFERENCES

1. Leavell, H.: Amer. J. Publ. Health, *61*:185, 1971.
2. Amer. J. Publ. Health, *59*:339, 1969.
3. San Bernardino County Health Department, San Bernardino, Calif.
4. South Carolina State Board of Health: 94th Annual Report, 1972–73.
5. *Toledo's Health Semi-Annual Report January 1,—June 30, 1964.* Ohio State Department of Public Health, p. 1.
6. Cornely, P. B., and Bigman, J. K.: Acquaintance with municipal government health services in a low-income urban population. Amer. J. Pub. Health, *52*:1877, 1962.
7. Blum, H. L., and Leonard, A. R.: *Public Administration—a Public Health Viewpoint.* New York, Macmillan, 1963, p. 255.
8. Rogers, K. D., and Reese, G.: Health studies of presumably normal high school students. Amer. J. Dis. Child., *108*:572, 1964.
9. Yankauer, A., and Lawrence, R. A.: Study of periodic school medical examinations. II. Annual increment of new defects. Amer. J. Publ. Health, *46*:1553, 1956.
10. Morbid. Mortal. Week. Rep., *11*:152, 1962.
11. Morbid. Mortal. Week. Rep., *12*:133, 1963.
12. Morbid. Mortal. Week. Rep., *12*:422, 1963.
13. Morbid. Mortal. Week. Rep., *11*:410, 1963.
14. Sliepcevich, E. M.: The school health education study: a foundation for community health education. J.School Health, *38*:45, 1968.
15. Fluoridation Reporter, Vol. XI, No. 2. Chicago, American Dental Association, 1973.
16. School Health Education Study: *Health Education: a Conceptual Approach to Curriculum Design.* St. Paul, Minn., 3M Education Press, 1967.
17. Haldeman, J. C.: Financing local health services. Amer. J. Publ. Health, *45*:970, 1955.
18. *It's Your Children's Bureau.* Washington, D.C., United States Department of Health, Education, and Welfare. Superintendent of Documents. Publication No. 357, 1964, pp. 38–46.
19. Freeman, R. B., and Holmes, E. M.: *Administration of Public Health Services.* Philadelphia, W.B. Saunders Co., 1960, pp. 471–76.
20. Declaration of the Presidents of America. Meeting of the American Chiefs of State. Ponta del Este, Uruguay, 1967, p. 22.
21. Hanlon, J.: *Public Health; Administration and Practice.* St. Louis, C.V. Mosby Co., 1974, p. 141.
22. Gunn, S. M., and Platt, P. S.: *Voluntary Health Agencies: An Interpretive Study.* New York, Ronald Press, 1945.
23. Roney, J. G.: *Public Health for Reluctant Communities.* River Edge, N.J., River Edge Printing Co., 1962, pp. 55–57.
24. American Social Health Association: *Why We Believe in United Giving.* American Social Health Association, New York, 1970.
25. Hanlon, J. J.: *Public Health Administration and Practice.* 6th ed. St. Louis, C. V. Mosby Co., 1974, p. 118.

SUGGESTED READING

Alford, R. R.: *Health Care Politics: Ideological and Interest Group Barriers to Reform.* Chicago, University of Chicago Press, 1975.

American School Health Association: *Directory of National Organizations Concerned With School Health.* 8th ed. Kent, Ohio, ASHA Publications, 1974.

Andreopoulos, S. (ed.): *Primary Care: Where Medicine Fails.* (Forum, Sun Valley, Idaho, June, 1973.) New York, Wiley, 1974.

Benson, E. R., and McDevitt, J. Q.: *Community Health and Nursing Practice.* Englewood Cliffs, N.J., Prentice-Hall, 1975.

Berkanovic, E., et al.: *Perceptions of Medical Care: The Impact of Prepayment.* Lexington, Mass., Lexington Books, 1974.

Bonvechio, R.: *School Health Curriculum Guide.* Dubuque, Iowa, Kendall/Hunt, 1975,

Brody, E. M. (ed.): *A Social Work Guide for Long-Term Care Facilities.* DHEW Publication No. (HSM) 73–9106. Rockville, Md., National Institute of Mental Health, 1974.

Burgess, A. W., and Lazare, A.: *Community Mental Health.* Englewood Cliffs, N.J.: Prentice-Hall, 1976.

Bygren, L. O.: *Met and Unmet Needs for Medical and Social Services.* Scandinavian Journal of Social Medicine, Supplementum 8. Stockholm, The Almqvist & Wiksell Periodical Co., 1974.

Cohn, V.: *Sister Kenny, the Woman Who Challenged Doctors.* Minneapolis, University of Minnesota Press, 1976.

Cull, J. G., and Hardy, R. E.: *Organization and Administration of Drug Abuse Treatment Programs: National and International.* Springfield, Ill., Charles C Thomas, 1974.

Demone, H. W., Jr., and Harshberger, D. (eds.): *Handbook of Human Service Organizations.* New York, Behavioral Publications, 1973.

Department of Health and Social Security: *Future Structure of the National Health Service.* London, H.M.S.O., 1970.

Douglas-Wilsont, I., and McLachlan, G.(eds.): *Health Service Prospects: An International Survey.* London, Lancet, 1974.

Durbin, R. L., and Springall, W. H.: *Organization and Administration of Health Care: Theory, Practice, Environment.* 2nd ed. St. Louis, C.V. Mosby Co., 1974.

Eisner, V., and Callan, L. B.: *Dimensions of School Health.* Springfield, Ill., Charles C Thomas, 1974.

Freymann, J. G.: *The American Health Care System: Its Genesis and Tranjectory.* New York, MEDCOM, 1974.

Fuchs, V. R.: *Who Shall Live? Health, Economics and Social Choice.* New York, Basic Books, 1975.

Gartner, A. (ed.): *The New Human Services Review.* New York, Behavioral Publications, 1975.

Ginzberg, E., and Yohalem, A. M. (eds.): *The University Medical Center and the Metropolis.* (Conference, New York, November, 1973.) New York, Josiah Macy, Jr., Foundation; Independent Publishers Group (distributor), 1974.

Hanlon, J. J.: *Public Health Administration and Practice.* 6th ed. St. Louis, C.V. Mosby Co., 1974.

Hobson, W. (ed.): *The Theory and Practice of Public Health.* New York, Oxford University Press, 1974.

HSMHA Hotline. U.S. Department of Health, Education and Welfare, Health Services and Mental Health Administration, Office of Communications and Public Affairs, Washington, D.C.

Illich, I.: *Medical Nemesis.* New York, Pantheon, 1976.

Interpreters' Services and the Role of Health Care Volunteers. American Hospital Association, 840 North Lake Shore Drive, Chicago 60611, 1974.

Leininger, M., and Buck, G.: *Health Care Issues.* Philadelphia, F.A. Davis, 1974.

Modern Management Methods and the Organization of Health Services. Public Health Paper No. 55. Geneva, World Health Organization, 1974.

Monroe, M., awd Yaller, B.: *A Practical Guide to Long-Term Care and Health Services Administration.* Greenvale, N.Y., Panel Publications, 1973.

Muller, C. F., and Jaffe, F. S.: *Financing Fertility-Related Health Services in the U.S., 1972–1978. A Preliminary Projection.* New York, Planned Parenthood Federation of America, Inc., 1972.

Murray, D. S.: *Blueprint for Health—A Multinational Portrait of the Costs and Administration of Medical Care in the Public Interest.* New York, Schocken Books, 1974.

National League for Nursing: *The Problem-Oriented System. A Multi-Disciplinary Approach.* Publication No. 20–1546, 1974.

Perlman, M. (ed.): *The Economics of Health and Medical Care.* (International Economic Association Conference, Tokyo, April, 1973.) New York, Wiley, 1974.

Planned Parenthood Federation of America, Inc.: *Major Federal Resources for Family Planning Services and Population Research.* New York, 1971.

Public Affairs Committee: Pamphlets. New York, 1974.

Rafferty, J. (ed.): *Health, Manpower and Productivity. The Literature of Required Research.* Lexington, Mass., D.C. Heath & Co., 1974.

Reed, L. S., et al.: *Health Insurance and Psychiatric Care: Utilization and Cost.* Washington, D.C., American Psychiatric Association, 1972.

Ruchlin, H. S., and Rogers, D.C.: *Economics and Health Care.* Springfield, Ill., Charles C Thomas, 1973.

Schulberg, H. C., and Baker, F.: *Developments in Human Services.* New York, Behavioral Publications, 1975.

Smith, V. K.: *Welfare Work Incentives.* Lansing, Mich., Michigan Department of Social Services, 1974.

Smolensky, J., and Bonvechio, R.: *Principles of School Health.* Lexington, Mass., D.C. Heath & Co., 1967.

Spiegel, A. D., and Podair, S. (eds.): *Medicaid: Lessons for National Health Insurance.* Washington, D.C., Aspens Systems Corporation, 1975.

Stevens, R., and Stevens, R.: *Welfare Medicine in America: A Case Study of Medicaid.* New York, Free Press, 1974.

U.S. Department of Health, Education and Welfare: *The Voluntary Agency and Community Mental Health Services.* Washington, D.C., U.S. Government Printing Office, 1974.

Wilson, F. A., and Nehauser, D.: *Health Services in the United States.* Cambridge, Mass., Ballinger, 1974.

Wren, G. R.: *Modern Health Administration.* Athens, Ga., University of Georgia Press, 1974.

CHAPTER 7

Chronic Disease

CHRONIC ILLNESS: A MAJOR PROBLEM

Chronic disease is a problem whose scope is as great as the total population of the country. Each member of the population is a potential victim and, to the extent that control is possible, the key to individual control lies with the individual. Although all people are possible targets of chronic disease, and the largest number of victims are under 65 years of age, older persons are more likely to be disabled by chronic conditions. In the population of the United States, the proportion of older persons is growing, and chronic diseases will become an increasing problem. The Commission on Chronic Illness defines a chronic disease as any impairment or deviation from normal that has one or more of the following characteristics: is permanent; leaves residual disability; is caused by nonreversible pathological alteration; requires special training of the patient for rehabilitation; or may be expected to require a long period of supervision, observation, or care.[1]

There is wide agreement that the major medical care problem in the country is chronic disease. One of every six persons is chronically ill; more than two-thirds of our deaths are caused by chronic illness. It is interesting to note that the chronic disease mortality trends are similar in most modern world countries. Three of every four hospital beds are occupied by victims of long-term illnesses. Many of these patients are chronically ill because they did not seek the attention of doctors early enough. Some patients would be better off at home if professional supplementary home care were available. Others who are incapacitated could learn to take care of themselves and with proper rehabilitation could learn to lead useful lives. As a result of these conditions, the chronically ill are consuming a disproportionate amount of time of already overworked doctors, nurses, and welfare workers, and they are overloading hospitals and other medical facilities. Other problems involved in chronic illness include expense and inadequacy of facilities for adequate early diagnosis and treatment, inequalities in distribution of physicians, mounting costs of medical care, and the insidious nature of the increase of chronic illnesses.

Prevention and treatment of chronic illness are community problems and affect each member of a community. Although two of every three deaths are caused by chronic diseases, the disability that results is of equal or greater importance. Consequences of prolonged disability from chronic diseases include medical expenses, loss in productive activity, and prolonged suffering of the patient. The major share of the financial burden for the care of the chronically disabled is usually derived from community, state, and federal taxes.

Age Group Affected

As an individual ages, his tissues undergo changes which increase his chances of becoming a victim of one or more chronic diseases. However, chronic diseases are not a problem confined to the older segment of the population. Chronic or degenerative conditions of cardiovascular disease and cancer cause more deaths among school age children than do all the infectious and parasitic diseases combined.[2] The degree to which individuals in the various age groups are affected by disability is illustrated partially by the following statement:

> It is true that the highest rate of prevalence of chronic disease and disability occurs among the older persons in the population, but, as the National Health Survey discovered, more than three-quarters of those with chronic illness and two-thirds of the invalids are between the ages of fifteen and sixty-four and more than half the chronic invalids are under the age of forty-five.[3]

One of every 7 men and 1 of every 8 women between the ages of 17 and 44 are limited in their major activity, their ability to work, keep house or go to school because of a chronic condition. Between the ages of 45 and 64, about one-fourth of men and one-fifth of women are limited in major activity because of a chronic condition. At ages 65 and over, nearly three-fifths of men and two-fifths of women are so handicapped. Approximately one-third of all people attributed their chronic illness to some disorder of the circulatory system, with heart disease the most frequent condition noted among men, and arthritis second.

One chronic disease case of every 6 involves a person under 25 years of age, and 1 chronic disease case of every 2 involves a person under 45 years of age. Cerebral palsy, which affects more than 500,000 persons, occurs most often before, during, or soon after birth. Rheumatic fever, which has crippled at least 750,000 Americans with rheumatic heart disease, almost always strikes for the first time during childhood. Rheumatoid arthritis most often strikes between the ages of 35 and 40. Diabetes and cancer are primarily diseases of middle and old age, but often strike earlier. Multiple sclerosis, a remissively progressive disorder of the central nervous system, characteristically affects persons between the ages of 20 and 40; onset is rare below the age of 12 or after 50 years of age. Muscular dystrophy, a disease that gradually wastes away all the voluntary muscles of the body, is a scourge of childhood and youth. Diseases of the heart or arteries, though concentrated in the years after 40, are distributed to some extent in every age group.[4]

It is estimated that about 3,000,000 persons under 20 years of age suffer from chronic ilness or physical impairment. Some of these young people can be treated successfully, but often at considerable expense. Others require special educational programs and placement services if they are to lead adjusted, useful lives. Each time the community allows one of these young people to spend his entire life in inactivity, nearly 50 man-years of productive effort and contented living are wasted.

PREVENTION

Modern medicine has successfully learned how to prevent the most devastating of the infectious diseases, as a result of the coordinated efforts of research workers and practicing physicians and the willingness of the public to accept preventive measures. With this record, an obvious question is why similar results have not been achieved for today's major causes of death, particularly cardiovascular diseases, stroke, and cancer, which together account for some 70 per cent of all deaths in the United States. Much time has passed since statistically proven risk factors for heart attacks were established, since it was demonstrated that treatment of hypertension leads to a reduction in the occurence of strokes, since cigarette smoking was shown to be related to lung cancer and a variety of other diseases, and since Papanicolaou first demonstrated the value of cervical smears in identifying early lesions of the cervix. Why, then, has this knowledge not been translated into effective health and social legislation to reduce the mortality and sickness associated with these events? Two leading physicians explain:

> A major reason is the apathy that exists among most human beings when it comes to anything for which the results are long delayed. Whether it is the health crisis or the energy crisis, man tends to live for today. In addition, many individuals are afraid that a visit to the physician will uncover an illness of which they are not aware. This public attitude is matched by a similar disinterest among most physicians for preventive measures. Traditionally, physicians are trained to deal with symptoms and find it difficult to adjust their thinking to conditions that are in an asymptomatic stage. That physicians have not learned to appreciate the statistics of probability is borne out by the fact that much of the medical profession

has not been willing to translate the known risks for an individual to develop a heart attack into a long-term preventive program. Although many learn by experience, physicians have not been trained in the psychological art of how to motivate people not to smoke, to modify their diets, or to take prescribed medication. America's hospitals are not geared to preventive medicine, and the fact that most of our insurance carriers cover principally therapeutic, and not preventive, care compounds the problem.[5]

The missing ingredient in successful prevention, however, is the fact that the public still reacts not to health, but to sickness. Periodic exams are postponed, and visits to a health professional are usually prompted only by an immediate, identifiable need. Prevention also makes good economic sense. Educating citizens in the health practices necessary to achieve these standards is an essential part of the responsibility of each health professional. Seeking to raise and maintain the quality of social, physical, and mental health and demonstrating and teaching established practices leading toward good health are responsibilities which should be shared by the State Department of Health and the health professionals. It may be that the most significant health challenge of the future is that of instilling in each person a strong sense of responsibility for his own health.

Prevention of chronic illness and disability requires mobilization of individual and public resources. Freedom from chronic illness can be achieved through united efforts toward individual health promotion, toward averting the occurrence of illness, and toward early detection of disease through health examinations and mass screening programs. At present, the prevention of severe forms of many chronic diseases depends largely upon early detection. Usually this implies the discovery of cases by means of screening procedures, examination, and diagnosis. There is evidence for the fact that severe forms of chronic disease and complications can be averted by early treatment. However, the majority of cases are already in severe or advanced forms when detected. Clinical and public health practices lag in utilizing the existing knowledge and measures for the prevention of chronic disease.

Chronic disease experts agree that there is no certain method of primary prevention at the present time for the following diseases or conditions: alcoholism, arteriosclerosis, degenerative joint disease, diabetes, epilepsy, essential or primary hypertension, multiple sclerosis, glaucoma, and rheumatoid arthritis. However, prompt and continuing application of known measures of primary prevention will result in a substantial reduction in the amount of and impairment by the chronic diseases shown in Table 7-1.

Periodic Health Examinations

Secondary prevention means halting the progression of a disease from its early unrecognized stage to a more severe one and preventing complications or sequelae of disease.[6] One of the best methods for detecting

Table 7-1 Prevention of Chronic Diseases

CHRONIC DISEASE	PREVENTION
1. Blindness	
Retrolental fibroplasia	Control of oxygen administered to premature babies
Congenital cataracts	Immunization with German measles vaccine
Cataracts	Protective goggles—safety equipment
Glaucoma	Early detection and treatment
Ophthalmia neonatorum	Silver nitrate or penicillin drops in new-born babies' eyes
2. Paralytic poliomyelitis	Immunization with Salk and Sabin vaccines
3. Cardiovascular diseases	
Rheumatic fever	Early detection and use of antibiotics
Atherosclerosis	Dietary control
Syphilitic heart disease	Early treatment
4. Cancer	Avoiding certain pollutants, excessive smoking, excessive radiation, chemicals and other irritants; early detection and treatment, know the 7 danger signs
5. Deafness, retardation	Immunization with German measles, mumps, and measles vaccine
6. Dental caries	Fluoridated water supply, periodic visits to dentist, good diet and personal hygiene

chronic disease is a periodic physical examination. A good periodic health examination should have four main sections: a complete medical hisory; a thorough and comprehensive medical examination; appropriate laboratory, x-ray, and other diagnostic procedures; and health guidance and follow-up. The periodic health examination represents only a partial solution to the problem of early detection of chronic disease. The weaknesses and limitations of the health examination are time, cost, personnel limitations, the cursory nature of some examinations, poor public acceptance, inability to detect all incipient disease, and limited facilities for diagnosis and treatment.

Though regular checkups are important for detecting health problems in youngsters and the elderly, or in people with obvious symptoms of illness, they appear to many doctors to be largely unproductive for the vast majority of the population. In general, according to Drs. Vickery and Fries, Americans should not waste their money on annual checkups but should rely instead on easy-to-perform tests that can often be done inexpensively by a nurse or paramedic.*

Screening Examinations

Screening is another method of secondary prevention. Finding chronic diseases in their early, treatable stages would be no problem if everyone in the United States could and would go to his physician for a complete health appraisal once or twice a year. For this reason, medical and health authorities have urged regular health checkups in order to detect early signs of disease. Since time, costs, personnel shortages, and other factors already mentioned preclude the possibility of regular comprehensive health examinations for the majority of the population, relatively simple and inexpensive procedures of other types are needed to sort out persons with probable evidence of chronic disease in order to refer them for diagnosis and medical care. To help solve this problem, a fresh and interesting idea is the multitest clinic. This clinic screens persons for two, six or twelve diseases at a time. One blood sample can be tested for signs of diabetes, anemia, and venereal diseases; the same chest x-ray can be inspected for signs of tuberculosis, lung cancer, and heart defects; the urine sample can be examined for diabetes and kidney disorders. Multiple screening is not intended to diagnose diseases, but to discover persons who have need of consulting their physicians for diagnosis and treatment. The results of the screening tests are sent to the individual's physician or to the doctor named by him. The process is inexpensive, flexible, and fast, and can be done by nonmedical personnel. The value of screening as a measure to prevent blindness from glaucoma is stressed:

> It is estimated that 2 per cent of all persons over 40 years of age suffer from glaucoma and, with the increasing proportion of aged persons in our population, the number of persons included in that 2 per cent is constantly growing. With early detection and treatment, glaucoma seldom progresses to blindness; yet at present, 12 per cent of all blind people are blind as a result of glaucoma. Obviously, we are not detecting and treating cases in time.
>
> Encouraging progress has been made in the development of tonometry and other detection techniques. However, there are 59 million Americans over 40 years of age who, ideally should be examined annually for glaucoma. The task is formidable, but a promising start is being made in a few communities through the use of mass screening, comparable to the mass casefinding programs that have proved so successful in the control of tuberculosis and venereal disease.[7]

A screening program will be most effective when it has the support of the medical association and voluntary and official agencies. A few effective screening tests are shown in Table 7-2.

The great advantage of screening is that it affords a means of bringing the benefits of early detection to large groups of the population. Selection of population groups for screening programs should include hospital patients, prisoners, members of industrial and labor groups, students, recipients of social and welfare services, members of group health plans, federal, state and local government employees, and members of the Armed Forces. Multiple screening is one way of detecting early signs of disease and of assuring speed, efficiency, and economy. Screening provides an excellent opportunity for health education, but it is not a panacea. Its ultimate value in the community will be achieved when it becomes an integral part of a well-rounded chronic disease program.

---

*Vickery, D. M., and Fries, J. F.: *Take Care of Yourself.* Reading, Mass., Addison-Wesley, 1976.

Table 7–2 Effective Screening Tests.

TEST	DISEASE DETECTED
1. X-ray	Tuberculosis (tuberculosis test) Heart defects Cancer Emphysema (breathing capacity test)
2. Visual field and tonometry	Cataracts Glaucoma
3. Audiometer	Hearing loss
4. Blood and urine tests	Diabetes Anemia Syphilis Kidney disorders
5. Cytology (especially uterine cervix)	Cervical cancer (Pap test)
6. Self-examination of breast	Breast cancer
7. Weight; blood pressure; cholesterol and triglyceride levels	Heart disease

Selected Screening Tests

Glaucoma. Glaucoma is the leading cause of preventable blindness in our country. It accounts for approximately 20 per cent of the blindness in the United States today. About 2 per cent of people over 35 have glaucoma and most of them don't know it. Glaucoma is caused by increased fluid pressure inside the eye. The pressure injures the nerves, causing a gradual loss of eyesight. In the early stages there is no pain or noticeable change in eyesight, but vision may be slipping away beyond recovery. With proper treatment and care, visual impairment due to glaucoma can be greatly delayed or even prevented altogether. Vision lost before glaucoma is discovered and treated cannot be restored. People over 30 and those with a family history of glaucoma are more likely to develop the disease.

Diabetes. Diabetes is a disease in which the body cannot use food properly. One adult in 60 in the United States has diabetes and most of them do not know they have it. In diabetes, the body cannot regulate the blood sugar level. The food we eat is digested into its component parts and then absorbed and carried in the blood stream. Insulin allows these substances, of which glucose is one, to be stored in fatty tissues and muscles for future use. The blood glucose level normally goes up as we eat and down as we work or play. In diabetes the blood sugar (glucose) remains high.

The screening test measures the blood sugar level under exact conditions. Anyone whose blood sugar level is found to be too high will be advised to see his own physician for further tests. With proper medical treatment, the blood sugar level can be controlled. Untreated diabetes is a leading cause of blindness and heart disease. It may also affect the kidneys and other organs. In the early stages there are no visible symptoms. People over 40 who are overweight or have a family history of diabetes are more likely to become diabetic.

Heart Diseases. The way we live can decrease our chances of heart disease. Maintain your correct weight. Keep your blood pressure down. Eat a diet low in animal fats. Exercise moderately each day. Limit or stop smoking. At the screening clinic, weight, blood pressure, cholesterol, and triglyceride level are determined as a means of assessing an individual's chances of developing heart disease.

Cancer. Cancer of the uterus (womb) and the breast are serious threats to women. Periodic medical checkups, testing, and breast self-examination lessen the risk. At the screening clinic, women are given a Pap Test (cervical cell test) and learn the technique of regular breast self-examination. Through movies and pamphlets, men and women also learn about other warning signs of cancer.

Lung Diseases. Emphysema is the major

chronic disease of the lungs. It is caused by prolonged inhalation of irritating substances (tobacco, smoke, and smog) and results in coughing, wheezing, and shortness of breath. The chest x-ray is not a good test for either emphysema or cancer. Although chest x-rays have been used for tuberculosis screening, the tuberculin (skin) test is the preferred test.

Prompt Treatment

Many chronic diseases can be minimized and even cured if detected early. If parents and teachers are able to observe the signs and symptoms of certain diseases, they should refer children to physicians quickly and therefore prevent chronic or disabling consequences. For example, a hemolytic streptococcal infection usually precedes rheumatic heart disease. If detected early enough, however, the streptococcal infection can be treated with penicillin to prevent the disease. Protective hormones such as cortisone and ACTH are often used to soften the effect of the infection.

Adequate Nutrition

"Lengthen the belt line and shorten the life line" can certainly be applied to specific chronic diseases. For instance, diabetes and heart disease are more prevalent in obese persons. Nutritional diseases and lowered resistance occur more often among those individuals who are unaware of the necessity of a wholesome and healthful diet.

Industrial Hygiene

Industrial hazards such as dust, chemicals, and radiation can lead to a variety of occupational diseases which are chronic in nature. These air pollutants are increasing at a dangerous rate; management and medicine working together have shown that the worker can be protected from these hazards. More and more industries have come to realize that promotion of the health of workers represents a sound investment, and there are many ways in which industry can play an important role. An increasing number of businesses and industries are establishing policies requiring the pre-employment and periodic medical examinations of workers, and many plants engage in superior health education programs. Rehabilitation programs also benefit business and industry.

Accident Prevention

Accidents kill more persons between the ages of one and 35 than any disease and rank fourth among the causes of death for all ages. Motor vehicle accidents and falls cause over 60 per cent of all accidental deaths yearly. Every year many more accident cases are added to the list of chronically disabled individuals. Developing safe behavior habits and attitudes in children and adults, initiating community safety education programs, creating community health and safety councils, and developing more and better safety equipment and regulations for industry are a few suggested preventive measures. Also important are employment of trained safety engineers, adoption and enforcement of more stringent traffic laws, and the addition of safety education in the school curriculum.

Education

Public education is of prime importance in conducting a chronic disease prevention program. The facts must be presented to all the people, and the people must be motivated to act accordingly.

FEDERAL AND STATE PROGRAMS

The Health Department Versus Blindness

Many health departments throughout the United States are undertaking special projects in an effort to prevent disease and accidents. Prevention of blindness in children and adults is a good example of one project being undertaken by many state health departments. The problem is magnified when we consider an increased aged population with corresponding increased blindness due to chronic conditions such as diabetes, cancer, and hypertension. However, early detection of certain eye conditions can prevent blindness. For example, glaucoma, which is most frequent among middle age persons, is second only to cataract as a cause of blindness, and accounts for about

14 per cent of adult blindness in the United States. Glaucoma, often called "tunnel vision," is a condition of increased fluid pressure within the eye which causes atrophy of the optic nerve and results in gradual loss of vision. Symptoms include blurred vision, headache, eye pain, and nausea; if detected early enough the disease can be cured. Community screening programs and education can prevent blindness from glaucoma.

Amblyopia, also known as "lazy eye" or "one-eye vision," is a condition of vision dimness leading to blindness and is most common among children. In most cases, if this condition is not discovered by the time the child is six years old, he will lose the sight of one eye. This can be prevented by preschool and primary vision screening programs.

The importance of vision defects in relation to public health is illustrated by the fact that World War II Selective Service rejections for visual defects ranked second; vision defects also rate high as a cause of rejection for industrial employment today. Furthermore, the problem is magnified when we consider administrative costs of state welfare aid to the blind, loss of productivity, taxes, and loss of purchasing power. Since early detection is the key to the prevention of blindness among adults and children, new ways must be found to reach these groups through education and case-finding.

Rehabilitation

Each of the 50 states, the District of Columbia, and Puerto Rico operate a rehabilitation program in cooperating with the Office of Vocational Rehabilitation. Under this federal-state plan, a handicapped person may apply for whatever help he may need to become self-supporting. About 60,000 men and women a year are being rehabilitated by this system. In most cases their disabilities are a result of illness. The Office of Vocational Rehabilitation estimates that between 1,500,000 and 2,000,000 Americans of working age are so severely disabled that they cannot support themselves, and that another 250,000 are disabled each year, primarily by chronic disease. The Office of Vocational Rehabilitation believes that most of these individuals could become self-supporting if Congress or the state legislatures, or both, voted enough money for rehabilitation. With present funds, the number of rehabilitants probably cannot exceed 60,000 a year. Once rehabilitated and working again, the handicapped person no longer needs support from community, state, and federal taxes. In fact, the person begins paying taxes again. Individual and family happiness contribute to the success of the rehabilitation program.

Community rehabilitation centers serving several hospitals, or established as part of one or more existing hospitals, have been very successful. The personnel required varies with the size of the community. A city with a population of 100,000, for example, requires the services of a psychologist, a social service worker, and a vocational counselor, as well as occupational and physical therapists. All programs and activities are supervised and directed by medical authorities.

Mental Retardation Program

The Mental Retardation Branch, Division of Chronic Diseases, is the only program that is solely concerned with providing assistance in the overall development of community health services for the mentally retarded. Its establishment reflects recognition of the ever-growing number of possibilities to capitalize on the rapid advances in medical and related knowledge in behalf of the mentally retarded. New avenues to prevention of mental retardation are opening up and growing wider. Greater amelioration of the handicaps often associated with mental retardation is now possible, thus enabling the mentally retarded to make the most of the potential they do have. Perhaps most important, care of the retarded in their home communities is increasingly accepted and sought—now often as the first choice of parents, families, and communities. Community health and other services for the mentally retarded will be increasingly needed as the retarded, like the rest of the population, reap the benefits of health advances and longer life.

The long-range goal of the Mental Retardation Program is to assist states and communities in ensuring the existence of comprehensive services for the mentally retarded throughout the United States. A major objective, therefore, is to stimulate the development and improvement of community health services for the mentally retarded in concert with related community services. The full range of these needed community health services would encompass the prevention and diagnosis of mental retardation, and continuing treatment for the retarded when they need it. The state planning now in progress gives state agencies unique opportunities to plan and work together to provide comprehensive services for meeting the total needs of the retarded. To attain these objectives, the Mental Retardation Program concentrates its energies and activities in the following areas:

1. Assistance in meeting professional training needs in order to improve the health services given by individual professional practitioners and by community agencies.
2. Improvement and expansion of preventive diagnostic treatment and medical rehabilitative services.
3. Improvement in communication of new knowledge about the health and medical aspects of mental retardation to the health and allied professions, interested groups, and to the general public.
4. Support of surveys and studies to determine the extent of problems and the availability of manpower, services, and facilities.

*The Regional Medical Programs (RMP)**

Regional Medical Programs are a formalized activity of the federal government. Public Law 89–239, enacted in 1965, authorized the establishment and maintenance of Regional Medical Programs to assist in making available the best possible patient care for heart disease, cancer, stroke, and related diseases. In the years preceding 1965, there was a trend toward regionalization of health resources, growth of a national biomedical research community of unprecedented size and productivity, and a change in the needs of society.

The specific purposes of the act are: (1) to act as a catalyst and stimulant to physicians, nurses, and other health professionals in speeding the use of the latest developments in prevention, diagnosis, treatment, and rehabilitation in these and related diseases (heart, cancer, stroke), (2) to shorten the time lag now existing between the discovery of new methods and their use on the patient, and (3) to make the highest type of service available to physicians for their patients no matter where they live, whether it be in the most isolated rural areas or in the heart of the inner city.

**Note:* Regional Medical Programs are now a part of the Comprehensive Health Planning Act.

COMMUNITY PROGRAMS

Many successful chronic disease programs have been developed in communities throughout the country. Home-care programs, for example, have been very successful in caring for the patients and making more hospital beds available for others. It has been estimated that 70 per cent of chronically ill individuals would be better cared for in their own homes, provided the homes maintained satisfactory facilities for nursing care. Chronically ill patients may also be cared for in privately operated nursing homes. Operators of these homes are encouraged to maintain high standards and to foster a close relationship between doctors, hospitals, and nursing homes. Also important is the willingness and ability of welfare agencies to pay adequate fees for impoverished invalids.

There is a need for more hospitals for chronic illness, qualified privately-owned nursing homes, and other similar facilities. Many communities or counties have established central services for their chronically ill. The first central service was established in Chicago in 1944 by the Institute of Medicine, the Welfare Council, and the Community Fund. Each program conducts some or all of the following activities:

1. Surveying the problem of chronic disease. In Chicago the central service knows the approximate number of persons affected, their ages, sex, financial status, diagnosis, degree of disability, and the amount and type of care needed. It also knows what facilities are available for various types of treatment and care at what cost, and what additional facilities are needed.
2. Referring disabled persons and their families to the institutions and agencies best able to serve them. A Milwaukee hospital was ready to discharge a 60 year old woman who had been admitted for a fractured hip. But where could she go to convalesce? Besides her hip trouble she had such a severe case of arthritis that she hadn't walked in five years. The Central Agency for the Chronically Ill referred the patient to a nursing home where Milwaukee's Curative Workshop helped with her rehabilitation at the request of her physician. Today she is back in her own home, not only taking complete care of herself, but also doing some of the housework.

3. Working to expand facilities for the chronically ill. Both the Milwaukee and the Chicago agencies have encouraged qualified persons to open nursing homes and have given practical advice on how to run them. The Essex County group in New Jersey has started a homemaker service to aid the chronically ill person at home.

4. Acting to stimulate community interest in every phase of the problem.[8]

Our state legislatures and municipal and other official bodies, influenced by expanding medical knowledge and a more informed public, are becoming more aware that conditions such as diabetes, heart disease, cancer, mental disorders, arthritis, rheumatism, glaucoma, and other chronic and degenerative diseases can be controlled through sustained and coordinated community-wide effort. Being aware of these problems, what can the modern American community do to meet its responsibilities to the well-being of its people? The most effective basis on which to organize a program to fight chronic disease is to integrate all phases and all stages of a community-wide attack—prevention, early detection, treatment, and rehabilitation—into programs that recognize and utilize the common denominators among chronic disabilities in various disease categories, age groups, and sources of service or funds in meeting the total need. Diagnosis and treatment of chronic illness must be an integral part of general medical care of high quality available not only to the indigent, or to those who can pay for services, but to all who need them.

At the heart of any successful community disease program is the private practitioner. Only with the help of local physicians who will assist in applying the full range of community resources to the need for expanding and improving health services can acceptable results be obtained in the early detection, prompt treatment, and maximal rehabilitation of those with chronic disorders.

Five processes by which the community may proceed toward the goal of providing a chronic disease program include health maintenance, prevention of disease or injury, detection and treatment of illness in its earliest state when cure is often feasible, limitation of disability to preserve the maximum normal function, and restoration of the capacity for the highest level of independent activity of which the patient is capable.

Our best hope for control of chronic disease in the not-too-distant future depends on the dedication of all community health resources to the comprehensive exercise of these control processes.[9] Federal, state, and local health agencies have stepped up their chronic disease programs. The key word—*prevention*—is stressed by all agencies. Their tools include legislation, education, research, and treatment, supported by coordination and cooperation. The current emphasis placed on treatment and control of chronic diseases is fully warranted.

CANCER

Cancer is uncontrolled abnormal cell growth. Mankind has been afflicted with cancer for centuries; tumors have been found in prehistoric animal skeletons and in human remains from very early civilizations. Today, no race, creed, or nationality appears to be free from cancer. The warning signs may be trivial or minor, and thus are frequently ignored or forgotten.

There has been a marked increase in the number of cancer cases and deaths since 1900. However, certain factors, such as increase in average life expectancy, increase in population, more accurate diagnosis, and increased use of radioactive elements and other possible cancer-producing materials may partially account for this increased cancer rate.

Cancer strikes 1 person in 4. Statistically, the chances of recovering from it are 1 in 3, but—depending on the site—chances of survival may be much higher if the cancer is detected early enough. Current cure rates for cancers of the stomach, lung, breast, colon, rectum, and uterus could be vastly improved through earlier detection of the disease.

The American Cancer Society urges individuals to have a medical checkup annually no matter how well they feel, to learn cancer's seven danger signals, and to go to a doctor immediately if any of these signs is detected. The seven danger signals of cancer are unusual bleeding or discharge, a lump or thickening in the breast or elsewhere, a sore that does not heal, a change in bowel or bladder habits, prolonged or severe hoarseness or cough, prolonged indigestion or difficulty in swallowing, and physical change in a wart or mole.

Reference Chart: Leading Cancer Sites, 1975*

SITE	ESTIMATED NEW CASES 1975	ESTIMATED DEATHS 1975	WARNING SIGNAL IF YOU HAVE ONE, SEE YOUR DOCTOR	SAFEGUARDS	COMMENT
BREAST	89,000	33,000	LUMP OR THICKENING IN THE BREAST.	ANNUAL CHECKUP. MONTHLY BREAST SELF EXAM.	THE LEADING CAUSE OF CANCER DEATH IN WOMEN.
COLON AND RECTUM	99,000	49,000	CHANGE IN BOWEL HABITS; BLEEDING.	ANNUAL CHECKUP INCLUDING PROCTOSCOPY, ESPECIALLY FOR THOSE OVER 40.	CONSIDERED A HIGHLY CURABLE DISEASE WHEN DIGITAL AND PROCTOSCOPIC EXAMINATIONS ARE INCLUDED IN ROUTINE CHECKUPS.
LUNG	91,000	81,000	PERSISTENT COUGH, OR LINGERING RESPIRATORY AILMENT.	PREVENTION: HEED FACTS ABOUT SMOKING, ANNUAL CHECKUP. CHEST X-RAY	THE LEADING CAUSE OF CANCER DEATH AMONG MEN, THIS FORM OF CANCER IS LARGELY PREVENTABLE.
ORAL (INCLUDING PHARYNX)	24,000	8,000	SORE THAT DOES NOT HEAL. DIFFICULTY IN SWALLOWING.	ANNUAL CHECKUP.	MANY MORE LIVES SHOULD BE SAVED BECAUSE THE MOUTH IS EASILY ACCESSIBLE TO VISUAL EXAMINATION BY PHYSICIANS AND DENTISTS.
SKIN	9,000***	5,000	SORE THAT DOES NOT HEAL, OR CHANGE IN WART OR MOLE.	ANNUAL CHECKUP, AVOIDANCE OF OVEREXPOSURE TO SUN.	SKIN CANCER IS READILY DETECTED BY OBSERVATION, AND DIAGNOSED BY SIMPLE BIOPSY.
UTERUS	46,000**	11,000	UNUSUAL BLEEDING OR DISCHARGE.	ANNUAL CHECKUP, INCLUDING PELVIC EXAMINATION WITH PAP TEST.	UTERINE CANCER MORTALITY HAS DECLINED 65% DURING THE LAST 35 YEARS. WITH WIDER APPLICATION OF THE PAP TEST, MANY MORE LIVES CAN BE SAVED, ESPECIALLY FROM CERVICAL CANCER.
KIDNEY AND BLADDER	43,000	17,000	URINARY DIFFICULTY. BLEEDING – IN WHICH CASE CONSULT DOCTOR AT ONCE.	ANNUAL CHECKUP WITH URINALYSIS.	PROTECTIVE MEASURES FOR WORKERS IN HIGH-RISK INDUSTRIES ARE HELPING TO ELIMINATE ONE OF THE IMPORTANT CAUSES OF THESE CANCERS.
LARYNX	9,000	3,000	HOARSENESS – DIFFICULTY IN SWALLOWING.	ANNUAL CHECKUP, INCLUDING MIRROR LARYNGOSCOPY.	READILY CURABLE IF CAUGHT EARLY.
PROSTATE	56,000	19,000	URINARY DIFFICULTY.	ANNUAL CHECKUP, INCLUDING PALPATION.	OCCURS MAINLY IN MEN OVER 60, THE DISEASE CAN BE DETECTED BY PALPATION AND URINALYSIS AT ANNUAL CHECKUP.
STOMACH	23,000	14,000	INDIGESTION.	ANNUAL CHECKUP.	A 40% DECLINE IN MORTALITY IN 20 YEARS, FOR REASONS YET UNKNOWN.
LEUKEMIA	21,000	15,000	LEUKEMIA IS A CANCER OF BLOOD-FORMING TISSUES AND IS CHARACTERIZED BY THE ABNORMAL PRODUCTION OF IMMATURE WHITE BLOOD CELLS. ACUTE LEUKEMIA STRIKES MAINLY CHILDREN AND IS TREATED BY DRUGS WHICH HAVE EXTENDED LIFE FROM A FEW MONTHS TO AS MUCH AS TEN YEARS. CHRONIC LEUKEMIA STRIKES USUALLY AFTER AGE 25 AND PROGRESSES LESS RAPIDLY.		
			IF DRUGS OR VACCINES ARE FOUND WHICH CAN CURE OR PREVENT ANY CANCERS THEY PROBABLY WILL BE SUCCESSFUL FIRST FOR LEUKEMIA AND THE LYMPHOMAS.		
LYMPHOMAS	29,000	19,000	THESE DISEASES ARISE IN THE LYMPH SYSTEM AND INCLUDE HODGKIN'S AND LYMPHOSARCOMA. SOME PATIENTS WITH LYMPHATIC CANCERS CAN LEAD NORMAL LIVES FOR MANY YEARS.		

*All figures rounded to nearest 1,000.
**If carcinoma-in-situ is included, cases total over 86,000.
***Estimates vary widely, from 300,000 to 600,000 or more, for superficial skin cancer.

INCIDENCE ESTIMATES ARE BASED ON RATES FROM N.C.I. THIRD NATIONAL CANCER SURVEY

Figure 7–1 Leading cancer sites. (From Cancer Facts and Figures, American Cancer Society, 1975.)

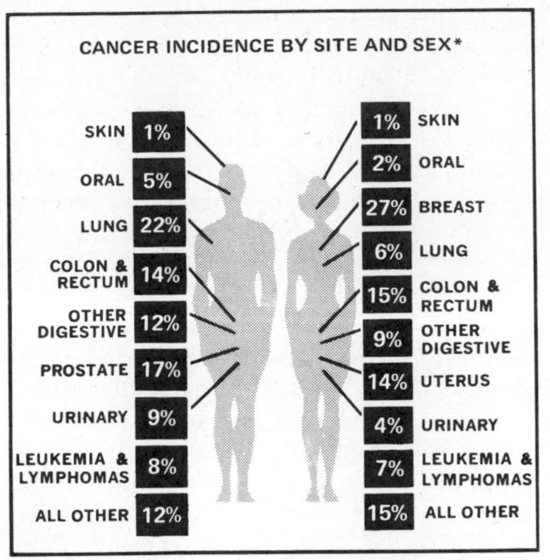

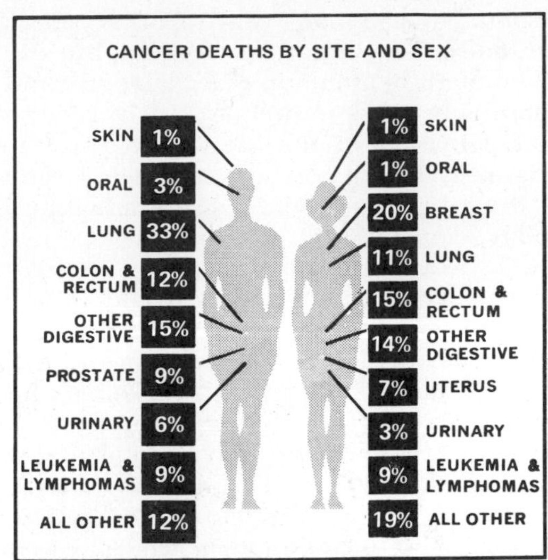

*Excluding superficial skin cancer and carcinoma-in-situ of uterine cervix.

Figure 7–2 Percentage of cancer incidence and deaths by site and sex. (From Cancer Facts and Figures, American Cancer Society, 1975.)

Early Detection

Perhaps the most crucial deficiency of modern cancer therapy is the difficulty of detecting new tumors at a stage of their development when therapy has a high chance of success. Largely as a result of delayed detection, cancer can now be cured in only 1 of every 3 afflicted individuals (where "cure" is defined as survival for five years). This represents an increase of nearly one-third as compared to the cure rate 15 years ago, but some scientists suggest that as many as 90 per cent of individuals with cancer could be cured with current techniques if tumors could be detected earlier.

A major problem, of course, is that many people receive irregular medical care and there is thus little opportunity for physicians to even attempt detection. By the time these individuals perceive overt symptoms of a tumor, it has generally metastasized (dis-

CANCER'S 7 WARNING SIGNALS

Change in bowel or bladder habits

A sore that does not heal

Unusual bleeding or discharge

Thickening or lump in breast or elsewhere

Indigestion or difficulty in swallowing

Obvious change in wart or mole

Nagging cough or hoarseness

If YOU have a warning signal, see your doctor!

THE 7 SAFEGUARDS URGED BY ACS

Lung: Reduction and ultimate elimination of cigarette smoking.

Colon-Rectum: Proctoscopic exam as routine in annual checkup for those over 40.

Breast: Self-examination as monthly female practice.

Uterus: Pap test for all adult and high-risk women.

Skin: Avoidance of excessive sun.

Oral: Wider practice of early detection measures.

Basic: Regular physical examination for all adults.

Figure 7–3 Warning signals and safeguards against cancer. (From Cancer Facts and Figures, American Cancer Society, 1975.)

seminated malignant cells to other sites in the body), and a cure is unlikely. But even when medical attention is available, the most commonly used techniques, such as x-rays and palpation of the breasts and prostate, require that a tumor be moderately large to be discerned, and there is a substantial probability of metastasis.

It would thus be extremely useful to have biochemical tests that would indicate the presence of a tumor. There are already some enzyme assays that assist in the diagnosis of cancer. The activity of alkaline phosphatase in the blood, for example, is increased in individuals with skeletal or liver tumors; the activity of acid phosphatase is increased in individuals with prostate tumors. Most assays, though, are less specific for organ site.

Dr. Bruce Ames of the University of California at Berkeley found that certain carcinogens were capable of causing mutations in bacteria. Mutogenic screening, which involves taking a sample of urine and introducing it into a culture of *Salmonella,* may soon be helpful in preventing cancer. Cervical and vaginal cancers have been detected using a new laser cell-sorting system.

A very important part of the health exam, and one too often neglected, is a rectal examination. This procedure is valuable, especially for older people, because over 70 per cent of all cancers of the large bowel can be touched by the examinating physician's finger. Elderly men will benefit particularly from a rectal examination, since this procedure will reveal most cases of cancer of the prostate.

Further information about the gastrointestinal tract can be obtained from chemical analysis of a small fragment of stool; such analysis is especially helpful in determining whether there is bleeding into the gastrointestinal tract and, if so, in determining where the bleeding is located.

Women should have a pelvic examination as part of their annual checkup. It takes only a few minutes and provides an opportunity for the physician to do a Pap smear at the same time. This painless procedure is named after its developer, Papanicolaou; it consists of gently swabbing the surface of the uterine cervix and examining the scrapings under a microscope. Any cancer cells in the smear can be detected easily by an experienced eye, and in this way cervical cancer may be diagnosed very early. Early cervical cancers often cannot be detected in any other way. Cervical cancers are not painful in the early stages, and they may not cause any change in normal secretions. Also, since it may take as long as five to seven years for cervical cells to progress through the stages of becoming atypical, then precancerous, they will eventually be detected at one yearly checkup, even if they were missed at the preceding examination.

If the precaution of having a pelvic examination seems unwarranted, one should consider the alternative. Early detection of a cancer usually permits an excellent chance of cure without removal of the uterus. Late detection usually reveals invasive cancer, which requires hysterectomy (surgical removal of the uterus) or deep x-ray therapy, which may disrupt generative functions. Moreover, there is usually only a 50 to 80 per cent chance of cure. Increasing use of the Pap smear has lowered the incidence of fatalities from cervical cancer by 38 per cent in 15 years, although only about half of all women in the United States are tested at regular intervals. The Pap test should properly include the cytologic detection of many other cancers of the body (male and female). For women, a yearly examination that includes a pelvic examination and special examination of the breasts will provide as much safety as possible.

Breast Cancer

Ninety thousand American women will discover this year that they have breast cancer. The American Cancer Society estimates that 1 out of every 15 women will develop breast cancer. Nine out of every 10 can expect to be alive in five years if their tumors are detected and treated at an early stage. Unfortunately, most women fail—out of fear or ignorance—to examine their breasts regularly for lumps and to get regular medical checkups, with the result that their tumors may not be discovered until the cancer has spread to other parts of their bodies. Because of this widespread neglect, the mortality rate for breast cancer has scarcely dropped at all in 35 years; in 1975 the disease killed approximately 33,000 women in the United States.

Although a majority of breast tumors turn out to be benign (noncancerous), the only way to find out for sure is through a

BREAST CANCER: DEFINITIONS OF TERMS

Mammography—A special x-ray technique designed to examine the soft tissues of the breast. It is less reliable for small, firm breasts than for large, fatty ones—the fatty tissue offers a dark background against which the cancer stands out as a white mass.

Thermography—an early diagnosis method that utilizes a heat-detection device. Since cancer cells give off more heat than normal cells, thermography can alert the doctor to "hot spots." (But thermography also reacts to the heat given off by any inflammatory breast condition.)

Simple Mastectomy—Removal of the entire breast, but not the muscles and lymph nodes. Sometimes called "total mastectomy."

Modified Radical Mastectomy—Removal of the breast, plus lymph nodes in the armpit, but not the muscles.

Radical Mastectomy—Removal of the breast, all lymph nodes in the armpit, and the pectoral (or chest) muscles beneath the breast.

biopsy—the examination of a small section of tumor under the microscope. Any woman can develop breast cancer,* but some women seem more susceptible to it than others. Statistically, the woman in the greatest danger is someone in her mid- to late 40's who began menstruating early and continued late, who never had children or did not begin having them until she was past 30, who is obese, and whose mother or sister had the disease. Recent studies strongly suggest that the increased risk of breast cancer for women with fewer children is due mainly to the late age at which the first childbirth occurs. Women with a first birth before the age of 18 had about one-third the breast cancer risk of those with first birth at age 35 or over. A second pregnancy showed little, if any, additional protective effect. Age is far less significant in the patient's prognosis than the stage at which the disease is diagnosed.

This does not mean that someone who fits most or even all of these categories is certain to develop breast cancer. Nor does it mean that the disease is hereditary; no concrete evidence has been found that genes for breast tumors are passed from generation to generation. But the disease does have a disturbing tendency to run in families. A woman whose mother or sister has had breast cancer is twice as likely to develop the disease as a woman with no such family history. If both her mother and sister have had breast cancer, her risk may be 47 times greater.

Despite years of research, doctors still know relatively little about the cause of breast cancer. There is no certainty about the role of viruses, despite the fact that they are known to cause breast cancers in animals; research has yet to establish that they can do the same in humans. Virus-like particles have been found in the breast milk of women with cancer and family histories of the disease. But viruses have also been detected in the milk of women who have not had cancer. Hormones produced by women during the menstrual cycle and pregnancy are also under suspicion, but no one has yet determined how they might cause breast cancer or be controlled to prevent it.

Diet has also been implicated as a factor in breast cancer, which appears to be more common in countries where people consume large quantities of animal fats. In the United States, the disease appears more frequently among the affluent and well fed than among other groups. Japan, where the traditional diet is low in animal fats, has the lowest breast cancer rate of 39 countries covered in a recent study. But even there the rate is rising as the Japanese forsake their old diet of fish and rice for a Westernized menu of meat and fats. Japanese women who emigrate to the United States have higher breast

* So can men, although breast cancer appears 100 times less frequently in males than in females.

cancer rates than those who remain in Japan, and their United States–born daughters have breast cancer rates approaching those of American women in general. How and why high-fat diets might trigger breast cancer remains a mystery.

About the only thing that doctors can say with certainty is that injuries to the breast do *not* initiate the disease. Researchers are also practically convinced that breast feeding has no influence—for good or bad—on breast cancer rates.

The chances of a breast cancer victim are markedly improved if the tumor is detected and a mastectomy performed before malignant cells spread to the lymph nodes. A study conducted by the American Cancer Society dramatically shows how earlier detection can be achieved. Doctors at 25 centers screened 75,000 women over the age of 35 for breast cancer. They used three techniques: physical examinations, thermography and mammography. Of those women who underwent biopsies to determine if suspicious growths were in fact malignant, 289 were found to have cancer. In 77 per cent of these victims, the cancers had not yet spread to lymph nodes under the arms. However, self-examination remains the technique by which 95 per cent of all breast cancers are now found. In more than half of such cases, the cancerous cells have already reached lymph nodes. Thus the early detection provided by professional screening can make a vital difference: a woman whose cancer has not reached the lymph nodes has at least an 85 per cent chance of being alive five years after her operation; if the nodes are involved, her chances decrease by half.

According to the American Cancer Society, every woman should thoroughly examine her own breast every month, just after her menstrual period if she is premenopausal. In addition, says the American Cancer Society, every woman should visit her gynecologist or family doctor at least once a year, and her checkup should include a Pap test to detect cervical cancer as well as a manual examination of the breasts. For women over 35 and those with a prevalent family pattern of breast cancer, the manual examination may sometimes be supplemented by mammography, a special tumor-sensitive x-ray of the breast, and thermography, a newer technique that measures small elevations in breast temperature produced by tumors.

With the discovery and successful operations of breast cancer in Shirley Temple Black, Happy Rockefeller, and Betty Ford, much of the reluctance, if not the fear, to face the disease is seeming to fade. Television commentator Barbara Walters educated—and startled—her viewers by demonstrating a breast examination (fully clothed) on the Today television show. Doctors' offices, hospitals, and clinics found themselves inundated with requests for examinations. Telephone operators at the American Cancer Society in Manhattan lost count of the requests for information. This open attitude is one of the greatest advances made in the past 20 years in the fight against breast cancer.

Viral Carcinogenesis

Scientists have grappled with the idea that viruses could cause human cancer for at least 70 years, but only within the last 10 years have they accorded it widespread respectability. The idea was suspect for so long because cancer in humans simply did not behave like other diseases of viral origin. It did not appear to be infectious, and there were no confirmable isolations of a causative virus. Over the years, however, a comparative handful of pioneers accumulated evidence that proved that viruses did in fact cause cancer in animals. So the recurring question was: If viruses can cause cancer in animals, then why not in humans?

Identification of a viral role in the etiology of cancer could initiate the development of a vaccine to prevent the cancer. Carcinomas—the type of cancer associated with herpes simplex viruses—are by far the most common, accounting for 85 per cent of human cancer.

If any type of human cancer is caused by a virus, it is probably leukemia. The virus may not be an infectious virus in the same sense as those that cause polio and measles, but strong evidence is accumulating that some form of virus is involved in the etiology of leukemia. There is, however, evidence indicating that many other factors, including environmental influences and genetic predisposition, are also involved.

Chemical Carcinogenesis

Chemicals—in industry, in the environment, and in the diet—may be the single most important cause of human cancers. Many scientists estimate that at least 60 per cent and perhaps as many as 90 per cent of the over 650,000 cases of cancer that will be discovered in the United States in one year will have been caused by environmental factors, mostly chemicals. Nearly 1000 chemicals have been reported to produce tumors in man or other animals, and many times that number are suspect. Yet despite these statistics, and despite all the research that has been carried out since chimney soot was first identified as a cause of cancer over 200 years ago, little is known about the mechanisms of chemical carcinogenesis. In part, this state of affairs results from the greater emphasis that has been placed on viral carcinogenesis. More important, it reflects the fact that, until recently and with only a very few exceptions, the field has been dominated by experimentalists who paint suspect chemicals on the skins of animals or feed the chemicals to animals to determine whether the chemicals induce tumor formation. This process has been useful in identifying carcinogens that should be removed from the environment, but it has been of limited value in showing the mechanisms of carcinogenesis or in revealing ways to inhibit or reverse the action of the chemicals. Some of the kinds of drugs (chemicals) that it is believed may be linked to cancer are:

Diethylstilbestrol (DES). Young women whose mothers received diethylstilbestrol, a synthetic form of estrogen, during pregnancy are involved in a study of the relationship between exposure to this hormone in the uterus and development of a very rare vaginal cancer. The relation of stilbestrol to cancer in young women was first suspected in 1971, when two physicians at Massachusetts General Hospital found the extremely rare cancer of the vagina (adenocarcinoma) in seven young women whose mothers had received stilbestrol during their pregnancies. Stilbestrol was administered to pregnant women with threatened or frequent miscarriage or certain conditions such as diabetes. The hormone is also used as a livestock feed supplement to promote growth. Documented incidence of stilbestrol-linked cancer in humans, however, is extremely small. At least 200,000 female offspring (perhaps far more) were exposed to the hormone and less than 100 cases of cancer have been reported to date.

Some "DES daughters" have adenosis, a condition in which the cells of the cervix and vagina remain as glandular tissue rather than developing as they normally would. Adenosis is not cancerous. The specific test for adenosis is iodine staining of the vaginal and cervical areas. If the test is positive, a colposcopic examination is advised. A number of physicians believe that women with adenosis should not take estrogen in any form because it may trigger abnormal cell growth in the adenosis tissue. Birth control pills and "morning after" pills, for example, contain estrogen.

Rauwolfia. Women aged 50 or over who take certain types of medication to relieve mild cases of high blood pressure run a threefold increased risk of developing breast cancer.* Ten to 20 per cent of all United States women in the over 50 age group have some degree of hypertension, and hundreds of thousands of them are being medically treated for the condition. Most of these patients take a small daily dose of reserpine or a related alkaloid, both extracted from the roots of the Indian shrub, *Rauwolfia serpentina.* The rauwolfia products have been in use for 20 years, have generally been well tolerated in the dosage used by most patients, and are inexpensive compared with newer medications for lowering blood pressure. Theories as to how reserpine-type alkaloids might influence breast cancer are as yet inconclusive. A leading United States cancer epidemiologist believes that the action is not to cause the cancer—that usually takes many years—but to stimulate or accelerate its development.

Alcohol. There is a significant relationship between excessive use of alcohol and certain cancer, according to the National Institute on Alcohol Abuse and Alcoholism. Cancers of the mouth, pharynx, larynx, and esophagus, and primary cancer of the liver, appear to be definitely related to heavy alcohol intake in the United States and other parts of the world where these cancers occur with high frequency among men. Heavy smoking and heavy drinking seem to be particularly implicated in cancers of the mouth, pharynx, and larynx, in which heavy intake of both alcohol and tobacco has not only an additive, but apparently a potentiating effect in increasing risk. The cause of cancer at any specific site is now generally viewed as probably involving the interaction of several fac-

*Since this writing, however, a major article in the Journal of the American Medical Association has shown this finding to be controversial and inconclusive.

tors; alcohol may be one of these factors in certain sites.

Epidemiological Aspects of Cancer

Many researchers feel that environmental factors contribute from 60 to 90 per cent of cancers. Potentially dangerous are such things as asbestos dust, cigarette smoke, pollutants of air and water, viruses, radiation, food additives, and the thousands of low-level insults to the body that are a part of contemporary life. When millions of people are exposed to tiny amounts of a cancer-producing substance, only a small percentage may be affected, but this can still lead to thousands of patients whose cancer could have been prevented. Researchers in the field of epidemiology seek to relate differences in the occurrence of cancer to an element or elements in the environment. Once key elements are isolated, research can move into the laboratory and the hospital to complete the picture and develop corrective steps. For example, one research project is comparing diets among peoples with very different rates of cancer of the rectum and colon. In their native land, the Japanese have a low rate of this cancer; if they move to the United States, their children tend to have the high incidence that we have here. Blacks in Africa rarely have this cancer, but black Americans have a high rate. The processing of much of our food, the removal of roughage, and a diet high in animal fats and proteins may be factors in the Western world's high rate of large-bowel cancer.

A striking example of what epidemiology can uncover is the effect asbestos was found to have on people exposed to even low levels of asbestos particles in the air. E. Cuyler Hammond, Sc.D., of the American Cancer Society, and Irving J. Selikoff, M.D., of the Mount Sinai School of Medicine, have found very high rates of lung cancer among unprotected workers in asbestos factories and among construction workers using asbestos to insulate pipes. Concern has led to the use of protective measures in the asbestos and construction industries. The incidence of lung cancer in asbestos workers who smoke cigarettes is nine times the already higher rate among cigarette smokers in general. In Japan, in 1972, Dr. Takeshi Hirayama completed a five-year study of 265,000 Japanese over 40 years of age living in one area. He found death rates for cigarette smokers much higher than for nonsmokers, demonstrating that the danger of cigarettes leaps the barriers of different diet and different lifestyles—differences that have sometimes been offered in defense of cigarette smoking.

Environmental Factors and Gastric Cancer. Gastric (stomach) cancer is a major concern in every country for which solid information is available. The extremely high and low incidence rates in certain areas predicate environmental factors as causative agents, as indicated by the following data:

1. Gastric cancer patients give a familial history of gastric cancer more often than do patients with primary sites, except those with skin cancer.

2. Phenol is a secondary carcinogen present in all smoke, soot, tar, and smoked foods. Smoked salmon and trout are staples in Icelandic and Finnish diets.

3. Two soft coal-mining counties in Utah, Carbon and Emory, have three times the incidence of gastric cancer as the rest of Utah.

4. Talc in talc-treated rice, which is popular among the Japanese, may contain the carcinogen responsible for the excess of gastric cancer among the Japanese.

5. Salt concentration had a cocarcinogenic effect in experimental gastric carcinogenesis. Salted fish is a staple in four of the countries that have a high incidence of cancer.

6. Nitrosamines may be carcinogenic, as indicated by the fact that many areas with high gastric cancer rates are agricultural, and sodium nitrate is used widely as fertilizer. Nitrate also is present in large concentrations in the water of these areas. Bacon, which is usually processed with sodium nitrate, is also under suspicion.

Prevention

Some cancers *can* be prevented. In the area of prevention, much is already known. At present, the types of cancer that can be directly related to known carcinogenic exposures are (1) *lung,* in its relation to cigarette smoke and certain other inhalation hazards (particularly asbestos, chromates, and radioactive materials); (2) *skin,* as it relates to a variety of crude tar products and radiation;

(3) *bladder,* in relation to aromatic amines and their derivatives; (4) *leukemias,* in relation to radioactive materials; and (5) *mesotheliomas,* as they relate to asbestos. Recent research has pinpointed the common plastic vinyl chloride as a cause of angiosarcoma of the liver in workers in certain chemical plants. It has also recently been found that aerosol spray products discharge fluorocarbons into the air, which in turn diminishes the protective ozone layer. Many scientists believe that the ozone layer is necessary to protect against ultraviolet rays and ensuing skin cancer.

An enormous amount of epidemiologic information has related cancer risk with sex, age, race, ethnic background, rural and urban differences, and diet. The risk of dying from lung cancer is 20 times greater in men and women who have smoked heavily for years than in nonsmokers. A high risk of breast cancer has been noted in women who are obese, who are from 40 to 60 years of age, who are childless or have had a child after the age of 30, and in those with a family history of cancer among blood relatives. Recent studies have shown that women whose husbands have prostate cancer have an increased risk of developing uterine and breast cancer. It is suggested that these women should be checked frequently. Women with a family history of breast or ovarian cancer, or with a personal history of menstrual difficulties should have a pelvic exam every six months. Some researchers feel that exogenous estrogens can be a cause of endometrial (uterine wall) cancer.

Additional characteristics of cancer risk by region are being sought in a compendium of cancer mortality data recently compiled for each county in the country for the period 1950 to 1969.

Patients with cancer of the breast, the colon and rectum, the lung, the oral cavity, the skin, or the uterus are most likely to survive, either by prevention or through early diagnosis and treatment. They add up to about 60 per cent of all cancer cases and almost 50 per cent of deaths. In recognition of this, the American Cancer Society has singled out these sites for emphasis in a massive effort to help save thousands of additional lives each year through intensification of its educational and service efforts at all levels of organization. Here, in brief, are the safeguards urged by the Cancer Society:

1. Breast. Monthly self-examination as regular female practice.
2. Colon and Rectum. Proctoscopic examination as routine in annual checkups for those over 40.
3. Lung. Reduction and ultimate elimination of cigarette smoking.
4. Oral Cavity. Wider practice of early detection measures.
5. Skin. Avoidance of excessive sun.
6. Uterus. Pap tests for all adult women.
7. Basic. Annual physical examination for all adult men and women.

Detection and Diagnosis

In the area of detection and diagnosis, the practicing physician is the first line of defense for the individual patient. *The best defense against death from cancer is early diagnosis.* The means for early detection of cervical cancer, for example, is readily available in the Pap test. Its importance cannot be overstated when we remember that cervical cancer could be largely eliminated through early detection, yet almost 10,000 women die from this type of cancer each year. Another example is breast cancer, which now can be diagnosed by mammography at a stage when the disease is still localized. A mass-screening study in which breast cancer was detected early through mammography and promptly treated resulted in a reduction of one-third in the death rate of patients over a five-year period. In a major cancer control activity, the National Cancer Institute and the American Cancer Society are cooperating in a joint national program in which more than two dozen demonstration screening centers will evaluate and demonstrate early breast cancer detection techniques of medical history, clinical examination, and use of mammography, thermography, and xeroradiography.

Although some lung cancers can be detected through sputum cell examination at an earlier stage than is possible by chest x-ray film, studies are under way to determine whether sputum cytology is a practical tool for early detection. If sputum cytologic evidence shows abnormal cells, a fiberoptic bronchoscope, a relatively new instrument, makes it possible to visualize and probe all the major areas of the lung, offering the possibility of locating a cancer that may be removable by surgery.

A recent report on a 25-year follow-up study of 18,000 persons more than 50 years old described the value of periodic examinations for colon and rectal cancer. Those who had received periodic proctoscopic examinations and had polyps and other precancerous conditions removed, had a colon cancer rate only 15 per cent of that expected if examinations had not been done regularly.

The National Cancer Institute's detection and diagnostic research focuses on early diagnosis of cancers of the lung, breast, large bowel, uterus, bladder, and prostate, which together encompass 60 per cent of all human cancers, excluding skin cancer. Much of the detection research is in the development and demonstration of screening techniques. The cooperation of physicians in motivating people to use these methods is invaluable.

QUACKERY—STILL A PROBLEM

Cancer quackery continues to be a serious menace. Men and women who capitalize on the despair of cancer patients and their families are still active in most states.

Because cancer quackery is against the law in many states, advocates of unproved and worthless remedies frequently persuade their victims to leave the state for treatment. The relatively few quacks who may still be operating underground are inexorably being eliminated.

It is vital that cancer patients and their families investigate carefully before acting in time of stress. Before jeopardizing the life of a loved one or exhausting the family's funds on worthless treatments, reliable sources of information should be checked. The American Cancer Society, in cooperation with state and local health departments, and the United States Food and Drug Administration have investigated many "cancer quacks" and have been successful in bringing about many court convictions.

Most health departments have an active cancer-control program, consisting of educating the public to the need for early detection; the training of laboratory technicians in techniques for early detection, such as the microscopic examination of cervical smears; conducting epidemiological studies of cancer; and the development and evaluation of cancer-control services within the various states.

A basic element of many cancer-control programs involves the tumor registry, in which is filed information about diagnosis and treatment of cancer cases, as well as some of the important characteristics of the patient. These registries provide a tremendous reservoir of information that is useful in evaluating the progress of cancer-control measures. The follow-up mechanism, by which reports are made on each case every year until time of death, helps keep patients under continuous medical supervision. This is as important in cancer as it is in tuberculosis and other chronic diseases. The registry supplies data for research and contributes to a better understanding of the epidemiology of cancer.

Treatment

Radiation and surgery are the most widely and successfully used methods of curing cancer. Newer equipment has been developed for radiation therapy, such as the linear accelerator, which emits a smaller and sharper beam, permitting deeper penetration into the involved area without affecting the overlying skin. More radiation energy can be delivered without harming the surrounding healthy tissue. Physicists are also developing a low-cost, compact machine that will emit high-energy neutron beams for treatment.

Chemical agents, drugs, hormones, and radioactive medications have also proved to be extremely valuable in treating certain types of cancer.

SMOKING AND DISEASE

For more than a decade, various government reports have linked cigarette smoking to lung cancer, emphysema, and other respiratory ailments. Investigations have also demonstrated a significant association between cigarette smoking and the incidence of angina pectoris. In 1971 the U.S. Surgeon

General issued a 488-page report to Congress which showed, among other things, that smokers who rely on pipes and cigars are not as safe as they imagine. According to the report, which detailed hundreds of studies on millions of smokers and nonsmokers, cigarette smokers are at least 20 times as likely to die of lung cancer as nonsmokers, and six to 10 times as likely to die of cancer of the larynx. They are also more susceptible to peptic ulcers, the delivery of stillborn babies, and cancer of the urinary tract.

In addition, the report cited experimental evidence that cigarette smoking causes a relative deprivation of oxygen in the heart muscle. It also contributes to circulatory problems by constricting arteries. The Surgeon General's conclusion was, "Cigarette smoking is a significant factor in the development of coronary heart disease."

Because pipe and cigar smokers rarely inhale deeply, they are only slightly more susceptible to lung cancer than nonsmokers. But pipe smokers can develop cancer of the mouth or lip. Many pipe puffers and cigar chompers do draw smoke down as far as the larynx. As a result, their chances of developing cancer of the throat are 3 to 7 times greater than those of people who avoid smoking of any kind.

Cessation of smoking reduces the risk of mortality and morbidity by 4 to 10 times in such diseases as lung cancer, heart disease, chronic bronchitis, and pulmonary emphysema. Statistics indicate that within three to six years after a smoker has quit the habit, the risk of dying from lung cancer approaches that of a nonsmoker. (A Smoker's Self-Testing Kit is available from the U.S. Department of Health, Education and Welfare, No. 74–8716.)

Effect of the Surgeon General's Report on Smoking

When the Surgeon General of the United States reported that nonsmokers in the vicinity of smokers were considerably affected by carbon monoxide, organizations such as ASH (Action on Smoking and Health), and GASP (Group Against Smokers Pollution), started campaigning for the rights of nonsmokers. Carbon monoxide in the blood stream inhibits the ability of the hemoglobin to pick up and carry oxygen. Many states now have laws that prohibit smoking in public places. Where there are no such state laws, cities have enacted their own laws. The purpose is to protect the health and comfort of nonsmokers, but smokers benefit also, because of the restriction on the number of places they can smoke.

Nonsmokers are concerned with the following inequities:

1. All cigarette advertising has been banned on television and radio. However that also stops equal time for effective anti-smoking messages—and no limits have been placed on newspaper and magazine advertising. In fact, over $300,000,000 per year are spent for cigarette ads.

2. Tobacco products are required to carry a printed warning that smoking is dangerous to health. But since it's been shown that 95 per cent of the populace now know that, the real effect of the notice is to protect tobacco companies from lawsuits.

3. Congress spends over $11,000,000 a year on agencies such as the National Clearinghouse for Smoking and Health. At the same time, though, it's spending more than five times that much on research to develop sturdier tobacco plants, inspection of tobacco leaves, and support payments to tobacco exporters.

4. Tobacco and alcohol are both related to political (vote-getting) and economic issues. Some congressmen from tobacco-growing states, for example, claim that heavy taxing of high tar and nicotine cigarettes would place an economic hardship on millions of their constituents. A few researchers have even suggested that some manufac-

CHILDREN AND SMOKING

The National Congress of Parents and Teachers (PTA) has published the pamphlet "His First Cigarette May Be a Matter of Life or Death," printed in both English and Spanish. These pamphlets are available in quantity, through your State Department of Health. A smoking and health education curriculum unit from grades K through 7 (Berkeley Project) is also available from the National Clearinghouse for Smoking and Health.

PUNCH A HOLE IN THE PROPER SPACE FOR EACH ANSWER. THEN TURN OVER TO GET YOUR SCORE

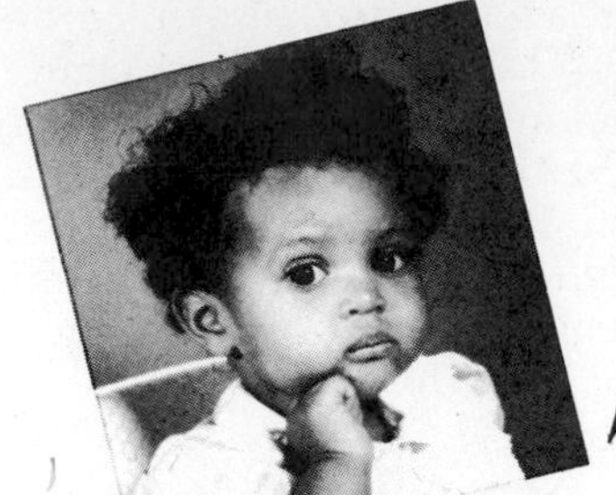

What's Your Cigarette Smoking I.Q.?

		TRUE?	
1	Scientific evidence shows that cigarette smoking shortens life.	YES	NO
2	Just one cigarette upsets the balance of air and blood in your lungs.	YES	NO
3	Smoking has no damaging effects on the heart.	YES	NO
4	Smoking two packs a day is no more harmful than smoking one pack a day.	YES	NO
5	Cigarette smoking heads the list of causes of chronic bronchitis.	YES	NO
6	Scientific research has not shown any association between smoking and emphysema.	YES	NO
7	Cigarette smoking is the major cause of lung cancer.	YES	NO
8	Non-smokers are sick just as often as smokers.	YES	NO
9	It's too late to stop smoking if you've smoked for 5 years or more.	YES	NO
10	Every year 1 million Americans quit smoking.	YES	NO

Your Christmas Seal association has a booklet that can help you kick the smoking habit . . . ask for it. If you have any special questions see your doctor or your Tuberculosis and Respiratory Disease association.

Figure 7–4 (Courtesy of the American Lung Association.)

COUNT 10 FOR EACH CORRECT ANSWER

See other side first!

YOU'RE WELL INFORMED	**100**
GOOD, BUT LEARN MORE	**80-90**
WHAT YOU DON'T KNOW MAY HURT YOU	**under 80**

NO	YES		
	X	1	For smokers, risk of shortened life is 70 per cent greater than for non-smokers.
	X	2	The imbalance of air flow and blood flow can be measured *immediately* after one cigarette.
X		3	Among smokers, the number of deaths from heart disease are almost double those of non-smokers.
X		4	The more cigarettes a person smokes, the greater his risk of disability and premature death.
	X	5	Smoking is the *most important* cause of chronic bronchitis.
X		6	Research has not yet shown smoking causes emphysema, but smoking is a contributing factor.
	X	7	The risk of death from lung cancer is 10 times greater for smokers than for non-smokers.
X		8	Smokers spend 88 million extra days in bed in comparison to non-smokers.
X		9	No matter how long you've smoked, some of the harmful effects of smoking begin to reverse themselves the minute you stop.
	X	10	There are now more than 21 million Americans who are ex-smokers.

1-70

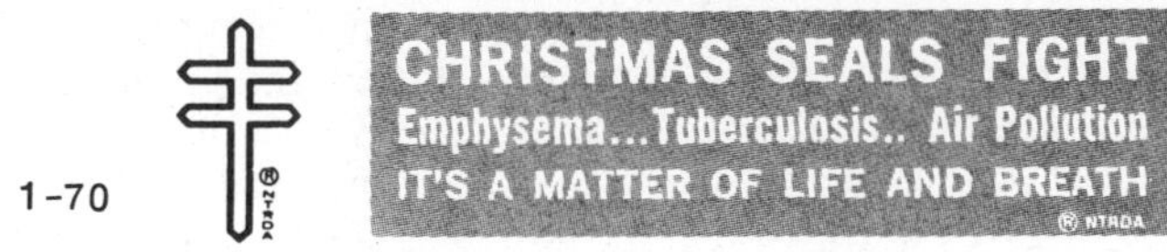

Published by the National Tuberculosis and Respiratory Disease Association

Figure 7–4 *Continued.*

turers are coercing various scientists around the country into questioning and challenging the findings of scientists who have found tobacco and alcohol to be serious health hazards.

5. Federal agencies have withdrawn from the market such safe and health-preserving agents as cyclamates. Yet they permit the greatest carcinogen in our society—cigarettes—to be sold in vending machines.

QUITTING TIPS FOR SMOKERS

1. Find a strong incentive to quit.
2. Tell your friends you're quitting.
3. Pick a date on which you will start to quit and get yourself mentally ready for it.
4. Try halfway measures like tapering off. This works for some people, whereas others have to stop completely.
5. Store up on temporary substitutes like low-calorie gum, celery, carrots, and so on.
6. Throw out visible signs of smoking, such as ashtrays, lighters, matches.
7. Sit in the non-smoking section of the movies, trains, planes, and buses. Don't go to the lobby during theatre intermission. Make it inconvenient to smoke.
8. If you have the urge to smoke, put it off 10 minutes...and 10 minutes again...and again.
9. Carry a single cigarette with you as security—that way you won't panic when the urge to smoke hits you, and you won't smoke because it's your last cigarette.
10. Avoid smoking-related activities (morning coffee, drinking, etc.) for the first few days of quitting.
11. Remind yourself often that you have CHOSEN not to smoke.
12. Re-program your thinking: "I am comfortable without a cigarette." "I don't want a cigarette."
13. Drink plenty of water.
14. Drink liquor slowly; without a cigarette, you may tend to gulp drinks.

Even though 65,000 people die every year from lung cancer and emphysema directly caused by smoking, there is no means of coding smoking as a diagnosis. The hospital index of the International Classification of Diseases codes around 7500 diagnoses, including over 275 designations for various dependencies such as heroin, alcohol, aspirin, and absinthe, but there is not one such coding for smoking or nicotine. Perhaps death certificates should be required to read "bronchogenic carcinoma due to cigarette smoking" and "emphysema due to smoker's bronchitis" whenever appropriate. Medical students should be taught to identify cigarette addiction as a problem whenever any patient inhales more than 10 cigarettes a day. No chart should be regarded as complete unless the smoking history is stated. As Dr. Richard C. Bates has stated:

> "Industrial physicians have every right to give cigarette smokers bad marks in pre-employment physical examinations. After all, smokers lose 45 per cent more days from work because of illness than nonsmokers do. They're also likely to be less productive at work and more prone to be injured on the job. Cigarette smokers, too, are more likely to be addicted to alcohol and other drugs. Thus a corporation that hired only nonsmokers would have a significant economic advantage over its competitors. Doctors in private practice should consider these points in hiring their own employees, too.[10]

What can be done to effectively deal with the problem? Most experts agree that the solution has four phases.

1. One phase is reducing the number of new smokers. This phase deals mainly with those in the 12 to 18 year age group, and the responsibility for carrying it out rests with parents and teachers. Most young smokers have parents who smoke. The generation gap is not an issue as far as cigarette smoking is concerned. Teachers and other educators can help by introducing an effective anti-smoking education program into the basic curriculum in grammar school through high school. For the rest of this decade, the end of the postwar baby boom will be reflected by the entry of relatively fewer teenagers into the population. Because of their small numbers, this age group could prove an easy

target for antismoking campaigns. If enough teenagers can be persuaded not to take up the habit, they will serve as an example to the younger children coming into this age bracket.

2. The second phase is to encourage smokers to quit. This might be done by behavior modification and counseling. Increased efforts are needed to make smoking less socially acceptable. (Some measures have already been taken to forbid smoking in planes, theaters, and restaurants.) Tentative findings reveal that smoking is more apt to be habit forming than addicting. Those who smoke to relieve nervous tension should be encouraged to seek other methods of dealing with their problems. Antismoking clinics have been formed in many cities throughout the nation. They have been somewhat effective for those who have sought their help.

The last two phases deal with the smoker who cannot or will not quit smoking.

3. One is the development of the safe cigarette. Some progress has been made in this area. Today's cigarettes contain on the average two-thirds as much tar and nicotine as those of 10 years ago. But nicotine seems to increase flavor and habituation (which sounds somewhat like addiction), and when sales decline for a certain brand, the company raises the nicotine content. Perhaps more federal regulations for tar and nicotine levels, are needed, but there is confusion as to who has the authority to do this. The development of the "safe cigarette" is further hampered by the fact that scientists don't

WOMEN AND SMOKING*

"Yes, there are a lot of good reasons for women to quit smoking. Find yours."

( ) I'm a mother. Children whose parents smoke are more likely to smoke than those whose parents don't.
( ) My closet smells rotten, my clothes smell rotten; I'm sick of it.
( ) Lung cancer deaths are twice as high among women who smoke.
( ) I'm pregnant. Smoking can affect the health of my baby. Smoking during pregnancy retards the growth of the baby, for one thing.
( ) I'm middle-aged. Women 45–54 who smoke have twice the risk of dying of coronary heart disease as those who don't.
( ) My niece imitates everything I do. I saw her pick up a pencil one day and imitate me smoking.
( ) I seem to be sick a lot. I also smoke a lot. Women who smoke have more chronic illness, lose more time from work, are sick in bed more often than those who don't smoke.
( ) I know my husband's been trying to quit. How can he with me still puffing away?
( ) I want to wake up feeling fresh and clean again. I've had it with nicotine hangover in the mornings.
( ) The thing that appeals to me most is: If I quit and stay quit, in most cases, it can be as if I never smoked. There's something about this that absolutely knocks me out. A clean slate; a real second chance. You just don't get many of those.
( ) I quit once for 10 days and, frankly, I felt pretty good about it. I like that feeling; this time I'm quitting for good. Lord knows, I've done a lot harder things in my life.
( ) So many people I know have quit, I'm beginning to feel stupid smoking.
( ) There's something very cool and self-assured about women who don't need ciagarettes.
( ) I thought it was hopeless; I quit once and went back. But someone told me a lot of people had to quit over and over before it took. I'm trying again. It can't hurt.
( ) If I quit, I'll save 50¢ a day. That's $3.50 a week, $14.00 a month, $182.50 a year. That buys almost a gallon of gas a day Five quarts of milk a week. Gas, electric, and 2 movies a month. After a year, I can take a vacation on cigarettes I didn't smoke.
( ) Somewhere in the back of my head I've been nursing the illusion that smoking is really only dangerous for men. I've just seen the latest statistics. The death rate for women who smoke is more than 20% higher than for women who don't. We've come a long way baby, but I'm not going any further.

All you need is help and encouragement.

*From Women and Smoking, Rockville, Md. 20852. U.S. Department of Health, Education and Welfare. (Free booklets available.)

know everything about the hazardous effects of smoking. Until they know what to eliminate, the task is useless. Research has been done with cellulose cigarettes, but it is not known whether inhaling cellulose is any less dangerous than inhaling tobacco.

4. The last phase deals with encouraging smokers to practice more healthful smoking habits. These include reducing the number of cigarettes smoked, smoking only half of each cigarettes, and taking fewer puffs. Smokers should make it a habit to have regular physical examinations so that certain diseases can be diagnosed and treated early. Other measures have been suggested to decrease the death rates from smoking-related diseases. One is to raise federal taxes, but this might encourage smokers to get the most out of the cigarette they can afford to buy. This means smoking down to the filter, which is a dangerous habit. A new warning has been assigned for use on cigarette packs. It reads, "Warning: Cigarette Smoking is dangerous to health, and may cause death from cancer, coronary heart disease, chronic bronchitis, pulmonary emphysema, and other diseases." If this warning were mandatory on all printed advertisements, and made to occupy at least one-fifth of the ads area, then the proportion of antismoking advertisements to cigarette advertisements would be equal to that on television before the ban and might cause a reduction in the number of American smokers.

Other suggested measures include the formation of an advisory committee similar to that which produced the Surgeon General's report in 1964. This new committee could spell out precise specifications for *substantial* reductions in the amounts of tar, nicotine, and other dangerous ingredients that cigarettes will be allowed to contain. In addition, cigarette manufacturers should be required, *by law,* to meet these specifications. Many experts estimate that such mandatory standards, imposed step-by-step over a 5-year period, would not cause undue hardship to the tobacco industry.

Since the Surgeon General's report was issued in 1964, more than a million people have died from lung cancer and emphysema directly attributed to cigarette smoking. This figure does not take into account the deaths from other smoking related killers. Furthermore, carbon monoxide given off by cigarettes is injurious to the health of others in the immediate vicinity of the smoker, according to at least one research study. Smoking is indeed a public health problem, one that has not received the attention it deserves.

CABBAGE CIGARETTES

Isn't it hypocritical to expound piously on the world food shortage and impending mass starvation while agricultural agencies the world over are aiding and promoting the growing of tobacco, "the most widely grown commercial non-food plant in the world"?* To be sure, tobacco does contribute to population erosion through emphysema and cancer, but this hardly seems a humane means of population control, and these diseases cause a great drain on medical resources and finances.

Since 44.8 per cent of the world's vast tobacco acreage lies in "starving" Asia,* would it not be humanitarian to offer economic inducements to farmers to switch from tobacco to food crops?

If people must smoke, let their cigarettes be made of a less toxic plant material—not a monopolizer of arable land, but a vegetable by-product of food crops, say, cabbage, lettuce, or papaya leaves."

*B.C. Akehurst: Tobacco. *Humanities,* New York, 1969.

CARDIOVASCULAR DISEASE

The leading cause of death in the United States today is diseases of the heart and blood vessels. Each year, heart disease is responsible for 1 of every 2 recorded deaths, killing nearly 1 million Americans. For each patient who dies, 11 others are chronically

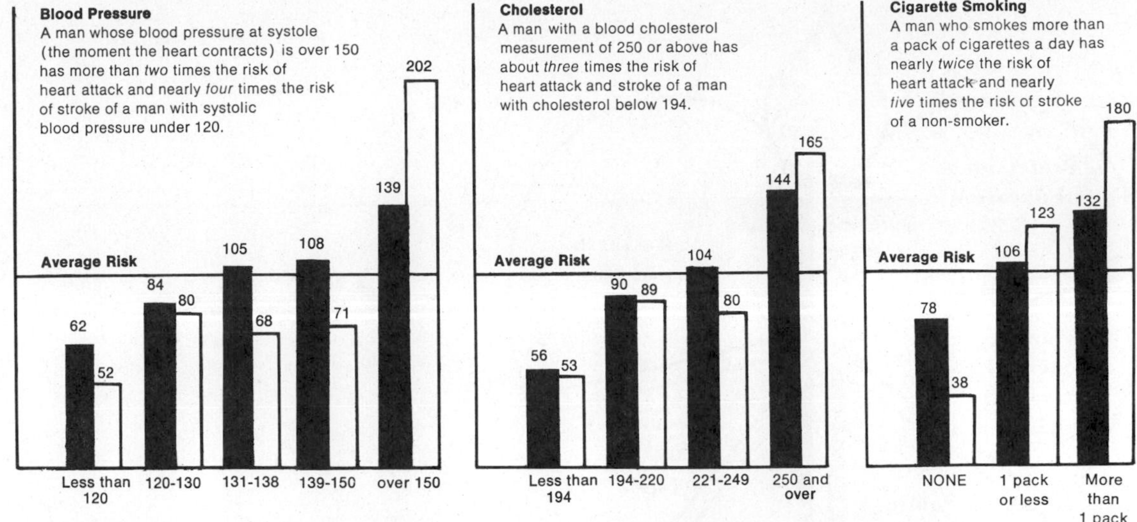

Figure 7–5 Risk factors in heart attack and stroke. (From Heart Facts 1975, American Heart Association, p. 19.)

ill, and many of them are afflicted in their most productive years. Cardiovascular disease is an important cause of disability for all ages above 15, and about 6 billion dollars is lost annually due to employee absenteeism. Each day, heart disease kills on the average of 1400 Americans, and cerebral strokes take another 500 lives. The death toll is more than one life a minute and hundreds of thousands are crippled every year. Diseases of the heart and circulatory system now cause nearly 71 per cent of all deaths in the United States.

Coronary heart disease is our leading killer, and the toll is increasing. The first heart attack is fatal to almost 40 per cent of

KNOW THE SIGNS

The Warning Signs of Heart Attack

- **Prolonged, oppressive pain or unusual discomfort in *center* of chest.**
- **Pain may radiate to shoulder, arm, neck or jaw.**
- **Sweating may accompany pain or discomfort.**
- **Nausea, vomiting and shortness of breath may also occur.**

The Warning Signs of Stroke

- **Sudden, temporary weakness or numbness of face, arm or leg.**
- **Temporary loss of speech, or trouble in speaking or understanding speech.**
- **Temporary dimness or loss of vision, particularly in one eye.**
- **An episode of double vision.**
- **Unexplained dizziness or unsteadiness.**
- **Change in personality, mental ability or the pattern of headaches.**

ACT IMMEDIATELY

Sometimes these symptoms subside, then return. When you experience one or more warning signs, call your doctor and describe these symptoms in detail. If he's not immediately available, get to a hospital emergency room at once. Be prepared to act. Instruct others to act if you cannot. Keep a list of numbers—doctor, hospital, ambulance or other emergency services and police—next to your telephone, and in a prominent place in your pocket, wallet or purse.

Figure 7–6 Warning signs of heart attack and stroke. (From Heart Facts 1975, American Heart Association, p. 20.)

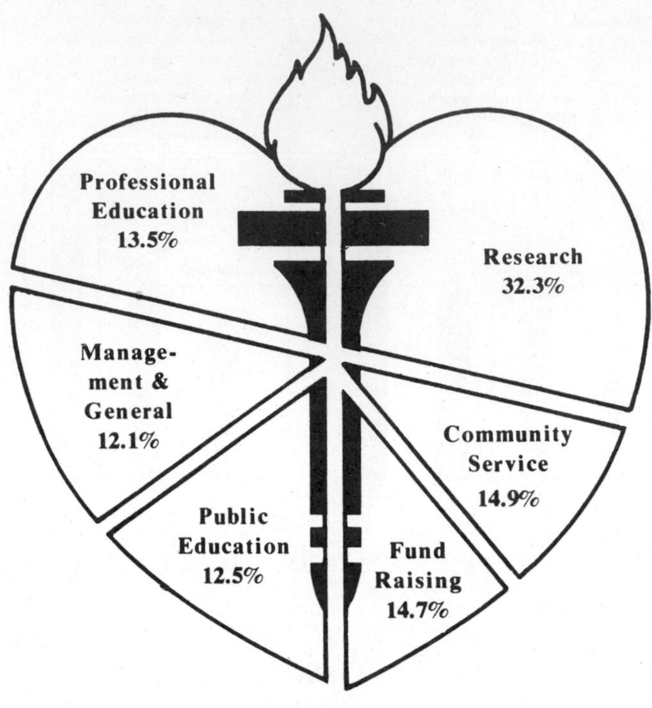

Figure 7–7 Where the heart dollar goes. (From Heart Facts 1975, American Heart Association.)

the victims. Death is either immediate or occurs as a direct result within six weeks. Almost 20 per cent die in the first hour.

The incidence of heart disease has increased among persons who are 30 to 60 years of age. Heart disease flourishes in our country in areas where modern urban industrial life is most developed and where changing physical habits, such as eating, exercising, working, and smoking, are most pronounced.

The heart diseases, in addition to their dominance as a cause of death, are the cause of widespread associated illness and disability in the United States. It is estimated that 14.6 million adults suffer from known heart disease, and nearly as many have suspected heart disease. Thus, nearly one-fourth the adult population already has or is likely to develop heart disease. The frequency of heart disease increases sharply with age. Fewer than 1 per cent of the population between the ages of 18 and 24 have definite heart disease, while 25 per cent of the population at 65 years old suffer from some known form of this disease.

Causes

Causes of the major cardiovascular diseases are unknown. Suggested possibilities include obesity, hormones, diet, exercise, overwork, occupation, cigarette smoking, emotional tension, environment, and social characteristics.

One study has suggested complicated relationships between drinking and heart disease: persons who never drank were found to have the same rates of coronary heart disease as those who drank at either light or heavy levels. On the other hand, former drinkers who had stopped were more than three times as likely to suffer a heart attack than the other groups. It is not clear why former drinkers have a higher rate of coronary heart disease. This group may include persons in poorer health than other groups, leading to greater susceptibility to coronary heart disease. While these data are by no means sufficient to establish a protective role for alcohol among persons with high coronary risk characteristics, it does seem that for most persons the use of moderate amounts of alcohol does not have detrimental effects leading to coronary heart disease.

The death rate of men from heart diseases exceeds that of women at all ages, but the greatest variation between the sexes is caused by the soaring rate among men aged 45 to 64. Furthermore, a man's chance of dying from a heart attack if he lives in New York State is more than twice as high as that of a resident of New Mexico.

What's Your Risk?

Stop. Take a moment to determine just exactly which factors in your diet and life are the ones which could be contributing to your risk of suffering prematurely from heart disease. Which ones could you (should you) change? The first three are inalterable. But the last eight are up to you!

OK. Add them up.

- A score of **4** or less means a very low risk. Only about 5 out of 100 people in this group will suffer heart attacks before the age of 65.
- **5-7.** Slightly below average. There is room for change.
- **8-10.** Average risk. Too high for comfort. 20 out of 100 average men suffer heart attacks in middle age.
- **11-13.** High risk. Make some changes in your lifestyle. Like today. If possible, get a medical checkup so that you can find out what your cholesterol level, triglyceride level, and blood pressure are.
- **Over 14.** One person out of every two in this group is likely to have a heart attack before the age of 65. Look through this paper for heart healthy suggestions and get a check-up! ♥

SEX: If you're a man, give yourself one point. Before the age of 60, the average man has a higher risk of heart attack than the average woman. ☐

AGE: If you've over 35, give yourself one point. The older you are the greater your risk. ☐

FAMILY: Give yourself one point if a member of your immediate family died of a heart attack before retirement age. ☐

CHOLESTEROL: An average person eats seven whole eggs a week, organ meats more than once a week, and red meat almost every day. If you eat about the average amount of foods high in cholesterol give yourself one point. More? Two points. Substantially less? No points. ☐

SATURATED FAT: The average person eats sausage two or three times a week; meat, whole milk, some butter and ice cream daily. Take one point if you are average. Two if above average. No points if you eat non-fat or low-fat dairy products and restrict your consumption of hard animal fat. ☐

SALT AND HIGH BLOOD PRESSURE: If you *know* that your blood pressure is higher than it should be or if you use a lot of salt . . . take one point. ☐

SUGAR: If you sugar your coffee, eat candy, or lots of sweets you can raise your level of triglyceride and you should take one point. ☐

SMOKING: Give yourself one point for each half pack of cigarettes you smoke each day. ☐

EXERCISE: If you get no real exercise . . . two points. Some . . . one point. No points if you exercise thoroughly at least three times a week. ☐

WEIGHT: If you are more than 10 pounds overweight . . . two points. Between 5 and 10 over . . . one point. ☐

TENSION: One point if your life is constantly full of deadlines and time pressures. ☐

TOTAL SCORE ☐

Figure 7–8 Factors contributing to heart disease. (From Your Heart Beat, Vol. 1, No. 1. Stanford, Calif., Stanford Heart Disease Prevention Program, 1975.)

Some defects may be present in a child's heart or great vessels at birth. For example, the pulmonary artery and aorta may be transposed and cause death soon after birth. Scarring and narrowing of the valves may be acquired later in life as the results of rheumatic fever. However, 90 per cent of all heart disease in the United States is due to arteriosclerosis and hypertension or high blood pressure.

AMBITION HARD ON THE HEART

The hard-driving, aggressive, deadline-conscious person runs a much greater risk of coronary heart disease than his more relaxed counterpart, according to a team of San Francisco scientists.

They surveyed more than 3000 men in a long-term study and concluded that personality may be a factor in determining who will develop heart disease. Personality Type A—the ambitious type—was found to develop heart disease at a rate nearly twice as great as the more passive individual, Type B.

In their study the scientists followed 3524 men, ages 39 to 59, employed by 11 California corporations. All were found free of heart disease when the project began in

1960. Since then, there have been 133 cases of coronary heart disease, with 94 found in the Type A group. Personality was determined by interviews with trained personnel.

A spokesman for the study said that the evidence "finally confirms the hypothesis that personality and behavior play a significant causal role in the development of coronary heart disease." This influence is exerted independent of any of the other risk factors apparent from the study.

Other factors found to be associated with heart disease susceptibility were a parental history of the disease; elevated blood pressure; physical inactivity; diabetes; level of education (the lower, the greater the risk); and cigarette smoking.[13]

The Risk-Factor Concept

One of the major studies aimed at learning more about heart disease and its prevention is the Framingham Heart Study, sponsored by the National Heart Institute, which is part of the federal government. This project, which began in 1959 in Framingham, Massachusetts, is a large-scale, prospective, epidemiologic study of over 5000 adults. The Framingham Study is investigating many factors that seem to be related, in varying degrees, to the development of heart disease. Some of the high-risk factors have been determined to be age, family history of the disease, sex, high blood pressure, cigarette smoking, EKG abnormalities, diabetes, gout, stress, low vital capacity, overweight, insufficient physical activity, high blood triglyceride levels, and high blood cholesterol levels. There is a slightly higher risk for women who are over 40 and for those who are on the Pill. The risk is multiplied for individuals who have more than one risk factor.

The scientists involved in these research projects have generally become convinced that changes in personal habits can lower the risks of contracting heart disease. Physicians who observe early signs of incipient cardiovascular disease in patients often prescribe changes in habit in order to reduce risk. Many of these scientists and physicians are so convinced of the dangers of the risk factors that they have changed their own habits to reduce the risk for themselves.

Reducing the risk of cardiovascular disease requires changes in basic behavior. Unfortunately, there is no magic pill that can be taken to accomplish the designed results. Instead, one must make changes in daily patterns of living; he must alter, for example, patterns of eating, exercising, and cigarette smoking, all of which may be quite difficult to change. Further revisions in behavior may be required as the results of additional research become available. No research is of value unless the knowledge that is gained is applied.

For example, the Heart Association rec-

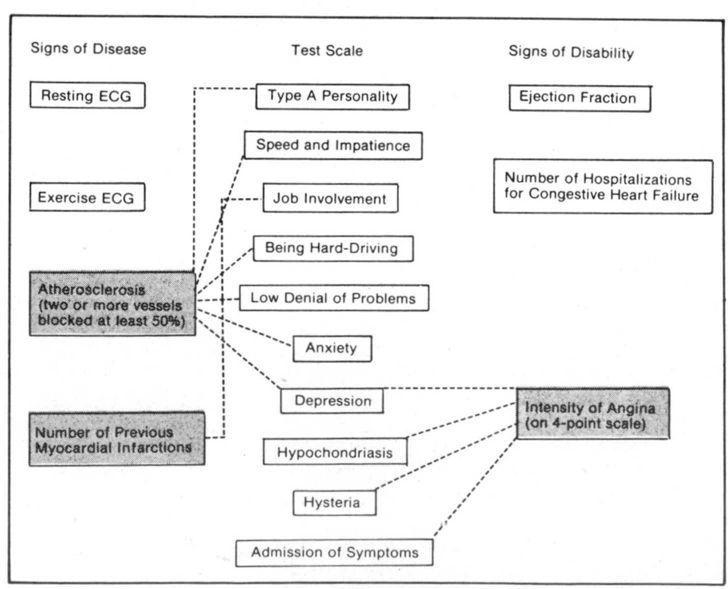

Figure 7–9 Some of the behavioral characteristics that, according to workers at Boston University Hospital, seem associated with cardiovascular and psychological findings. (From Medical News, JAMA, *232* (7): 696, May 19, 1975.)

ommends the following dietary principles to help reduce risk: (1) adequate intake of protein, vitamins, minerals, and other nutrients, (2) maintainence of desirable weight by limiting calories, and (3) limiting intake of foods containing saturated fats and cholesterol, substituting polyunsaturated fats when possible.

COMMON FOODS AND THEIR CHOLESTEROL CONTENT [2]

The tabulation below shows the cholesterol content in milligrams of 100-gram (3½-ounce) portions of common foods:

Food	mg	Food	mg
Beef, raw	70	Ice cream	45
Brains, raw	2000-plus	Kidney, raw	375
Butter	250	Lamb, raw	70
Caviar or fish roe	300-plus	Lard and animal fat	95
Cheddar cheese	100	Liver, raw	300
Creamed cottage cheese	15	Lobster meat	200
Cream cheese	120	Margarine, vegetable fat	0
Cheese spread	65	Margarine, ⅔ animal fat	65
Chicken, raw	60	Milk, whole	11
Crab	125	Milk, skim	3
Egg, whole	550	Mutton	65
Egg white	0	Oysters	200-plus
Egg yolk, fresh	1500	Pork	70
Egg yolk, dried	2950	Shrimp	125
Fish fillet	70	Sweetbreads	250
Heart, raw	150	Veal	90

Stress

It is difficult to know what creates stress in a person. The cave man, for instance, lived in continual fear of the sabertoothed tiger. Nowadays our enemy seems to be the very civilization we live in. The individual who finds it hard to keep up with today's pace of life runs more risk than the person who adapts to this pace.

It is known that emotional or psychological stress has profound effects on the cardiovascular system. The heart rate increases, blood pressure goes up, there is a rise in fatty acids in the blood, and the viscosity and the coagulability of the blood increase. Even though it is known that these cardiovascular effects occur under stress, the importance of these effects on the development of cardiovascular disease has not been conclusively established.

The work of Friedman and Rosenman is especially noteworthy because they have identified a type of person who is "coronary-prone," and they have developed methods of testing for personality characteristics. Their coronary-prone person is found to be a hard-driving, aggressive individual who is habitually rushing to meet deadlines. If deadlines are not an inherent part of his job, he creates self-imposed deadlines, which constantly place him under pressure. He is impatient with objects or people who do not move rapidly enough to match his speed and may find it necessary to run over them to get things done. This person is referred to as the "Type A personality."

The "Type B personality" is the converse of Type A. He is slower moving, does not impose or attempt to meet unreasonable deadlines, and manages to cope with his environment without the apparent urgency exhibited by Type A. The results of this study indicate that Type A is much more likely than Type B to develop heart disease. At least one researcher's findings do not agree with this study. Other researchers, although confirming a personality pattern of anxiety and stress, believe that there may be additional coronary-prone personality types.

ARE YOU A TYPE A?

Yes No

- ☐ ☐ Do you have a habit of explosively accentuating key words in your ordinary speech or of finishing your sentences in a burst of speed?
- ☐ ☐ Do you always move, walk, or eat rapidly?
- ☐ ☐ Do you feel (and openly show) impatience with the rate at which most events take place? Do you find it difficult to restrain yourself from hurrying the speech of others?
- ☐ ☐ Do you get unduly irritated at delay—when the car in front of you seems to slow you up, when you have to wait in line, or wait to be seated in a restaurant?
- ☐ ☐ Does it bother you to watch someone else perform a task you know you can do faster?
- ☐ ☐ Do you often try to do two things at once (dictate while driving or read business papers while you eat)?
- ☐ ☐ Do you often find your mind wandering when listening to someone else?
- ☐ ☐ Do you habitually bring the subject of conversation around to your own concerns and interests?
- ☐ ☐ Do you find yourself attempting to schedule more and more in less and less time?
- ☐ ☐ When you meet an aggressive or competitive person, do you find yourself compelled to "challenge" him?
- ☐ ☐ Do you constantly evaluate your own and other people's activities in terms of numbers (money earned, hours spent, etc.)?
- ☐ ☐ Do you almost always feel vaguely guilty when you relax and do absolutely nothing for several days (even several hours)?

Other stressful behavior and environment patterns have been implicated as causes in increasing the risk of heart disease. Some stress-oriented studies have discovered the following: urban dwellers have a higher incidence of heart disease than do rural dwellers; white-collar workers have a higher incidence than do agricultural workers and blue-collar workers; persons who change residence frequently have higher rates than those who do not move; and men who change jobs frequently have a higher rate than those who are stable in their jobs. Some physicians attempt to modify these behavioral patterns in normal patients on the premise that the modification is a logical way to reduce risk. Other physicians do not feel that there is sufficient evidence at the present time to warrant these changes for the person who has no clinical symptoms of heart disease.

There is general agreement that a person who has heart disease should reduce his life stresses. In treating persons who have heart disease, physicians usually attempt to identify sources of emotional or psychological stress and then try to help the patient reduce that stress. The additional load that the stress places on the cardiovascular system may have deleterious effects on the already damaged system.

"Training to Relax" Lowers Serum Cholesterol Levels

A new program called Cardiostress Management Training has helped patients experience a decrease in cholesterol and triglyceride levels. There are two parts to the program: Anxiety Management Training, and Visumotor Behavior Rehearsal. Patients learn to manage stress, including the stress associated with trying to change their behavior patterns. According to Dr. Suinn, Director, Colorado State University, the entire training process takes only one four-hour session. During the first 20 minutes, the patients are taught to relax particular muscle groups. They perform a series of exercises similar to isometrics to tense, then relax, areas of the body. Once they have learned this, the patients identify situations associated with stress, such as increased work loads and demands, personality conflicts at work or at home, and family pressures. The idea is to know exactly which situations induce stress.

The next step is imagery. The patients visualize stressful situations so they can reexperience the stress response. They are asked to focus on the physical cues to stress, such as increased heart rate, sweating, and muscle tension. Next they are instructed to "switch off" the stress with relaxation. When the cues reappear, the patient recognizes them and, more important, is capable of dealing with them. In some patients the relaxation reflex becomes automatic, while in others it remains a deliberate action. The patients eventually learn to use imagery to practice new ways of dealing with stressful situations by "trying on" new solutions. The training is being tried as a preventive measure for type A individuals who have not had myocardial infarctions – yet.

Causes of Stress: Loss and Threats

There are two major types of stress. One type involves *loss* (of a loved one, a job, or the loss of self-esteem that comes when a person's level of aspiration is impossibly high and he feels incapable of reaching it). The other type of stress involves *threats* (to the individual's status, goals, health, and security). Such stresses can generate symptoms of depression, anxiety, or both.

In a study conducted by Thomas Holmes, it was revealed that patients who experienced the more serious life crises (or too much change) also were more likely to get the serious chronic diseases (see chapter on Mental Health). Perhaps the activity of coping with too many crises can lower resistance to disease, particularly when one's coping techniques are faulty or when they lack relevance to the type of problems to be solved. Research also has revealed that persons in other cultures, groups, and communities have varying degrees of differences in the weight assigned to some life events. For example, the Japanese give far more allegiance to structured family life than do Americans. Also, different cultures have different views of ethical conduct. Americans emphasize internal Christian moral values, placing guilt above humiliation as a guide to ethical conduct, whereas the Japanese rank humiliation first.

The study also detected family-structural differences between different cultures. The American family, for example, tends to be an isolated grouping of one or two parents with children; Japanese family members are likely to be part of a much larger family circle.

In addition, new studies are appearing that help to identify the high-risk stress personality type. (See chapter on Mental Health.)

Each period in life has its own set and degrees of stresses. Many psychiatrists agree that children need the opportunity to confront various problems when they are young and learn to cope with them. Parents, by intervening prematurely, may prevent their children from developing tolerance for problems or acquiring problem-solving mechanisms. Society's concern with time, speed, anxiety, frustration, conflict, and taking the "easy way out" complicate and intensify the process.

A great deal of stress can be prevented in various ways: by reducing changes; maintaining satisfactions, balance, and variety in life; finding a friend, expressing and sharing your feelings; talking about inner worries and feelings; reevaluating values and set priorities; ignoring the unimportant; and striving for movement, duration, and purpose. Stress and anger are closely related. Most psychiatrists now agree that everyone gets angry, and that the way we handle anger may make the difference between sickness and health, senseless destruction and constructive activity, despair and happiness. The important thing is to *know* that we are angry, recognize that anger is normal, find out what we are angry about, don't let anger accumulate, and find appropriate ways of working off anger. In any case, we each have our own way of dealing with stress: individual analysis; help from friends, neighbors, or professionals; hobbies; athletics; yoga or transcendental meditation; biofeedback or relaxation response.

Cigarette Smoking

Nearly 75 per cent of all men in the United States and over 40 per cent of the adult female population have smoked cigarettes regularly at one time or another. According to the most recent figures, 52 per cent of all men and 34 per cent of all women currently are smokers.

Is cigarette smoking associated with a higher death rate from coronary heart disease? Definitely yes. There has been a convergence of several types of evidence – statistical, clinical, and pathological – to give strong support to this conclusion. In men aged 45 to 64, the overall cardiovascular death rate for smokers is nearly double that for non-smokers.

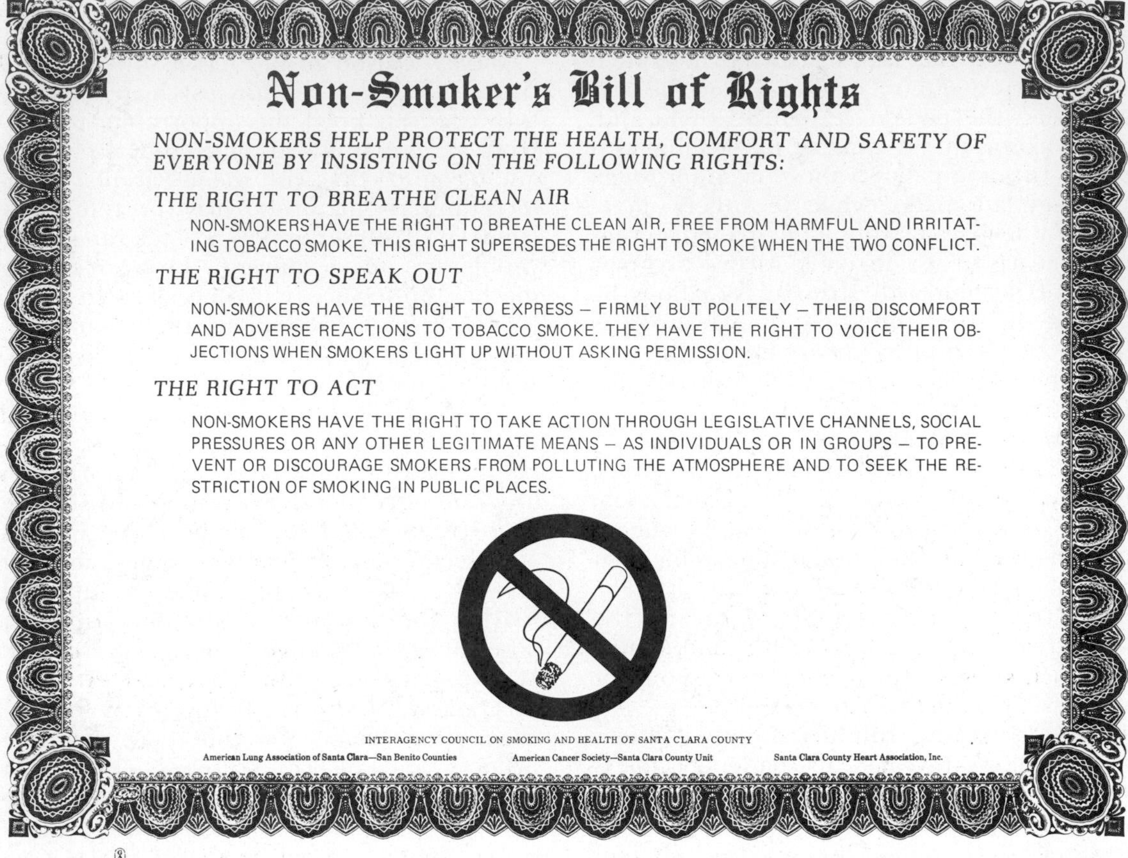

Figure 7–10 Antismoking campaign. (Courtesy of Interagency Council on Smoking and Health of Santa Clara County, Santa Clara, Calif.)

Heart disease is only one of several disorders associated with cigarette smoking. Among the most important of the others are lung cancer, emphysema, and bronchitis. Generally, the evidence indicting cigarettes falls into three categories:

1. Statistical evidence. Numerous statistical studies support the conclusion that cigarette smoking is an important factor in the occurrence of cardiovascular diseases. These surveys have been remarkably consistent; studies at Framingham, Mass. and Albany, N. Y. produced findings in very close agreement. A study of 290,000 veterans, conducted by the National Heart Institute, found a 61 per cent higher death rate from coronary heart disease among cigarette smokers as compared with nonsmokers or occasional smokers. In England, two researchers reported twice as high a death rate from coronary disease among male smokers than among nonsmokers aged below 65.

2. Clinical evidence. Consider, for example, the peripheral vascular disorder known as Buerger's disease, which causes gangrene of the fingers and toes. For years this disorder has been known to occur only in cigarette smokers. Two of the most widely known respiratory disorders, bronchitis and emphysema, with prevalence enormously higher among smokers than nonsmokers, have a standard remedy throughout the world, namely, a directive to stop smoking.

There are other changes taking place in the human body and its chemistry as a result of cigarette smoking. These involve such abnormalities as a temporary increase in blood pressure, an acceleration in blood clotting, and an increase in the carbon monoxide in the circulating blood.

3. Pathological evidence. A number of pathological studies strengthen the case against cigarettes. Typical is one undertaken at New Orleans, where investigators examined coronary arteries taken from 645 males at autopsy. Those who smoked more than 25 cigarettes a day showed fatty deposits about twice as great as those found in nonsmokers.

Types of Cardiovascular Disease

Cerebral Hemorrhage or Stroke

Cerebral hemorrhage is one form of cardiovascular disease and is listed as the third

SMOKE LESS
CHOOSE A CIGARETTE WITH LESS TAR AND NICOTINE
HELP YOUNG PEOPLE NOT TO START
RESPECT RIGHTS OF NON-SMOKERS
FIND YOUR WAY TO QUIT
YES! THERE ARE 5 THINGS YOU CAN DO ABOUT SMOKING

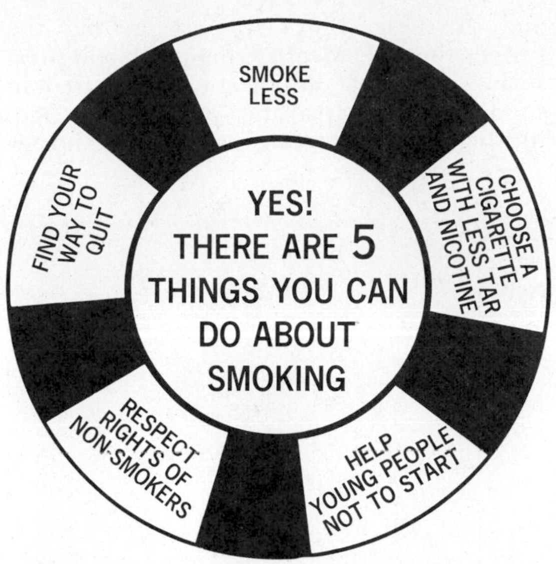

Figure 7–11 Five things to do about smoking. (From Heart Facts 1975, American Heart Association.)

leading cause of death in the United States. Among physicians, a disorder of the blood vessels in the brain is called *C.V.A.*, or cerebral vascular accident. To the layman, however, any C.V.A. is known as a stroke or apoplexy. The term encompasses all kinds of C.V.A.'s and all degrees of severity, with or without paralysis. Four causes of strokes are: hemorrhage in the brain caused by the bursting of a blood vessel (this type is usually severe and causes paralysis), thrombosis or clotting in the affected artery, embolism or traveling clot, and spasm of an artery. In any case, a stroke may or may not irreparably damage that part of the brain where nerve centers controlling sight, hearing, speech, memory, and skilled acts are located.

Rheumatic Fever

Rheumatic fever—usually thought of as a childhood disease—most frequently strikes between the ages of 5 and 15. It is always preceded by streptococcal infection, usually a sore throat. But not all "strep" infections lead to rheumatic fever. After an initial attack, rheumatic fever is apt to recur. That is why it is important for those who have suffered rheumatic fever in childhood to remain on long-term penicillin or other antibiotic therapy. This can prevent recurrence of strep infection and resultant rheumatic fever and rheumatic heart disease in which the heart valves become scarred and deformed. Since the mid-1940's mortality from rheumatic heart disease has declined sharply in the 5- to 24-year age group, largely because of the use of antibiotics to prevent strep infection. Although generally a preventable disease, rheumatic heart disease was the cause of an estimated 14,130 deaths in 1971. Rheumatic heart disease afflicts an estimated 100,000 children and 1,600,000 adults.

Rheumatic heart disease can not only shorten life, it can also seriously impair the quality of the patient's life. Although rheumatic fever and rheumatic heart disease are preventable, incidence rates remain far too high, particularly among lower-income groups. The problem is to motivate those most at risk to seek prevention and to ensure that effective preventive measures are available to them.

Rheumatic fever has its highest incidence in school-age populations, although attacks are also seen in young adults, particularly those who have had a previous attack. In urban areas, incidence rates have been shown to be higher in blacks than in whites. Major social and economic improvements are probably essential for the complete prevention of this disease. However, until such far-reaching changes are effected, much can be done. The first step in primary prevention is identification of streptococcal infection. This requires education of parents, patients, school nurses, clinic personnel and physicians. It also requires access to reliable laboratories where streptococcal identification can be accomplished at reasonable cost. The second step is effective treatment for streptococcal infection. This also requires lay and professional education and motivation. Low-cost penicillin is generally available, as are substitute drugs for patients sensitive to penicillin. The prevention of rheumatic heart disease depends on the effective prevention of rheumatic fever. Prevention of recurrent attacks of rheumatic fever requires motivation of the patient to persist with long-term prophylaxis and continued medical care to monitor and reinforce this prophylaxis.

Hypertension

Hypertension, or high blood pressure, is no respector of age or sex, and is probably the single leading factor in disability and death in the United States today. The American Heart Association believes that less than half of all hypertensives know that they have high blood pressure. Only half the hypertensives who are aware of their illness are under treatment to control their blood pressure, and of these, only half are getting the proper therapy. Measurement of blood pressure is the most important factor used in predicting life expectancy at any given age: the higher the blood pressure, the shorter

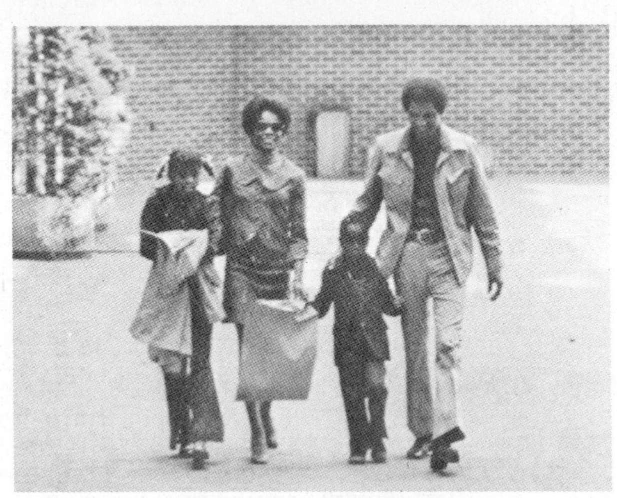

High Blood Pressure: A Major Cause of Death Among Black Americans

The Silent Killer

High blood pressure kills. It can cause strokes, heart failure, kidney disease and more. It's called the "Silent Killer" because you might not even know you have it. Usually there's no pain or other sign of trouble.

High Blood Pressure—A Big Problem For Blacks

It's a fact—high blood pressure is one of the biggest causes of Black deaths in the United States. Doctor's don't know why, but Blacks get high blood pressure more often than other Americans.

Who Gets High Blood Pressure?

Anybody. You can feel good, look fine, and still have it. It hits young and old, men and women, easy-going and up-tight people. But if you're over 40, there's an even bigger chance you have high blood pressure.

Now For The Good News

Blood pressure can be checked quickly—without pain. And most times high blood pressure can be treated—often just by taking medication. Then, when it's under control, you usually can lead a normal life.

Figure 7–12 (From National High Blood Pressure Education Program. Bethesda, Md., National Institutes of Health, May, 1975.)

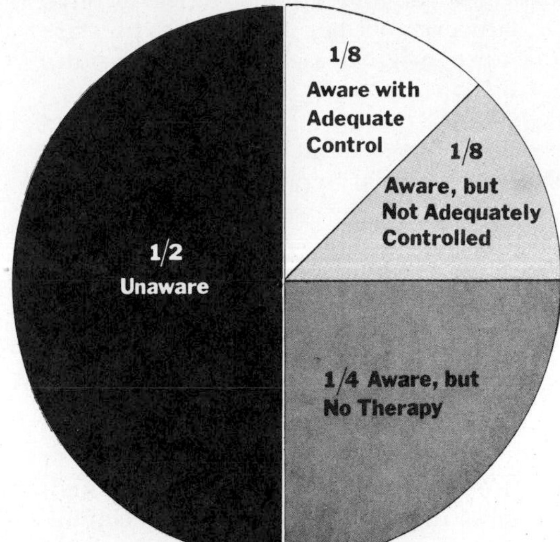

Figure 7–13 (From Heart Facts 1975, American Heart Association, p. 4.)

the life expectancy. Generally, a person is considered to have high blood pressure if his reading is persistently higher than 140/90.

Heart attacks and strokes kill more Americans than all the other leading causes of death combined, including cancer and accidents. High blood pressure alone is listed as the primary cause of only 60,000 deaths a year. But hypertension, which rarely appears on death certificates, is the underlying cause of hundreds of thousands of other deaths. Heart disease claims an estimated 600,000 Americans per year, and hypertension is the major contributor to heart disease. Strokes kill about 200,000 per year, and hypertension is the leading cause of stroke. Kidney disease may account for as many as 60,000 deaths per year; hypertension is the major contributor to kidney disease. An untreated hypertensive is 4 times as likely to have a heart attack or a stroke as someone with normal blood pressure and twice as likely to develop kidney disease. Thousands of Americans will have their eyesight impaired, suffer from internal hemorrhages, or miss work because of hypertension.

STAMP OUT FOOD FADDISM

Food faddism is indeed a serious problem. But we have to recognize that the guru of food faddism is not Adele Davis, but Betty Crocker. The true food faddists are not those who eat raw broccoli, wheat germ, and yogurt, but those who start the day on Breakfast Squares, gulp down bottle after bottle of soda pop, and snack on candy and Twinkies.

Food faddism is promoted from birth. Sugar is a major ingredient in baby food desserts. Then come the artificially flavored and colored breakfast cereals loaded with sugar, followed by soda pop and hot dogs. Meat marbled with fat and alcoholic beverages dominate the diets of many middle-aged people. And, of course, white bread is standard fare throughout life.

This diet—high in fat, sugar, cholesterol, and refined grains—is the prescription for illness; it can contribute to obesity, tooth decay, heart disease, intestinal cancer, and diabetes. And these diseases are, in fact, America's major health problems. So if any diet should be considered faddist, it is the standard one. Our far-out diet—almost 20 per cent refined sugar and 45 per cent fat—is new to human experience and foreign to all other animal life....

It is incredible that people who eat a junk food diet constitute the norm, while individuals whose diets resemble those of our great-grandparents are labeled deviants.[14]

A small percentage of the cases of hypertension stem from kidney disease, pinching of the aorta, and tumors on the adrenal gland. However, 95 per cent of the cases are of unknown origin (essential hypertension). Hypertension has been detected in children as early as 12 months of age. Researchers have discovered several factors that may be involved in essential hypertension:

1. *Obesity.* Excess weight, whether it is only a few extra pounds or many, may bring an increase in blood pressure.

2. *Heredity.* Most researchers feel that heredity plays some role in high blood pressure.

3. *Diet.* Modern studies have strengthened the connection between salt intake and pulse changes. Tribesmen in Africa, who eat almost no salt, rarely if ever develop high blood pressure. But in northern Japan, where people eat approximately 50 grams of salt a day, half the population dies of strokes, a common complication of high blood pressure (Fig. 7–14).

4. *Race.* For reasons that remain to be fully determined, blacks are particularly prone to hypertension. According to the American Heart Association 1 out of every 4 adult black Americans has high blood pressure, compared with 1 out of 7 adult whites. Some scientists theorize that blacks are genetically incapable of handling the large amounts of salt that are found in a diet rich in pork and highly seasoned soul food. Others suggest that the pressures of being black in America alone are enough to cause the disease.

5. *Stress.* Though many of those with apparently complete control over their emotions have high blood pressure, researchers have found that there is a relationship between stress and hypertension. Blood pressure normally rises with excitement or alarm. In most people, the pressure drops when the excitement is over. But according to one theory, in many people the level drops by smaller increments, eventually stabilizing at a higher level than before.

6. *Smoking.* The incidence of stroke in the hypertensive person who smokes is 16 times that of the hypertensive person who doesn't smoke.

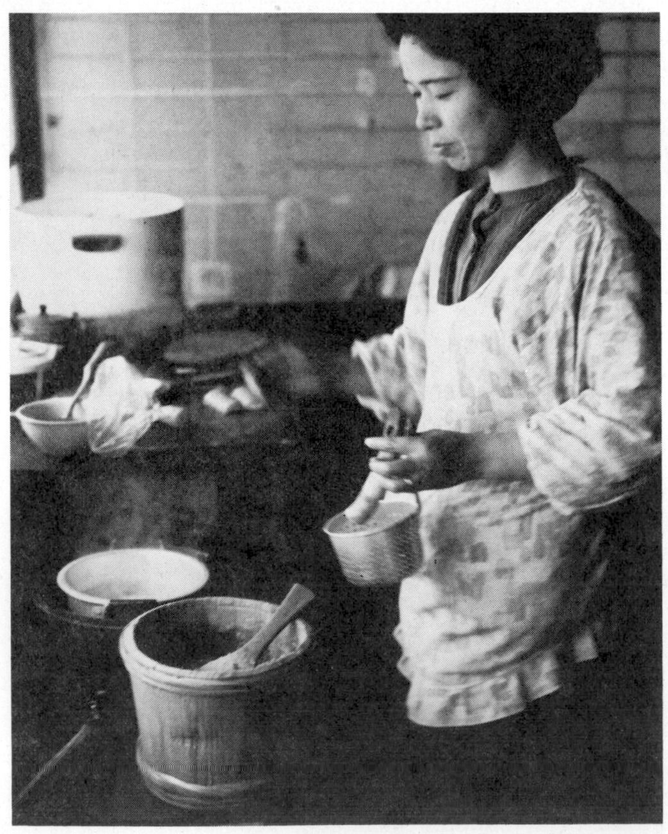

Figure 7–14 Unlike the Eskimos, people in the northern part of Japan eat large quantities of salt, and among them, hypertension is common. Doctors are accordingly recommending a low salt diet. (From Stamler, J.: Nutrition and the present epidemic. World Health, August–September, 1970, World Health Organization.)

WOMEN AND HEART DISEASE

(1) Although an American woman's risk is half that of an American male in middle age, it's still high. For example, it's five times as great as the risk for Japanese men:

(2) While heart attack rates for men have stabilized, the rate among middle-aged American women is rising—probably because (a) they now smoke more cigarettes, and (b) housework now involves less of the hard labor that once helped to keep women fit, and (c) women's liberation has given many women equal job opportunities and equal stress.

(3) After menopause, a woman's risk increases sharply. If she wants to avoid a heart attack in her 60's, she should start preventing the buildup of atherosclerosis in her 40's, at the latest.

(4) Women suffer almost as many strokes as men. Most strokes occur because the arteries to the brain become obstructed by deposits of atherosclerosis. We can reduce the risks of strokes in the same way we reduce the risk's of heart disease: by not smoking, watching our diet, controlling our weight, and exercising.

In any case, drugs are the therapy of choice. Research in this area has advanced rapidly. Other treatment includes exercise, diet, biofeedback*, and relaxation response (a kind of transcendental meditation technique). Preventive programs include massive education efforts to help potential victims reduce their risks by giving up smoking, losing weight, reducing cholesterol intake, resting and relaxing more, and controlling blood pressure. No one method works for all; individual treatment is necessary. Public aid for hypertensives includes sending blood pressure mobile units to canvas the streets giving free hypertension tests to all; setting up testing equipment in supermarkets, colleges, and industrial plants; and having dentists and dental technicians take patients' pressure. All screening programs should include adequate medical follow-up.

*A technique that employs electronic monitoring devices to help patients learn how to control autonomic nervous system functions such as heartbeat and blood circulation.

Prevention

The specific measures currently directed toward the prevention of infectious diseases

HOW TO MURDER YOUR HUSBAND

Consider these 10 socially accepted methods for accelerating the advent of merry widowhood. They are scientifically designed to help you cut down your husband in his prime, without risking capital punishment, jail, or even the tacit disapproval of your social circle. And you can do most of it under the guise of wifely devotion, and with the loving indulgence of your spouse.

(If you really love and cherish your husband, however, take the opposite course to my advice. It may postpone his departure by many years, give you a vigorous and grateful companion for the autumn years, and ensure that your children's children will have a grandfather, for which they, too, will thank you.)

1. Fatten him up.
2. Keep him liquored up.
3. Keep him sitting down.
4. Feed him saturated fats.
5. Get him used to heavily salted food.
6. Fill him up with coffee.
7. Offer him cigarettes.
8. Keep him up late.
9. Don't let him go on vacation.
10. Nag him and worry him.[15]

should be expanded and applied directly to heart disease control. There are many categories of cardiovascular diseases in which infectious diseases play an important etiologic role. A specific example is the relationship between rubella infection during the first trimester of pregnancy and congenital heart defects of the baby, such as patent ductus arteriosus. A specific public health program in the community aimed at immunizing youngsters can help prevent this problem. Such a program could include the exposure of nonimmunized girls to German measles before puberty and the use of gamma globulin in pregnant women exposed to the infection.

Other viral infections during pregnancy and certain nutritional and vitamin deficiencies can lead to congenital abnormalities in the body. Public health programs aimed at prevention of such infections or deficiencies can ultimately reduce the incidence of many types of congenital defects of the heart and blood vessels. Such programs, which are "routine" to most local health departments, must be encouraged, supported, and expanded.

In rheumatic fever and rheumatic heart disease also, effective public health action will greatly lower incidence in the community. The relationship of beta hemolytic streptococcal infection and the development of rheumatic fever and rheumatic heart disease has been established for many years. Systematic public health programs aimed at early detection and treatment of streptococcal throat infection among school children can aid in preventing rheumatic fever and, consequently, rheumatic heart disease. Such a program could have the following components:

1. Detection of streptococcal infection by routine examination of school children, with utilization of throat culture and newer laboratory methods, such as fluorescent antibody technique, for early and prompt diagnosis.
2. Early administration of antibiotics (penicillin) in proper dosage and for proper duration, as has been recommended by the American Heart Association.
3. In children with rheumatic fever, an effective public health program that will provide means for adherence to the prophylactic measures described by the American Heart Association should be initiated. Such adherence to prophylaxis and the regular use of antibiotics (penicillin) will prevent the recurrence of rheumatic fever and, in most cases, will prevent the development of rheumatic heart disease. The local health department is an ideal setting to help the local practicing physicians and the community with such a problem by providing followup service through its public health nurses and public health educators.

Subacute bacterial endocarditis is another disease in which public health activities can prove effective and essential in preventing many premature deaths and disabilities. An effective public health program in this field can be initiated with advocation of systematic use of antibiotics (penicillin) before dental or minor medical surgery in patients with heart disease and with public and professional education aimed at bringing the sequence of events in development of subacute bacterial endocarditis into focus and encouraging the necessary prophylactic measures known to the medical and dental professions.

Venereal disease control programs of local health departments can be strengthened to bring syphilis under complete control and consequently to prevent luetic heart disease.[16]

The local health department and the local branch of the American Heart Association joined forces long ago to combat heart disease by providing research, professional and public education, and community service. At the national level, the American Heart Association and the National Heart Institute of the United States Public Health Service have cooperated in the development of a single-focused attack on cardiovascular diseases.

Research grants include studies concerned with such problems as the movement of metals across cell walls, the effects of stress on bodily absorption of fats, the electrical forces of heart muscle, the pattern of life that leads to heart disease, and the role of diet (coffee, for example), physical exercise, occupation, cigarette smoking, stress, obesity, the taking of drugs, such as aspirin, and cholesterol levels in heart disease. Epidemiologic studies of various kinds are necessary to help find the causes of this disease.

Here are the recommendations of the American Heart Association to reduce the risk of heart attack:

1. Eat fewer saturated (animal) fats, getting a larger portion of your fat requirements from polyunsaturated (vegetable) fats, and avoiding high-cholesterol foods.

2. Don't smoke cigarettes. Men who are heavy cigarette smokers have over twice the risk of nonsmokers of suffering a heart attack. Women also have a higher risk.

3. Maintain normal weight. Middle-aged men who are grossly overweight run a substantially greater risk of fatal heart attack than middle-aged men of normal weight.

4. Adopt a program of regular exercise that is compatible with your age and physical condition.

5. See your doctor regularly for a physical check-up, enabling him to begin prompt treatment if high blood pressure or diabetes is present.

There are certain uncontrollable factors. Perhaps the most important of these is genetic inheritance. Fortunate indeed is the male with two long-lived grandfathers and a family record of longevity. Obviously, one can do nothing about a choice of ancestors. Sex is a matter one has no choice in, but men are far more susceptible to coronary artery disease than are women. This is especially true below the age of 50. Another uncontrollable factor is age; the risk of heart attack increases as one grows older.

Cardiopulmonary Resuscitation (CPR)

Many communities are conducting programs to meet a vital need in coronary care. More than half of the 700,000 Americans who die of heart attacks each year never make it to the hospital, where their lives might have been saved through modern techniques. These unfortunate victims have generally suffered a severe disturbance in heart rhythm, which can lead to brain damage and death if not corrected within minutes.

Citizens are being trained by heart associations and fire departments to administer instant first aid to any heart attack or stroke victim. This effort is backed up by mobile fire department paramedic squads equipped to provide sophisticated monitoring and treatment while the victim is en route to the hospital. If CPR is started within 1 minute after an attack, the chance of recovery is 98 per cent.

Programs

Since the problem of cardiovascular disease is so broad in scope, every health jurisdiction should be able to find some area of particular interest for positive action. Many local health departments are already engaged in various public health activities that can be expanded to encompass a wider range of achievements in the field of cardiovascular diseases. Obviously, the local community must determine its needs and plan positive and effective programs to meet these needs. The Heart Disease Control Program of the State Department of Public Health works closely with local health officers, local physicians, local chapters of the Heart Association, and community leaders to provide assistance so that each community can make a thoughtful appraisal of its needs in the following ways:

1. To focus attention on the problem as it exists in each local community.

2. To scrutinize the related existing public health program activities to see whether they are adequate.

3. To formulate a plan of action acceptable to that particular community, and also to meet the community needs more adequately in the field of cardiovascular diseases.

4. To fill the gap between our presently available knowledge and its application in the public health programs serving the community.

Although no two communities are identical in terms of the problems or resources, there are several activities that are, nevertheless, applicable in most communities. In general, the program activities of a local health jurisdiction in the field of heart disease control include prevention (primary and secondary), detection and case-finding programs, diagnostic services, ancillary services, rehabilitation, community research, health education, and evaluation.

In planning community service and demonstration projects and epidemiologic investigations, at least two points deserve consideration by agencies. First is the necessity for obtaining the cooperation and support of local medical societies and heart associations. This is important to the success of any heart disease program. Every cardiovascular control program should be presented to these societies and their appropriate committees in the early planning stage, and they should be asked to make recommendations on the program. If the heart association and medical society officials, who are usually leading practicing physicians in the community, have shared the responsibility of planning the control program, then that program has an excellent chance for success. Second, there is always the question of funds and financial support for these programs. Today persons and agencies with sound, well considered plans for improving health services or for demonstrating new approaches in disease control can usually find financing. Local health agencies can apply for support to the National Heart Institute of the National Institutes of Health (United States Public Health Service), the Heart Disease Control Program of the United States Public Health Service, and the Heart Disease Control Program of the State Department of Public Health.

Advances in Diagnosis and Treatment

Diagnosis by Echocardiography

Ultrasonic examination of the heart is a new, developing examination modality that has attracted considerable attention and offers promise as an important diagnostic tool in cardiac disease. Its popularity stems directly from its noninvasive, nonionizing nature, which permits easy examination, even at the bedside if necessary. The unique ability of ultrasound to differentiate solid structures of the heart from the blood without the use of contrast agents can be used to obtain crucial information about cardiac structure. Records of the movement of cardiac elements also offer important information about heart function.

Congenital heart disease is one of the newer areas in which echocardiography has been put to use. Common conditions such as tetralogy of Fallot, transposition of the great vessels, and hypoplasia of the left side of the heart can be readily diagnosed ultrasonically. Recognition of other conditions by echocardiography appears to be progressing rapidly. Echocardiography today is an established and reliable diagnostic tool. It offers a well-defined service to physicians caring for patients with cardiac disease.

Treatment

Advances in the treatment of heart disease are given in Table 7–3.

As the list indicates, many new advances include surgery, antibiotics, the heart-lung machine, replacing diseased arteries with nylon arteries, and the use of radioactivity and electronics in aiding rapid and efficient diagnosis. Individual surgeon skills and smooth cooperation of the operating team account for a great deal of success in this area. Also important is hypothermia or bathing the patient in ice water to lower the temperature as much as 20 degrees, thus reducing the need for blood and oxygen. With the body "hibernating" in this manner, for example, the aorta can be closed long enough to permit replacement of the diseased section without damaging vital nerve cells.

Many other advances can be expected in the diagnosis and treatment of heart disease in the near future. Considering present limitations, reasonable predictions might include the following:

1. Surgical techniques will continue to make dramatic advances: Heart transplants will be increasingly successful as specific factors are discovered that insure success. Artificial devices that can replace all or part of the heart and various portions of the vascular system will be developed. Heart muscle that is damaged by heart attacks will be replaced with new materials that will restore the function of the heart. Damaged blood vessels will be replaced surgically before a heart attack or stroke occurs.
2. Heredity will be controlled, perhaps through alteration of genes, so that inheritance of "coronary proneness" will not occur.

TABLE 7–3 Advances in the Treatment of Heart Disease

DEFECT OR DISEASE	ADVANCE OR TREATMENT
Syphilis	Penicillin
Diphtheria	Immunization
Subacute bacterial endocarditis	Antibiotics
Rh negative baby	New blood supply; Rho Gam
Hypertension	Drugs
Arteriosclerosis	Surgery; drugs
Rheumatic fever	Penicillin
Heart and blood vessel defects	Surgery
Heart transplant	Surgery

3. Pregnancies will be managed more carefully in order to eliminate congenital heart malformations.

4. The specific process of rheumatic fever will be determined, and means will be developed to eliminate the disease and, consequently, rheumatic heart disease.

5. The exact causes of high blood pressure will be discovered and the ways of controlling it will be improved.

6. Additional increments in knowledge will be made about all of the elements that are related to atherosclerosis—cholesterol, hypertension, hormones, exercise, smoking. Ultimately, the whole process of atherosclerosis will be understood, and understanding will be followed by control measures that will prevent the disease from developing.

Some of these predictions may become realities rather quickly. Others may require years of effort, and progress may be agonizingly slow. Given enough time and support, medical researchers will probably produce the solutions to the seemingly insurmountable problems of cardiovascular disease.

Community services for heart patients have two major objectives: to develop and improve facilities that will assist the physician in the total management of the cardiac patient; and to help the patient and his family, through organized community effort, to cope with many personal, social and economic problems caused by cardiac disease. One of the most important phases in the treatment of patients with coronary artery disease is rehabilitation. It is vitally important that these patients return to gainful employment as soon as feasible. Work records indicate that these patients make an excellent adjustment, are good workers, and have a low rate of absenteeism. They seem to be less prone to emotional instability if they return to work early.

OTHER CHRONIC DISEASES

Emphysema

Emphysema is a disease of the lungs characterized by a thickening of the lung tissue and excessive secretion of fluids in the lungs. Victims of emphysema are usually between 50 and 70 years old. Both sexes are susceptible, but more men suffer from this disease than women; the ratio is about 10:1. A high percentage of the victims of emphysema are or have been heavy smokers. The disease is often a late effect of past chronic infection or irritation of the bronchial tubes. Some physiological changes that occur when the bronchi become irritated are: obstruction of the airways, trapping air in the lung beyond them; a tearing of the tiny air spaces, resulting in less contact between blood and air; and an overstretching of the lungs, causing a less efficient exchange of oxygen and carbon dioxide. The victim has trouble getting enough air, is short of breath, is subject to chronic respiratory infections, and has difficulty sleeping because of cough and shortness of breath.

The changes occurring in emphysema may also interfere with the passage of blood through the small blood vessels to the lung. This makes the heart work harder to pump blood, and the heart may enlarge under the strain. Those with emphysema should obey the following rules:

1. See your doctor. Do not treat the disease yourself.

2. Don't smoke. A high percentage of those who contract emphysema are heavy smokers, and continued smoking makes it worse.

3. Exercise and watch your diet. Keeping fit not only helps prevent emphysema and other diseases, it also speeds recovery.

4. Avoid polluted air. Do not expose yourself unnecessarily to dust or fumes of any kind.

5. Try to avoid colds or respiratory disorders and see your doctor if you are infected.

Chronic emphysema not only kills more people than ever before, but it makes respiratory cripples of many otherwise strong and hard-working persons. Further studies on physical and vocational rehabilitation of those affected by emphysema are badly needed.

Dust Diseases

The name of each different pneumoconiosis or dust disease is related to the dust that produces it. Dust diseases are usually associated with occupational exposures. Each of the following is considered a dust disease and can cause chronic illness:

1. *Silicosis* comes from inhalation of silica or quartz dust. Quartz is found in many kinds of rocks. Miners usually dig through quartz to get gold or coal.

2. *Anthracosilicosis* is also known as coal worker's pneumoconiosis and is caused by inhaling a combination of coal dust and silica. This can be a serious disease.

3. *Asbestosis* is caused by inhaling asbestos fibers.

4. *Berylliosis* is caused by inhaling the dust from beryllium salts. This can be a very serious disease.

5. *Bagassosis* is caused by breathing the dust from pressed stalks of sugar cane, called bagasse. It is not too serious a disease.

6. *Baritosis* is caused by inhaling the dust of barium oxide. It is usually not serious.

7. *Siderosis* is caused by inhaling the dust of iron ore or arc welding fumes. It is not too serious.

8. *Stannosis* is caused by inhaling the dust of tin ore. It is not too serious.

The lungs are protected against dirt or mineral dust in the atmosphere by tiny hairs called cilia, which line the nose and the bronchial tubes. Over the cilia is spread a thin mucus to help trap foreign particles before they enter the lungs. This mechanism works well most of the time, but even nature's defense can fail when exposed to high and prolonged concentrations of contaminants. The cost from dust disease in sickness and death, in broken families, in lost manpower, and in money for treatment has been very large. However, public health and other agencies are promoting preventive measures to combat the dust diseases. High levels of dust can be combated by the use of face masks. Clean air piped into a closed hood over the worker's head or the removal of dust by suction as it is produced is effective. The wetting down of dust-producing materials before they are worked on also helps. The seriousness of a dust disease is very often determined by how much dust is inhaled and for how long. A job change may be required to effect a cure, or the hazard may be reduced by avoiding the breathing of dust and proper medical treatment.

Arthritis

Ten million Americans are victims of arthritis to some degree and about 150,000 are completely disabled by this disease. Arthritis costs Americans about $100 million a year. It causes more personal discomfort and disability than any other chronic disorder. Arthritis is not a killer, but it disables the individual for long periods. There are several types of arthritis, but only the most common are described here.

Rheumatoid Arthritis. Inflammation and swelling of the joints occur. This type of arthritis is about three times as common in women as in men. The usual symptoms are sensations of pain in the extremities, fatigue, loss of weight, and swelling of the joints. If treatment is delayed, crippling results. The treatment usually includes a balanced diet, heat therapy, rest, and special exercises. Aspirin is the most commonly used medication.

Osteoarthritis. This type of arthritis is a degenerative softening of the bone ends at the joints, believed to be a result of aging. Causative factors may include overweight and hard usage of the joints. Osteoarthritis of the spine is common and seems to be more prevalent in certain families, suggesting genetic factors. X-rays often indicate a considerable degree of osteoarthritis of the joints of elderly people who are without symptoms of rheumatism. Treatment includes hydrotherapy. Reduction of joints is sometimes useful, but in general it is less effective than exercise. Use of salicylates is the most important method of treatment. Steroids and hormones are used by some specialists.

Gout. Swelling of the extremities is the most important symptom of gout, which is caused by metabolic imbalance usually brought on by improper diet. It usually begins as an acute arthritis. The toes or the entire foot may show some swelling with pain. The disease results from deposits of uric acid in the joints, owing to the high uric blood level. The salicylates and many modern drugs help to reduce the high level of uric acid in the blood.

Bronchitis

Bronchitis is the inflammation of the membrane that lines the bronchial tubes, and it is classified as acute or chronic. The acute form is characterized by inflammation of the trachea and the bronchi. It usually accompanies severe respiratory infections. Such infections cause the person to be more susceptible to bacteria already present in the respiratory tract. These bacteria cause the irritation to the lining of the lung.

Chronic bronchitis is characterized by prolonged coughing and excessive expectoration. The cough is more or less continuous and often unnoticed by the victim. This disease is also called catarrh or secondary bronchitis. The principal cause is prolonged irritation of the bronchial mucosa. Air pollutants, smoking, or dust inhalation can cause the mucous glands and cells to overproduce and the ciliated membrane lining the bronchial tubes to thicken.

The individual is usually requested by his physician to give up smoking, to keep physically fit, and to practice good nutrition. Antibiotic drugs and bronchodilators may be used under the supervision of the physician.

Diabetes

Diabetes is a metabolic disease in which the ability of the body to oxidize carbohydrates (sugars) is lost. If untreated, it can lead to loss of other metabolic functions, coma, and death. It is calculated that there are more than 26 million diabetics in the world today. There are more than 3,000,000 known cases in the United States.* Diabetes may appear at any age. It is liable to produce complications in the kidneys and urinary tract. Symptoms include extreme fatigue, loss of appetite, and excessive urination and thirst.

Diabetes has been linked with a recessive gene. A family history of diabetes is found in 10 per cent of nondiabetic individuals, but in more than 50 per cent of diabetics. For example, when both husband and wife are diabetics, and there are four offspring, chances are that two will be diabetic and two will carry the diabetic gene.

Diabetes appears to be related to age level in the United States. It is rare in persons younger than 21 years of age. It strikes more frequently in people between 21 and 45, and more than 50 per cent of the cases develop in people between the ages of 45 and 60. The disease is found in twice as many women as men. In the United States, the incidence is equal among blacks and whites. High caloric intake favors diabetes, obesity is often associated with the disease, and diabetes and hypertension frequently occur in the same patient.

There may be related causes of physical inactivity and dietary habits. In Japan and China, there are few diabetics among the poor, and even among the rich it is less common than in the West.

Controlling Measures. Health education, normal diet, regulation of body weight, care and treatment in pregnancy, control of hypertension, and measures to combat atherosclerosis are very important in the control of diabetes. At the same time, the education of the diabetic must be emphasized. Books, pamphlets, special classes, and lectures can be used. There are camps for diabetics. In the United States, the American Diabetes Association, founded in 1940, has approximately 52 branches throughout the United States.

Employment with great physical or nervous demands is unsuitable for the diabetic. The diabetic should be careful of infections and should refrain from alcohol.

Treatment includes a low-calorie diet to correct glycosuria and hyperglycemia and to reduce the patient's weight until a near-normal body weight is achieved. Insulin is used under the supervision of a physician. The dose is adjusted to individual needs to keep glycosuria to a minimum and hyperglycemia to levels between 120 and 200 mg./100 ml.

Ordinary symptoms of this disease should be remembered: loss of weight, increased thirst, frequent urination, and skin infections. Vision is often impaired because of excess sugar in the fluids of the eyes. The longer the disease is untreated, the more difficult it is to bring it under control.

QUESTIONS FOR DISCUSSION

1. What is the difference between chronic disease and communicable disease?
2. Which age groups are affected by chronic disease? Which chronic diseases are most prevalent in these age groups?
3. Are the number of chronic disease cases in the nation increasing or decreasing? How does this affect community health programs?
4. List five different examples of how we can prevent five specific chronic diseases.
5. Explain the difference between primary prevention and secondary prevention.
6. In what ways can we develop successful chronic disease programs in communities throughout the country?
7. Have the number of cancer cases and fatalities increased since 1900? Explain.
8. "Until there is definite proof that tobacco causes lung cancer, why not continue smoking?" Discuss this statement.
9. Discuss three new community approaches to cancer prevention.
10. (a) What part does the local health department play in cancer prevention?
    (b) State health department?
    (c) United States Public Health Service?
    (d) Local cancer society?
    (e) State cancer society?
11. List and briefly discuss five reasons why people fail to obtain periodic physical examination.
12. What type of legislation concerning cigarette labeling do you favor?

*It is estimated that there are at least this many more diabetics who are *undetected*.

13. Is research relating to heart disease and cholesterol conclusive?
14. What is the relationship between exercise and heart health?
15. Discuss the problem of emphysema during the past five years.
16. Describe a coronary thrombosis; a myocardial infarction.
17. What are the most common types of arthritis?
18. What is arteriosclerosis? Stroke?
19. What are the coronary arteries? What is their function?
20. Describe ulcers, gout, senile dementia, glaucoma, cataract, diabetes, allergies.
21. Define tumor, benign tumor, malignant tumor, metastasis.
22. What is leukemia? Discuss its importance.
23. How can one prevent heart disease?
24. Discuss quackery and cures for cancer and for arthritis.
25. Describe the voluntary health agencies and their role in chronic disease programs.
26. How does physical exercise affect heart disease? One's life span?
27. What have been the recent advances in cancer, heart disease, and arthritis?
28. Discuss the National Institutes of Health and their research into chronic diseases.
29. List the most common kinds of heart disease. Discuss the physiology of and prognosis in each of them.
30. List the most common types and sites of cancer, and discuss the prognosis in each.

QUESTIONS FOR REVIEW

1. How does the Commission on Chronic Illness define a chronic disease?
2. In what age group does cerebral palsy most often occur?
3. What is secondary prevention?
4. What four main points should a good periodic health examination cover? What are some of the limitations of even a good examination?
5. List two methods of secondary prevention.
6. Give one prevention measure for congenital cataracts.
7. Name an important measure that would help prevent blindness from glaucoma through early detection.
8. Describe glaucoma; amblyopia.
9. What is the long-range goal of the Mental Retardation Program?
10. What are two alternatives to hospitalization for chronically ill patients?
11. What are five processes by which a community may create a local chronic disease program?
12. What is the most crucial job in relation to chronic disease prevention?
13. What are the seven danger signals of cancer?
14. List the seven types of cancer that patients are most likely to survive with and the safeguards that should be taken to prevent them or detect them early.
15. What are the two most widely used methods of curing cancer?
16. What is the leading cause of death in the U.S. today?
17. What are some suggested possibilities for causes of major cardiovascular diseases?
18. What three health conditions cause 90 per cent of all heart disease?
19. What are the usual warnings of a heart attack?
20. What are the characteristics of the "Type A" personality? "Type B"?
21. What are the three general categories of evidence that indicate cigarettes as a cause of disease?
22. What are four causes of a stroke?
23. What are certain uncontrollable factors in relation to chronic disease?
24. What are the two major objectives of community service for heart patients?
25. Describe the characteristics of emphysema. What are five rules that people with emphysema must follow?
26. Which of the dust diseases is caused by inhalation?
27. Describe the characteristics of arthritis. What are the three most common types of this condition?
28. What are some of the symptoms of diabetes? List some measures that can be taken to control diabetes.

REFERENCES

1. Commission on Chronic Illness: *Chronic Illness in the United States. I. Prevention of Chronic Illness.* Cambridge, Mass., Harvard University Press, 1957, p. 4.
2. Kahn, H. A.: Changing causes of death in childhood. Publ. Health Rep., *66*:1246, 1951.
3. National Health Assembly: *America's Health: a Report to the Nation.* New York, Harper and Brothers, 1949, p. 85.
4. Yahraes, H.: *Something Can Be Done About Chronic Illness.* New York, The Commission on Chronic Illness, Public Affairs Pamphlet No. 176, 1954, p. 4.
5. Wynder, E. L., and Peacock, P.: The practice of disease prevention. JAMA, *229*(13):1743, September 23, 1974.
6. Commission on Chronic Illness: *Chronic Illness in the United States. I. Prevention of Chronic Illness.* Cambridge, Mass., Harvard University Press, 1957, p. 28.
7. Burney, L. E.: *Address Before the House of Delegates.* Indiana State Medical Association, October, 1956, pp. 5 and 6.
8. Yahraes, H.: *Something Can Be Done About Chronic Illness.* New York, The Commission on Chronic Illness, Public Affairs Pamphlet No. 176, 1954, p. 26.

9. Knott, L. W.: Components of a chronic disease program. Am. J. Pub. Hlth., *52*:2082, 1962.
10. Bates, R. C.: Smoking. Medical Economics, May 12, 1975, pp. 81–85.
11. Morton, J. F.: Cabbage cigarettes? Science, May 16, 1975.
12. Miller, B. F., et al.: *Freedom from Heart Attacks.* New York, Simon & Schuster, 1972.
13. Heart Disease linked to aggressiveness. Today's Health, March, 1969. Published by The American Medical Association.
14. Editorial. *Nutrition Action,* March–April, 1975.
15. Mayer, J.: *Your Heart Beat.* Stanford Heart Disease Prevention Program, Vol. 1, No. 1, p. 1, 1975.
16. Borhani, N. O.: Heart disease control in California. California's Health, *20*:113, 1963.

SUGGESTED READING

Abrams, R. D.: *Not Alone with Cancer: A Guide for Those Who Care, What to Expect, What to Do.* Springfield, Ill., Charles C Thomas, 1974.

Austin, D. F., and Werner, S. B.: *Epidemiology for the Health Sciences: A Primer on Epidemiologic Concepts and Their Uses.* Springfield, Ill., Charles C Thomas, 1974.

Bates, B.: *A Guide to Physical Examination.* Philadelphia, J. B. Lippincott Co., 1974.

Bouhuys, A.: *Breathing: Physiology, Environment and Lung Disease.* New York, Grune & Stratton, 1974.

Brams, W. A.: *How to Live with Your High Blood Pressure.* New York, Arco Publishing Co., 1974.

Browning, P. L.: *Mental Retardation: Rehabilitation and Counseling.* Springfield, Ill., Charles C Thomas, 1974.

Brulé, G., et al.: *Drug Therapy of Cancer.* Geneva, World Health Organization, 1973.

Clipson, C. W., and Wehrer, J. J.: *Planning for Cardiac Care: A Guide to the Planning and Design of Cardiac Care Facilities.* New York, Health Administration Press, 1973.

D'Cruz, I. A.: *All About High Blood Pressure.* New Delhi, Orient Longman Ltd., 1974.

Dinman, B. D.: *The Nature of Occupational Cancer.* Springfield, Ill., Charles C Thomas, 1973.

Doll, R., et al. (eds.): *Host Environment Interactions in the Etiology of Cancer in Man.* Geneva, International Agency for Research on Cancer, World Health Organization, 1974.

Dunn, W. L., Jr. (ed.): *Smoking Behavior: Motives and Incentives.* Washington, D.C., Winston (distributor, Halsted [Wiley], New York), 1973.

Eliot, R. S. (ed.): *Contemporary Problems in Cardiology: Stress and the Heart.* Vol. 1. Mount Kisco, N.Y., Futura Publishing Co., 1974.

Frank, M. J.: *Cardiovascular Physical Diagnosis.* Chicago, Year Book Medical Publishers, 1973.

Fritschler, A. L.: *Smoking and Politics: Policymaking and the Federal Bureaucracy.* 2nd ed. Englewood Cliffs, N.J., Prentice-Hall, 1974.

Gordis, L.: *Epidemiology of Chronic Lung Disease in Children.* Baltimore, Johns Hopkins University Press, 1973.

Gunzburg, H. C. (ed.): *Experiments in the Rehabilitation of the Mentally Handicapped.* (Study Group, London, July, 1972.) Scarborough, Ontario, Butterworth, 1974.

Holland, J. F., and Frei, E. (eds.): *Cancer Medicine.* Philadelphia, Lea & Febiger, 1973.

Hutchinson, J. C.: *Hypertension: A Practitioner's Guide to Therapy.* Flushing, N.Y., Medical Examination Publishing Co., 1975.

Illich, I.: *Medical Nemesis.* New York, Pantheon Books, 1975.

International Union Against Cancer: *Health Education Theory and Practice in Cancer Control.* Geneva, UICC, 1974.

Jukes, T. H.: Laetrile for cancer. JAMA, *236*:1284, September 13, 1976.

Kaplan, N. M.: *Your Blood Pressure: The Most Deadly High. A Physician's Guide to Controlling Your Hypertension.* New York, MEDCOM, 1974.

Maugh, T. H., and Marx, J. L.: *Seeds of Destruction.* New York, Plenum Press, 1975.

Pickering, G.: *Hypertension: Causes, Consequences and Management.* 2nd ed. Edinburgh, Churchill Livingstone, 1974.

Pomeroy, L. R., et al. (eds.): *New Dynamics of Preventive Medicine.* Vol. 2. New York, Stratton Intercontinental Medical Book Corp., 1974.

Public Affairs Committee, New York (pamphlets).

Rosenbaum, E. H.: *Living With Cancer.* New York, Praeger, 1975.

Schottenfeld, D.: *Cancer Epidemiology and Prevention: Current Concepts.* Springfield, Ill., Charles C Thomas, 1975.

Shaper, A. G., et al. (eds.): *Cardiovascular Disease in the Tropics.* London, British Medical Association, 1974.

Stephenson, H. E., Jr.: *Cardiac Arrest and Resuscitation.* St. Louis, C. V. Mosby Co., 1974.

Tarizzo, M. L. (ed.): *Field Methods for the Control of Trachoma.* Geneva, World Health Organization, 1973.

Tizard, J. (ed.): *Mental Retardation: Concepts of Education and Research.* London, Butterworth, 1974.

World Health Organization: *IARC Monographs on the Evaluation of the Carcinogenic Risk of Chemicals to Man.* Vols. 4 and 5. Geneva, 1974.

World Health Organization: *WHO Expert Committee on Tuberculosis.* 9th report. WHO Technical Report Series No. 552. Geneva, 1974.

CHAPTER 8

Communicable Disease

Public health officials point with pride to the decrease in incidence of communicable disease during the past 70 years; it is remarkable and encouraging. We now have considerable understanding of the three primary tools for the control of infectious diseases. These are sanitation (preventing the spread of disease organisms from one person to another); immunization (putting a barrier within a person to make him less susceptible to an infection; and case finding followed by antibiotic treatment (when sanitation and immunization are not adequate). However, there are thousands of germs of many different kinds, and they are all tough, prolific, insidious, patient, and continually moving about, looking for a new home. In addition, when disease rates drop, governmental funds for control of those diseases frequently drop. Also, the decline of one variety of germ usually shows an increase in a new or different type of germ, such as the virus of infectious hepatitis. Thus, communicable disease continues to remain a major health problem.

IMMUNIZATION LAWS

Compulsory immunization, specifically smallpox vaccination, was required in some states not long after this country became a nation. Vaccination now keeps smallpox under control in most of the world. The last case in the United States occurred in 1949, and massive reductions in cases have occurred in Africa, South Asia, and Central and South America. Worldwide smallpox eradication programs have been so successful that the hazards of vaccination now exceed those of acquiring smallpox. Thus, routine vaccination in smallpox-free areas such as the United States are no longer recommended. However, the Public Health Service, the American Academy of Pediatrics, and the Amreican Medical Association still recommend smallpox vaccination for all health personnel and all travelers to and from areas where smallpox still exists.

Legislation specifically designed to require immunization of children before entry to school has a direct correlation with the development of poliomyelitis and measles vaccines. Therefore, many states have amended old vaccination laws and enacted immunization laws that increase their scope, requiring immunization against diphtheria, pertussis, tetanus, poliomyelitis, measles, mumps, and rubella.

There is good reason to believe the immunization level of the American people against many diseases has dropped to a dangerous low. For example, the U.S. Immigration Survey conducted by the Center for Disease Control shows that only 60 per cent of American children aged 1 to 4 years have been adequately immunized against poliomyelitis. A continuing check and vigilant attention to the immunization of the population, particularly children, is essential to the improvement of public health.

A combination of legislation with proper regard for minority rights that do not infringe on community safety, together with educational efforts to interpret the facts and to motivate action, is the appropriate choice in free society, where the individual rather than the state is the primary consideration. In emergencies, whatever action is necessary

DPT — DIPHTHERIA—PERTUSSIS—TETANUS

Requirement*

At least *4 doses* of DPT vaccine, with the last dose being *within 3 years* preceding admission are *required* for first entry into primary school. Children who enter California schools for the first time at age 7 years or older are exempt from the pertussis (whooping cough) requirement. These latter children are considered adequately immunized if they have had *at least 3 doses* of DPT or Td (Tetanus and Diphtheria toxoid), with the last dose *within 10 years* preceding admission.

Conditional Admission

— A child who has had no DPT or Td immunizations has 2 weeks to begin immunizations.

— A child has 30 calendar days from the date when a dose becomes necessary (see chart below for immunization intervals) to obtain each of the required subsequent doses.

POLIOMYELITIS

Requirement*

A child has fulfilled the polio vaccine requirement for school entry if he or she has either:

a. Had 3 injections of Salk polio vaccine. (This vaccine has not been routinely used in this country since the mid-1960's and currently is not readily available.)

b. Had at least 2 doses of trivalent oral polio vaccine. This vaccine, also known as Sabin type vaccine, is usually given by drops on a sugar cube. Current recommendations are that at least 1 booster dose following the primary series of 2 doses is necessary for adequate protection.

Conditional Admission

— A child who has had no polio immunization has two weeks to begin immunizations.

— A child with partial polio immunizations has 120 calendar days from first admission to complete the requirements.

MEASLES (RUBEOLA)

Requirements*

A child has fulfilled the measles vaccine requirement for school entry if he or she has either:

a. Had measles disease (Although not required, the diagnosis should have been made by a physician.) or;

b. Had measles vaccine either alone or in combination with rubella (German measles) vaccine and/or mumps vaccine.

Conditional Admission

— A child who has had no measles vaccine or has not had measles has 2 weeks to receive measles vaccine.

*Where special circumstances require an individual determination, the local Health Officer or a designated representative shall make this determination.

Exception from these requirements is possible for medical reasons and also if immunizations are contrary to a family's beliefs.

RECOMMENDED IMMUNIZATION GUIDE

IMMUNIZATION	STARTING AGE(S)	INITIAL SERIES	BOOSTERS
DIPHTHERIA TETANUS PERTUSSIS (Whooping Cough) There is a 3-in-1 type vaccine called DPT and a 2-in-1 type called Td.	Ages 6 weeks through 6 years of age get DPT vaccine. (Many physicians stop giving DPT at about age 5 or 6.)	3 IMMUNIZATIONS One month apart. 4th IMMUNIZATION One year after 3rd.	5th IMMUNIZATION Upon entering school.
	Children 7 years of age and older get Td vaccine.	2 IMMUNIZATIONS One month apart. 3rd IMMUNIZATION One year after 2nd.	Td booster every 10 years.
POLIO (Live Sabin Trivalent Oral Vaccine)	Begin: 1 to 2 months of age.	2 DOSES Two months apart. 3rd DOSE 8 months after 2nd.	Booster upon entering primary school.
MEASLES (Rubeola) (Live-Virus Vaccine)	12 months or older.	One immunization.	No booster needed.
RUBELLA (3 Day German Measles) (Live-Virus Vaccine)	12 months of age to puberty.*	One immunization	No booster needed.
MEASLES/RUBELLA (Combined Live-Virus Vaccine).	12 months of age to puberty.*	One immunization.	No booster needed.
MUMPS (Live-Virus Vaccine)	12 months of age to puberty.	One immunization.	No booster needed.
MEASLES/MUMPS/RUBELLA (Live-Virus Vaccine)	12 months of age to puberty.*	One immunization.	No booster needed.
SMALLPOX	Smallpox vaccinations are only recommended for those persons traveling to countries where the disease still exists, or those persons in certain health professions.		

*Females past puberty should be evaluated by a physician prior to receiving rubella vaccine.

Figure 8–1 Immunization requirements for first entry into primary school in California. (Courtesy of State of California Department of Health.)

must obviously be taken; at such times, the good citizen is willing *temporarily* to subordinate his individual preferences to the public welfare.[1]

Alarmingly, although there are known effective procedures for the prevention and control of tuberculosis, syphilis, poliomyelitis, and encephalitis, these diseases continue to take lives. We now have immunization to protect against German measles, measles, and mumps. Too often, however, the immunization level of a community is low. The solution to this complex problem involves reinforced mass health education; intelligent use of existing knowledge; development and improvement of techniques, methods, and materials; and continued research. In addition, active surveillance consisting of prompt diagnosis, reporting, and epidemiologic investigation of individual cases is a most important public health measure. Communicable diseases are a major cause of absenteeisms in school and industry, and some can cause crippling physical, mental, and economic impairment. The economic loss is great to industries, school districts, and individuals; enormous expenditures are required for treatment and hospitalization.

Current Immunization Procedures

The availability of new attenuated live virus vaccines has led to re-examination of immunization recommendations. In the first year of life, DPT (diphtheria, pertussis, and tetanus) and polio immunization are currently recommended. Vaccines for measles, mumps, and rubella should not be given earlier than one year of age, because of both lower take rates and potentially higher adverse reactions. It is not clear whether or not boosters will be necessary for all of these live virus vaccines. Recent information indicates that tetanus antibody persists for a long time. Routine tetanus boosters are being given too frequently, and adverse hypersensitivity reactions have been increasingly reported. The current recommendation for tetanus boosters after a primary series is every 10 years. If a dose is administered as part of wound management, then the 10-year interval is determined from that date.

VACCINATION SCHEDULE
(Recommended to its member physicians by the American Academy of Pediatrics)

AGE	PREVENTIVE(S)
2 months	DPT—combined diphtheria-pertussis (whooping cough)-tetanus injection—and TOPV—trivalent oral polio vaccine, covering the three viruses that can cause this disease
4 months	DPT and TOPV
6 months	DPT and TOPV
12 months	MMR—combined measles-mumps-rubella injection—and TB (tuberculosis) skin test
18 months	DPT and TOPV
5 years	DPT and TOPV
15 years	DT—DPT minus the "P"

Figure 8–2 Vaccination schedule. This schedule is a flexible guide that may be modified by the physician to fit individual situations.

The physician must remain flexible in his immunization recommendations to adapt to the new information concerning vaccine administration.

COMMUNITY EDUCATION

Education is fundamental to the application of all other control measures. This involves dissemination of appropriate and feasible information, communication, and intrinsic motivation. Too often local and official health agencies assume that they must merely provide vaccines or medical services; they neglect the adequate planning and preparation necessary to launch a community education program. Parents and children must be continually and emphatically informed of the need for disease protection. In many instances, parents are apprehensive about immunizations because of reports of reactions and failures, indifference, or fear of the needle. Too often motivation for immunization is extrinsic; for example, a sudden rise in the number of poliomyelitis deaths and cases in a city usually results in a rise in the number of persons requesting polio immunization in that city.

Education is necessary to help prevent most diseases (see Table 8–1).

LEGAL ASPECTS OF DISEASE CONTROL

Primary responsibility and authority for public health is vested in the states. The first state health departments were established primarily for the prevention and control of communicable disease. State disease-control functions range from consultation and advisory services to the direct operation of complex statewide programs. During the past half-century, much of the states' responsibility for public health services has been delegated to local health departments; the state continues to supply technical advice, consultation services, and emergency assistance. The federal government has necessarily assumed responsibility for communicable disease control in three broad functional areas: preventing introduction of disease from abroad; limiting the spread of disease across state lines; and assisting states when health problems exceed state resources. As far as possible, federal activities for disease control are integrated with activities at state and local levels.

TABLE 8–1 Diseases Prevented by Education

DISEASE	PREVENTION BY EDUCATION
Typhoid fever	Personal hygiene
Bacillary dysentery	Personal hygiene
Infectious hepatitis	Personal hygiene
Botulism	Proper home canning procedure
Salmonellosis	Keep food hot or cold
Poliomyelitis	Immunization
Encephalitis	Eliminate mosquito breeding areas
Trichinosis	Cook pork
Syphilis	Eliminate promiscuity; blood test
Tuberculosis	Periodic chest x-ray, Mantoux test
Rabies	Vaccinate dogs

Each state has adopted laws relating to the health and safety of its citizens. These laws are basic minimum requirements and standards that must be met by each local health department. However, local officials and citizens may enact additional health legislation to meet the changing and increasing health needs in their area. Usually the enforcement of these laws is no problem, but occasionally the services of the local sheriff or chief of police are necessary to protect the health and safety of the citizens within a community. Examples of these situations would be a recalcitrant patient with active tuberculosis, a restaurant owner who consistently refuses to comply with the suggestions of the sanitarian and health officer, and a farmer who refuses to pasteurize his milk before distribution to the public. Sanitarians are plagued with nuisance calls, most of which can be tactfully and diplomatically solved. It must be stressed, however, that education, tact, and diplomacy are the keys in promoting public health efficiency, coordina-

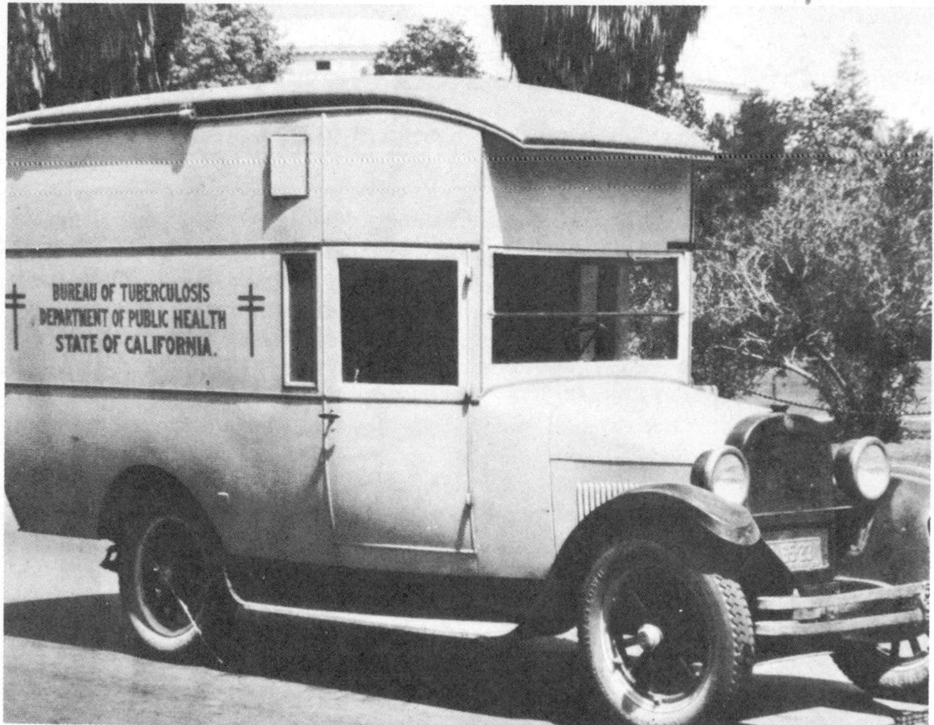

Figure 8–3 Traveling sanitation unit covers inspection of automobile campgrounds, summer resorts, roadhouses, and other places patronized by the traveler. (From Healthnews, August, 1973, p. 6. California Department of Health, Sacramento, Calif.)

TABLE 8–2 Content of the Course for Public Health Inspectors on Public Health Law*

Title	Content	No. of Sessions
An Introduction to the Nature, Function and Structure of the Canadian Legal System	Emphasis placed on the structure of the court, the British North America Act, the division of power between the federal and provincial governments, and the federal-provincial-municipal responsibility in the public health area.	2
Formulation and Enactment of Public Health Law	How health legislation is initiated, drafted and amended; what diverse interests are considered and who makes the final decisions and on what basis; the role that Public Health Inspectors can play in the continuing development of this area of the law.	1
Public Health Laws and Regulations	A review of federal, provincial and municipal public health law, rules and regulations.	1
The Courtroom—Effective Enforcement of the Law	An introduction to criminal law and evidence; investigation and preparation of a case; testimony and courtroom manner.	2
Personal Liability of the Public Health Inspector	Public rights versus private rights.	1
When Not to Enforce the Law	The Public Health Inspector's prime function is to preserve the public health. The law is one of the tools at his disposal. It should be used when other methods are ineffective. Discussion and examples as to when to enforce the law and when to educate the public.	1

*All lectures were given by members of the legal profession except the last, which was given by a public health physician. One instructor is qualified in both law and medicine. From MacKenzie, C. J. G.: The continuing role of the university in the education of public health workers. Canad. J. Publ. Health, *55*:493, 1964.

tion, and cooperation. Public health laws are utilized only when less severe measures have failed.

The Department of Continuing Medical Education of the University of British Columbia, in cooperation with the Department of Preventive Medicine and the Faculty of Law, has sponsored a course in public health law since 1963. The content of the course is given in Table 8–2.

SELECTED COMMUNICABLE DISEASES

Statistics and information on selected communicable diseases follow.*†

*For a complete analysis and community management of 117 communicable diseases of the world, refer to: *Control of Communicable Diseases in Man,* published periodically by the American Public Health Association. The American Academy of Pediactrics publishes an authoritative reference on currently accepted procedures for diagnosis, treatment, and prevention of infectious diseases in children. Write to P.O. Box 1034, Evanston, Illinois.

†Statistics and case histories of the various communicable diseases printed in small type in this chapter have been derived from *Morbidity and Mortality Weekly Report,* U.S. Public Health Service.

Cholera

Cholera should no longer exist. Modern sanitation can eliminate the primary causes of this highly infectious disease—i.e., waste-contaminated water supplies—and advanced medical techniques can effectively treat it. Yet cholera continues to spread and to take lives.

Even a single case of cholera must be viewed seriously. The disease can strike any community almost anywhere on earth where sanitation is poor and the germ is imported by someone who carries the vibriocholerae—the tiny comma-shaped microbe that causes the illness.

Reports from the World Health Organization during the past few years have placed cases in 60 nations in Asia, Africa, and various parts of Europe. In Africa alone, where cholera is a relative newcomer, the disease has struck more than 80,000 persons in little more than two years and killed at least 20,000.

Cholera has been a scourge of mankind for thousands of years. Ancient Sanskrit writings describe epidemics that were probably cholera. It has been a persistent fact of

A

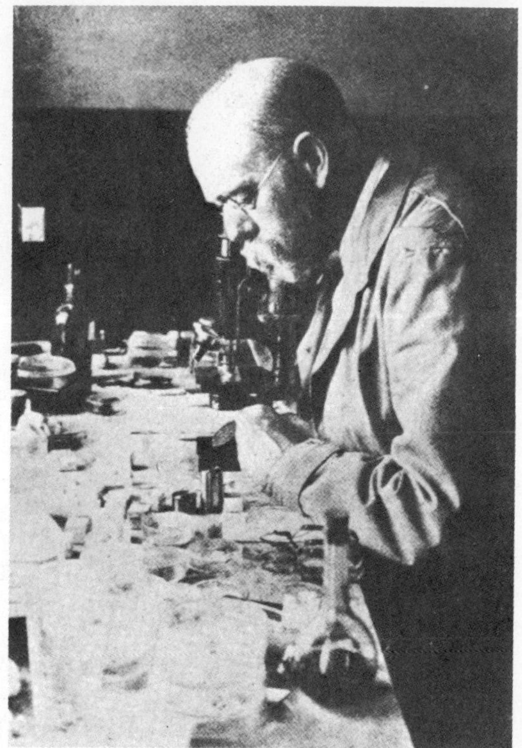

B

MINISTÈRE DES AFFAIRES ÉTRANGÈRES.

PROCÈS-VERBAUX

CONFÉRENCE SANITAIRE INTERNATIONALE

OUVERTE A PARIS

LE 27 JUILLET 1851.

PARIS.

IMPRIMERIE NATIONALE.

Figure 8–4 *A,* Robert Koch (1843–1910) made possible the isolation of different kinds of bacteria in pure culture. In 1882 he discovered the bacillus of tuberculosis, and two years later announced from Calcutta, India, that he had identified the causative organism of cholera. Although, at the time, many scoffed at his claims, history has fully vindicated him. *B,* A historic document: the proceedings of the first International Sanitary Conference. (From World Health, April, 1973, p. 5.)

life and death in the Indian subcontinent for centuries.

The germ passes from person to person indirectly, usually through water contaminated by human excrement. It can survive for weeks in sea water. Contaminated shellfish have been blamed in some outbreaks.

The disease does not directly poison the body but causes such a copious outflow of fluid because of diarrhea that the patient may die within hours as a result. The standard treatment today is primarily to replace the fluid and the lost salt and other minerals. The fluid is either infused into a vein or, in milder cases, taken by mouth. In the latter case a little sugar is added to the salty water because it helps the fluid pass through the intestinal wall into the blood stream. Antibiotics also are used in treating cholera because they shorten the period of illness. They do not cure the disease, however.

Simple as the treatment sounds, the massive amounts of fluid needed in treating cholera victims make care difficult when the outbreak occurs in a place remote from good medical facilities. The cholera patient may lose as much as a quart of fluid an hour over a period of several days, and this fluid must be replaced at the same rate.

Dr. John Snow, the nineteenth century London physician who became famous for showing the link between contaminated water and the then mysterious disease in the mid-1850's, first noticed cholera's dramatic dehydration effect. In his day, however, replacement of the fluid fast enough and for a long enough period of time was impossible, and as a result, as many as three-quarters of the victims of cholera died.

Today, with proper treatment more widely available, the death toll is small. There is also a vaccine against cholera, but its protection is too imperfect and too short-lived to eradicate the disease. There is no sure way of eliminating a major outbreak except by rigorous attention to sanitation of food and water.

Anthrax

Anthrax primarily affects animals such as cattle, sheep, goats, horses, and pigs, but it can also be contracted by humans. It is caused by a bacillus that produces a spore highly resistant to disinfection. These infectious spores may persist on a contaminated item for many years. Although human infection in the United States and most industrialized nations is infrequent, Haiti has had an endemic anthrax problem for many years. Since the contamination in goatskin drums was discovered in 1974, all products from Haiti made in whole or in part from untanned goatskin have been banned from this country. Any products such as drums, rugs, pitchers, and so on, purchased from Haiti in past years should be regarded as potentially infectious. Most Haitian products in the United States were purchased in Haiti by travelers. There are only a few retail outlets for these products in this country, mainly located in Florida and New York. Persons having Haitian drums or other items made with untanned goat hide should double-wrap them in plastic bags and call their local health department for advice on proper disposal methods.

Encephalitis

Acute encephalitis is a major problem in California, Texas, North Dakota, Illinois, and many other states. The mosquito transmits the virus from infected birds to horses and to man (Fig. 8–5). Encephalitis fatality is high, and serious and permanent neurological consequences may develop in a patient. With the development of many thousands of additional acres of irrigated land the great increase in the volume of commercial and industrial waste waters, the mosquito problem is magnified in many states.

The western equine type of encephalitis (horse to mosquito to man) usually occurs in early to mid-summer and is more likely to affect younger individuals. The St. Louis variety (bird to mosquito to man) occurs later in the year and seems to affect mostly the older age groups.

An epidemic of Venezuelan equine encephalomyelitis (VEE) worked its way northward from South America and crossed the border into Texas in 1971. This strain killed thousands of horses, but fortunately it is rarely fatal to humans.

Mosquito Control Programs

Mosquito control programs have three possibilities to work on:

Physical Control. Drain or fill mosquito breeding beds, or build permanent ponds to eliminate seepage areas. This approach is best, but it is slow and expensive to implement.

Biological Control. Breed mosquito-eating fish in all possible water-filled containers and impoundments. *Gambusia affinis,* which resembles a guppy, is the fish of choice, and is provided free to all takers by the local control agencies. It first was imported from Texas in 1922, and has given yeoman service in mosquito control work ever since.

Chemical Control. Regrettably, this continues to be the major activity. DDT was introduced in copious amounts in 1946. It was the "wonder chemical" that was supposed to solve all of the world's pest problems. By 1952, mosquitoes were breeding strains that proved impervious to DDT, so newly available phosphate compounds were used. Aircraft dusting with a low-volume, high-concentration technique gives good results, and the chemical deteriorates into a nontoxic, inert form within several weeks.

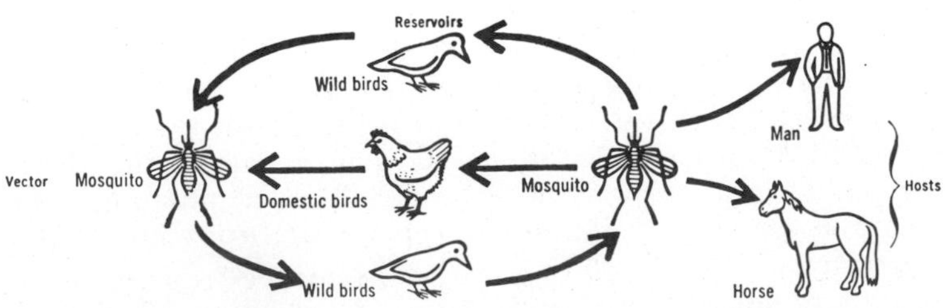

Figure 8–5 Man and the horse—accidental hosts of encephalitis. The three types of arthropodborne encephalitis—St. Louis, western and eastern—are maintained primarily by bird-mosquito-bird infection chains. Neither man nor horse is the usual reservoir, as was once believed. Many types of mosquitoes carry the virus, and it may reside temporarily in various domesticated animals and rodents. Where the virus is maintained (unobserved) during interepidemic periods remains a mystery. (From *Patterns of Disease.* Parke, Davis & Co., July, 1960.)

YOU MAY BE RAISING MOSQUITOES IN YOUR BACKYARD!

MOSQUITOES breed only in water . . . and water standing just a few days can produce a crop of mosquitoes!

IF there are any places around your house where water collects, such as tin cans, temporary water containers and ponds—YOU MAY BE RAISING MOSQUITOES!

LET'S CHECK YOUR BACKYARD...

YOU SHOULD . . .
Flatten or dispose of tin cans. Empty barrels, buckets, and other containers and stack them upside down.

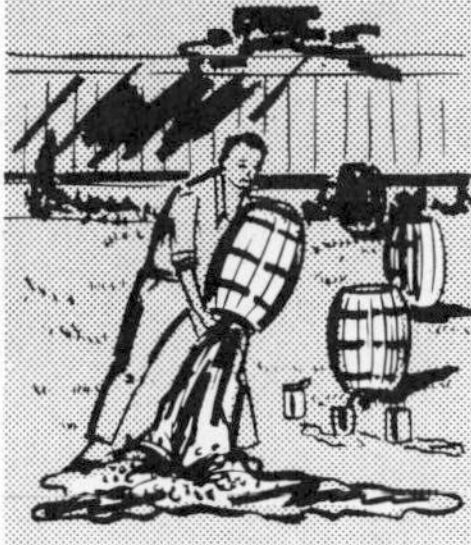

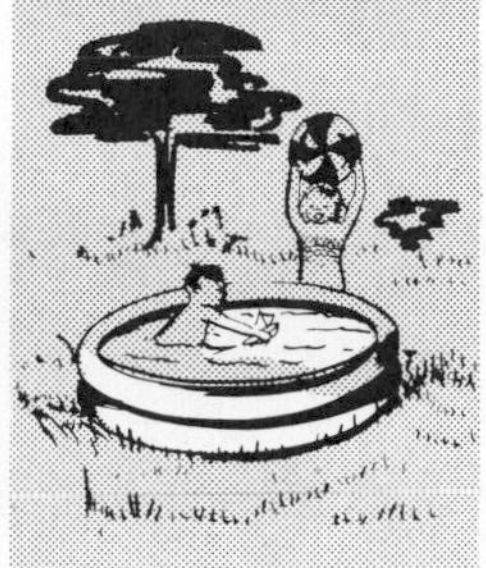

YOU SHOULD . . .
Empty your plastic swimming pool frequently and store it inside during the winter.

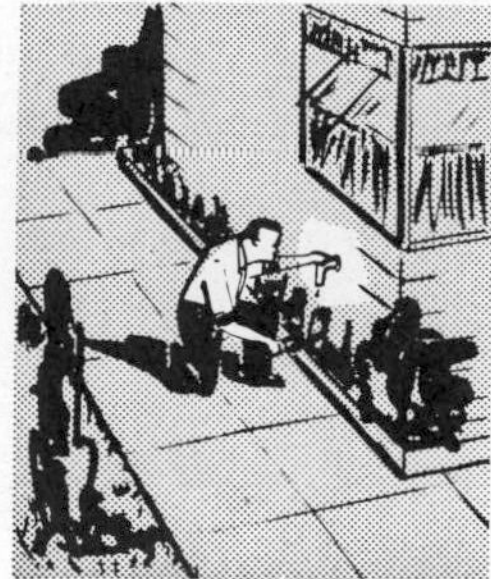

YOU SHOULD . . .
Avoid over irrigating, especially near the house. Repair leaky pipes and outside faucets.

YOU SHOULD . . .
Repair and seal cesspools and septic tanks so that mosquitoes cannot enter.

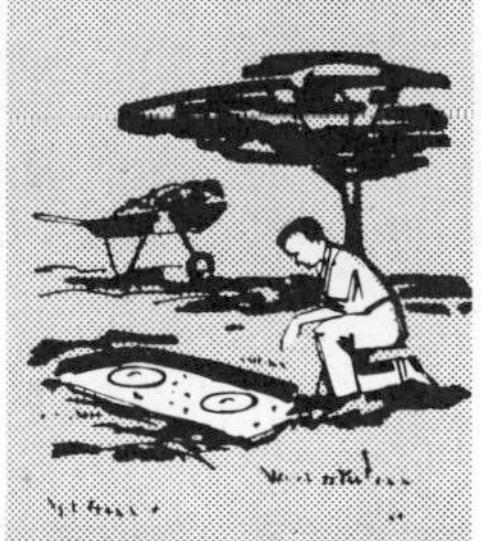

AND REMEMBER

. . . besides being vicious biters, MOSQUITOES can carry several serious diseases such as MALARIA and SLEEPING SICKNESS (ENCEPHALITIS)!

Figure 8–6

MANNING THE MALAY MOSQUITO TRAP

Kuala Lumpur

For all of 24 years, a Kuala Lumpur municipal employee has been sleeping on the job! And nobody minds it at all. For R. Veerappan is human bait in a mosquito trap.

Every night, from 6 until midnight, he mans a mosquito traphouse about three miles from downtown Kuala Lumpur, one of 13 stations in the city, to guard against malaria.

Mosquitoes feed on humans, so if you want to catch mosquitoes give them human bait.

When Veerappan takes up his post each evening, he lights an oil lamp to attract the mosquitoes, opens the doors on either side of the 10 foot by 7 foot trap-house and goes to bed on a bunk under a mosquito net.

Every hour he gets up and closes the doors, trapping the mosquitoes inside the house. Its walls and ceilings are screened with insect mesh.

He catches the mosquitoes, puts them in a test tube, opens the doors, and goes back to bed.

At midnight another trapper takes over and Veerappan can get six hours of uninterrupted sleep until it is time to report at the health department with his night's catch, which is usually about 20 mosquitoes.

When all 25 trappers have handed over their catch, the mosquitoes are sent to the Institute for Medical Research for classification.

If a malaria-carrying *Anopheles* mosquito is found, the health department's special survey squad is notified and the hunt begins.

The seven-man squad goes to the traphouse where the mosquito was caught and searches the area until the mosquito-breeding spot is found. The area is then sprayed to eliminate the malaria menace.[2]

Further mosquito abatement programs, new and more effective insecticides, and continued research and health education may yet win the battle against encephalitis. Education programs must stress the fact that certain mosquitoes may carry disease germs and that mosquitoes lay their eggs in stagnant water.

German Measles (Rubella)

Rubella epidemics surge across the nation every six to nine years. The 1964 epidemic caused an estimated 30,000 stillbirths. Another 20,000 infants born to mothers who contracted rubella during pregnancy suffered defects ranging from heart abnormalities to mental retardation.

Several strains of rubella vaccine have proven effective. Since these vaccines have been licensed, many parts of our country are carrying out mass immunization of prepubertal boys and girls in order to increase the immunity in the individual and reduce the potential for an epidemic spread to susceptible adolescents and young adults. Although young children are thought to be the major cause of transmitting the virus, it is also spread by older children and, on occasion, by adults. The embryopathic potential of the vaccine virus is not known. Because of this, the vaccine is contraindicated in pregnant women, and vaccine administration to any postpubertal females must be approached with caution. At present, the U. S. Public Health Service has recommended that children in Kindergarten and the early grades of elementary school deserve initial priority for vaccination. Outbreaks are most common among unvaccinated high school students.

Some physicians, however, are in doubt about the effectiveness of the new vaccine. They maintain that its immunity has not yet been proven to last more than four years, so that most of the young girls inoculated now could later be susceptible to the disease anyway; that only immunizing part of the population would not stop the spread of the virus enough to justify the program; that such a mass program might prevent the population from building up a natural immunity to the virus, which many researchers and doctors claim 85% of the people accomplish.

Any persons wishing to be inoculated can do so by going to their private doctor, or to any of the regular clinics maintained by the county health department throughout the county.

Some states now require rubella antibody tests of female applicants for marriage licenses. The purpose of the rubella test is to identify women who have no detectable antibodies and are thus susceptible to the infection and would be at special risk of having a defective infant if infection should occur during the first trimester of pregnancy. Exceptions may include females over 50, females who have had surgical sterilization, and females who present lab evidence of immunity to rubella.

Genital Herpes

The painful blister-like vesicles of genital herpes, similar to common cold sores or fever blisters of the mouth and lips, have been quietly disrupting sexual relationships for several hundred thousand Americans every year. The awareness that these infections are not trivial nuisances was triggered by three major discoveries in the past decade:

1. It was firmly established that the herpes simplex virus (HSV) primarily responsible for lesions around the oral area (type 1) differed from the virus affecting the genital area (type 2).

2. A major difference between the two viruses was found to be in their means of transmission, HSV-2 being spread primarily through venereal means.

3. A growing body of evidence pointed to a probable association between HSV-2 infections and the development of cervical cancer.

Additionally, the significance of HSV infections in pregnancy has only recently been appreciated, with reports indicating high rates of neonatal death or neurological damage among infected infants.

There is some debate as to the prevalence of HSV-2 infections. Physicians have not been required by law to report cases, as they are for such bacterially caused diseases as syphilis and gonorrhea. Controversy centers on disparate claims for the efficacy and safety of various treatment methods. Freezing lesions with liquid nitrogen, x-ray therapy, inoculations of vitamin B, repeated smallpox vaccinations, and many other approaches are described by Dr. Allan Lorincz, of the University of Chicago Medical School, as "clinical witchcraft," with sparse evidence that such methods prevent recurrences.

More recently, a dye-light or photoinactivation procedure, developed at the Baylor University College of Medicine, has gained popularity. The procedure involves application of proflavine dye at the onset of lesions, which are then repeatedly exposed to incandescent or fluorescent light over an 18- to 24-hour period.

Researchers have long postulated that cervical cancer may be caused by a venereally transmitted virus. Recent seroepidemiologic studies continue to support a growing body of evidence that HSV-2 may well be that virus. The evidence suggests a relationship between 6 and 10 times that attributable to chance. Whether the relationship is one of cause and effect remains to be proven.

Much additional research effort is being expended to develop and test "vaccines" that could provide protection for infants and sufferers from either primary infections or the painful, infectious recurrences.

Hepatitis

Hepatitis, a disease which was virtually unknown to the average person 10 years ago, has increased so alarmingly in recent years that there is widespread concern about it. The disease occurs in two forms: *infectious hepatitis,* which arises from direct contact with the waste products of an infected person or by the use of contaminated food or water, and *serum hepatitis,* which is caused by the use of contaminated medical instruments, or by receiving a transfusion of infected blood. In terms of how they affect the patient and the type of treatment they require, the two types of hepatitis are quite similar—each is a viral disease which specifically affects the liver, damaging and sometimes destroying the cells of that vital organ.

Why is this debilitating and often persistent disease on the increase? Not all the reasons for this trend are fully understood, but many doctors have reported an increase in serum hepatitis among young persons taking drugs. Obviously, needles used for such injections are not likely to be properly sterilized. Another possibility is that increased pollution of water is contributing to this health problem. Several Michigan residents became ill when a septic tank overflowed and polluted well water. In a Mississippi town, a number of persons suffered hepatitis after eating oysters that were taken from contaminated waters.

Most patients recover from hepatitis, but the illness can be very prolonged and discouraging; if it is not promptly and properly treated, chronic liver trouble can develop. Fortunately, this is not a common complication.

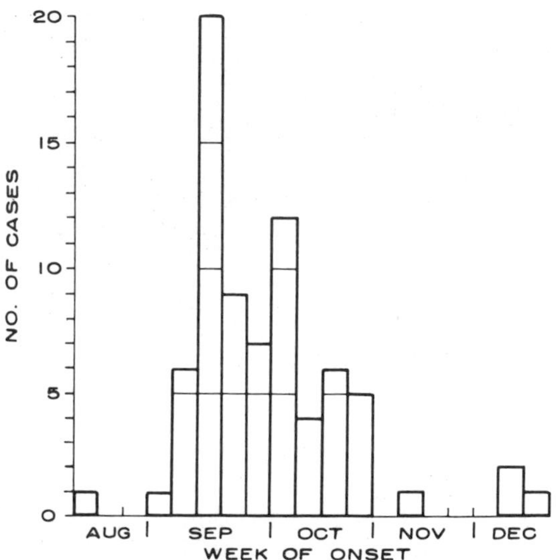

Figure 8–7 Hepatitis cases traced to an Oregon bowling alley from August to December in 1961.

Hepatitis usually starts with an array of symptoms that *could* mean the onset of a number of diseases—symptoms such as fever, chills, aches, pains, and gastrointestinal distress, including nausea, vomiting, diarrhea, and a pronounced loss of appetite. The fact that the liver is enlarged and tender to the touch and that the patient develops the yellowish tinge of jaundice provides the doctor with a significant clue that the patient's misery and weakness are caused by hepatitis. This suspicion can readily be confirmed by blood studies.

Like almost all viral infections, hepatitis cannot yet be effectively treated by medication. Patients are encouraged to rest and adhere to a high-protein diet, avoiding fats if (as often happens) they cannot be tolerated.

Dear Parents:

The ______________________ School District and the Santa Clara County Health Department will be conducting a rubella immunization clinic at ______________________ on ______________________. The vaccine will be offered to girls in the 5th and 6th grades. Immunizations for other children in your family may also be obtained from your private physician or Health Department clinic.

German measles (rubella or 3-day measles) is the disease that causes birth defects if women get it during the first three months of pregnancy. This immunization is not for the same disease as the measles shot that has been available for several years. That shot is for red measles (rubeola or 10-day measles).

By having your daugher immunized now, you will help protect her from having a rubella-damaged baby when she becomes a mother. The Santa Clara County Medical Society and the Santa Clara County Health Department recommend that girls in the 5th and 6th grades receive this protection.

Even if you think your daughter has had German measles she should have this immunization. German measles can be very hard to diagnose and is, therefore, often mis-diagnosed.

YOUR CHILD SHOULD NOT BE GIVEN A SMALLPOX, RED MEASLES (RUBEOLA) OR GAMMA GLOBULIN IMMUNIZATION FOR ONE MONTH BEFORE OR AFTER THE SCHEDULED GERMAN MEASLES IMMUNIZATION. YOUR CHILD SHOULD NOT RECEIVE THIS IMMUNIZATION IF SHE IS ALLERGIC TO DUCKS, RABBITS, DOGS, AND NEOMYCIN.

If you wish to have your child receive this immunization, please complete and sign the attached form. This must be returned to the school by ______________________.

- -

I request that my child ______________________ who is in the ______________________ grade/class, room # ______________________ at ______________________ School be given a rubella immunization, and hereby give my consent.

Signature ------------------------------ Date ------------------------------
Address ------------------------------ Phone ------------------------------

In some instances, medication may be given to suppress vomiting, and some patients require intravenous feeding. The overall aim of treatment is to keep the patient in as sound a condition as possible until the infection has run its course.

If a person in the home has hepatitis, there is a dual responsibility: (1) for the patient, and (2) for the well-being of other members of the household. To protect other members of the family, the patient's dishes, soap, and towels should not be shared. Injections of gamma globulin are often advised for persons who have been exposed to the disease; they should be given as early as possible, and—even if they do not prevent the disease—they may reduce its severity.

Many doctors also advise injections of gamma globulin for persons who are traveling to foreign countries where the standards of sanitation are dubious. In addition, the traveler should be very cautious about what he eats and drinks while visiting such countries . . . bottled water for drinking, brushing teeth . . . avoid uncooked vegetables and fruits, unless they have unbroken skins . . . avoid using ice, it may have been made with contaminated water.

What preventive measures can the individual take? — Always wash hands after using the toilet — keep flies away from food — insist on proper standards of sanitation, in the home and throughout the community.

Hepatitis — Oakland County, Michigan

During 1969, 163 cases of viral hepatitis were reported to the Southfield Office of the Oakland County Department of Health, a marked increase over the 91 cases reported in 1968 and the 57 cases in 1967. This health department serves a middle and upper socioeconomic suburban area adjacent to Detroit, with a population of approximately 565,000 people in 20 towns.

Epidemiologic case histories were obtained by public health nurses on 147 of these 163 reported cases. No clustering of cases was evident with respect to month of onset. Analysis by age and sex, however, showed a marked increase in cases for both sexes in the age groups from 15 to 24 years, with 99 cases (68 in males and 31 in females) occurring in these age groups. Of these 99 persons, 47 (32 males and 15 females) were suspected or admitted parenteral users of drugs.

The 47 drug-associated cases represented a sharp increase over the totals of drug-associated cases for 1968 (9 cases) and 1967 (0) and were spread throughout the year with a preponderance (30) occurring in the last 6 months. These cases were reported from towns which had not had in the past high rates of drug-associated hepatitis. There were no known deaths in this group.

Interviews were conducted among individuals selected from the age groups 15 to 24 years who had hepatitis in 1969. The following conclusions were made from these interviews: 1) the majority of the hepatitis cases within this age group were associated with parenteral use of drugs; 2) an estimated 1 to 3 percent of the high school age population used drugs parenterally; 3) the increased number of hepatitis cases seemed to represent relatively high attack rates within several isolated small groups who shared needles; 4) approximately 50 percent of the patients with drug-associated hepatitis have been hospitalized; 5) there appears to be considerable underreporting of drug-associated hepatitis cases.

Infectious Hepatitis in Oregon

An outbreak of infectious hepatitis, apparently waterborne, was traced to a bowling alley in Marion County, Oregon. Between August and December, 73 individuals closely associated with a bowling alley became ill. Fifty cases were icteric and 23 anicteric. All cases occurring after September were thought to be secondary. Food and beverage histories revealed that only two items were consumed by all who became ill — tap water and an orange drink made from a concentrated fruit syrup and tap water. Beverage histories were obtained on 61 persons who had bowled at the center within 30 days preceding the first known case. The data suggest that water may have been the vehicle of transmission.

Confirmatory evidence was supplied by two patients who had minimal exposure at the bowling alley. One was a small boy who had accompanied his mother to the bowling alley and was given an orange drink; the second was an older boy who had stopped in for a drink of water while on a bicycle trip.

The possible source case was an individual with onset of hepatitis on August 11, who spent many hours, up to 18 each day, on the bowling alley premises during the prodromal and early infectious period of his illness (August 4–18). During this time, the bowling center toilet facilities were used by this patient for the disposal of excretory wastes.

Water for the bowling establishment was supplied by a well that had been drilled five years earlier. There was a history of repeated troubles from excess amounts of air and lowered water pressure in the water lines. Persons interviewed told of dirty and foul-smelling water obtained from all facets, including the drinking faucet. Water samples from all outlets showed contamination for both *Escherichia coli* and *Streptococcus faecalis*.

The sewage disposal system consisted of a 1000 gallon tank located on the opposite side of the building from the well and an effluent line of unknown construction to a tile field located in a former orchard behind this building. The tile field reportedly consisted of four tile lines, each 100 feet long. The exact location was not determined but was assumed to be at least 50 feet from the well.

Influenza

One of the most serious respiratory diseases is influenza, for it is able consistently to attack people of all ages throughout the world. Incidence frequently is highest in young adults. Influenza has increased in virulence throughout the years, although since 1942 it seems to have become milder again.

Influenza has periodically been epidemic in the United States. Several tragic worldwide pandemics have occurred. One of the most dreadful was the 1918–1919 outbreak, in which some 20 million cases of influenza and pneumonia caused approximately 850,000 deaths. Like pneumonia, it is one of the leading causes of death in the United States.

Influenza is an acute disease of the respiratory tract that affects the whole body. It is characterized by sudden onset, with chills, fever around 102° (it may rise to 104°), headache, muscular pains, prostration, sore throat, and cough. Like the common cold, it paves the way for secondary infections caused by hemolytic streptococci and pneumonia. Most deaths are due to complications from pneumonia. Recovery usually takes four to five days.

The causative agent is classified in the myxovirus group of viruses. There are four different types of influenza virus: influenzas A, B, C, and CA. Influenza C and CA parainfluenza are rare varieties causing mild forms and are not as important as A and B. Influenza A breaks down into four different strains, referred to as sets or families. The A type has occurred in the northern hemisphere every year or so in epidemic form. Epidemics caused by type A influenza viruses are more frequent and are generally more severe than those caused by type B. These viruses have caused influenza on a worldwide basis since 1947.

A vaccine containing the new Asian strain of type A was developed and proved safe and effective. It is the only preventive measure against the disease. Immunity against influenza is specific for each type and each strain. The virus of one type does not seem to produce antibodies against another type. This seems to be the reason that individuals can have second attacks in a year or two; according to serologic tests, an attack of influenza confers a relatively longlasting immunity to the specific virus. The 1957–1958 epidemic and the 1976 mass national immunization (swine flu) were the first times in history that physicians, public health workers, laboratory workers, and others were ahead of the influenza epidemic. The quick identification of the Asian A strain, the alertness of health personnel, and the stepped-up production of vaccine were significant factors in controlling the disease in the 1957 epidemic. In any case, possible benefits versus costs and risks are usually weighed.

Influenza is spread by direct contact, by droplet infection through the air, and possibly by contact with inanimate objects contaminated with fresh virus. Sneezing, coughing, and talking are common ways of transmitting the virus from person to person. It quickly spreads from one part of the country to another and to other countries because of modern transportation. The incubation period of influenza is short, ranging from 24 to 72 hours. The early stages are the most contagious.

Several studies of mass immunization have shown the importance of immunization as a control measure in epidemics. However, because of the numerous strains of the virus and the necessity of having a particular vaccine for each strain, vaccination is not an absolute control procedure. Influenza control through widespread vaccination of the general population is not currently a public health objective for several reasons: the variable effectiveness of short-lived antibody levels with available influenza vaccines; the relatively low attack rates of influenza in community outbreaks; and the low frequency of serious complications from the disease in healthy people in the general population. So far, no one has developed one single vaccine that will be highly successful against all types of virus. Quarantine is not effective as a control measure during influenza epidemics. Prompt bed rest and good medical care are recommended measures for preventing serious complication and for early recovery.

Influenza is considered a serious illness only for certain high-risk groups, such as those with chronic lung, heart, renal, and metabolic diseases and the elderly (especially persons over age 65). However, absenteeism can be very serious in industry and schools and can hamper the operations of hospitals if large numbers of employees become ill at the same time. It therefore seems reasonable for employers to encourage employees to obtain influenza vaccinations. Others should discuss this with their personal physicians and decide whether or not they want this protection. Influenza vaccinations should be started as soon as September 1. Those vaccinated previously need only a single booster; others need two vaccinations, two months apart.

Malaria

Malaria has been responsible for huge mortality and morbidity rates and great economic losses for centuries. In 1955, the World Health Organization undertook the greatest public health venture of all time. It initiated an eradication program against malaria. The campaign was started with DDT spraying to kill the mosquitoes, and with the use of antimalarial drugs for those already infected. The program has made significant progress, although in many countries 10 to 15 per cent of infant deaths are still caused by malaria.

The malaria eradication program is an awesome task. An army of almost 200,000 doctors, engineers, spraymen, and entomologists, among others, are involved in this extensive undertaking. In Mexico, mortality due to malaria has decreased markedly as a result of the program. In Nicaragua, similar results have been recorded.

Unfortunately, many public officials involved in the program have become complacent, and malaria has returned to certain areas, such as South Asia, with a vengeance. Quinine, which is used to treat malaria, is in short supply in some areas; India, for instance, has not encouraged cultivation of the cinchona trees from whose bark the drug is obtained. The malaria parasite is showing a rising resistance to the drug chloroquine, a synthetic substitute for quinine. Furthermore, rising petroleum prices have sent the costs of insecticides much higher, placing another burden on the tenuous economic situation in that area.

The Vietnam War and jet travel provided vehicles for a fresh invasion of malaria in the United States. More than 2000 Vietnam veterans were afflicted with malaria after returning stateside in 1970.

Malaria remains the world's leading infectious disease, afflicting over 50 million persons a year, mostly in Asia, Africa, and Central and South America. The disease is caused by a one-celled organism of the *Plasmodia* family. The parasites begin their life cycle in the *Anopheles* mosquito. The mosquito carriers then inject immature *Plasmodia* into the blood when they bite. After maturing in the liver, the *Plasmodia* reenter the blood, where they destroy the red blood cells and multiply. Typically malaria becomes a chronic disease with recurrent episodes of fever, chills, and anemia. In its most severe form, malaria can cause death through damage to the brain, kidneys, and lungs.

Severe malaria became a serious threat in Vietnam when U.S. troops engaged the Viet Cong in the jungles of the central highlands. To prevent malaria, GI's took weekly doses of antimalarial drugs and were told to continue the medication for at least eight weeks after returning home. But some men failed to follow the regimen, and some parasites survived the drug therapy and entered the U.S. Since the *Anopheles* mosquito is prevalent in most parts of the nation, the disease could spread.

An Alabama case involving three teenagers was the first sign of a minor outbreak. All responded quickly to drugs and were soon sent home. Epidemiological studies were conducted. Through interviews, the investigators learned that the three youngsters had attended movies at an open-air drive-in one weekend. Next, they learned that a 15-year-old girl from Rochester, New York, who had gone to the same theater during a visit to Alabama, had also contracted malaria after returning home. Moreover, an entomologist at Auburn University reported that there had been a large population of *Anopheles* mosquitoes in the area, which embraces the big U.S. Army Infantry Center at Fort Benning, Georgia. And finally, it was revealed that several Vietnam veterans who developed malaria had gone to the movies at the Alabama drive-in.

The likelihood of widespread outbreaks of malaria in the U.S. remains remote. The disease doesn't spread from person to person as easily as smallpox and flu do. Malaria requires a "critical level" of carriers and mosquitoes before an epidemic can get started. So far it hasn't happened.

Preventive Measures

1. Application of residual insecticide (chlorinated hydrocarbons such as DDT, benzene hexachloride, or dieldrin) in suitable formula and dosage on the inside walls of dwellings and on surfaces upon which vector anophelines habitually rest will generally result in effective malaria control, except where resistance to these insecticides has appeared. When resistance occurs, the chlorinated hydrocarbons can be replaced by organophosphates (such as malathion) or carbamate compounds. These are effective in residual application, but may be more toxic to man in certain formulations (such as Arpocarb). Entire communities should be

treated in a spraying project, to be carried forward year after year until malaria ceases to be endemic, after which surveillance activities may be carried out to eliminate the residual parasites in man. Countrywide effort over at least four consecutive years followed by adequate surveillance has in some instances eradicated malaria in local regions.

2. Where residual insecticide is not available, nightly spraying of living and sleeping quarters with a liquid or an aerosol preparation of pyrthrum or other space sprays is useful.

3. In endemic areas, install screens in living and sleeping quarters and use bed nets.

4. Insect repellents (such as diethyltoluamide 50 per cent solution or dimethylphthalate; or 2-ethylhexane-diol, 1, 3—commonly called "612") applied to uncovered skin and impregnanted in the clothing of persons exposed to bites of vector anophelines are useful.

5. Sanitary improvements, such as filling and draining to eliminate breeding places of vector anophelines, should not be neglected. Larvicides (such as oil and Paris green) are now not commonly used where residual spraying is effective, but may be useful under special conditions. The chlorinated hydrocarbons are not recommended as larvicides, but organophosphorus compounds such as Abate or Fenthion may be of value. Effectiveness of antilarval methods varies with the particular vector species involved.

6. Regular use of suppressive drugs in malarious areas.

7. Effective treatment of acute and chronic cases is an important adjunct to malaria control and essential in attempted eradication, with case detection methods to locate those still infected.

8. Blood donors should be questioned for a history of malaria or possible exposure to the disease, and should be rejected if they have a history of malaria at any time, or of drug prophylaxis within the preceding two years.

Fatal Malaria—Wisconsin

On Nov 7, 1969, a 21-year-old serviceman returned to the United States from Vietnam on emergency leave to attend his father's funeral. He had brought no malarial suppressive drugs with him. Three days later, he experienced an episode of fever, chills, and anorexia. On November 18, he consulted a physician because of persistence of these symptoms, was told he had "flu, and was sent home. Two days later, he consulted a second physician who told the patient that malaria was a possibility, but the patient refused both a blood test and hospitalization.

On November 21, he was admitted to a civilian hospital with fever, chills, tachycardia, and restlessness and was treated with penicillin, digitalis, aspirin, and diazepam. Three days later, a peripheral smear showed a very heavy infection with *Plasmodium falciparum,* and therapy was begun with oral quinine and chloroquine. Intravenous quinine, whole blood transfusions, and sedatives were given because the patient demonstrated hypotensive episodes, a hematocrit of 22 percent, and neurologic abnormalities which included altered states of consciousness and pathologic reflexes. He expired on November 27.

Measles

Although measles is treated lightly by most people throughout the world, the disease may cause brain injury and is often fatal. The virus is sometimes the direct cause of fatal pneumonia, but more often it is the precursor of a bacterial infection. Measles also has a tendency to attack the middle ear, which may lead to permanent deafness. The disease can also cause encephalitis or brain inflammation, with a high (10 per cent) mortality rate and a higher rate of permanent damage. Most deaths occur among infants under three years of age. Measles vaccine is most effective in preventing this disease.

Pneumonia

Pneumonia is not one disease, but several diseases characterized by inflammation in one or more lobes of the lungs. These diseases rank first among the communicable diseases in the list of the most common causes of death. Everyone can be susceptible to pneumonia, although young children, the aged, and alcoholics are most susceptible. In the 15- to 34-year age group, there has been about a 95 per cent reduction in the mortality rate since 1900.

The pneumonias are classified into three major types: pneumococcal acute lobar pneumonia, bacterial pneumonia other then pneumococcal, and primary atypical pneumonia (virus pneumonia).

Onchocerciasis

Onchocerciasis (river blindness) is prevalent in tropical Africa as well as in the central portions of South America. Tiny flies (*Simulium*) transmit the disease by carrying microscopic young forms of worms. These are transmitted to the human bitten by the fly. In the human, when the worms reach the adult stage, they produce subcutaneous nodules in which they develop hundreds of thousands of young. These microscopic worms then invade the tissues of the skin and eyes, with blindness a frequent outcome. The disease is often referred to as river blindness because of its high incidence in river valleys. The fly that transmits the disease is known to reproduce best in this type of environment. New drugs have been developed for the successful treatment and control of the disease. In some areas, spraying with insecticides (DDT) has been effective in exterminating *Simulium* (the transmitting agent). In 1945, a survey in Kenya showed that 36 per cent of the children below the age of 6 were infected. By 1953, after a campaign against this disease, not a single child below the age of 6 was infected. However, more than 250,000,000 people are still affected by onchocerciasis, and attempts are being made to organize mass programs for its eradication.

Preventive Measures:

1. Avoiding bites of *Simulium* flies by covering body and head as much as possible; use of insect repellents, such as diethyltoluamide.
2. Control of vector larvae in rapidly running streams and in artificial waterways by DDT or other insecticides, and sometimes of adult *Simulium* by aerial spray; feasibility depends on vector and terrain.
3. Provision of facilities for diagnosis and treatment.

Polio Vaccine

The widespread use of polio vaccine is a dramatic example of how a once dread paralytic disease can be virtually eliminated from a country in less than a lifetime. Paralytic polio cases declined from 18,308 in 1954 to 19 in 1971. Nevertheless, low immunization rates still prevail in certain disadvantaged urban and rural groups, particularly for infants and children born since the mass immunization program of 1958–1962. Most polio cases in recent years have been among those groups.

Today, the oral vaccine has become standard because it is easier to administer than the injection. A three-dose immunization series is required. It should be started at 6 to 12 months of age in an infant, commonly with the first dose of the DTP vaccine. The second dose of polio vaccine should be given about 8 weeks later. The third dose should be administered 8 to 12 months after the second. Routine immunization of adults against polio is not necessary for those residing in the continental United States, where there is little likelihood of exposure. However, an unimmunized adult who has been exposed to a polio case or who will travel to areas where polio is epidemic or occurs frequently should be vaccinated. People who work in hospitals or other places where they might be exposed to polio should also be vaccinated.

Psittacosis (Parrot Fever)

Although parakeets and parrots are probably the most common source of human psittacosis, infections have been traced to pigeons, ducks, chickens, turkeys, canaries, sea gulls, egrets, and road runners. Parakeets are the usual source of human cases because of the growth in popularity of this bird. Prevention includes education and health legislation establishing a control program for banding and recording all birds that are sold commercially.

Rabies

Rabies is probably the most feared of the viral zoonoses. Once the symptoms develop, rabies is always fatal to animals and to humans. If the long, expensive, and sometimes dangerous Pasteur treatment is begun early enough, however, rabies may be prevented. The Pasteur treatment consists of 14 or 21 consecutive doses of rabies vaccine. There is a new vaccine type that requires only three injections at intervals of three to four days, but it is not available everywhere. The seriousness of rabies in this country cannot be measured by the small number of cases in man—only about 5 to 10 annually.

Approximately 60,000 persons receive

injections of rabies vaccine each year because of bites by rabid animals. Although the cat, wolf, fox, skunk, and bat may transmit rabies, dogs seem to present the greatest problem to children and adults. It is interesting to note that children under 15 years of age account for over 50 per cent of all human rabies deaths. This is attributed to higher inherent susceptibility and greater opportunities for severe exposure. Perhaps teachers and parents should better inform children as to the inherent dangers in petting strange dogs and catching or playing with wild animals. Children should be told to inform their parents immediately about any animal bites inflicted upon them.

Rabies is on the rise throughout the world. It is being spread by vampire bats and cattle in Latin America, by the fox and dogs in Europe, by stray dogs in Asia, and by monkeys in Africa. The problem is magnified when we consider the tremendous loss of livestock and the time and money spent by state and local health departments to combat this problem.

Rabies in Animals

Of note is the change in distribution of rabies in animal hosts, for the overall decrease is due to the reduced number of cases in domestic animals, particularly in dogs. Since 1960, rabies cases in wildlife have exceeded those in domesticated animals. Nationwide, no progress in reducing the number of rabies cases in domestic animals has been achieved for several years. On this basis, it appears that further reductions in the incidence of rabies will come only after measures are found to control the disease in wildlife.

The incidence of fox rabies has declined during the past decade, whereas that of skunk rabies has increased. Since the initial isolation of rabies from an insectivorous bat in Florida in 1953, a large number of rabid bats have been found throughout the United States, many in areas reporting few or no cases of rabies in other host species. In contrast, the significant increase of racoon rabies is the result of a highly localized epidemic, which first appeared in Florida and has since moved slowly northward.

Rabies in Humans

Prevention of human deaths from rabies depends on programs of animal bite investigation, destruction of rabid animals followed by strict quarantine of the victim, prophylactic treatment of exposed persons, and control of domestic and wild animals. Control of rabies in dogs is based upon registration, vaccination, adoption and enforcement of strict leash ordinances, prohibition of cross-breading dogs with wolves, impounding of unlicensed dogs, and control of stray dogs. The adoption of dog vaccination ordinances by local government officials is a major preventive measure. Wildlife control is based on poisoning and trapping. Poisoning is dangerous to people and domestic animals, and trapping is slow and impractical. Controlling rabies in dogs is much sounder and more feasible than wildlife controls. These measures must be supported by intensive health education programs aimed at the total population.

Rabies Death in Kentucky

The patient, a 74-year-old resident of Powell county, died on June 26, 1964. Approximately five weeks previously he had investigated a commotion in his chickenhouse and had found a fox under the shed. In attempting to chase the fox away, he was bitten on the left thumb. The fox was killed and discarded. The man refused rabies vaccination initially, but after two calves died within the following two weeks of apparent rabies, he assented to vaccination. He received 14 doses of duck embryo vaccine, the last, three days before onset of symptoms.

On June 22, he experienced tingling on his left side, followed subsequently by progressive paralysis, photophobia, hydrophobia, and death. Postmortem examination revealed Negri bodies in brain material.

Snail Fever (Schistosomiasis; Bilharzia)

The World Health Organization says the incidence of snail fever is rising, constituting a grave public health problem despite many years of chemical, biological, and ecological control efforts. The disease flourishes in developing countries because of irrigation and dam-building programs that build up new water areas. Some authorities predict, for example, that the economic benefits of the Aswan Dam in Egypt will be canceled by the further spread of this disease.

Snails are a host for the disease. They give off larvae that live in the water and that penetrate the skin of a person who is working, swimming, or wading in the water.

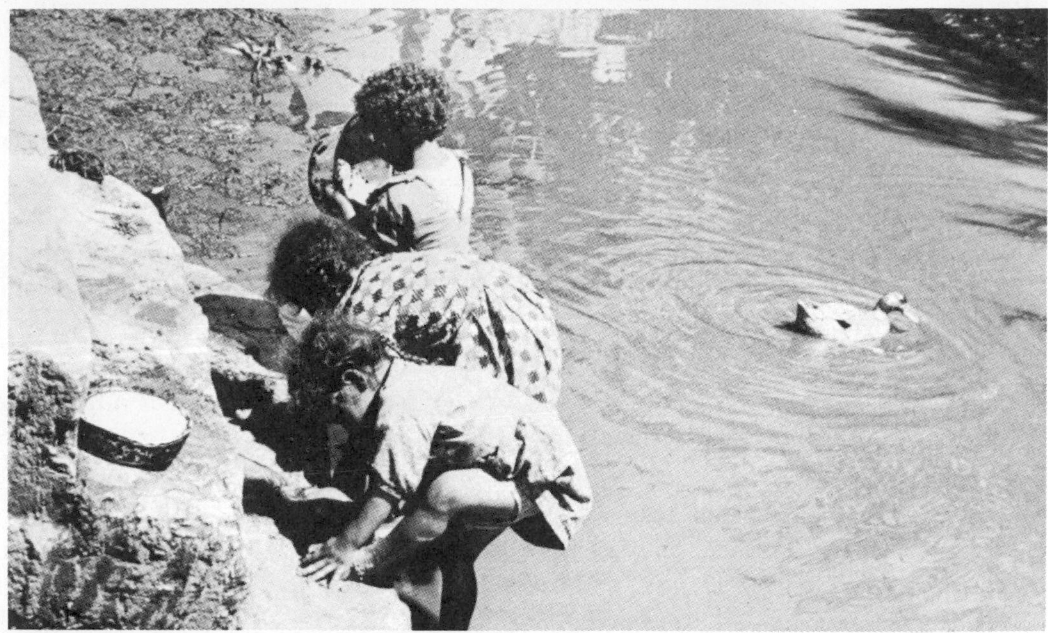

Figure 8–8 Water snails play an essential part in the transmission of schistosomiasis. The disease is common in Egypt, where children and adults are often in contact with water in canals and in the Nile. According to Egyptian specialists, schistosomiasis may be a predisposing factor for cancer of the bladder. (From World Health, February–March, 1970, p. 46.)

Then the larvae enter the blood, are carried to blood vessels of the liver, develop to maturity, and migrate to the veins of the abdominal cavity. The disease is chronically debilitating and sometimes fatal. If often seriously injures the liver, the intestine, and the urinary tract.

Snail fever isn't a significant health problem in the United States, but it is prevalent in Latin America, Africa, the Philippines, the Far East, and the Middle East. There is currently a drug called Hycanthone that will protect against the disease.

Preventive Measures

1. Disposal of feces and urine so that eggs will not reach bodies of fresh water containing snail intermediate host. Control of animals infected with *S. japonicum* is desirable but usually not practical.
2. Improved irrigation and agricultural practices; drainage and reclamation of swamps.
3. Treatment of snail breeding places with molluscicides.
4. Provision of water for drinking, bathing, and washing clothes from sources free from cercariae.
5. Provision of cercaria-repellent or protective clothing for persons required to enter contaminated water.
6. Education of people in endemic areas regarding mode of transmission and methods of protection.
7. Mass treatment of infected persons in endemic areas, which may help to reduce transmission through lessened severity and duration of the disease; unfortunately, in the past this has not materially reduced prevalence.

Tetanus

In contrast to diphtheria, tetanus has declined remarkably slowly in the past two decades despite extensive immunization, particularly of children. Over half of all cases of tetanus in the United States occur in adults. Of cases among adults, females account for the greater proportion among all age groups up to 50 years. Beyond age 50, cases are more frequent among males. The extensive tetanus immunization program carried out during World War II in the military appears to have conferred durable immunity to those immunized.[3] Although cases are reported somewhat more frequently from the southern states, tetanus occurs throughout all regions of the country. Recorded deaths due to neonatal tetanus, however, are confined almost exclusively to the southern United States. Two cases of tetanus, both fatal and diagnosed clinically, were reported from New Jersey in April, 1964. In neither case was the history of previous tetanus immunization known.

Case 1. A 29-year-old Negro female consulted a physician April 2, because of a three day history of nuchal rigidity and increasing trismus to the extent that she could not open her mouth. The patient gave no history of cuts, infections, or lacerations during the three months prior to onset. No evidence of such could be found on physical examination.

She was admitted to a hospital, where laboratory studies, including spinal tap and blood cultures, were unrevealing. A throat culture grew streptococci. A diagnosis of tetanus was made on the basis of clinical evidence.

The patient was treated with 100,000 units of tetanus antitoxin intravenously daily, 10,000,000 units of penicillin daily, sedatives and muscle relaxants. On April 3, a tracheostomy was performed because of respiratory difficulty; breathing was assisted with a respirator. On April 6, the patient developed bronchopneumonia. A broad spectrum antibiotic was added to the above regimen. The patient became opisthotonic on April 7, and died later that day.

At autopsy, there were no abnormal findings on gross examination. The uterus showed no evidence of pregnancy; the diagnosis of septic abortion appears doubtful. A postmortem vaginal culture was negative for *Clostridia.*

Case 2. A 58-year-old Negro female sustained a six-inch cut on her left knee after falling on outdoor stairs April 2. She was taken to a hospital, where the cut was cleaned and repaired with catgut and wire suture. She was given tetanus toxoid and penicillin. Four days later, the patient saw a private doctor, who described the wound as red and inflamed. He treated her with a broad spectrum antibiotic and Varidase, hot soaks, and elevation of the extremity. On April 7, the patient complained of trismus and nuchal rigidity; she was hospitalized and a diagnosis of tetanus was given.

On admission, the wound was opened and bathed with hydrogen peroxide solution. She received 20,000 units of tetanus antitoxin intramuscularly and an equal amount intravenously, administered over a 12-hour period. She also received 1,200,000 units of penicillin. In the evening the patient was sedated. She died the following morning, April 8. The patient had no respiratory difficulty or seizures during her hospitalization.

Gross examination at autopsy showed minimal cerebral edema and basilar congestion in both lungs. A smear of the wound taken at autopsy showed gram-positive rods; *Clostridium welchii* was grown from a culture. *Clostridium tetani* could not be identified.

Trachoma

Trachoma and infectious conjunctivitis represent a leading cause of blindness in the world, affecting some 400,000,000 people. Trachoma is particularly prevalent in North Africa, where in certain regions practically the entire adult population is infected. The rate of infection among preschool-age children in these areas runs between 70 and 90 per cent. Other regions of the world also suffer a high incidence. A study conducted in India revealed a 78 per cent infection rate among rural school children. A pilot project on Taiwan uncovered a 48 per cent incidence among its children. Sulfonamides and particularly antibiotics are effective in clearing up the condition. Mass campaigns on a national level are being encouraged to bring this disease under control.

Preventive Measures

1. Provision of adequate case-finding and treatment facilities, with emphasis on preschool children.
2. Health education of the public in the need for personal hygiene, especially the risk in common use of toilet articles.
3. Improved basic sanitation, including availability of soap and water.
4. Epidemiological investigations to determine important factors in occurrence of the disease in each specific situation.
5. Experimental vaccines; these are currently under trial, but their efficacy has not been established.

Trichinosis

Trichinosis is a major public health problem, even though the simple measure of thoroughly cooking pork and pork products will prevent the disease. It is estimated that every American consumes three servings of infested pork a year, and that 25,000,000 to 50,000,000 Americans carry trichina larvae in their muscles and internal organs. Between 200 and 300 human cases are reported each year despite the fact that trichinosis is not reportable in most states. The practice of feeding hogs raw garbage has kept the disease prevalent in pork.

What happens after infested pork is ingested by humans? Live worms, freed by digestion of the meat they infest, travel into the intestines, where they grow and reproduce, causing upset stomach, vomiting, and diarrhea. Young worms, born fully formed, move into the lymphatic system and the blood stream, and finally invade muscles where they grow for about three weeks before coiling up inside a cyst that they form in the muscle.

This can lead to swelling or hemorrhages under the skin, headaches, fever, and difficult breathing. There is no drug that kills trichinae after they enter the blood stream or muscle. Doctors can treat symptoms and prevent complications like pneumonia, but they cannot cure the disease. The seriousness of the disease depends on how heavily the pork was infested and how much was eaten. Most victims recover.

TRICHINOSIS FROM BEAR MEAT

Twenty-three people were involved in an outbreak of trichinosis due to ingestion of bear meat. Of 18 persons who ate uncooked meat, 12 developed fever, myalgia, periorbital edema, and eosinophilia. All had positive skin tests, and 10 had positive bentonite-flocculation tests (BFT's). Of the 11 asymptomatic patients, including all 5 who had eaten only cooked meat, 6 had tests negative to both and 5 had positive skin tests or BFT's or both.[4]

TRICHINOSIS AMONG THAIS LIVING IN NEW YORK CITY

Two outbreaks of trichinosis occurred among recent Thai immigrants to New York City. The first outbreak occurred in 1971 and involved three members of one family who had eaten raw pork. The second outbreak occurred in 1973 and affected 20 individuals, all of whom had eaten portions of the same raw pork preparation. In Thailand, raw pork dishes are commonly eaten but, owing to the absence of the infection in domestic swine, human trichinosis is rare. Thai immigrants, who are unaware of the dangers of eating raw pork in this country, are a high-risk group for trichinosis.[5]

Preventive measures against trichinosis include legislation requiring that hogs be fed only cooked garbage, and education programs that stress the importance of cooking pork at 140° F. for at least 30 minutes per pound.

Circumstances relating to the occurrence of trichinosis in a Wisconsin University graduate student provided a unique opportunity to demonstrate the source of the infection: contaminated pork chops.

About October 1, two graduate students who shared cooking facilities purchased two thick pork chops at a local market. Hasty preparation resulted in inadequate cooking of the chops. Both chops were sampled but then refrigerated. One of the students consumed one of the chops on the following day.

Three weeks later, he experienced anorexia and nausea without vomiting or diarrhea, followed by aching muscle pains in the chest and back, malaise, nonproductive cough, chills, and fever to 103°. His eyelids became swollen and he developed severe, throbbing headaches and boring eye pain. He was admitted to the hospital on November 3. A trichinella skin test was positive; biopsy of the gastrocnemius muscle revealed *Trichinella spiralis.* He recovered uneventfully. The second student experienced similar but milder symptoms. His skin test was equivocally positive. After discharge, the patient brought the remaining, now six week old, pork chop to the State Laboratory of Hygiene. Microscopic examination revealed encysted *T. spiralis* in the meat.

Trypanosomiasis

Trypanosomiasis (sleeping sickness) is a disease found in most of Africa south of the Sahara Desert. Several types of protozoa are responsible for trypanosomiasis. The disease is transmitted by the tsetse fly, and animals as well as humans are susceptible to the illness. Some trypanosomes (protozoa causing the disease) are harmless to animals but dangerous to man. The animals in these cases act as reservoirs of infection. The tsetse fly, by first biting the animal and then man, transmits the disease. The opposite is sometimes found to be true where some trypanosomes are harmless to man but fatal to the animals. In these cases, the people are deprived of animals which are needed as a source of protein or to help cultivate the land for the growth of crops. Either directly or indirectly, the disease is a source of hardship to man. Insecticides are now used in many areas to eradicate the tsetse fly. Drugs

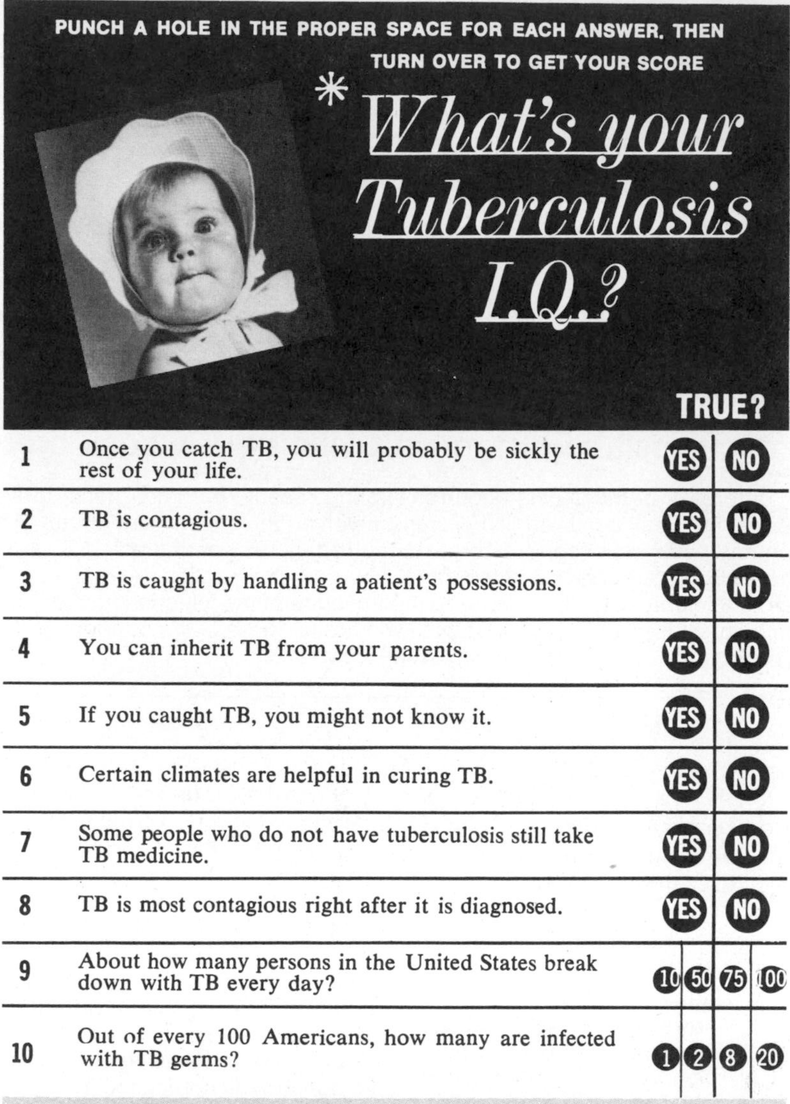

Figure 8–9

are also used to treat people who have contracted the illness. In the past, sleeping sickness was invariably fatal, but it can now be cured if treated in the early stages. Programs of prevention and treatment of the disease need to be continued and further extended.

Preventive Measures

1. Provision of adequate facilities for disposal of feces.

2. Education of all members of the family, particularly children, in the use of toilet facilities. Encouragement of satisfactory

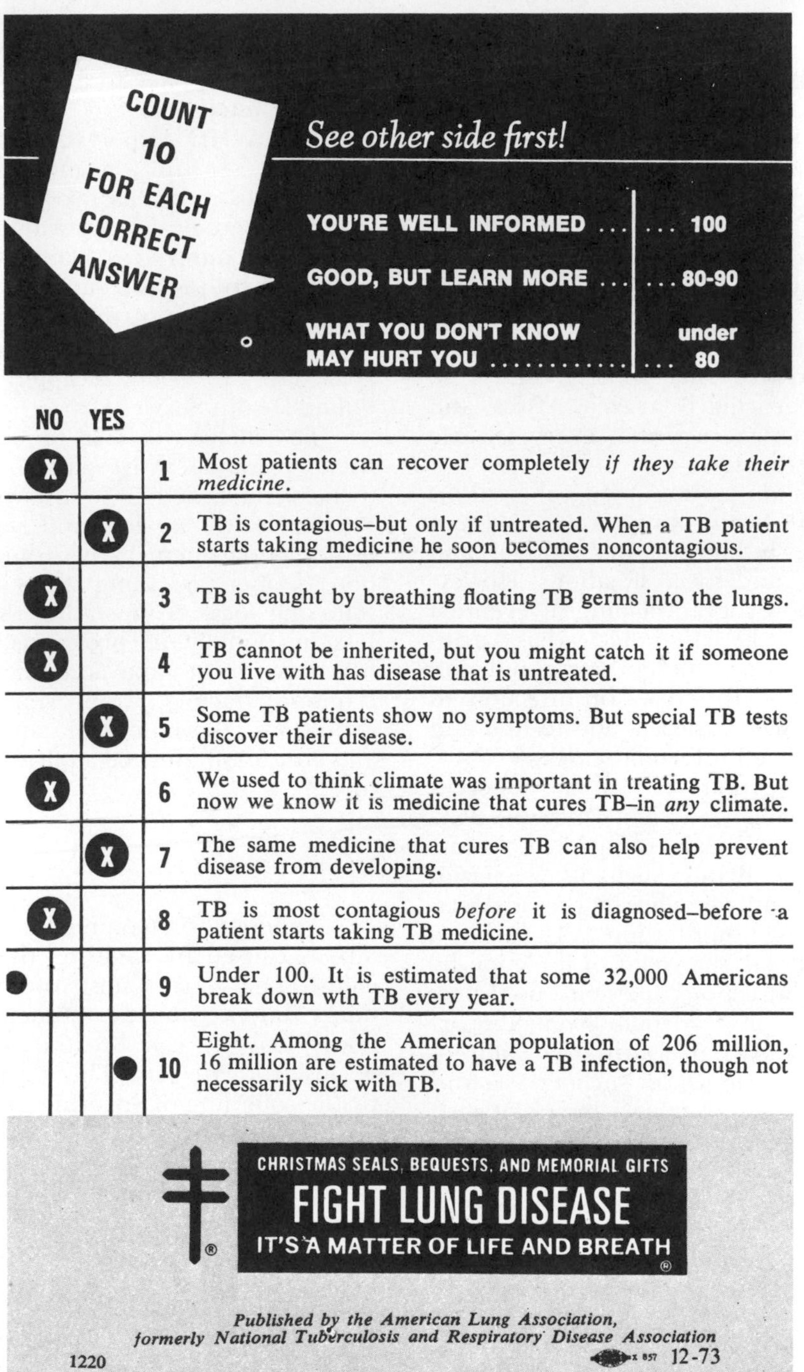

COUNT 10 FOR EACH CORRECT ANSWER

See other side first!

YOU'RE WELL INFORMED ...	... 100
GOOD, BUT LEARN MORE ...	... 80-90
WHAT YOU DON'T KNOW MAY HURT YOU	... under 80

NO	YES		
X		1	Most patients can recover completely *if they take their medicine.*
	X	2	TB is contagious–but only if untreated. When a TB patient starts taking medicine he soon becomes noncontagious.
X		3	TB is caught by breathing floating TB germs into the lungs.
X		4	TB cannot be inherited, but you might catch it if someone you live with has disease that is untreated.
	X	5	Some TB patients show no symptoms. But special TB tests discover their disease.
X		6	We used to think climate was important in treating TB. But now we know it is medicine that cures TB–in *any* climate.
	X	7	The same medicine that cures TB can also help prevent disease from developing.
X		8	TB is most contagious *before* it is diagnosed–before a patient starts taking TB medicine.
		9	Under 100. It is estimated that some 32,000 Americans break down wth TB every year.
		10	Eight. Among the American population of 206 million, 16 million are estimated to have a TB infection, though not necessarily sick with TB.

CHRISTMAS SEALS, BEQUESTS, AND MEMORIAL GIFTS
FIGHT LUNG DISEASE
IT'S A MATTER OF LIFE AND BREATH

Published by the American Lung Association, formerly National Tuberculosis and Respiratory Disease Association

1220 12-73

Figure 8–9 *Continued.*

hygienic habits, especially in the practice of washing the hands before handling food.

Tuberculosis

Tuberculosis is one of the most serious public health problems in the world. Conservatively estimated, at least 15 million people have active tuberculosis, and more than 3 million die annually. In India alone, between 3 million and 5 million people are estimated to have the disease. In Latin America, there are 600,000 known cases of active tuberculosis, and probably three times as many undetected cases. There are 30 thousand new cases in America every year.

Clearly, the inadequacy of statistical information in the less developed areas of the world makes it practically impossible to define the dimensions of the global tuberculosis problem precisely. Nevertheless, the fact is inescapable that tuberculosis is so widespread, particularly in Asia, Africa, and parts of Latin America, that every feasible effort must be made to control it.

The methods used to fight tuberculosis necessarily vary from country to country and no doubt are influenced by national and local economic and social situations. However, any control program aiming at eventual eradication must be based on two basic principles: to protect as much of the population as possible from the risks of infection to which they may be exposed, and to find and treat adequately all infectious cases.

Effective weapons to combat tuberculosis are available. Vaccination with BCG (Bacille Calmette-Guérin) can protect against infection,* and drugs such as isoniazid, streptomycin, and *p*-aminosalicylic acid can render patients noninfectious. To achieve this goal—to break the chain of infection by making the infectious patient noninfectious—flexibility and adaptability in the organization of control measures are required. In some parts of the world, such as Asia and Africa, the problem of tuberculosis is of such magnitude that approaches used in the United States or Western Europe are inapplicable. In India, for example, the pattern of treating patients with drugs at home is widespread, because the available hospital beds are far too few, and there is neither time nor money to provide enough beds for the large number of patients.

Equally important is the development of efficient community-wide services. These must be adapted to the particular needs and situation of a given country. Involved in such a development is the proper training of physicians and auxiliary workers of all kinds. Knowledge and tools exist; the challenge is to use them fully and effectively. This challenge does not apply solely to the developing countries; it applies to all countries, including the United States.

The WHO Expert Committee on Tuberculosis set up a standard by which a country can judge its progress toward control of tuberculosis. According to the committee, no country can claim to have eliminated tuberculosis as a public health problem until the number of tuberculin-positive children under 14 is less than 1 per cent. This goal has also been accepted by the U.S. Public Health Service.

To achieve this goal requires the fullest use of the cooperative pattern of control activities established by official agencies (U.S. Public Health Service, and state and local-health departments), the voluntary associations (American Lung Association and its state and local groups), and the health professions. Finally, all programs to control tuberculosis must take account of social and economic factors. Improvement of living conditions, economic situation, nutrition, and education must be a part of the total picture.

Identification of TB

Tuberculosis (commonly referred to as TB) is caused by a germ—the tubercle bacillus. The germ most often attacks the lungs, but it can affect other parts of the body. Anyone can breathe in tuberculosis germs from the air. The germs are spread by the coughing or sneezing of a person who have live TB germs in his or her sputum. A person can be ill with the disease and can be spreading it to others without even knowing it. Some of the symptoms of tuberculosis are frequent coughing, feeling tired and weak, unexplained loss of appetite, and losing weight. Spitting up blood is a sign that the disease has developed well beyond the early stages.

Most people who develop tuberculosis

---

*Use of the BCG vaccine, however, is still controversial; see discussion on page 265.

illness today, however, were infected years ago when the disease was much more widespread. They breathed in germs from someone who had the disease, but their bodies' defenses were stronger than the germs and encased them in calcium. When the body's defenses weakened years or decades later, the barriers began to crumble and the TB germs escaped and multiplied. Symptoms of tuberculosis illness then developed.

Taking pills specific for the tuberculosis germ can cure the disease. During treatment, in fact, most people today can carry on normal, active lives at home and at work. In some cases, short hospital stays may be necessary, but many patients are not hospitalized at all. Those who have TB germs in their sputum can become noninfectious rapidly by taking tuberculosis medicines. People who harbor tuberculosis can prevent the illness from developing by taking medication for up to a year.

Incidence of TB in the United States

Tuberculosis cases and deaths in the United States have declined steadily since reporting began in the nineteenth century. Data for 1974 showed approximately 14.3 new cases and 1.8 deaths per 100,000 population. Since 1975, tuberculosis cases reported to the Center for Disease Control have been defined as persons who have one or both of the following characteristics: (1) positive bacteriology; (2) treatment with two or more antituberculosis drugs. Included are persons who had disease at some time in the past and who have disease again with one or both of these characteristics. This change in reporting practice was approved by the Association of State and Territorial Health Officers. These rates are 46 per cent and 58 per cent lower than the corresponding rates of 1964. The rate of infection, judged by the prevalence of positive tuberculin skin tests, has also declined, particularly for susceptible groups, such as young children.

The incidence of tuberculosis cases varies broadly among different segments of the population and in different localities. For example, the failure of the tuberculosis case rate to decline rapidly in Massachusetts is attributable to (1) an influx of high-risk population into the state, (2) high unemployment rates and continuing decline in the standards of inner-city housing, and (3) the ever-present problem of alcoholism and other forms of self-abuse.[6] Cases occur twice as frequently in males as in females. Rates increase sharply with age in both sexes and in all races. More than 80 per cent of reported new cases are in persons over 25 years of age, most of whom were infected in the past. Reported cases are generally typical post-primary pulmonary disease. The risk of infection is greatest for those who have repeated exposure to persons with unrecognized or untreated sputum-positive pulmonary tuberculosis. Chemotherapy rapidly reduces the infectiousness of cases. Efforts to control tuberculosis in the United States are directed toward the early identification and treatment of cases and preventive therapy with isoniazid for infected persons at high risk of developing active disease. Here BCG (the Bacillus of Calmette and Guérin) has been used mainly for selected groups of persons who live or work where they have an unavoidable risk of exposure to tuberculosis.

BCG Vaccines

The Bacillus of Calmette and Guérin (BCG) was derived from a strain of *Mycobacterium bovis* attenuated through years of serial passage in culture by Calmette and Guérin at the Pasteur Institute, Lille, France. It was first administered to humans in 1921. Thorough application of modern methods of case detection, chemotherapy and preventive treatment can be highly successful in controlling tuberculosis. One of the objections to the use of BCG is that the value of the tuberculin test would be lost. Nevertheless, an effective BCG vaccine may be useful under certain circumstances. In particular, BCG may benefit uninfected persons with repeated exposure to infective cases who cannot or will not obtain or accept treatment.

Specific Recommendations

1. BCG vaccination should be seriously considered for persons who are tuberculin skin-test negative and who have repeated exposure to persistently untreated or ineffectively treated sputum-positive pulmonary tuberculosis.

2. BCG vaccination should be considered for well-defined communities or groups of an excessive rate if new infections can be demonstrated and the usual surveillance and

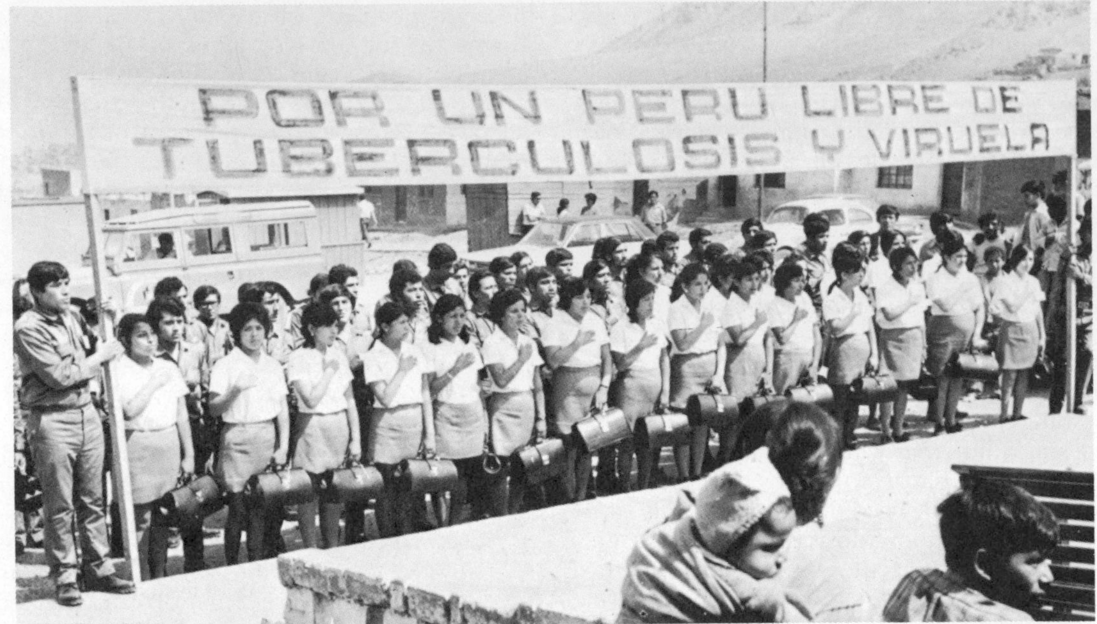

Figure 8–10 Many countries have combined the smallpox eradication program with BCG vaccination activities to combat tuberculosis. Shown here is a group of vaccinators of the combined program in Peru. (From Disease control and evaluation. Gazette, Pan American Health Organization, 6(3):6, July–September, 1974.)

treatment programs have failed or have been shown not to be applicable. Such groups might exist among the socially disaffiliated and those without a regular source of health care, possibly including some alcoholics, drug addicts, and migrants. Groups such as health workers who may be at particular risk of exposure to unrecognized pulmonary tuberculosis should, where possible, be kept under surveillance for evidence of newly acquired tuberculous infection. It must be recognized that only the occurrence of new infections reflects whether transmission is actually occurring.[7]

Attempts to use BCG vaccine in immunotherapy are continuing, and results in treating stage II melanoma (regional lymph node metastases) are encouraging.

TB Screening

Modern tuberculosis screening programs attempt to identify people who may have the active disease and therefore need treatment. Certain target groups found to have a high incidence are regularly screened. Screening also attempts to identify those who have tuberculous infection without active disease. These are the people who need chemoprophylaxis; chest x-rays alone are not now recommended as a mass screening procedure for detecting chronic, non-infectious lung disease. When there is no reason to suspect that the tuberculous infection rate is high, a tuberculin test screens out those with negative reactions.

The tuberculin skin test is one measure of the biological variability between persons who have been infected with Mycobacterium tuberculosis and those who have not. Any other causes of variability interfere with the accuracy of the test and are therefore undesirable. Unfortunately, many such variables do exist, usually resulting in false-negative readings.

Preventive Therapy

Antimicrobial drugs, which have revolutionized the therapy of tuberculosis, can also be used to prevent disease in the infected individual. Preventive therapy (chemoprophylaxis) presumably acts by diminishing the bacterial population in "healed" or roentgenographically invisible lesions of the person taking the drug. It is, in reality, treatment of infection and can prevent progressive tuberculosis from developing. A substantial and growing body of scientific data testifies to the value of isoniazid (INH) in prevention of the disease tuberculosis. The extensive trials conducted by the United States Public Health Service show a consistent reduction of morbidity in treated groups; it seems reasonable to expect that preventive therapy can substantially reduce future morbidity from tuberculosis in high-risk groups.

Every person who shows a positive tuberculin skin test is at some risk of developing tuberculous disease and can benefit from preventive therapy. Since the risk of developing disease is lifelong, the benefit from preventive therapy is greater the younger the age and the longer the life expectancy. The risk of contracting hepatitis, the most serious complication of INH therapy, increases with age. The risk of hepatitis is exceedingly low in the under-20 age group and reaches a peak among persons over 50. Priorities must be set for preventive therapy, taking into consideration not only the risk of developing tuberculosis compared with the risk of INH toxicity but also the ease of identifying and supervising persons for whom preventive therapy is indicated, and their likelihood of infecting others.

The following groups are listed in order of priority:

1. Household members and other close associates of persons with recently diagnosed tuberculous disease.

2. Positive tuberculin skin test reactors with findings on the chest roentgenogram consistent with nonprogressive tuberculous disease, in whom there are neither positive bacteriologic findings nor a history of adequate chemotherapy.

3. Newly infected persons.

4. Positive tuberculin skin test reactors in special clinical situations.

5. Other positive tuberculin skin test reactors. The risk of tuberculosis is highest in infancy, high again in adolescence and early adult life, and continues at a lower rate for a lifetime.[8]

Patient Follow-up

Because modern drugs can cure rather than merely arrest tuberculosis, federal and other medical experts are recommending abandonment of traditional lifetime follow-up for those ex-tuberculosis patients who successfully complete their drug therapy. For patients, the new recommendations mean they will no longer need to check periodically with the physicians to make certain their disease has not reactivated. For physicians, discontinuing lifetime follow-up means releasing medical personnel and clinic funds to provide better care for the 30,000 Americans discovered with new active tuberculosis each year and for other needed tuberculosis services. In February, 1974, the Center for Disease Control (CDC) Public Health Service recommended discharging from medical care tuberculosis patients who complete adequate drug therapy. The CDC recommendation comes at the end of the 20-year steady decline in the tuberculosis case rate. Health departments have been finding it difficult to obtain funds for tuberculosis control in the face of increasing competition from other medical problems.

Recommendations for Health Department Supervision of Tuberculosis Patients

The following statement has been developed as the official position of the Center for Disease Control, based on the recommendations of the Tuberculosis Advisory Committee.

Tuberculosis patients who complete adequate chemotherapy should be considered cured. The have no need for routine lifetime periodic recall for x-ray or examination. Indeed, perpetuating lifetime follow-up of such treated patients diverts clinic personnel and resources from the crucial task of providing services for those who really need them. Highest priority should be given to prompt and thorough treatment for newly diagnosed patients with tuberculosis. Medical supervision is most important during the early months of outpatient chemotherapy, whether treatment begins at home or with a brief period of hospitalization. Patients known to have had tuberculosis without chemotherapy, who are still being followed, should receive preventive treatment. Contacts of patients with newly diagnosed tuberculosis and other high-risk infected persons should be sought and should receive preventive treatment.

Persons who have responded well to treatment and have completed the recommended course of therapy should be told to expect their recovery to be permanent. The diagnosis of treated tuberculosis becomes part of their medical history. These persons should be discharged with instructions not to return unless they develop symptoms that could be caused by tuberculosis, such as a cough of longer than two weeks' duration, significant weight loss, persistent fever, or prolonged respiratory infection. Persons who have completed preventive therapy should also be discharged with similar instructions to return if they develop symptoms.

If a patient has not responded well to drugs or has had an irregular course of treatment, efforts should be made to complete adequate therapy. Special treatment programs, such as directly administered ambulatory therapy, should be considered for such patients. Continuing periodic chest roentgenograms and bacteriologic examinations should be considered only for persons in whom all attempts at therapy have failed. If such persons are in occupations where infectiousness may have serious consequences (such as some school and hospital personnel) they should be examined more than once a year or, if feasible, transferred to areas where there are minimal consequences to contacts if the person becomes infectious.[9]

Case Report: Outbreak of Tuberculosis in South Carolina

In January 1969, far-advanced active tuberculosis with cavitation was diagnosed in a 34-year-old man in Charleston County, South Carolina. Fourteen weeks earlier, he had seen his private physician because of "pain in abdomen" and because he was "unable to work" and "unable to keep down food." He was started on antacid therapy. The patient returned to work, but in January his employer requested assistance for him from the local health department. The public health nurse saw him and noted weight loss, constant coughing with heavy expectoration, and fever; he was hospitalized, and tuberculosis was bacteriologically confirmed by a positive sputum culture.

Because he worked in a closed area in a tire and battery shop and lived in a crowded, heavily populated poor community on James Island, his household, work, and community contacts were tuberculin tested in January. Of the 147 persons who were tuberculin tested, 58 had reactions of 10 mm. or more duration (positive), 86 had reactions of 0 to 9 mm. induration (negative and doubtful), and 3 tests were not read. Following X-ray of the 147 contacts, 6 active cases and 2 inactive cases were diagnosed; all 8 had positive tuberculin tests. Two patients with active tuberculosis were hospitalized, and the other 4 were placed on triple chemotherapy and are being followed on an outpatient basis. The 2 with inactive tuberculosis as well as the other 50 positive reactors were placed on isoniazid.

In August 1969, follow-up tuberculin tests on 77 of the 86 persons with negative reactions in January showed that 4 persons had converted. Two were placed on isoniazid. The other 2 had not been x-rayed as of December, 1969. No additional cases were found.*

*Report in Morbidity and Mortality (U.S. Dept. of Health, Education and Welfare).

Bovine Tuberculosis

The gentle dairy cow was once the cause of the severely crippling bone and gland disease called bovine tuberculosis. The scrofula—great masses of neck glands—and the hunched backs from infected vertebrae were but a few manifestations of this common zoonosis transmitted by raw milk. Fortunately, such is not the case today. Regular testing of cattle for tuberculosis and removal of infected animals from the herd is now required by law.

Case Report

On February 9, 1974, a cow culled from a milking herd and sent to slaughter in Detroit, Michigan, was diagnosed by a meat inspector as having generalized bovine tuberculosis. The herd of origin of this cow was then tested by veterinarians from the Michigan Department of Agriculture; 181 of 182 animals had positive reactions. The only nonreactor was a newborn calf. Eighty-seven milking cows were in the herd, and 34 of them were found to have generalized disease on slaughter in mid-March; the remainder either had localized disease or no gross lesions. Several of the 34 had extensively infected supramammary lymph nodes, indicating the strong possibility that they were excreting tubercule bacilli in their milk. One of the 87 milking cows, obviously ill when loaded on the truck at the farm for slaughter, was dead when the truck arrived at the slaughterhouse and was found to have generalized tuberculosis. Specimens from the cattle are being cultured in the Michigan Department of Agriculture laboratory and at Michigan State University.

Seven family members live on the farm: the father and his wife, their son and his wife, and the son's three children (all under 5 years of age). The father and son run the farm, and all seven drink unpasteurized (raw) milk from the herd. Chest x-rays on all seven family members were normal; Mantoux skin tests revealed one positive reactor—the son—who had a 30 mm. induration. All seven members have been placed on antituberculosis therapy.

This is the largest single herd outbreak of bovine tuberculosis recorded by the Michigan Department of Agriculture. The epizootiologic aspects of this outbreak are under investigation at this time. (Reported by John Quinn, D.V.M., Michigan Department of Agriculture; Norm Keon, Tuberculosis Program, and Donald B. Coohon, D.V.M., M.P.H., Chief, Division of Disease Control, Michigan Department of Public Health; and R. M. Scott, D.V.M., United States Department of Agriculture, Lansing.)

Editorial Note

Infection with either Mycobacterium tuberculosis or Mycobacterium bovis can be transmitted from man to cattle or cattle to man. In the past, contaminated raw milk was not an unusual vehicle of transmission of tuberculosis to man by the gastrointestinal route. Tuberculin testing of cattle and slaughter of reactors, as well as pasteurization of milk, have reduced the transmission of tuberculosis from cattle to man in the United States to minimal levels. However, as indicated by this outbreak, bovine tuberculosis may still present an occasional health hazard, especially in persons who live on farms and who drink unpasteurized milk. This outbreak also emphasizes the need for postmortem examination of cattle for gross evidence of infection with tuberculosis.[10]

Typhoid Fever

Communicable diseases are divided into nine or more classes and one of these includes diseases of gastrointestinal origin, closely associated with poor sanitation. These include the enteric diseases, of which typhoid, the dysenteries, and bacterial food poisoning are examples. Here community and individual sanitation constitute the important bulwark against infection. Protection of water and milk supplies and proper sanitation of public eating places are essential. Vaccination is of value in the case of typhoid fever, but a need for its widespread use may be evidence of failure in the task of environmental sanitation. Epidemiologic investigation of all cases and outbreaks is important, and typhoid fever offers one of the few examples of a disease in which the control of chronic carriers is essential.

The role of the carrier in the spread of typhoid fever has long been known. After Sopher's discovery in New York City in 1907 of the first and probably best known carrier—"Typhoid Mary"—health authorities were alerted to search for these individuals. In California in 1912, Sawyer identified the second known carrier in the United States. Since that time, records of carriers have been collected and maintained in the files of all Departments of Public Health. With the decline in the number of cases traced to water and milk and the general improvement in community sanitation, the individual typhoid carrier has assumed an increasingly important place in the control of this disease.

There are still approximately 800 cases of typhoid fever in the United States each year. Most of the current cases occur in groups within a single family after grandma (who is a typhoid carrier) has moved in to help care for the younger generation. Although acute cases can be cured with chloramphenicol, most elderly women refuse treatment (the drug may have serious side effects). Letters of agreement from typhoid carriers emphasize food handling precautions (Figs. 8–12 and 8–13).

Typhoid Fever in Texas

An outbreak of 6 cases of typhoid fever due to *Salmonella typhi,* Phage type E, was traced to well water apparently contaminated by a carrier. The 6 patients were among 20 relatives who had attended a family gathering near Raywood, Texas, for a few hours on July 4. Fifteen to 17 days later, 3 of the children, 2 of the women, and 1 of the men attending this gathering became ill with symptoms suggestive of typhoid fever. Two of the patients lived in Louisiana, 2 in Houston, Texas, and 2 in Raywood, Texas. The Houston patients were confirmed by blood and stool cultures, which demonstrated *S. typhi,* Phage type E. The remaining four cases were clinically consistent with the diagnosis of typhoid fever.

Although no food had been consumed at the reunion, it was learned that the women and chil-

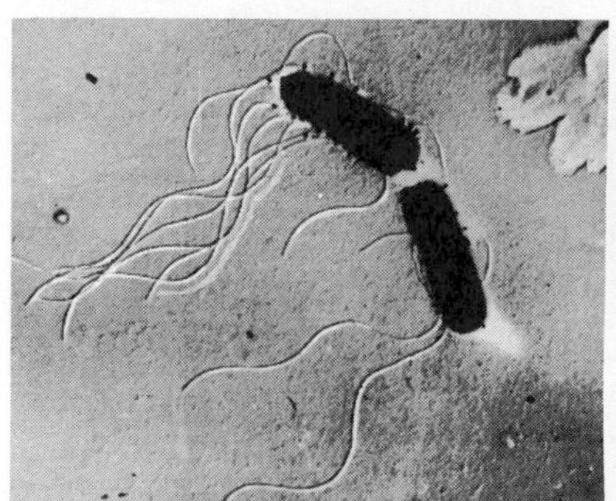

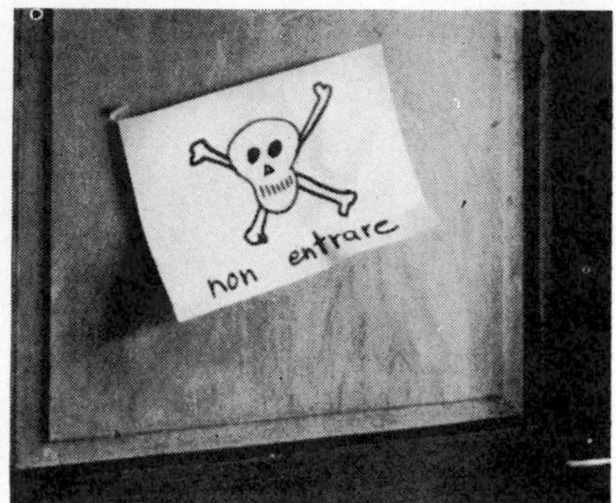

Figure 8–11 *A,* Typhoid bacteria, magnified 10,000 times. *B,* Infected hotel rooms are sealed. (From McCarry, C.: Typhoid. Saturday Evening Post, May 25, 1963.)

TYPHOID CARRIER AGREEMENT

Address ____________________

Date ____________________

Giles S. Porter, M.D., Director
State Department of Public Health
Sacramento, California

My dear Doctor Porter:

I have been informed that my excreta contain typhoid bacilli and that unless unusual precautions are taken persons will contract typhoid fever from me. Realizing this danger, I hereby agree to observe the precautions stated below, that I may be permitted to remain in free communication with other persons.

1. I shall take no part in the preparation or handling of milk or other food which will be consumed by other persons than my own immediate family. I shall not participate in the management of a dairy or other milk distributing plant, boarding house, restaurant, food store or in any occupation involving the preparation or handling of food.

2. I shall inform the local health officer of any contemplated change of residence so that he can notify the State Department of Public Health and obtain their approval.

3. I shall submit specimens for examination when requested by the State Department of Public Health or its authorized agent.

Respectfully,

____

Signature

Figure 8–12 A typhoid carrier letter of agreement. (From Beck, M. D., Hollister, A. C., et al.: *Typhoid Fever Cases and Carriers, an Analysis of the Records of the California State Department of Public Health from 1910 through 1959.* California State Department of Public Health, 1962.)

dren had drunk water from a private well. Only one man consumed water, and he contracted typhoid fever. The well was 16 ft. in depth, with a 1½ inch pipe imbedded in sand. The surrounding hole was much larger than the pipe, thus easily allowing surface drainage to enter. Investigation of the suspected premises revealed human feces strewn in the yard from slop jars used during the night, and feces deposited behind trees and out-buildings. Although an outside toilet was available, it apparently was rarely used. Of fecal specimens obtained from occupants of the house, *S. typhi,* Phage type E, was isolated from an asymptomatic male member of the family. Cultures of the well water revealed *S. typhi* E. Texas health officials concluded that the male host, an unsuspected typhoid carrier who had never been known to have had the disease, had probably contaminated the well water.*

The Zermatt Typhoid Incident

One of the most dramatic serious epidemics to occur in the world in many years occurred in the little Alpine ski resort of Zermatt, Switzerland, in March 1963. At least 350 confirmed or suspected cases of typhoid were traced to Zermatt visitors from Switzerland and eight foreign countries. Deaths included three local citizens and a British tourist. Public health officials discovered that a barmaid in one of Zermatt's largest hotels was a typhoid carrier. Carriers or active cases were found in every bakery in town; in one bakery all four bakers and the cook were infected. Public health officials recalled that Zermatt's drinking water had not been chlorinated for a 24 hour period between March 8 and March 10, 1963, and a pipe carrying drinking water had broken at a point near an open sewer. In addition, the River Visp, which runs through the heart of the village, was saturated with untreated sewage and garbage. Many persons believe the unnecessary delay in investigation was linked with "the intentional suppression of news about the presence of a contagious disease for reasons of financial gain."[11]

Epidemiologic Notes and Reports: Outbreak of Typhoid Fever in Connecticut and Massachusetts

Four cases of typhoid fever have been traced to a grinder (submarine, hero, poor boy) sandwich shop in Hartford, Connecticut.

*Report in Morbidity and Mortality (U.S. Dept. of Health, Education and Welfare).

OFFICE OF THE DIRECTOR

STATE OF CALIFORNIA
Department of Public Health
2151 BERKELEY WAY
BERKELEY 4, CALIFORNIA

Malcolm H. Merrill, M.D., Director
State Department of Public Health
Berkeley, California

TYPHOID CARRIER AGREEMENT

My dear Doctor Merrill:

I have been informed that my excreta contain typhoid bacilli and that unless unusual precautions are taken, persons will contract typhoid fever from me. Realizing this danger, I hereby agree to observe the precautions stated below, that I may be permitted to remain in free communication with other persons.

1. I shall take no part in the preparation, serving or handling of milk or other food which may be consumed by any person other than members of my own immediate family.
   I shall not engage in any occupation which brings me in contact with milk, milk products, milk bottles or milk utensils.
   I shall not participate in the management of a dairy or other milk distributing plant, boarding house, restaurant, food store or any place where food is prepared or served or in any occupation involving the preparation or handling of food.
   I shall encourage the members of my family to be immunized against typhoid fever.
2. I shall wash my hands thoroughly with soap and hot water after using the toilet and before handling food for my immediate family.
   If modern flush toilets are not available, I shall dispose of my excreta according to the instructions given me by the local health officer to prevent access of flies and/or contamination of drinking water.
3. I shall report to the local health officer immediately any case of illness suggestive of typhoid in my family or associates.
4. I shall inform the local health officer of any contemplated change of address or occupation so that he can notify the State Department of Public Health.
5. I shall notify the health officer or have the hospital notify the health officer when hospitalization is required for any personal illness.
6. I shall communicate with the local health officer before submitting to any type of treatment intended for the cure of my carrier condition.

I have been informed that the local health officer and the California State Department of Public Health will keep the information confidential that I am a carrier unless I violate this agreement in some way and action for protection of the public becomes necessary.

Witnesses:
(1) ______________________ ______________________ Signature of Carrier

(2) ______________________ ______________________ Address

______________________ (date)

Figure 8–13 A typhoid carrier letter of agreement. (From Beck, M. D., Hollister, A. C., et al.: *Typhoid Fever Cases and Carriers, an Analysis of the Records of the California State Department of Public Health from 1910 through 1959.* California State Department of Public Health, 1962.)

The first case was identified on August 8 following isolation of *Salmonella typhi* from a stool specimen of a 22-year-old woman in Hartford; she had become ill with fever and headache on July 11 and subsequently developed diarrhea. On August 25, in Springfield, Massachusetts, 2 other cases in siblings, ages 10 and 9 years, who had become ill on July 11 and 18, respectively, were identified. These children had visited their aunt in Wilson, Connecticut, a Hartford suburb, on June 27 and 29. The fourth case was in a 24-year-old man who regularly ate at the shop and who became ill in October.

When the first 3 cases were found to be due to *S. typhi,* phage type F–1 (a relatively uncommon type in New England), an investigation was begun. It was learned that the three patients had eaten in several of the same eating establishments in the Hartford area. Stool specimens were obtained from all employees of these restaurants; *S. typhi* phage type F–1 was isolated from three specimens of a 50-year-old cook working at a grinder shop near Hartford. She had come to the United States from Lebanon 12 years ago and had begun working in the shop in March 1969. She gave a history of a febrile illness of 1 month's duration requiring hospitalization 19 years ago in Lebanon. Her 21-year-old son, who helped make the grinders, was found to have *S. typhi* phage type F–1 in a second specimen. He gave no history of recent illness and no past history of typhoid fever, and a third specimen from him

American Victims

"We had been to Zermatt before and loved it," says Mrs. Walter Braun, wife of a shoe manufacturer in Beverly Hills, California. "But when we started to get sick I went to our concierge and looked him in the eye and said, 'We've heard something is going around called the Zermatt fever.' He said, 'I don't know what you're talking about.'

"A week after we came home I started to feel punk. I took my temperature—I had 102 to 105, up and down every five hours. It's a very disagreeable sickness. It's like someone taking a baseball bat and beating you all over, and when you wake up you can hardly move."

What Betty Braun had was not Zermatt fever but typhoid. Like Mrs. Braun, most of the 11 American victims did not know what was wrong until they returned home.

"One of the doctors in Zermatt," says Mrs. Braun, "told a friend of ours: 'You don't have Zermatt fever. Your temperature isn't high enough. Besides, only women and children get it.'" Another American tourist reports that when his daughter began suffering from an upset stomach, "the hotel said there were two doctors there for setting bones—but for stomach sickness, drink tea."

Typhoid is not as lethal as it used to be, but it's not much fun. "I had a very high temperature, and my lungs were filling up, so they put me on antibiotics for four or five days," says one victim, a 47-year-old construction executive. "Then I had to be taken off the antibiotics so they could make tests. Then they put me in the hospital when my temperature went up again, more antibiotics, then out two weeks, then you're down again."

After all this, the victims also suffered large medical bills. "It cost us roughly $2,000," Mrs. Braun estimates. "The medical bill was more than my whole trip for my wife and myself," says another victim. And there are other difficulties. Anyone found to have typhoid must keep in touch with the local health department for six months.

"My Lord, people treat you like a leper," complains an airline stewardess from Santa Monica, California. "I've had to move out of my apartment because my two roommates have to go on flying. I'm at a friend's home. I'm just not permitted to touch food. It's a demoralizing thing."

Hospitalized and helpless, the Zermatt victims are also hopping mad. "I think it's criminal," says the stewardess. "I'm damn mad," declares another victim. "I think they pulled a dirty trick."

—Roger Vaughan

Figure 8–14 (From McCarry, C.: Typhoid. Saturday Evening Post, May 25, 1963.)

shortly after the second was negative. Both the mother and son were placed on long-term ampicillin therapy and were not to work at the shop until follow-up stool cultures were negative.

*Medical Milestone: Mary Mallon, "Typhoid Mary"**

Typhoid Mary has made her final appearance in the nation's news. Her death this month at the age of 70 brought to an end a much-publicized period of nearly 30 years' isolation in a New York City institution. Although she may appear no more in the news, Mary Mallon will live forever in medical annals.

Engineer-Detective

Mary owed her fame to a sanitary engineer, George A. Soper. Studying several outbreaks of typhoid fever in suburban New York homes in the early 1900's, Soper found the water and food supplies to be beyond suspicion. As an engineer, he might well have concluded his investigation at this point. But in his search for factors that might be common to typhoid-stricken house-holds, Soper looked beyond the end of his nose and found that one Mary Mallon had served as a cook in many of the afflicted homes and that the disease always followed but never preceded her engagement. Bacteriological examination of her feces showed Mary Mallon to be a chronic typhoid carrier. Interestingly enough, Mary seems to have sensed this before anyone else because when typhoid appeared in the family she served, although she had no M.D. or D.P.H. degree, she

*Reprinted with permission from the November 1968 issue of *HEALTH NEWS*, a copyrighted monthly publication of the State of New York Department of Health.

thought it best to leave at once, without giving a forwarding address.

Typhoid Mary strikingly illustrated the importance of the chronic carrier in causing typhoid fever. She was largely responsible for the important public health procedure of making thorough search for a carrier among those who have been in intimate association with, or who have prepared food for, the typhoid patient. Like 20 per cent of all typhoid carriers, Mary never suffered from any illness recognized as typhoid fever. Her case demonstrated the fact that a considerable number of carriers might be overlooked if a search for carriers were confined to those persons giving a history of previous typhoid fever.

From 1907 to 1910, while incarcerated by health officials, Mary sought release by legal means. The New York Supreme Court upheld the community's right to keep her in isolation. In recent years it has not been necessary to confine a typhoid carrier, modern control methods being based on frequent supervision of the carrier in his home. However, the established right of the community to require isolation has been applied to other chronic contagious diseases, notably in cases of careless or dangerous tuberculosis patients.

Back in the Kitchen

Perhaps because of popular sentiment in her favor, Mary was released from confinement in 1910. She promptly disappeared. In the next couple of years typhoid fever occurred in a New Jersey and a New York hospital, affecting more than 200 people. Typhoid Mary had returned to her old occupation of cook and had worked at both hospitals under an assumed name. This experience taught health officials that a typhoid carrier must always be kept under close supervision and never be permitted to handle food or drink intended for public consumption.

Chronic Carriers

Since 1911 typhoid carriers have been legally declared to be such, and out of the experience with Typhoid Mary have grown the regulations forbidding carriers to care for children or to handle food, milk and dairy products for other than members of the immediate family. Health officers visit upstate New York's 419 typhoid carriers at least once in every three months to insure enforcement of such regulations. Of course, family members are endangered by the presence of the carrier in the home, typhoid being forty-two times as prevalent in such homes as in the general population. Considerable hope is offered the families of typhoid carriers by knowledge that typhoid vaccination will reduce risk by 80 per cent.

Former cooks and milk handlers are very common on the roster of typhoid carriers maintained by the State Department of Health. This is only natural since nearly three-quarters of the carriers were discovered by investigation which centered about those who handled milk or food consumed by the typhoid fever patient. Nearly all of the remaining carriers were added to the list by routine examination of "release specimens" from all recovered cases of typhoid. About one out of forty typhoid patients becomes a chronic carrier and probably remains such for the rest of his life unless special curative means are employed. The law considers the typhoid fever patient guilty until he is proved innocent. That is, after recovery he must obey typhoid carrier regulations until, if he is among the thirty-nine out of forty who clear up spontaneously, bacteriological examination shows he is not a carrier. This requirement has been in effect in upstate New York only since November 1929. As time goes on, and all cases are required to submit specimens for release, there will be few unknown typhoid carriers in the population free to engage as cooks or dairymen; they will be only the few who, like Typhoid Mary, develop into carriers through becoming infected with the germs of typhoid fever without becoming ill or at least without developing an illness recognized as typhoid fever.

Forbidden Occupations

To be found to be a typhoid carrier means little or no inconvenience or financial sacrifice to the clerk or factory worker, but to the cook it may mean a loss of job and livelihood, and to the dairyman a substantial loss of income. No doubt Typhoid Mary sought work as a cook under an assumed name in 1910 because she needed a livelihood and cooking was the only occupation she knew. The State Legislature recognizes that considerable loss of income may tempt a typhoid carrier surreptitiously to engage in forbidden occupations, and, to remove such temptation, annually appropriates money to compensate carriers who were formerly food or milk handlers and who are unable to make a living at the new occupations they must seek.

The later years of Typhoid Mary's isolation were largely voluntary. If she wished she might have availed herself, as many other carriers have, of the knowledge that there is at least a 60 per cent chance that a carrier may be cured by removal of the gall bladder. The state extends financial aid to those carriers who wish to have the operation but are unable to pay for it themselves.*

Some years ago when it was learned that there were many other carriers like Typhoid Mary unrecognized in the population, many people thought that every food and milk handler should be examined to learn if the individual were a typhoid carrier. There are many food handlers but few typhoid carriers in the general population, with the result that many thousands

---

*The intent of this legislation was to assist carriers until they were trained in a non-restricted occupation. This effort was, for the most part, a failure—funds became just a "hand-out" and the Legislature discontinued the appropriation.

of people were examined needlessly and very few carriers were found. The cost was tremendous, often as high as $100,000 for the detection of a single carrier. This expensive, outmoded practice is still being carried on in a number of cities. A much smaller amount, spent for the services of a trained epidemiologist, will accomplish a great deal more. The requirement of reliable release specimens from all recovered typhoid fever patients with prompt reporting of cases by physicians and prompt investigation by the health officer or epidemiologist will detect many times the number of carriers that will be found by routine examination of all food and milk handlers, and at a much lower cost. The city that wishes to be free of typhoid should employ an epidemiologist, not a costly and grossly inefficient dragnet.

Requiem

Rest in peace, Typhoid Mary Mallon. Yours was the ill fortune to bring illness directly to hundreds. Yet because of the drama of your life, your compulsory and self-imposed confinement—features that attracted and focused the glare of publicity on the role of typhoid carriers in the occurrence of disease—you have been the agent for formulation of public health procedures which have and will continue to prevent many times the number of typhoid cases that you caused.

Undulant Fever (Brucellosis; Malta Fever; Bang's Disease)

At the same time as tuberculosis testing, cattle are examined for any evidence of Bang's disease, or brucellosis, also called undulant fever, Malta fever, or Mediterranean fever when infecting man. Human outbreaks of this disease occur when precautionary measures are neglected. Pasteurization is one such precaution. *Brucella abortus,* the germ which causes the disease in cattle, and *Brucella militensis,* the goat strain, are killed in the process of pasteurization. Transmitted to man primarily by unpasteurized milk from infected cows and goats, the disease has stricken whole farm families. The symptoms begin from 7 to 21 days after exposure, with chills, fever rising to perhaps 104° F., drenching sweats, severe headaches, and aching muscles and joints. The disease is called undulant fever because the fever is remittent or undulating, coming and going in waves. Early treatment may prevent the acute stage wherein the liver and spleen enlarge and other complications develop.

Undulant fever is not known to pass from person to person. However, one does not have to ingest milk from infected animals to contract it. Veterinarians, dairymen, butchers, and others who come into direct contact with the placentas of aborted cows or infected pigs may also contract the disease. Peculiarly, infants seldom are affected with undulant fever, even though all of their nourishment comes from milk. One or more of the antibiotics usually is effective in curing man of the disease. The campaign to stamp out brucellosis in cattle has been so successful that the disease may disappear entirely within a decade, the United States Public Health Service predicts. The same cannot be said of a brucellosis-like disease in swine which is presently on the rise. The infection is spread to man, specifically veterinarians, farmers, and butchers who come into close contact with the flesh of infected pigs. Currently, preventive measures call for the immunization of swine, particularly in areas where the disease has been found.

Venereal Diseases

For many years syphilis has been accepted as a public health responsibility, and its management has been concentrated to a greater extent than that of most diseases in public health clinics supported entirely or partially by public health funds. This can be explained by the fact that a large number of patients are in the lower socioeconomic groups and by the fact that the epidemiology of infectious syphilis is a public health responsibility. Under these circumstances, it is inevitable that control of the disease depends largely on the adequacy of public health programs and is best conducted by public health personnel. However, no program of disease control can be successful without the cooperation of the entire medical profession. The diagnosis and treatment of syphilis have never been confined to clinics; like other diseases, syphilis has always been a responsibility of general medicine.

Venereal diseases continue to head the list of reportable communicable diseases in most states. Gonorrhea leads them all.

One in 10 persons under 25 will have VD this year and this age group will have half of all reported VD cases. In all, five venereal diseases occur in the United States—gonorrhea, syphilis, chancroid, lymphogranuloma venereum, and granuloma inguinale. The last three, termed the minor venereal diseases, occur in such relatively small numbers that they do not pose a serious health problem. Gonorrhea accounts for the major rise in VD.

PREVENTION—THE KEY TO HALTING THE VD EPIDEMIC

It is high time we admit that our public health program to control venereal disease is a colossal failure; yet we persist in acting as if more of the same would solve the problem. The incidence of both infectious syphilis and gonorrhea has increased nationally almost continuously since the federally sponsored programs were initiated. Despite the knowledge that control of a communicable disease requires prevention, not just treatment, our national and statewide programs are almost entirely directed toward case finding and treatment of infected contacts. Both our syphilis epidemiologic program and our gonorrhea mass screening effort are intended to discover and treat the infected individual and generally ignore people not already exposed. Neither program directs any attention at all to the many other sexually transmitted infections.

The truth is that we have no preventive methods that can be applied on a community-wide basis to control venereal infections—no vaccines, no chemoprophylaxis proven suitable for mass or continued use, no public environmental controls. Successful prevention of VD today demands individual initiative and responsibility, and depends entirely on measures that each susceptible person must take for himself or herself. Yet in our limited public educational efforts we have tried not so much to tell the truth about venereal disease prevention as not to offend anybody, for education about sexually transmitted diseases has proven to be an emotionally charged topic. Some parents, educators, and even physicians have complained that to tell young people how to prevent VD is to promote sexual promiscuity and encourage youngsters to experiment sexually (though provision of services to prevent pregnancy has become mandatory). At times, indeed even in medical circles, we seem more intent on stamping out sin (extramarital sex) than disease (venereal infection). Trying to control disease by fear and failure to inform people on how to protect themselves is, I believe, immoral. Still, we loudly proclaim that VD education is not sex education, and we teach about symptoms, complications, and where to go for treatment, glossing over (or omitting) the fact that it is sexual behavior that determines exposure and prevention.

What needs to be done? First, we need to admit that treating cases will not ensure control of these communicable diseases, although finding infection and treating it is certainly necessary. Secondly, we need a massive campaign to improve our capability to prevent venereal infections—research on vaccines, on the use of antibiotics for prophylaxis, on the efficacy of local methods such as vaginal creams, tablets, or foams. Thirdly, we must initiate or expand preventive education, telling people that only by their own health behavior can sexually transmitted disease be controlled.[12]

Gonorrhea

The first record of gonorrhea is in the Old Testament, book of Leviticus (about 1500 B.C.), in which symptoms of the disease are described in detail. The Greek physician Hippocrates (400 B.C.) stated that gonorrhea resulted from "excessive indulgence in the pleasure of Venus," the goddess of love. Another ancient Greek physician, Galen (A.D. 220), mistakenly believed that gonorrhea was caused by an involuntary loss of male semen. Galen named the disease from the Greek words *gonos* (seed) and *rhoia* (a flow). Eventually, the true nature of the transfer of gonorrhea from person to person was understood. In the year 1161, brothels in London were forbidden by law to house prostitutes "suffering from the perilous infirmity of burning" (the burning pain felt on urination by most men and women with gonorrhea).[13]

Today, the large numbers of syphilis and gonorrhea cases are not the only concern. Gonococcal resistance to penicillin and other antibiotics is increasing; more men with asymptomatic gonorrhea are being identified; gonococcal pharyngitis is mounting; once relatively rare complications from untreated gonorrhea are being seen more frequently; and the incidence of congenital syphilis is increasing. Systemic gonorrhea is becoming more common; both symptomatic and asymptomatic rectal gonorrhea are appearing; and some strains of gonorrhea are showing increased resistance to antibiotics.

Many social, economic, and cultural reasons are cited for the rapid rise in gonorrhea, such as changing values and lifestyles of society, increasing sociosexual activities, the use of the pill, increasing mobility in society, inadequate venereal disease education, increase in population, unawareness of symptoms, shame and embarrassment inhibiting visits to doctors or VD clinics and naming contacts, misunderstandings and misinformation, and inadequate diagnosis and treatment by physicians. Sociosexual activity has increased, particularly in the middle and upper classes where "Victorian" morality has gradually declined. With the acceptance of the equality of the sexes has come the recognition that women have sexual needs and sexual rights. The good girl–bad girl dichotomy has become less distinct; premarital petting and coitus have become more common. Other reaons for the increase of gonorrhea include the following:

1. The short incubation period, which fosters rapid spread.
2. Poor reporting by physicians.
3. The increase in cases is not matched with enough budget and manpower to interview the cases, locate contacts, and get them treated.
4. Failure of physicians to provide epidemiologic treatment to contacts.
5. Asymptomatic reservoirs with inadequate screening procedures to detect them. Most women and patients with rectal gonorrhea are unaware of infection.
6. There is no simple blood test for gonorrhea comparable to the VDRL test for syphilis.
7. Resistance of some strains of gonococci to penicillin and other antibiotics.
8. Lack of immunity to gonorrhea. One can be infected again and again, and no immunizing agent has yet been discovered.
9. Poor acceptance of mechanical prophylaxis (the use of condoms), washing with soap and water, and urination after intercourse.
10. Spotty and inadequate venereal disease education. As mentioned in number 5 above, there is a huge reservoir of women who have gonorrhea and do not know it. About 8 out of 10 females with gonorrhea have no symptoms. These females can unknowingly spread the disease to their sex partners and allow their own infection to develop into serious complications.

Cause: The Gonococcus

Although gonorrhea is one of the oldest diseases known to man, the causative agent was not identified until 1879, by the German bacteriologist Neisser. Scientifically named *Neisseria gonorrhoeae,* the bacteria are commonly called gonococci or "diplococci," because they usually appear in pairs. These bacteria penetrate mucous membrane surfaces lining the genitourinary and digestive tracts, where they find the conditions of warmth, moisture, and lack of oxygen under which they can survive. The gonococcus may also survive in the tissues around the eyes of newborns and in the immature vulvar tissues of prepubescent girls. While gonococci stain readily with most dyes, the Gramstain, which retards the growth of other organisms (overgrowth) and provides necessary nutrients, is the method of choice. An atmosphere of from 5 to 10 percent CO_2 and a temperature of 35° F. is required for the optimum growth of the gonococcus.

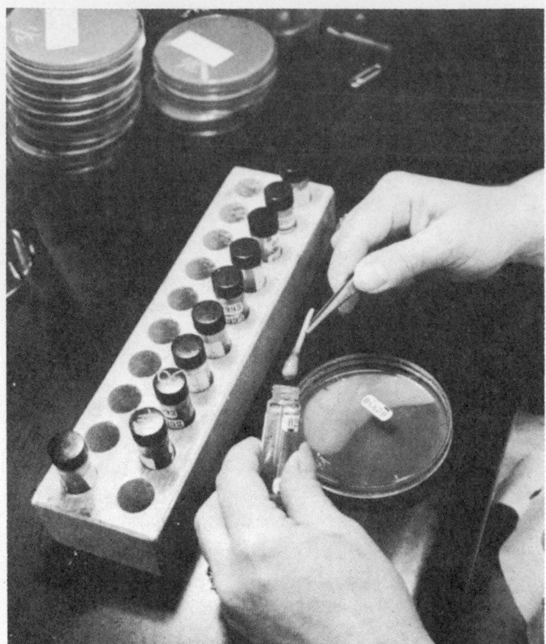

Figure 8–15 Taking a gonorrhea culture. (From Healthnews, April, 1975, p. 8. California Department of Health, Sacramento, Calif.)

Transmission

Gonorrhea is transmitted through sexual relations, including homosexual practices, and occasionally from an infected mother to the eyes of her newborn baby as the baby passes through the birth canal. Combined treatment with silver nitrate and penicillin has reduced the occurrence of the latter.

Symptoms

Because of differences in anatomical structure, men and women are affected by gonorrhea in quite different ways. In about 85 per cent of infected males, symptoms are noticed within seven days, most within two to four days. For symptomatic males, the disease begins with an inflammation of the urethral canal, causing a sharp, burning pain on urination. The white blood cells called to destroy the gonococci form a discharge from the penis. The discharge (exudate) is thick and purulent in the beginning and later becomes thin and watery. These symptoms usually subside after two or three weeks, when the infection may reach the prostate gland and the testicles, making them inflamed and tender. If involvement of the testicles is not treated, the passage of sperm is blocked and sterility results. Only 20 per cent of infected females are symptomatic and 80 per cent are asymptomatic, according to recent studies. This fact severely handicaps women who unknowingly allow the gonoccal infection to run rampant in their abdomens. For those fortunate few with symptoms, the disease may begin with a mild burning or smarting in the genital area, with or without slight discharge. Examination at this time may reveal a mild inflammation of the vagina and cervix. Usually after one or more menstrual periods, the infection ascends the reproductive tract. It may involve the fallopian tubes and ovaries, or spill into the abdomen, causing pelvic inflammatory disease (PID). At this time, pain and fever may be severe, or mild enough to be passed off as a stomach upset. Recent observations suggest that the infection may develop quickly, before a menstrual period has passed. Pelvic inflammatory disease has been found in 10 per cent of females with *N. gonorrhoeae* cultured from the cervical site. In addition, incidence of gonococcemia (pimple-like lesions on the extremities), once seldom seen, appears to be rising.

Infection subsides after a few weeks. It is followed by a chronic infection which may last for years and cause extensive damage to the reproductive tract. The most frequent serious damage is sterility. Tubal pregnancy sometimes occurs. Adhesions and fibroids may be secondary complications. Other complications which may occur, but are not frequent, include the inflammation of the joints and membranes surrounding the tendons (arthritis), spinal cord, and brain, and inflammation of the heart lining and valves.

Unfortunately, in the majority of cases, the symptoms of infections are slight or mild, arousing little or no concern. Consequently a doctor is not consulted, and gonorrhea in females usually goes undetected until the person is named as a contact. For this reason, venereal disease clinics in the area should be encouraged to interview infected males for their contacts. A study of 3600 male volunteer gonorrhea patients interviewed for sex contacts resulted in the identification of 1158 infected females, of whom 862 (74.4 per cent) were asymptomatic.[14]

Gonorrhea Screening

The most important tool available to us in identifying these asymptomatic females is routine gonorrhea screening. This has been demonstrated by several recent studies. In a study sponsored by the Public Health Service, involving 305,929 female tests obtained from a selected sample of clinic sites across the nation, venereal disease clinics had the highest positive rate—over 24 per cent. Although the number of positive results declined rather sharply after that, family planning clinics had a significant average yield of nearly 4 per cent positives. A large number of pelvic examinations are already being performed on females from high-risk groups in health department non-VD clinics, free clinics, OEO clinics, jails, migrant health clinics, and private medical clinics. But many of these examinations do not include cultures for gonorrhea. The objective of gonorrhea screening, therefore, is to encourage these facilities to include gonorrhea cultures as a routine part of all pelvic examinations they perform; thereby finding and treating many asymptomatic females who would otherwise have gone undetected.

Objectives

In order to achieve the long-term objective of reducing the prevalence of gonorrhea, the following gonorrhea screening objectives have been established by some state health departments:

1. The establishment of clinic sites statewide to do gonorrhea cultures as a routine part of pelvic examinations.

2. The culturing of females of childbearing age (15–44) throughout the state, with emphasis on serving women in high-risk categories (e.g., the educationally deprived, clients of agencies serving the poor and youth health care services).

3. The installation of a statewide gonorrhea surveillance network to control and evaluate the screening program, to rapidly disseminate vital

information, and to coordinate a cohesive statewide effort to control gonorrhea.

4. To keep physicians constantly updated about the latest techniques of diagnosing gonorrhea.

5. To alert the public—especially women—to the need to be tested for gonorrhea if they are sexually active.

Women today are taking greater responsibility for their own health. They should request a gonorrhea culture test as a part of their routine physical examinations. If there is any suspicion that they have had a sexual partner who has gonorrhea, they should go immediately to a physician or a health department venereal disease clinic and request a culture test for gonorrhea.

Legislation

In all but two states, 18-year-olds do not need parental consent to get most pregnancy-related health services, including abortion. And all 50 states allow anyone over 18 to be treated for venereal disease on their own. Most states are now extending medical rights to those under 18. In all states but Wisconsin, younger teenagers already have the right to get treatment for venereal disease without telling their parents. Some states are also making other medical services available to the under-18 group. In an attempt to meet the needs of its floating population of youngsters, many of them runaways, California enacted its "emancipated youth laws" in 1968. These statutes permit anyone over 12 to get venereal disease treatment and allow anyone over 15 who is living apart from his parents to get many types of treatment on his own. There seems to be growing, if reluctant, acceptance of the fact that in a changing society legal rights and measures relating to health treatment and services of youth are necessary. Sexual activities and sex-related activity among teenagers have increased enormously in recent years, and so have sex-related problems.

Syphilis

Syphilis is the most serious of the venereal diseases. It is caused by a spirochete called *Teponema pallidum,* which enters the body during sexual relations, reproduces at a rapid rate, and promptly invades every organ and body tissue through the blood stream and lymphatic system. There are three stages as the disease continues to spread: primary (first), secondary, and tertiary (third).

Primary Syphilis. Primary syphilis is the first stage of the disease. A sore or chancre (pronounced "shanker") usually appears in 8 to 30 days at the point where the spirochete entered the body (the cervix, the vagina, the area around the vagina, the penis, the mouth, the anus, or a break in the skin), where it frequently remains unnoticed because it is painless. Unfortunately, in women the sore may be located where it is very hard to see and can easily be missed. Enlarged lymph nodes may eventually draw attention to its presence. Diagnosis is made strictly on a laboratory basis, through examination by a special dark-field microscope of scrapings from the chancre, identifying the spirochete. Blood tests for syphilis usually become positive within four weeks after the sexual contact, but until then diagnosis can be made only by finding the causative spirochete. The chancre will disappear completely in a few weeks even without treatment, but this does not mean that the disease is cured.

Secondary Syphilis. Secondary syphilis typically develops two to six months following the sexual contact. There may or may not be accompanying signs. The most obvious sign of secondary syphilis is a rash which may appear all over the body, characteristically including the mouth, the genital organs, the buttocks, the palms, and the soles of the feet. Accompanying signs and symptoms are fever, aching, persistent sore throat, patchy loss of hair from the scalp and latter portion of the eyebrows, and widespread lymph gland enlargement. Secondary syphilis also disappears without treatment, giving the patient unjustified optimism, but again, this does not mean the disease is cured.

Latent Stage. The first two stages of early syphilis are highly infectious. They are followed by a "latent" period when the disease becomes noninfectious and is not transmitted to a sex partner. A positive blood test is the only means of diagnosis during this latent stage, because there is no evidence of the disease on physical examination and the patient has no symptoms. During the next four years (especially the first two) there can be periods when the disease is again highly infectious because the spirochete becomes active in the blood stream.

The spirochete may invade the central nervous system. A laboratory examination of the spinal fluid will detect this condition early, before damage starts. Early discovery of syphilis of the central nervous system and adequate treatment can prevent permanent damage to the brain and the spinal cord.

Tertiary Stage. After the fourth year, the disease enters the tertiary or third stage, which is noninfectious but very serious. The most serious and common complications of syphilis late in this third stage are those involving the heart and large blood vessels, the brain, and the spinal cord, any of which may be fatal. Insanity and blindness may also occur, and any organ of the body may be affected. Only very sophisticated laboratory tests can detect syphilis in this late stage.

Transmission to Unborn Child

Syphilis may be passed on from a mother to her unborn baby during any of these three stages, if her syphilis has been untreated or inadequately treated. At any time after the third month of pregnancy, any syphilis spirochete that still exists in the mother can be passed to the baby through the umbilical cord. Severe infection causes premature delivery, with a poor chance of survival for the baby. With less severe infection, the baby will not be premature but will be born with the disease—then called congenital syphilis.

The baby with congenital syphilis may develop a runny nose, enlarged liver and spleen, generalized enlargement of lymph nodes, anemia, jaundice, and nervous system changes. Because of the danger of transmitting syphilis to unborn babies, every pregnant woman should have a blood test for syphilis well before the third month of pregnancy. This blood test is always done as a part of prenatal care by the physician who takes care of the mother during her pregnancy.

Treatment

Penicillin is the best treatment for syphilis. Other antibiotics can be substituted for patients who are allergic to penicillin. The earlier therapy is instituted, the better the results. Early treatment cures syphilis. If treatment is begun later, the disease is cured, but the damage to vital organs will be permanent. Syphilis is a disease that involves the whole body. Everyone who contracts it should have lifetime follow-up physical and laboratory examinations, because early detection of the late signs and effects may halt the disease and be lifesaving. Patients with infectious syphilis should be sure that all their sexual contacts are notified, as they deserve and need immediate examination and treatment. Local public health departments are anxious to help the patient find all sources and contacts.

Venereal syphilis is a disease that has been created by the development of human society. It is clear that we cannot eliminate this disease by a simple attack on the orga-

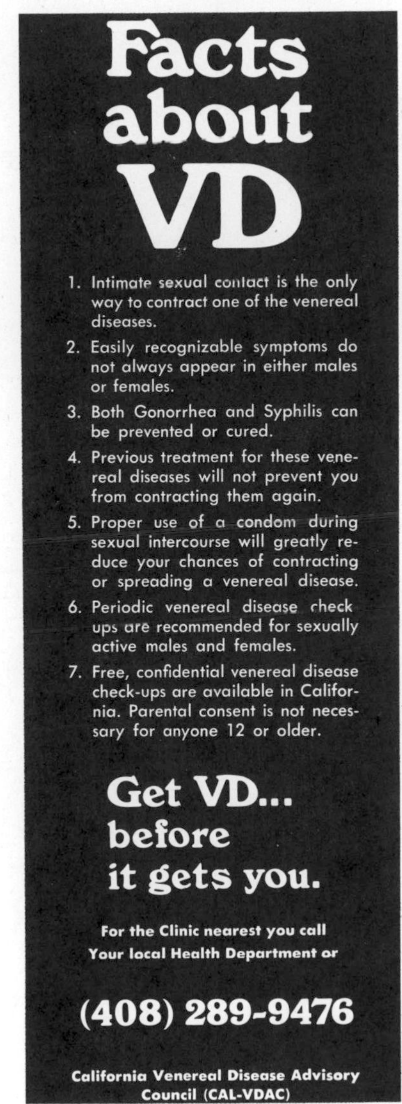

Figure 8–16 Facts about VD. (Courtesy of California Venereal Disease Advisory Council.)

	SYPHILIS	GONORRHEA	CHANCROID	LYMPHOGRANULOMA VENEREUM	GRANULOMA INGUINALE
Etiology	Treponema pallidum	Neisseria gonorrhoeae	Hemophilus ducreyi	LGV Virus	Donovania granulomatis
Incubation Period	7-90 Days (Usually 3 weeks)	2-14 days (Usually 3 days)	2-6 days	5-30 Days	Probably 8-90 days
Contact Examination (All sex contacts exposed within the following time periods)	Primary—3 months (Plus duration of symptoms) Secondary—6 months (Plus duration of symptoms) Early latent—1 year All Syphilis—Family contacts as indicated	2 weeks (Male) 1 month (Female)	1 month	2 months	3 months
Clinical Characteristics	Primary—Chancre Present Secondary—Rashes or Mucous Patches Latent—No symptoms, reactive serology Relapse—Recurrence of infectious lesions after disappearance of secondary lesions Late—Cardiovascular, central nervous system, gummata	Discharge Burning, pain Swelling of genitalia and glands	Pustular ulcer on genitalia or inguinal region Suppurative inguinal lesions	Vesicle on genitalia Enlarged inguinal lymph glands Fistula with pus	Eroded papule on genitalia Inguinal or perineal ulcers
Diagnostic Procedures	Darkfield Examination Serologic Tests for Syphilis Spinal Fluid Test X-Ray of longbones of infants Clinical and contact histories	Culture Smear Clinical and contact histories (Serologic test for syphilis)	Microscopic for Ducrey Bacillus Clinical and contact histories (Serologic test and darkfield examination for syphilis)	Frei skin test Serologic test for L.G.V. Clinical and contact histories (Serologic test and darkfield examination for syphilis)	Tissue scraping or biopsy Clinical and contact histories (Serologic test and darkfield examination for syphilis)
*Treatment	Penicillin Broad spectrum antibiotics	Penicillin Broad spectrum antibiotics	Broad spectrum antibiotics including streptomycin	Broad spectrum antibiotics	Broad spectrum antibiotics

* Write local or State Health Department for specific current recommendations on treatment and follow-up.

Figure 8–17 Chart of venereal diseases. (Courtesy of California Department of Public Health.)

nism. *Treponema pallidum* has managed to survive every previous attack for tens of thousands of years, including the development in this century of penicillin. The only way that we will be able to eliminate syphilis from our midst is to change those social conditions that permit it to exist.[15]

Other Sexually Transmitted Diseases

For an important discussion on other widespread venereal diseases, the reader is urged to refer to Sager, C. J. (Consultant): Sexual medicine today. *Medical Tribune,* February 4, 1976, p. 17.

Recommendations

1. Joint efforts by county and state medical services to keep physicians updated about diagnosis, treatment, and reporting techniques.
2. Public efforts to alert the public—especially sexually active women—about the importance of lab tests.
3. Mass health education programs in schools and communities. Neighborhood drugstores could disperse information about prevention and treatment; a national telephone "hot-line" could be established.
4. Support of laws allowing anyone of any age to buy condoms at the drugstore. Proper use of a condom greatly reduces the chances of acquiring venereal disease.
5. Ensuring that treatment is kept strictly confidential, so that guilt and shame will not prevent people from seeking required treatment.

Venereal Disease Division—Health Department

The Venereal Disease Division within a health department is responsible for implementing and maintaining a program of statewide control of the venereal diseases, and for upholding the state legislation in regard to these diseases. In Texas, for example, laws provide for:

1. Reporting and control of venereal disease cases.
2. Prenatal examination for syphilis.
3. Protection of the newborn.
4. Premarital examination for venereal disease.
5. Minor's capacity to consent to treatment for venereal disease.
6. Reporting of venereal disease laboratory tests.

QUESTIONS FOR DISCUSSION

1. Compare and contrast infectious diseases and communicable diseases.
2. Is infectious hepatitis a problem in your community? Your state?
3. How is tuberculosis transmitted or spread? What organs are affected by the germ?
4. Is tuberculosis a problem in your community? State? Explain.
5. Discuss the prevention and present treatment of tuberculosis.
6. Is tuberculosis increasing among the elderly? Why?
7. What is the value of large-scale tuberculin testing among preschool and school groups?
8. Briefly discuss the relationship between tuberculosis community education programs and the socioeconomic aspects of the community.
9. What is the function of your local tuberculosis and health association? What is the function of the local and state health department in connection with tuberculosis?
10. In what way does the public health nurse help in the fight against tuberculosis?
11. Discuss the major issues involved in the use of the BCG vaccine.
12. Is venereal disease a major problem in your community? State? Is it a major problem on your campus?
13. Is venereal disease increasing among adolescents? If so, why?
14. Discuss the differences between syphilis and gonorrhea in terms of etiologic agent, signs and symptoms, prevention, mode of transmission, number of cases, number of deaths, and methods of control.
15. How can we strengthen venereal disease control programs in our communities? What is being done by the health department to educate the public about VD?
16. How does syphilis relate to mental illness and prenatal health?
17. Discuss briefly the relationship between venereal disease community education programs and the socioeconomic aspects of the community.
18. What do we mean by "breaking the link in the chain of infection?
19. Discuss the prevention and present treatment of venereal disease.
20. What is the function of the local and state health department in connection with venereal disease?
21. Collect the Communicable Disease Summary for each month (get them from your local or state health department). Report on your findings.

22. What antibiotics are used today to combat disease?

23. Fill in the blanks concerning the following communicable diseases:

	ETIOLOGIC AGENT	NO. DEATHS PER YEAR IN U.S.	AGE RANGE OF GREATEST INCIDENCE	OCCURRENCE (WORLD)	VACCINE (YES OR NO)	TRANSMISSION
Bubonic plague						
Encephalitis						
Gonorrhea						
Infectious hepatitis						
Influenza						
Malaria						
Measles						
Pneumonia						
Psittacosis						
Rabies						
Rubella						
Sickle Cell anemia						
Snail fever						
Syphilis						
Tetanus						
Tuberculosis						
Trichinosis						
Tularemia						

QUESTIONS FOR REVIEW

1. What does the solution of the problem of low immunization levels of a community involve?
2. What is the earliest age that vaccines for measles, mumps, and rubella should be administered to a child? Why?
3. With whom does the primary responsibility and authority lie for public health?
4. In what three broad functional areas of public health has the federal government assumed responsibility?
5. Describe encephalitis. How is it transmitted?
6. What are the three possible types of mosquito control? Which is the major method of control today?
7. What are the reasons for some physicians doubting the effectiveness of the rubella vaccine?
8. Name the two types of hepatitis and list their causes.
9. How can hepatitis be treated?
10. What is the world's leading infectious disease?
11. What are the more serious results of the measles virus?
12. Which groups of people are most susceptible to pneumonia?
13. Name one of the most serious respiratory diseases and tell why it is so serious.
14. What are the four types of influenza virus? Which occurs most frequently?
15. What is the most common source of human psittacosis?
16. How can rabies be prevented?
17. What can the higher incidence of rabies in children under 15 years of age be attributed to?
18. Explain how snail fever is contracted. Where is this disease most prevalent and why?
19. What are two preventive measures of trichinosis?
20. What two principles must any control program for tuberculosis have?
21. What is the present public health procedure toward a chronic carrier of typhoid fever?

REFERENCES

1. Hein, F. V., and Bauer, W. W.: Legal requirements for immunizations. Arch. Environ. Health, *9*:82, 1964.
2. Manaff, A.: Manning the Malay mosquito trap. San Francisco Chronicle, 1970.
3. Axnick, N. W., and Alexander, E. R.: Tetanus in the United States, a review of the problem. Amer. J. Pub. Health, *47*:1493, 1959.
4. Wand, M., and Lyman, D.: Trichinosis from bear meat. JAMA, *220*(2):245, April 10, 1972.
5. Imperato, P. J., et al.: Trichinosis among Thais living in New York City. JAMA, *227*(5):526, February 4, 1974.
6. Massachusetts Department of Health: *Annual Report 1973*, p. 14.
7. Recommendation of the Public Health Service Advisory Committee on Immunization Practices, BCG vaccines. Morbidity and Mortality (U.S. Dept. of Health, Education and Welfare), *24*(8), February 22, 1975.
8. Preventive therapy of tuberculous infection. Morbidity and Mortality (U.S. Dept. of Health, Education and Welfare), *24*(8), February 22, 1975.
9. Recommendations for Health Department supervision of tuberculosis patients. Morbidity and Mortality (U.S. Dept. of Health, Education and Welfare), *24*(8), February 22, 1975.

10. Epidemiologic notes and reports, bovine tuberculosis—Michigan. Morbidity and Mortality (U.S. Dept. of Health, Education and Welfare), *23*(18), May 4, 1974.
11. Freitag, J. L.: Treatment of chronic typhoid carriers by cholecystectomy. Publ. Health Rep., *79*:567, 1964.
12. Riggs, M.: Prevention—the key to halting the VD epidemic. Healthnews, *2*(6):10, April, 1975.
13. Cherniak, D., and Feingold, A.: *VD Handbook,* 1972, p. 14. (Available by writing to P.O. Box 1000, Station G, Montreal, Quebec, Canada.)
14. Millar, J. D.: The Venereal Disease Problem in the United States. Paper presented at the National Venereal Disease Conference, Atlanta, Ga., November, 1971, p. 7.
15. Cherniak and Feingold, op. cit., p. 14.

SUGGESTED READING

Beers, R. F., Jr., et al. (eds.): *The Role of Immunological Factors in Viral and Oncogenic Processes.* Baltimore, Johns Hopkins Press, 1974.

Buxbaum, K. L., and Lindenmayer, S.: *What You Should Know About Venereal Disease.* New York, Harcourt Brace Jovanovich, 1975.

Faust, E. C., et al.: *Animal Agents and Vectors of Human Disease.* 4th ed. Philadelphia, Lea & Febiger, 1975.

Fry, L., and Seah, P. P. (eds.): *Immunological Aspects of Skin Diseases.* New York, Wiley, 1974.

Glasser, R. J.: *The Body Is the Hero.* New York, Random House, 1976.

Gordon, S.: *Facts About VD for Today's Youth.* New York, John Day Co., 1973.

Hall, L.: *I've Been Tested for Sickle Cell Anemia. Have You?* New York, Planned Parenthood Federation of America, 1972.

Horne, R. W.: *Virus Structure.* New York, Academic Press, 1974.

Hubbert, W. T., et al. (eds.): *Diseases Transmitted from Animals to Man.* 6th ed. Springfield, Ill., Charles C Thomas, 1975.

Krugman, S., and Ward, R.: *Infectious Diseases of Children and Adults.* St. Louis, C. V. Mosby Co., 1973.

Lasagna, L.: *The VD Epidemic.* Philadelphia, Temple University Press, 1975.

Mausner, J. S., and Bahn, A. K.: *Epidemiology: An Introductory Text.* Philadelphia, W. B. Saunders Co., 1974.

Pamphlets from Public Affairs Committee, New York.

Robbins, S. L.: *Pathological Basis of Disease.* Philadelphia, W. B. Saunders Co., 1974.

Sickle Cell Anemia: What It Is, What Can Be Done. A summary for health workers and community agencies. U.S. Government publication.

Soulsby, E. J. L. (ed.): *Parasitic Zoonoses: Clinical and Experimental Studies.* New York, Academic Press, 1974.

Top, F. H., and Wehrle, P. F. (eds.): *Communicable and Infectious Diseases.* 7th ed. St. Louis, C. V. Mosby Co., 1972.

CHAPTER 9

Mental Health

MENTAL ILLNESS—WHAT IS IT?

Mental illness is a disturbance of the mind and emotions. The illness may be so mild that it is unrecognized, or so severe that it is tragically disabling. Doctors have found that more than one-half of all persons who consult their family or school physicians for treatment of a physical ailment suffer from emotional difficulties.

There are two main categories of mental disease—the neuroses and the psychoses. The chief characteristic of neuroses is anxiety, and it is directly felt or unconsciously controlled by the use of various psychological defense mechanisms. The neurotic person does not lose contact with reality and does not display gross disorganization of personality. He may carry on his business and social affairs as a seemingly normal person; yet inwardly he may be suffering from anxiety, resentment, fear, or hostility that destroys his capacity for normal, happy living. Actually, there is a fine line between the neurotic individual and the so-called normal person, and experts disagree about where that line is to be drawn.

The psychotic person loses contact with reality. The chief characteristic of this illness is personality disintegration with disorientation for time, place, or person; hospitalization is usually required. The psychotic person may live in a dream world, perhaps unaware of his own identity or surroundings, or he may be unable to control his behavior. He may have fantastic ideas (delusions), or he may misinterpret what he sees and hears (illusions). He may see, hear, feel, taste, or smell things that are not there (hallucinations). Two common psychoses are schizophrenia and the severe depressive psychoses. Schizophrenia (reality disturbance) accounts for about one-half of the hospitalized cases of mental illness; most victims are young adults. The schizophrenic withdraws and has daydreams, delusions, and hallucinations; he suffers from disorganized thinking, and impairment of emotional response. The depressive suffers from feelings of worthlessness, guilt, and anxiety; an inability to find pleasure in normal activities; constipation; fatigue and weight loss; sleep disturbances; and occasionally serious considerations of suicide; 80 per cent of suicides have had a recent depression.

Possible contributing factors to mental illness include emotional experiences in infancy and childhood, increasing pressures in a fast age of insecurity, genetics, and certain chemical changes in the body. Most authorities agree that there is insufficient evidence to single out one factor.

Stress

Many scientists agree that stress may be as serious and as deadly as any communicable or chronic disease. Dr. Hans Selye, researcher in this area, reveals that stress causes a rise in blood pressure and sugar levels, an increase in stomach acid, and constriction of the arteries. If this sort of imbalance continues long enough, man reaches a state of exhaustion, and serious diseases or death may ensue.

There are two major types of stress. One involves personal *loss* (of a loved one, a job, or of self-esteem). The other kind of stress results from *threats*—to one's status, goals, health, security, and so on. Stress can generate symptoms of depression or anxiety, or both. Today statistics indicate that severe

Rate *Your* Stress Level This Year

In 1967, Thomas H. Holmes, M.D., first published his "Social Readjustment Rating Scale" which was developed as a means of quantifying the stress the ordinary person may be subjected to over a given period of time. Before devising the scale, Dr. Holmes, professor of psychiatry and behavioral sciences at the University of Washington School of Medicine, spent more than 15 years researching the potential relationship between change and ill health.

To take the test, check any of the events listed that have occurred in your life in the past 12 months. Your total score measures the amount of stress you have been subjected to in the one-year period and can be used to predict your chances of suffering serious illness within the next two years.

For example, a total score less than 150, means you have only a 37 percent chance of becoming ill in the designated period. If your score is between 150 and 300, you have a 51 percent chance of suffering poor health. If your score is more than 300, you are facing odds of 80 percent that you will become sick—and as the score increases, so do the odds that the problem will be serious. We caution you, however, to remember that a high score is *not* a guarantee of illness, it is simply an indication, according to Dr. Holmes, that because of the stress you have been subjected to, there is a chance of becoming ill.

Event	Value	Your Score
Death of spouse	100	
Divorce	73	
Marital separation	65	
Jail term	63	
Death of close family member	63	
Personal injury or illness	53	
Marriage	50	
Fired from work	47	
Marital reconciliation	45	
Retirement	45	
Change in family member's health	44	
Pregnancy	40	
Sex difficulties	39	
Addition to family	39	
Business readjustment	39	
Change in financial status	38	
Death of close friend	37	
Change to different line of work	36	
Change in number of marital arguments	35	
Mortgage or loan over $10,000	31	
Foreclosure of mortgage or loan	30	
Change in work responsibilities	29	
Son or daughter leaving home	29	
Trouble with in-laws	29	
Outstanding personal achievement	28	
Spouse begins or stops work	26	
Starting or finishing school	26	
Change in living conditions	25	
Revision of personal habits	24	
Trouble with boss	23	
Change in work hours, conditions	20	
Change in residence	20	
Change in schools	20	
Change in recreational habits	19	
Change in church activities	19	
Change in social activities	18	
Mortgage or loan under $10,000	17	
Change in sleeping habits	16	
Change in number of family gatherings	15	
Change in eating habits	15	
Vacation	13	
Christmas season	12	
Minor violation of the law	11	
Total		

Figure 9–1 "Social Readjustment Rating Scale," developed by Thomas H. Holmes as a means of quantifying the stress the ordinary person may be subjected to over a given period of time. (From Today's Health, January, 1975, p. 60.)

depression or anxiety may involve 20 per cent or more Americans at one point or another in their lives.

Each period in life has its own set of stresses. In early life, the child has to cope with his immediate family and the demands of school. The college years bring the stresses involving economic independence, academic superiority, shifting family relationships, and psychosocial adjustments. Children need the opportunity to confront various problems when they are young, and learn to cope with them. Parents, by intervening prematurely, may prevent the child from developing tolerances for problems or acquiring problem-solving mechanisms.

Today, the extra stress placed on individuals by a modern, permissive, mobile, industrialized, affluent urban society and the fading of the family concept (which leads to "impersonal" living and difficulty in relating to society) are frequently cited as causes of the erosion of the psychic stability and self-esteem of individuals.

Perhaps we dwell too much on the scope or depth of "mental illness" *vs.* "mental health." At least one psychiatrist, Tom Szasz, claims that mental illness is largely a myth. He claims that psychiatrists are in the business of manufacturing mental illness rather than helping people with the ethical and moral conflicts in their lives. He maintains that mental illness is a "lucrative business" perpetuated by a powerful mental health lobby that deprives people of their individual rights.

Quantifying Stress: Life Changes

The larger the life change, the more serious the illness. Life changes include job changes, marital status, births, and deaths. The stress model shown in Figure 9–2 looks like a series of optical

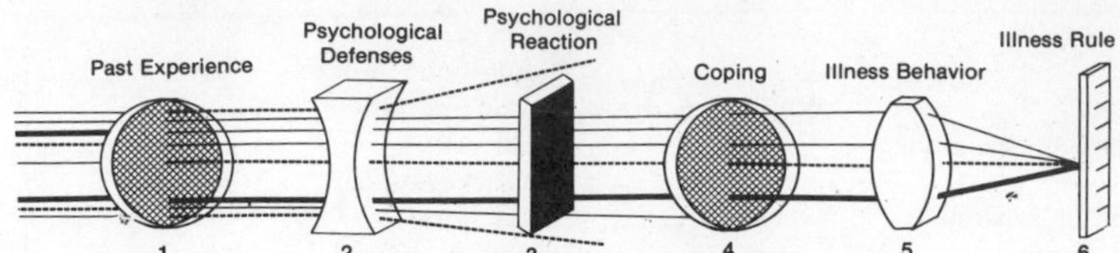

Figure 9-2 (From Medical News: A start at quantifying stress in life. JAMA, *232*(7):699, May 19, 1975.)

lenses, with life stress indicated by light rays of various intensities. The first step is a sort of polarizing filter where a person's past experiences alter the significance of this recent life change. Next, at step two, the individual uses ego defense mechanisms (such as denial) that may "diffract away" the event's impact. If the event is not diffracted, it may bring about any of a multitude of psychophysiological responses represented by a "black box" (step three). A person aware of his problems may respond by mood shifts, headaches, or muscle tension, but an individual unaware of his problems may respond by elevated lipid and blood pressure levels, or lowered blood glucose content. Certain responses are coped with or absorbed (step four) by muscle relaxing or physical exercises. However, unabsorbed or prolonged psychophysiological activation eventually leads to organ dysfunction and bodily disease perceived by the individual as symptoms that he may or may not report to medical personnel. His tendency to report the symptoms is called "illness behavior" and is the fifth step in the optical model, symbolizing the subject's attempt to focus his attention on his body symptoms. Medical diagnosis composes step six or the "illness rule."

By measuring the intervening variables and the time intervals between life changes and illness symptoms, it may be possible to learn how some subjects—despite severe life stresses—manage to remain in good health.[1]

Physiological Changes Due to Stress

In animals under emotional stress, fats are drawn from body deposits, emptied into the blood, and deposited along arterial walls; presumably the same thing happens in man, producing arteriosclerosis and coronary artery disease. Relaxation, exercise, and moderation help to relieve stress. Although a certain amount of stress is essential in life, hatred, frustration, boredom, and anxiety can cause many problems. Environmental stresses, such as noise and crowded highways, restaurants and recreational areas add their toll.

Advances and Problems in Treating Mental Illness

Mental illness is one of the most challenging unsolved public health problems today. The growing size of the mental-illness problem, the suffering it causes, and the staggering cost of care and treatment make the search for more effective preventive measures an urgent necessity. An estimated 20,000,000 Americans are now suffering from some form of mental illness; 3,000,000 men, women, and children are treated in mental hospitals, at psychiatric clinics, or by private psychiatrists each year. While new treatments are shortening the period of hospitalization, more than 50 per cent of the nation's hospital beds are occupied by psychotic patients, particularly schizophrenics. At least 800,000 more mental patients need hospital treatment, but have not been admitted to the already overcrowded institutions. It is estimated that 1 out of every 10 babies born today will be hospitalized with mental illness at some time during his lifetime. Because many emotionally disturbed persons do not see a doctor, there are no reliable statistics on the number of Americans with psychoneurotic problems like depression, anxiety, acute lack of self-confidence, hypochondria, and hysteria. The number of people so afflicted is large and may be growing as a result of the stress and unpredictability of modern life, as mentioned earlier. Another reason may be that mental illness is being detected earlier, and patients are seeking help earlier.

The proportion of elderly people in our mental hospitals is increasing at an alarming rate. Of all patients admitted to mental hospitals, 40 per cent are over 60 years old; 30 per cent are over 65 years of age. Many over 65 will remain in the hospital until death. Although many of these older persons have had a mild stroke or may be senile due to cerebral arteriosclerosis, many of these patients are simply custodial cases with no place else to go and no family to care for their simple needs; they are not treatable and are not really mentally ill. In order to cope with this problem, Kentucky, Ohio, and several other states, spurred by a combination of humanitarian motives and a desire to save tax money, are screening patients and are placing elderly persons who are not mentally ill in boarding and nursing homes. This program saves the state money because the patients promptly become entitled to federal old-age benefits, and the federal government also shares the cost of operating the nursing homes. Although the increase in the number of older age persons may be a factor in this problem, perhaps the nature of our present competitive, restless, mobile, status-seeking society may be involved.

The increase in the number of youngsters afflicted with mental illness parallels the problem of the aged. The rise in mental illness among children is probably due to more accurate diagnosis, as well as increased stress and less opportunity for the "modeling" on older siblings that was common in the large family units of old. In the past, many of these mentally ill youngsters roamed the streets or were sent to reform school. It is estimated that more than 10 per cent of the nation's public school children are emotionally disturbed and need guidance. Many juvenile delinquents are found to have learning disabilities that may have contributed to their inappropriate school behavior. Children as young as five years of age may develop schizophrenia.

In the 15 to 25 age group, which includes school and college students, three of the first five causes of death are essentially psychogenic in origin: accidents, suicide, and murder. It is the mind rather than the body that requires preventive and curative treatment in these cases. (The other two principal causes of death in the 15 to 25 age bracket are heart disease and cancer.) Emotional disorders, or psychiatric complaints, are among the principal medical problems of college students. It is estimated that perhaps 10 to 15 per cent of college students sometimes seek psychiatric help, although even higher figures have been recorded at some colleges.[2] It has been observed that there is a higher incidence of psychiatric complaints in college students than in their peers who go to work in more or less routine and stable working environments immediately after high school. Many college physicians are of the opinion that there is a greater likelihood of *emergence* of psychiatric problems in college students because of the recurrent challenges of their broad and constantly changing collegiate environment. In other words, the emotional problems, if any, come out sooner. This has its favorable aspect in that these patients receive relatively early treatment, which offers a greater possibility of success in a shorter period.

Great strides have been made through the years in the prevention of mental illness. For example, patients suffering from pellagra once filled mental hospitals in the South. Today, pellagra patients have practically disappeared because it was discovered that the disease is caused by a dietary deficiency. Another important example is the tremendous reduction in admissions to mental hospitals from advanced cases of syphilis since penicillin treatment was instituted in 1943.* Furthermore, much has been done to prevent brain damage (encephalitis) caused by unnecessary exposure to lead, cadmium, and other heavy metals by certain workers. A few large cities are conducting screening programs to detect brain-damaged children who ingested lead in the form of paint peelings from the walls and ceilings of older homes; these homes are also being sought out and condemned until the hazards are removed. There are far fewer mental cases following accidental injuries than formerly. Even with these advances, however, there has been a steady increase in the mental hospital population. Factors contributing to the increase in mental illness are the country's increased urbanization and industrialization, the higher proportion of older persons in the population, and the greater longevity of mental patients.

During the past 30 years, the growth of mental health clinics has been of great importance. They serve as mental first-aid stations where the public may obtain help for emotional problems before these problems become too serious. The clinics play a particularly vital role in preventing mental illness at the source or in formative years of childhood. Early recognition and prompt treatment are as important in mental illness as they are in physical illness.

---

*Nevertheless, in 1975 the cost was 47 million dollars a year for maintaining the syphilitic insane confined in publicly supported mental hospitals.

A number of surveys of public opinions and attitudes about mental illness have revealed that there has been advancement in terms of better public understanding of mental illness and greater tolerance or acceptance of the mentally ill. It appears that the American public does not universally reject the mentally ill, nor is it thoroughly defeatist about the prospects of treating mental illness. Research data have helped illuminate certain important aspects in this area; for example, several surveys over the years confirm that the higher the educational and occupational level, the more enlightened the opinions about mental illness. Certainly, any program of public education must seriously take into account the strong likelihood that there are many varieties of public opinions and attitudes about mental illness in the total population and that these are far from static. Nevertheless, we must continually strive to educate the public in an effort to change public attitudes and concepts of responsibility.

There is a particular need for well-supported and carefully planned research on all aspects of mental health. Prevention of mental disease may revolve around the same epidemiological principles utilized in preventing other diseases. For example, we must determine how many persons have the disease, what kind of people they are, and under what conditions they get the disease. This information can then furnish clues for intensive investigation of the causes.

Preventive Measures

1. Making adequate medical care available to all expectant mothers. (A relationship is known to exist between mental illness and inadequate prenatal, obstetrical, and early infant care.)
2. Working to change environmental factors that create unendurable stress.
3. Improving people's understanding of individual behavior, and avoiding attaching illness labels to behavior.
4. Having education programs available to those who would benefit from them, and continuing research aimed at identifying new and effective mental health education programs.
5. Making early identification of emotional or mental disorders through proper diagnosis, followed by quick, appropriate, and adequate treatment to remove or control an emotional problem before it develops further.

Treatment

Perhaps three potent forces are most responsible for the optimism that has developed during the past two decades regarding the treatment of mental illness. These forces are psychoanalysis, psychotropic drugs, and psychosocial therapy, including group therapy, the therapeutic community, and the open hospital. These three main areas of progress have contributed to the evolution of new treatment approaches, including crisis intervention techniques, day care centers, halfway houses, and a series of effective alternatives to hospitalization. The proliferation of these alternatives to hospitalization may eventually show actual bed hospitalization to be required for only a very small minority of even the sickest mental patients. Large state mental institutions are slowly closing.

Other important advances and promising research include the use of lithium carbonate ($LiCO_3$) to prevent the depressive phase of the manic-depressive syndrome; Ritalin (or methylphenidate hydrochloride), which may help certain children with certain learning or behavioral disabilities* and the hyperkinetic child; megavitamin therapy, which may help certain children with childhood schizophrenic or autistic tendencies; availability of long-acting, injectable drugs (such as phenothiozines) and tranquilizers for schizophrenics; and blood tests performed at birth to detect certain enzyme imbalances that may lead to mental deficiency (for example, phenylketonuria and galactosemia). Various programs involving behavior modification principles are of major importance in working with many emotionally disturbed children.

Depression involves changes in an individual's way of relating to his environment, in his physiology and neurochemistry, and in his psychic functioning. Treatment therefore involves a healthy environment (milieu), nor-

*Minimal brain dysfunction (MBD) is meant to refer to children with certain learning or behavioral disabilities, ranging from mild to severe, which are associated with deviations of function of the central nervous system.

mal physiology (chemotherapy), and a functional apparatus (psychotherapy). Healthy behavior (independence, assertiveness, and verbal expression of feelings) is encouraged and primed. Electroshock therapy, although condemned by many, is effective in certain types of depression. Generally, the patient is taught to be appropriately assertive and responsible for his own feelings and actions, and to become increasingly in charge of his own life. Additionally, the patient is encouraged to develop new interests and activities to the extent that he desires.

COMMUNITY MENTAL HEALTH PROGRAMS

We now have a great increase in outpatient resources, a considerable increase in trained personnel, improved treatment techniques, including drug therapy, and the development of pre and aftercare programs, and of programs and facilities concerned with alternatives to hospitalization.

The Short-Doyle Act of California defines community mental health services as:

1. Outpatient psychiatric clinics for those who are unable to obtain private care, including referrals by physicians and surgeons.
2. Inpatient psychiatric services in general hospitals and in nonprofit psychiatric hospitals affiliated as the psychiatric division of or with a general hospital for those who are unable to obtain private care, including referrals by physicians and surgeons.
3. Rehabilitation services for patients with psychiatric illnesses for those who are unable to obtain private care, including referrals by physicians and surgeons.
4. Informational services to the general public and educational services furnished by qualified mental health personnel to schools, courts, health and welfare agencies, probation departments, and other appropriate, public or private agencies.
5. Psychiatric consultant services to public or private agencies for the promotion and coordination of services that preserve mental health and for the early recognition and management of conditions that might develop into psychiatric illnesses.

The inadequacies of state hospitals have long been recognized. For 20 years or more there have been loud public demands for something better. It is only within the last decade, however, that any real attempt has been made to provide this alternative. In 1963, Congress passed the Community Mental Health Centers Act. For the first time, federal support was authorized for direct mental health services. In 1965, the first federal grants were made, and now there are more than 500 local mental health programs that have been awarded grants providing federal assistance.

In part, these federal funds have been important because they have brought new services to people who need them. Of much greater importance, however, is the fact that these funds have served to stimulate local interest and local action in the field of mental health. The federal grants have really been most significant as catalysts for the organization of new local services. The grants are awarded on a matching basis and, as a result, they have stimulated efforts to find local money to meet the matching requirements.

The fact that local groups take responsibility for their own mental health services is one of the most significant features of the community mental health approach. The availability and accessibility of services are certainly a function of geography, and patients are clearly much more likely to make use of services that they and their families can get to easily. On the other hand, geography is only one small part of the accessibility story. It is obvious that a mental health service must be psychologically accessible as well as being geographically accessible. Indeed, this psychological accessibility is essential to the success of any health service. The patient and his family must feel comfortable about his going to the service for help. They must feel that this behavior has the support and the endorsement of their friends and neighbors. In other words, they have to feel reasonably certain that the members of their own community approve of their seeking this kind of help.

As required by the federal program, each community mental health center must offer five basic services, and four of these are direct treatment services. These are inpatient care, outpatient care, day hospital care, and emergency services. Inpatient and outpatient care have long been part of the mental health center; however, these services take on a new aspect. Traditional mental health services have emphasized long-term care. In the setting of the community mental health center, on the other hand, inpatient and outpatient care are designed to offer short-term care for acute mental illness. Intermediate-length care and some long-term care are provided, but the primary goal is the treatment and resolution of the patient's problem in its acute phase.

Problems

Very few, if any, communities now have all these services and facilities. The lack of coordination in our communities in relation to resources now available for treating the mentally ill is one of the most serious obstacles to satisfactory psychiatric care today.

Other problems and complaints include the following: many mentally ill hospital patients discharged to certain local communities for treatment are not receiving treatment; some patients are placed in nursing or foster homes where conditions are poor; some centers provide more mental health positions but remain inaccessible or irrelevant to large segments of the community; many facility operators lack relevant education training or significant experience in the operation of a residential care home; some mental hospitals have closed too abruptly, thereby unleashing a minimally functioning population before the separate communities had time to prepare compensatory programs; location board and care homes have been opposed by local citizens; withdrawal of federal funds from programs for the mentally ill.

The problem becomes a political one because many state hospitals are the economic strength of many communities. State mental health workers' unions would almost certainly oppose a rapid closing of state hospitals.

Many nonprofit community mental health agencies are providing comprehensive social and vocational rehabilitation for mentally disturbed adults. A variety of programs are offered for mental patients, and contracts with state and county governments help pay some expenses. Programs include on-the-job training, community activities, and independent living training. If a client can hold a job, live independently, and establish social relationships, then he has made a beginning toward living a creative and personally enriching life.

Unfortunately, many people still feel that mental illness of any kind carries some kind of social stigma. As a result, they are reluctant to seek help even when they need it desperately. The best way to overcome this reluctance is for the community as a whole to show its support for mental health services, and the best way to show this support, obviously, is for the community as a whole to organize and establish its own local mental health service.

The development of facilities in the community for the care of severely ill patients does not necessarily mean that hospitalization for mental illness will become either unnecessary or undesirable. These facilities have been established in recognition of the need for close collaboration between community agencies and mental hospitals, for a frame of reference in which the mental hospital is considered one facility and one resource, in the whole chain of the community's armamentarium for dealing with mental and emotional illness.

New Concepts

The development of several new concepts has, in addition, helped to point up the importance of active and interlocking community activity in order to promote mental health in the broadest possible sense. Some of these include the growing awareness of the importance of social relationships in the etiology and treatment of mental illness, the increased interest in the study of the mental hospital as a social institution, the recognition of the importance of a therapeutic environment in the hospital and the community, the introduction of public health concepts in the plans for treating and rehabilitating the mentally ill, and the recognition of the special needs of the aged, the alcoholic, and the mentally retarded.

Crisis intervention programs in many communities have wisely utilized trained volunteers plus the telephone in an effort to help the lonely and sometimes needy senior citizen, the frightened drug abuser, the potential suicide, and the pregnant girl in need of counseling and guidance.

The future will demand major alterations in the attitudes of many groups of people toward the mental illnesses. Some of these changes will occur as the natural result of a changed situation. As more people receive help in their own communities for all gradations of the mental illnesses, the attitudes of the patients, their families, and the communities will gradually become more realistic, less based on outmoded negative stereotypes on the one hand and falsely optimistic hopes on the other. Other changes in attitudes will be brought about partially, at least, through carefully thought-out information and education programs.

Because of the multiplicity of social and community factors involved in the promotion of mental health and the amelioration of mental illness, and because use of existing resources is essential in the development of a community program for the reasons just discussed, the organization of forces and agencies into a combined effort is essential if mental health is to be effectively promoted. Communities differ considerably in actual assignment of responsibilites to groups and agencies for services to its citizens. The return of primary responsibility to the community from the remote state hospital implies the necessity for mobilization of medical, educational, social welfare, recreational, and spiritual agencies to an unprecedented degree.

COMMUNITY MENTAL HEALTH SERVICES

Community Mental Health Centers and contract services are established in many health departments, to offer help to children, adults, and families who are unable to afford the full cost of private care. Any fees for treatment are based on the ability to pay. People who desire information or services relative to mental health are invited to contact their nearest Health Department.

Services Designed to Prevent Mental Illness and Promote Individual and Community Mental Health

Treatment Services

1. Emergency psychiatric service. Help is available for anyone faced with an emotional crisis who may do harm to himself or to others, or is incapable of caring for himself. Immediate appointments given.

2. Suicide and crisis telephone service. Suicide prevention and crisis service is available 24 hours a day. Someone is always waiting to listen and help. All calls are confidential.

3. Hospital services. A psychiatric ward for persons needing short-term hospitalization is located in County Hospitals.

4. Outpatient treatment. People whose emotional problems do not require hospitalization may receive a short-term counseling, treatment, and referral assistance at all Mental Health Centers. Treatment may involve individual, family, or group psychotherapy.

5. Child and family treatment. Both children and entire families may be accepted for treatment if this is the approach that seems best for them. This is a part of outpatient services. Also included are group, family, and play therapy.

6. Alcoholism control program. Treatment and rehabilitation services are provided for people with alcoholic problems. Counseling is offered to their families. Consultation and education are available to individuals and community groups.

7. Drug abuse control programs, including methadone clinics. A drop-in outpatient clinic for information and patient screening is available. Outpatient treatment, limited hospitalization, counseling, education, and consultation regarding drugs are offered.

8. Rehabilitative services. Day treatment programs are available for patients needing extended psychiatric treatment. Occupational and recreational therapy, patient group activity, drug therapy, and group therapy are included in this service.

9. Family stress prevention service. This service provides counseling for families in which child abuse has occurred.

Preventive Services

1. Mental health consultation. Consultation by the mental health professional staff is offered to the personnel of schools, welfare, and other agencies to help handle the mental health problems of their clients, recognize early signs of trouble, and deal with the social conditions which may contribute to mental illness.

2. Information and education. Upon request by individuals and groups, information is given and programs are conducted on such subjects as local mental health services, mental illness and its treatment, and mental health principles in relationship to everyday living.

Goals

The County Health Department's Mental Health Program has the following goals: prevention of mental illness, promotion of individual and community mental health, and treatment and rehabilitation of people with mental illness and mental retardation. Mental Health Services are provided through the Mental Health Centers by a professional staff of psychiatrists, clinical psychologists, psychiatric and clinical social workers, and other personnel, and through contracts to pay community hospitals, clinics, and other agencies to extend their services to people unable to afford the full cost of care.

Needs

The primary need in community mental health services is for a systematic organization of the delivery system which will:

1. Identify relevant community needs for services.
2. Fill gaps in services in order to meet those needs.
3. Eliminate duplication of services.
4. Evaluate ongoing programs.
5. Modify programs to better meet needs.
6. Develop linkages among programs.
7. Provide continuity of care through coordinated treatment plans.
8. Better utilize private mental health resources.
9. Be integrated with the other systems providing human services.

The need for systematic organization of the delivery system applies to services for both children and adults. However, both the services for children and adolescents and the resources allocated to provide those services are insufficient. On the other hand, there is a wealth of services for the adult mentally disordered, but there is a need for determining true needs and for shifting resources to meet them more effectively.

A mental health care system, in order to maintain the dignity of the individual, must be accessible, continuous, and comprehensive. Every available mental health (or related) resource should be used in developing a comprehensive mental health program. Funding of proposed mental health programs should be based on (a) the demonstrated need and lack of existing resources to meet that need; and (b) the demonstrated willingness and ability of the proposed program to coordinate efforts with the existing mental health services in the community.

Youth centers and clinics sponsored either by official or voluntary agencies have helped many troubled young people. Aid has ranged from individual counseling to rap sessions, legal counseling, providing of drug information, runaway intervention, and free medical clinics. All facilities are free to the young people; the only requirement is that a youngster must seek help on his own. The three key words at most centers are *free, voluntary,* and *confidential.* Volunteers from all walks of life offer their time and help.

CRISIS INTERVENTION

Emergency services in mental health settings have increased greatly over the last several years. They are a required part of federally funded mental health centers; emergency services, including crisis intervention services, are widely advocated as providing alternatives to psychiatric hospitalization. A number of different terms are used loosely to designate emergency services, but two major categories include suicide prevention programs and crisis intervention programs.

In the course of the everyday events, situations occur which threaten the gratification of people's needs. As a rule, these upsets are temporary, and equilibrium is soon reestablished. There are, however, situations that create a series of problems which seem unresolvable and unbearable. Whatever the cause, they are upsetting and anxiety-producing, and often result in impaired functioning. Such a period of severe emotional disturbance is frequently referred to as a crisis. Often a crisis creates a change in a person's status or relationship to people and the community. When a change of status or relationship is sufficiently maladaptive or inappropriate by psychological and social standards, the person is said to have become "mentally ill." While intervention will likely alleviate the crisis, the lack of intervention may aggravate the crisis, and the result may be impulsive, irrational, and, in some instances, self-destructive behavior. An individual who is experiencing a "crisis" or "mental illness" requires appropriate intervention based on full use of community resources. There needs to be an emphasis on the development and utilization of programs in a community to serve as alternatives to hospitalization.

Crisis intervention based on crisis theory aims at restoring the individual to at least the previous level of equilibrium, and hopefully to a better one. Briefly, the intervention consists of identifying an emotionally hazardous precipitating event and determining why and how existing coping mechanisms are no longer sufficient to deal with the situation. Experience shows that once the individual achieves a better cognitive awareness of the nature of the problem and can express appropriate affect, there is a reduction in tension resulting in potential for a more adaptive resolution.

Suicide in Adolescence

A major study on suicide among young people brought out the following facts:

> In most countries throughout the world, suicide in adolescence has doubled over the past 10 years and now ranks between second and third among the leading causes of death during the teenage to young adult years. To some degree, this increase may be due to better and more accurate reporting on the part of coroners on death certificates. But better record keeping by no means accounts for the over 100 percent reported increase in suicides in young people. Many suicidologists feel that even more adolescent suicides are not reported as suicides but as accidental or undetermined deaths because of stigma to the family.
>
> The extent to which the adolescent lives in a continuous state of turmoil has long been recognized. Developmental psychologists have pointed out that the internal pressures in adolescence are perhaps greater than in any other period of human development.
>
> Today, we recognize that young people live under a great variety of pressures, including the stresses that result from the phenomena of adolescence, from the high expectancies of early adulthood and from those strains of competition and achievement that are unique to young people.
>
> Only in recent years has the seriousness of the problem of suicides in youth begun to appear in the professional literature. The studies of suicidal behavior on the college campus, for example, have led to the conclusion that suicide is a serious public health problem and, in the college setting, ranks as the second or third leading cause of death.
>
> There is no single answer as to why a young person wishes to put an end to [his] life. The reasons are multiple and complex. Research on this topic has been extensive, yet there is a need for much more to be done. Explaining why a young person turns to death as the only alternative includes such factors as family problems and pressures; loss of a loved one; despair at the threatened loss of an important relationship; financial pressures; identity problems (the transition from adolescence to the adult world); increased availability of drugs, including alcohol; high academic competition; and overpopulation, which has resulted in too many people wanting too many things that are not available. All these things contribute to feelings of anonymity and isolation.[3]

SUICIDE: MYTH VS. FACT

Myth	*Fact*
A person commits suicide without warning.	Although suicide can be an impulsive act, it is often thought out and communicated to others, but people ignore the clues.
People who talk about suicide never kill themselves.	Most suicides—8 out of 10—have given definite clues and warnings about their suicidal intentions.
Suicide is a random happening; there are very few cases.	Suicide is the 10th leading cause of death among all adults in the U.S.A. There are twice as many suicides as homicides.
Suicide is the "rich man's" curse.	Suicide shows little prejudice to economic status. It is represented proportionately among all levels of society..
More women than men commit suicide.	Although women *attempt* suicide twice as often as men, men *commit* suicide twice as often as women.
Suicidal persons really want to die, so there's no way to stop them.	Suicidal persons are often undecided about living or dying right up to the last minute;

	many gamble that others will stop them before it's too late.
A suicidal person can never be saved; he'll do it eventually.	People who want to kill themselves feel that way only for a limited time; the "crisis period" passes.
If a person really wants to kill himself, no one has the right to stop him.	No suicide case has only one victim: wives, husbands, children, friends, all suffer from the loss of someone who commits suicide.
Most suicides are caused by a single dramatic and traumatic event.	Precipitating factors may trigger a suicidal decision; more typically the deeply troubled person has suffered long periods of unhappiness, is withdrawn, depressed, helpless to cope with life, has little self-respect, and no hope for the future.
Suicide is inherited; it "runs in the family."	Suicide is a highly individual matter—there is no genetic predisposition to self-destruction.
Once stopped, the suicidal person is "cured."	Four out of 5 persons who kill themselves have tried at least once before.
It's morbid to talk about suicide to a person who is unhappy.	Depressed individuals need attention and emotional support; encouraging them to talk about their suicidal feelings can be therapeutic as a first step.

SUICIDE PREVENTION

The number of Suicide Prevention Centers are increasing throughout the country. The growing number of these agencies and the large number of calls for help suggest that they fill urgent needs. They appear to offer a valuable service not only to the suicidal persons who call upon them, but also to the public service agencies of the community.

The initial procedures in dealing with persons at risk of suicide fall into a general pattern: when a suicidal person calls, the suicide prevention worker tries to establish rapport, to evaluate the client's potential for suicide, and to decide upon a course of action.*

A large proportion of the clients who call the suicide prevention agencies in a crisis are referred for treatment to general hospitals, physicians and psychiatrists in private agencies, outpatient clinics, community agencies, clergymen, or other community resources. Sometimes the worker recommends that a client get in touch with nonprofessionals—the police, members of his family or close friends. The worker makes several follow-up calls to see if the caller has contacted the designated community resource. The programs of all suicide prevention agencies must be evaluated to determine the effectiveness of their goals and methods. The Center for Studies of Suicide Prevention (National Institute of Mental Health) is conducting such follow-up studies.

Suicide prevention agencies receive cooperation from most community agencies to which they refer callers; such cooperation is necessary if effective community health services are to be provided. Suicide prevention agencies should use every appropriate community resource that furthers their aims. Sometimes when one agency seeks the cooperation of another, it fails at first to obtain a favorable response. The reason may be that the staff members of the initiating facility have failed to appreciate the other organization's goals and problems.

Staffs of the suicide prevention agencies should be instructed in referral methods and should be familiar with the available community resources. The goals, functions and problems of other organizations, including the restrictions under which they operate, should be made explicit. Likewise, the other organizations in the community need to have this kind of knowledge about the suicide prevention agency.

Also, the public needs more information about suicide prevention agencies and mental illness. These agencies' efforts are still often restrained by prejudices, such as the belief that mental illness is disgraceful. Too

*For further information on suicidal processes and therapeutic techniques, refer to Faberow, N. L., and Shneidman, E. S.: *The Cry for Help*. New York, McGraw-Hill, 1965.

frequently people regard those who commit suicide, or who try to do so, as weak and useless. If the prevention agencies are to accomplish their aims, they will need not only increased financial support, but also the help of newspapermen, radio and television producers, publishers, and community leaders as shown below and on the following page.

PREVENTION OF MENTAL ILLNESS

Mental illness can be prevented. Prevention depends partly upon providing a healthful environment during childhood and partly upon helping the emotionally disturbed child early in his life. Other primary preventive measures include protection of the central nervous system from damage, facilitating the development of strong and mature personalities, providing help at critical periods in one's lifetime, e.g., puberty, military service, marriage, and retirement, and alleviating stress in the home, in school, or on the job.

The National Association for Mental Health lists the following 10 signs of good mental health:

1. A tolerant, easygoing attitude toward yourself as well as others.
2. A realistic estimate of your own abilities—neither underestimating nor overestimating them.
3. Self-respect.
4. Ability to take life's disappointments in stride.
5. Liking and trusting other people and expecting others to feel the same way about you.
6. Ability to give love and consider the interests of others.
7. Feeling part of a group and having a sense of responsibility to your neighbors and fellow men.
8. Acceptance of your responsibilities and doing something about your problems as they arise.
9. Ability to plan ahead and formulate realistic goals for yourself.
10. Putting your best efforts into what you do and getting satisfaction out of doing it.

Certain guide lines are essential for maintaining good relations and mental health in community work. They are:

1. Basic honesty—relate personal matters openly and relieve yourself of such pent-up emotions as love, hatred, and insecurity.
2. Attention and interest—be sympathetic and a good listener; maintain a sincere and genuine interest in people; try to understand a person's actions, reactions, and interests.
3. Attempt to understand yourself and others in interaction with you.

Initial Procedures Used in Preventing the Caller from Committing Suicide

Suicide Prevention Center, Los Angeles, Calif.

1. Establish contact and rapport.
2. Evaluate lethality by talking to patient about suicide (plan, specificity of time and method, prior attempts, etc.) and evaluating resources (intrapsychic and interpersonal).
3. Involve significant others.

Fulton-DeKalb Suicide Prevention Center, Atlanta, Ga.

Establishment of rapport, encouragement to discuss and delineate the precipitating events, urging to participate with the worker in finding alternatives, referring to treatment resources if available.

We Care, Inc., Orlando, Fla.

Crisis intervention worker tries to draw out the caller, to find out his problem; reassures caller that we do want to help, feel that we can if caller will tell worker what is bothering him; if caller is determined to go ahead with suicide, regardless of our help, we dispatch police or sheriff's department to intervene, take gun, etc., then we follow up.

Citizens for Mental Health, Buffalo, N.Y.

The caller is evaluated as to the seriousness or emergency nature. Depending on this, the caller would be:

1. Counseled over phone
2. Visited in person
3. Taken by police or rescue squad to hospital
4. Referred to clinic, hospital, social service agency, or clergyman.

Wyandotte County Guidance Center, Inc., Kansas City, Kans.

A quick assessment of the suicidal potentiality is the first approach to every call. What action is to be taken depends on the seriousness of the situation.

Emergency Mental Health Service, Phoenix, Ariz.

Keep them on the line and keep them involved. Find out if friends or relatives are close by. If no one is there, notify police, who will make a check. They (the police) are much more mobile than any other group or organization.

Santa Clara County Suicide Prevention Center, San Jose, Calif.

Obtain information, assess and evaluate information, and propose action.

Suicide Prevention Center, San Francisco, Calif.

Ours is a telephone "first aid" service for suicidal people. In emergency situations, our staff calls the necessary emergency facilities in the community to give the caller immediate aid. In all cases we win the caller's confidence in order to make the most appropriate referral for his particular problem.

Contra Costa County Suicide Prevention Center, Walnut Creek, Calif.

We ask, "May I help you?" and then play it by ear. Each caller responds somewhat differently depending on many variables.

Suicide Prevention Service, Eau Claire, Wis.

Personal attention, psychotherapeutically oriented.

Suicide Prevention, Inc., St. Louis, Mo.

Sympathy, attempt to understand, evaluation of risks, referral to appropriate resources, follow up to see they enter treatment.

Suicide Prevention Center, Denver, Colo.

When a call comes, we attempt to program a plan of action, whether it is to see the person in our program or to call on some other agency.

Mental Health Center, Suicide Prevention Service, Pasadena, Calif.

Name, telephone number. How do you plan to kill yourself? Why do you want to kill yourself? How will that help? Have you thought of something else to solve your problem other than killing yourself—death is forever.

Friends Organization, Miami, Fla.

We provide sympathetic listening, then evaluate the seriousness of the caller, and direct the caller to an agency or person where he can be helped.

National Save-A-Life League, New York, N.Y.

Your wish to help them; willingness to make possible contacts with relatives, friends, etc.; supportive help of all kinds; pastoral counseling, psychiatric, etc.

Suicide Prevention of Tarrant County, Fort Worth, Tex.

The question "Can I help you?" first; one requirement for prevention worker is a warm friendly voice; by skillful questioning and listening in particular, stress is reduced. If suicide is in progress—poison taken, etc.—trained police are called.[4]

Researchers have been investigating new and controversial methods of electroshock and psychosurgery. Scientists have learned how to analyze blood flowing through the living brain; this may lead to important discoveries. It is thought by some that the adrenal glands of the schizophrenics do not function as do those of normal people; certain chemicals produce false psychotic symptoms. The immediate future may belong to the biochemists and pharmacologists.

Other factors involved in preventing and solving our mental illness problem include our fast pace of life and the fact that many persons do not take the time to formulate a philosophy and to determine objectives in life. Once a person has established his objectives, he fails again if he does not strive to attain those goals. In this respect, one famous psychiatrist commented that the truth of the matter is that most Americans today exist without purpose and without significance. They have no articulate philosophy; they do not live within any frame of reference. To counteract this situation, a number of "consciousness cults" have developed in recent years: transcendental meditation (TM), biofeedback, yoga, encounter groups, and relaxation response groups, to name just a few.

Some people are able to achieve their goals by themselves, but for a great many people religious faith plays an increasingly important role. Religious leaders, physicians, teachers, counselors, social workers, parents, and others are beginning to emphasize the importance of integrating all the factors of personality, environment, and emotional status when dealing with children and adults. They are also beginning to understand and inform others about the meaning of the preamble to the constitution of the World Health Organization—"Health is a complete state of physical, mental, and social well-being and not merely the absence of disease or infirmity." The disturbed person must be considered as a complex unit of physical, mental, and emotional factors, subject to unique personal, family, and social influences.

As with every health problem, when the citizens become fully aware of the need, the battle is half won. The outlook for a concentrated attack on the problem of mental illness looks promising in most states; interest is gaining, and more people are openly facing the problem.

Many persons are joining hands in an effort to become more aware of themselves and others. Awareness groups, for example, strive to become totally involved in sensory perceptions, experiences, and interrelationships; this makes them more aware of objects and persons around them. Encounter groups examine individual feelings and attitudes by sharing and defending their beliefs. Primary-care physicians are becoming more aware of mental illness and thus are in a position to initiate *early* treatment.

Coed living helps students learn how to have friends. As community spirit grows, students don't have to pair off as lovers to get to know each other. They form brother-sister relationships, and take on large groups of friends. The main activity of these newly-made friends is talking with each other. The Friday night date is replaced by the Friday night identity crisis. Dormitory talk sessions often take the form of painfully intense public confessions. Nobody is expected to be at ease with the world or with himself. Sprawled in corridors and on the floors of rooms, they ask each other, "Who am I?", "Why can't I relate?", "Am I really unhappy?", and then furnish interminable answers. They test themselves daily, not just in the classroom.

PRINCIPLES FOR MENTAL HEALTH PROGRAM PLANNING[5]

Stress. Psychiatric disorder may be thought of as reflecting an individual's inability to cope with stress. Conversely, mental health is manifested by the ability of the individual to cope with life's stresses, external and internal. The symptoms of mental and emotional disorder are expressions of persons' attempts to deal with stress. While mental disturbance and deficiency are not related solely to stress, it is a useful concept for mental health program planning to think in terms of stress and disequilibrium in the face of stress.

Basic Goal. In these terms, the basic goal of mental health programs is the development, maintenance, and restoration of social and personal equilibrium despite emotional stress.

Practical Limitations. Established goals should be reasonably possible to attain. Even though planning may be for a decade ahead, the stated objectives should be limited to conform to the knowledge and resources available in relation to the problem at hand. Therefore, although well-being and recovery are desired whenever possible, the primary aim of programs planned at this time should be limited to assisting individuals in their release from or adjustment to stress and the restoration to a *reasonable operating level* of persons mentally incapacitated. The broad aim for the next several years cannot be general and complete emotional well-being and happiness, nor can it be complete cure. The problem at hand is large and the resources of knowledge and skilled manpower limited; this must be realized in the planning.

Disease Exists in a Culture. No state of disequilibrium exists in a vacuum; no problems of health or disease exist in isolation. Mental health depends on more than one factor—on physical, biological, social, economic, and other factors. Hence for a thorough understanding of a person's mental health or mental illness or deficiency, the person must be understood as a social, psychological, and biological member of a family and a community. Disequilibrium in an individual threatens the equilibrium of the family and the community.

Availability of Range of Psychiatric Services. There is a range of psychiatric services, direct and indirect, corresponding to the variety of needs. Included are services to patients, to their families, and to agencies that intervene in times of stress. An adequate program of mental health services requires that the whole gamut of psychiatric services be available. "Available" means that the services exist and are physically and financially accessible to individuals and agencies needing them.

Local Availability. As part of such availability, psychiatric services should be obtainable within the living radius of the recipient. Past practice often isolated the psychiatric patient from his family and friends, his job, and his community. Disruption of normal ties seriously interferes with the process of restoring health. To provide minimum dislocation, mental health services should be physically accessible to those needing them; the service should be where the recipient is.

Financial Availability. The results of mental disequilibrium are costly in human and financial terms to the individual and to society. Prevention and early effective treatment and rehabilitation will reduce this cost, but as is true of other services, will not eliminate it. Appropriate and adequate methods of financing mental health services are necessary; if a service cannot be purchased, it is not available.

Problem Identification. In coping with psychiatric problems, the problem should be identified and delineated from the concomitant problems affecting the individual, his family, and his community. Only in this way can help for the psychiatric component be selected with precision. Only in this way can treatment be chosen that is specifically suited to the problem; and the skill that is applied *should* be suited to the problem. Indeed, the *intervention,* treatment or otherwise, should be suited to the clearly identified problem.

Generic Services. When needs can be met by general health, welfare, education, etc., programs or services rather than by specialized psychiatric services, this should be done. Whenever generic services *can* adequately meet the identified needs, they are to be preferred over more specialized services.

Importance of Basic Services. In an individual's normal development, sound health, education, recreation, and similar programs are important in the promotion and conservation of mental health; in the event of mental disorder, they are important in treatment and rehabilitation. In addition, those engaged in providing the basic services are in most frequent contact with persons under abnormal stress and usually see them first. It is, therefore, important that they understand the mental health implications in the management of stress situations and have access to specialized assistance. Their absence may contribute to a vulnerability to stress.

Psychiatric Treatment. Psychiatric treatment should be provided as early as possible, with as much continuity as possible, with as little dislocation as possible, and with as much social restoration as possible.

Basic Program Elements. The elements required to implement a mental health program include manpower, knowledge, skill, and physical facilities.

Goal Centered, Subject to Measurement, Economical, and Efficient. Mental health programs, as other programs, should be based on clearly defined needs and should have stated objectives. This is necessary for effective channeling of resources, it aids public understanding, and is an essential ingredient of any effort to measure program efficiency. Provision for measurement in terms of effectiveness and economy should be routinely built into every mental health program. Programs should be needed, feasible, and as economic as is consistent with efficiency.

Public Responsibility. Many persons, including those who pay the costs, are affected by mental health services. They, therefore, have an interest in mental health planning and should have a voice in determinations that are made. Although many decisions are technical, based on clinical evidence, others are not. Mental health programs can and should be responsive to the needs and wishes of those affected; their development is not the sole province of those administering the activities. To achieve such responsiveness, suitable participation in planning and evaluation is a requisite.

MENTAL HEALTH ORGANIZATIONS AND SOCIETIES

Various professional organizations are endeavoring to meet the problem of nervous and mental disease. The American Psychiatric Association sets up standards for care in psychiatric hospitals and encourages the training of psychiatrists, psychiatric nurses, and psychiatric aides. It furthers psychiatric education and research and devotes much time and effort to the development of outpatient clinics and all other agencies concerned with the social and legal aspects of mental disorders. The Committee on Hospital Care, a branch of the American Hospital Association, is encouraging the development of psychiatric wards in general hospitals. Training centers are being established to train psychiatrists and nurses. One such center is the Menninger Foundation School of Psychiatrists at Winter General Hospital and the Topeka State Hospital, both located near Topeka, Kansas.

State and local societies for mental health and other citizen groups are active in expanding facilities in their local communities for the treatment and care of the mentally ill. Many of these local mental health organizations are sponsored by the Community Chest and may include an adult and child guidance clinic, a family service agency, a day center for the aging, and community service organization. There is usually a long waiting list applying for these services. Some state societies are organized by professional persons; in others laymen carry on the work. In many communities various organizations, clubs, lodges, parent-teacher associations, and churches have programs that are concerned either directly or indirectly with mental health. These programs include presentation of facts, exchange of ideas, problems and their partial solutions, and surveys to discover local mental health problems. Each group actively cooperates in an effort to solve its problems. Such groups also work for the improvement of mental institutions, strive for enlightened legislation, help to establish centers for prevention and research, and educate others regarding the steps leading to good mental health.

National organizations have developed programs of public education for the improvement of services to the mentally ill. The National Committee for Mental Health works for the conservation of mental health, the reduction and prevention of mental disorders and defects, improved care and treatment of persons suffering from mental diseases, special training and supervision for the feeble-minded, and provision of reliable information concerning these subjects. The National Mental Health Foundation sponsors a nationwide program of public education to create a better understanding of mental disorders, and methods of prevention and cure. Its purpose is to correct false beliefs about mental ailments, to cooperate with other agencies in stimulating research and training, to provide better care and treatment for the mentally afflicted, and to replace outmoded laws with enlightened legislation.

Mental health is a problem of the entire world; this fact precipitated the adoption of international measures for mental health. The Expert Committee on Mental Health of the World Health Organization had its first meeting in 1949 to formulate and agree upon principles and priorities in mental health work. In view of the tremendous needs and the present shortage of psychiatric personnel and facilities throughout the world, the Committee decided that it would be impossible to provide therapeutic facilities for all the needy people in the world. The Committee therefore suggested preventive measures for the ultimate solution of the mental-illness problem. The group emphasized the importance of public health and community programs to promote mental health.

Other international organizations involved in promoting mental health include the UNESCO (United Nations Educational, Scientific, and Cultural Organization) Project on International Tensions, which is probably the most elaborate international project involving psychiatric factors, and the World Federation for Mental Health, which is a group of nongovernmental organizations concerned with promoting mental health.

RECOVERY INC.

Recovery Inc. is a nonprofit organization offering a proven method of self-help after-care to prevent chronicity in nervous patients and relapses in former mental patients. The group is nonsectarian, even though a meeting place may be in a church or synagogue. Recovery Inc. was organized in 1937 by a small group of patients of the late Abraham A. Low, M.D., Associate Professor of Psychiatry at the University of Illinois Medical School. Dr. Low developed the Recovery techniques after many years of research study and treatment of patients. The self-help after-care method is based on Dr. Low's book, *Mental Health Through Will Training.*

Recovery helps those who want to help themselves. Regular attendance at meetings, study of the literature, and practice of the techniques are all a necessary part of the Recovery training. In weekly group meetings, which last about two hours, members help each other by giving examples of how they have practiced the Recovery Method in facing and handling specific difficulties. The meetings are conducted by veteran members who have received extensive training in demonstrating the Recovery Method. Recovery offers no quick and easy method that will immediately banish your symptoms and fears. However, those who have patiently practiced Recovery's self-help methods and have participated regularly in the group meetings have proved that the Recovery Method really works.

Any fear you may have about attending your first Recovery meeting is average. You may think that you are the only person in the world who suffers from these fearful thoughts and feelings, but you will begin to feel more secure when you meet others who have had, or are now having, similar difficulties. People are not expected to participate in the meeting until they have read a portion of Dr. Low's book. Even then, participation is voluntary. Feel free to have a friend or relative accompany you to Recovery meetings. Recovery does not supplant the physician. Each member is expected to follow the authority of his own physician or other professional. The Recovery Method supplies training in self-help and self-leadership. It does not offer advice, diagnosis, treatment, or counseling. Recovery is a program for adults—available to those 18 years of age or older.

It is impossible to "explain" Recovery in an information letter of this kind. It is also impossible for you to "understand" Recovery by attending one meeting. Attend Recovery meetings regularly in order to give Recovery a fair trial and yourself this opportunity to regain and maintain good mental health. For information concerning meeting locations and a list of literature write:

Recovery Inc. Headquarters
116 South Michigan Avenue
Chicago, Illinois 60603

Regional Centers for the Mentally Retarded

California's Regional Centers culminate many efforts to resolve a problem: when a family is unable to care for a person with mental retardation, should the state provide a single alternative—placement in a state hospital away from home and family? State hospitals do provide countless services. They must act as a school, a boarding home, a sheltered workshop, and a way station before transfer to a foster home or other community facility. However, more than half of the retarded persons do not need hospitalization. What they usually need is a variety of resources in the community to enable the individual and his family to obtain the best care and to maximize the retarded person's capabilities, at a cost and convenience his family can afford. Regional centers provide not only other alternatives, but a system to overcome some of the difficulties experienced by families of a retarded person.

For parents eager to keep their retarded child at home, or at least in the community, searching for answers can be a full-time occupation. Community resources are being developed constantly. The typical family, uncertain and harried, may consult several physicians seeking diagnostic confirmation, treatment, genetic counseling, therapists, school, and recreational and vocational avenues. They want respite from continuous responsibility. They must decide what care or service is needed, and then find someone to provide it. And, in all cases, the burden of paying for so many specialized types of care falls originally on the family (certain handicaps or degree of retardation are ineligible for much federal or state financial assistance). For most families, the cost of caring for a mentally retarded person can eat up savings as well as income. Ultimately, the family must seriously consider the question, "Who will care for my child when I am no longer able to?"

PROBLEMS OF THE VERY YOUNG AND THE VERY OLD

The very young and the very old have many similar physical and emotional characteristics and problems. Both are striving for independence, security, self-esteem, attention, and love. Since this text does not allow for a full discussion of all aspects of mental health, the author has chosen these two important and often neglected age groups to examine in detail.*

Child Guidance

From the moment of birth, a child begins to cope with his environment in an effort to maintain an equilibrium of constantly varying and changing forces. In a state of absolute stability there would be no growth or development, either physical or psychological. Conflict usually begins and exists for a time outside the child before it becomes internalized. Emotional disorders are due to the inevitable and characteristic conflicts associated with the various stages of psychological development. They are usually temporary, and within certain limits are regarded as phenomena of general development. Emotional health involves adapting or functioning in one's environment, forming ap-

---

*For a more thorough discussion, refer to Smolensky, J.: *A Guide to Child Growth and Development.* Dubuque, Iowa, Kendall/Hunt, 2nd edition, 1977.

propriate relationships with people, being able to perceive and evaluate the world of external reality, and fulfilling one's ability and individuality.

Psychological disorders, which are manifestations of internal emotional illness, are serious and difficult to treat. Conflicts exist within the personality structure, as it has developed out of the interaction of the child and his environment. Through the mental mechanisms of identification, the attitudes and traits of the parents and other significant persons in the child's life normally become internalized to form parts of the ego (sense of reality) and superego (conscience and ideals). As long as the state of tension or the psychological equilibrium of the child is kept within reasonable limits and he gains mastery over the disturbing experiences that inevitably occur in the course of development, the internalization tends to take place gradually and results in a reasonably harmonious internal personality structure.

If, however, the infant or young child experiences too much tension, he internalizes the images derived from his experiences too quickly and unselectively. Although this internalization is aimed at regaining psychological equilibrium, it tends to set up conflicts between the id (primitive urges, drives, and needs), the ego, and the superego in various combinations. For example, a child who feels that his mother is unduly harsh during toilet training may internalize her punitive attitudes to avoid further conflict with her. These attitudes now become a part of his superego, which as a result is set at odds with his normal aggressive drive and his normal id needs for pleasure and gratification; these features are damaging to his developing self-image and self-esteem, which are in the realm of the ego. Thus, what was formerly a conflict with the external world (his mother) has now become an internal or intrapsychic conflict.[6]

The basic images—those of the mother and the self—begin to be established gradually during the symbiotic phase of development. The acute anxiety occurring normally by about 8 or 9 months of age is presumed to be due to the acquisition of sufficiently clear images of mother and self for the infant to realize that his mother is not part of him. It seems probable that it takes a further period, extending well into the period between 12 and 24 months of age, until these first images (both perceptual and emotional) have become sufficiently stable so that the child can call forth a memory of his mother as a kind of reassurance when she is absent from him. Thus he has attained an important step in his psychological independence. Before these images of mother are available from memory, traumatic experiences tend to be felt as a threat or fear of loss of the love object, i.e., the mother. If the traumatic experiences during this period are severe, or if there is unduly prolonged or too-frequent separation from the mother, the effect on the child is proportionately severe.

Rule One:

Severe traumatic experiences occurring in this early period of development cause a psychosis at the time of the trauma, or can predispose the infant to the development of a psychotic disorder at a later age.

After the establishment of reasonably stable and constant images of the mother, traumatic experience causes fear of loss of her love. This is a lesser threat than the threat of losing that love object itself. Ego development and the establishment of basic identity have had a good beginning; the developing personality is well integrated; the child has confidence in people and seeks to continue receiving love from them; and his good relations with the outside world facilitate his adaptation. Now, when he and his environment are in conflict, his wish to continue receiving love causes him to attempt to control and modify the impulses and feelings that are bringing him into conflict with his parents. But since the traumatic experience has caused an excessive amount of conflict and tension, he cannot manage himself by normal defensive and adaptive techniques, and he exhibits symptoms.

Rule Two:

Traumatic experiences occurring after the establishment of stable images and reasonably adequate relations with people either cause neurosis at the time of the trauma, or predispose to the development of a neurotic disorder at a later age.[7]

Another concept pertaining to the child's ability to cope with the environment is that of "phase-specificity." This concept holds that an experience will be particularly traumatic if it happens to impinge on those developing functions which characteristically are most heavily instinctually and psychically energized (libido) in the particular stage during which the child suffers the experience. For example, a fracture of the jaw in an 11-month-old infant at the time he is being weaned, which forces him abruptly to give up his oral gratification, could be severely traumatic. On the other hand, the same injury in a child 3 years of age is not likely to have the same effect, because he is beyond the oral stage of development. An operation performed on a child 5 or 6 years of age, who at that age is normally greatly concerned about injury to his body or his genitals, is likely to have threatening implications that it might not have when the child has reached the age of 9 or 10 years. It is because of the concept of phase-specificity of trauma that the psychologically oriented physician may advise postponement of certain surgical or medical procedures (provided postponement is not detrimental to health) until the child has entered another stage of development.

In general terms, the kinds of environmental influences to be considered are (1) understimulation, (2) overstimulation, (3) emotional deprivation, (4) overindulgence, (5) overprotection, (6) too little challenge, (7) undue pressure, (8) inconsistency, either in the same parent or between the parents, (9) excessive conflict and tension in the home atmosphere, (10) unconscious approval by the parents of behavior that they consciously disapprove of (the child acts in accordance with the unconscious or true attitude of his parents).

It is important and necessary to differentiate between environmental influences and innate personality factors that exist in the child and/or parent. The most crucial qualities in the make-up of the child are the following, as suggested by Anna Freud. These important qualities are determined both by constitution and by environmental influences and experience.

Intensity of Drives and Needs. The needs of the undemanding child may go unrecognized and therefore unmet. The overdemanding child, on the other hand, because he is difficult to satisfy and to manage, may cause anxiety or other feelings in the parent, which secondarily will disturb the parent-child relationship.

Ability to Tolerate Frustration. The child who can tolerate frustration has less need to resort to the use of pathologic defenses.

Willingness to Accept Substitutes. The child who cannot accept a substitute, whether this is a substitute parent such as a babysitter, or substituted food, toys, or activities, remains tied to the frustration, and tensions increase.

Ability to Tolerate Anxiety. The ability to tolerate tension and anxiety and to control urges and feelings without repressing them and making them unconscious enables the child to face difficulties, to learn to interpose thought between the urge to act and action, to give and take and to negotiate with his parents and other people.

Most juvenile delinquents, for example, have not been able to properly develop and balance their primitive urges (id), their sense of reality (ego), or their conscience and ideals (superego). Their inability to cope with certain environmental problems and to resolve internal conflicts results in inappropriate behavior. One or more of the following four traits are often seen in dealing with delinquents:

1. Immaturity—"I want it now!"
2. Impulsiveness—striking out.
3. Passivity—seldom completes work or tasks.
4. Aggressiveness—destructive, high-amplitude behavior.

It has been said that neurotic adults were neurotic children. For example:

1. Jim, a 30-year-old bachelor, was raised by an overprotective mother, who did everything for him. He is now set in his ways and is looking for a girl who typifies his mother, but simultaneously dislikes what his mother has done to him. Finally he marries, and now "spoils" his newborn baby girl, giving her all the affection he couldn't give to other women.

2. Jack's mother often commented, "No girl is good enough for my little boy." Jack was hypercritical of all women, and when he finally did marry, he frequently and overtly criticized his wife.

3. Sue, having marital problems, sought security in her children. Her children fulfilled her needs, but unfortunately the children never acquired independence, nor were they allowed to fulfill their own needs.

4. Some women, who as children lacked attention and affection from their fathers, must now prove their femininity.

5. Some men, who as children were "put down" by their fathers and thus devel-

oped feelings of inadequacy and insecurity, must now prove their masculinity. Their idea of a "real man" involves physical and athletic prowess, and unfortunately much in our society today reinforces this concept.

Many children with behavior problems have not been exposed to consistent limits or adequate structure. They have failed to learn that freedom necessitates responsibility; limits and boundaries foster security. Limitations are necessary to anchor the child to reality. Appropriate structure is necessary (especially today in this era of confusion) for a child to deal with things commensurate with his capabilities. Without an external structure and set of standards, frustration, inner conflict, and poor self-image join forces to create a child with inappropriate behavior. These children must then be guided, with firmness, trust, and confidence, through a program that sets definite limits and structures for them.

In order to understand the activities and reactions of a child, the therapist must have three fundamental attributes: (1) patience, (2) faith in the child's ability to solve his own problems, and (3) the ability to see the problems through the child's own eyes.

The number of children and young people seeing psychiatrists and counselors has increased dramatically during the past decade. This doesn't necessarily mean that today's young are more confused or reflect the turmoil and unrest of the 1960's and 1970's. There are many reasons for this increase:

1. Parents and allied health professionals are more aware of and more knowledgeable about emotional disorders of children.
2. It is more acceptable for parents to seek help for their children today.
3. A variety of mental health facilities are currently provided within the community.

Self-Esteem

The most important goals to be achieved by the growing child are a sense of self-esteem, individuality, and recognition that people are important to each other. These characteristics become most valuable in later life in dealing with the responsibilities of college, work, marriage, and parenthood. This self-sufficiency does not simply appear with increasing age, but is the outcome of the successful handling of the child's changing needs and his mastery of the challenges of his environment. We are continually positively reinforcing and guiding the child toward independence, balance, and security within his potential. Meanwhile, we are cultivating his natural desire to learn.

The feeling of personal worth plays a crucial role in human happiness and effectiveness. Clinicians are well aware in a general way that many of the disturbed patients who come to them for treatment feel themselves to be incompetent and socially rejected. It is universally recognized that self-confidence and an optimistic assessment of one's abilities contribute markedly to business success and the formation of friendships. There is also a popular belief, less firmly based, that the development of self-esteen depends on physical attractiveness, ability, social status, and material welfare. Perhaps the most important thing any parent can do for any child at any age is to try to give him a good self-image. The idea of his own self, how he sees himself and feels about himself, in large part determines what he will attempt to achieve and the degree of his success. It is important that parents have good images of themselves; this encourages children to improve their self-image.

Self-esteem is based chiefly on two concepts: "I am lovable" and "I am worthwhile." It isn't so much what we say to our children that influences their feelings of self-acceptance as it is a matter of how we treat ourselves. One important principle is to make only reasonable demands (with regard to age and individuality) that children can fulfill. This helps the child make reasonable demands of himself. A child, however, must be able to handle failure before he can enjoy success. Some general rules on what parents should *not* do are as follows:

1. Don't reason with your child to show him that he shouldn't be disappointed at his failure.
2. Don't put him off with clichés, such as "everything's for the best."
3. Don't point out to him how you would have acted differently.
4. Don't try to improve his personality by telling him how he should have behaved.
5. Don't minimize the situation, as if his failure really didn't matter.
6. Don't immediately try to cheer him up. Give him a chance to express his disappointment and sorrow.

If a parent can learn to meet and accept his child's failure comfortably, chances are the child will come to terms with his problem. However, the parent who meets a failure with disappointment, chagrin, and anger—all expressed directly or indirectly, whether knowingly or not, by words and actions—can quite likely guarantee a repetition. The parent's own fear of failure—in his role as a parent, or in his fear of his child's repeating his mistakes—is basic to the problem of assuring the child's success or failure.

The 2-Year Old (Autonomy)

In the early months of the second year, the baby who trusts himself and the world is ready to concentrate on the next stage in personality growth, the development of autonomy. He is mobile, feeds himself, expresses himself with a few choice words, and has many choices to make. The sense of being unique and having the freedom to make choices is a vital part of being human. Choosing involves taking or leaving, holding onto or letting go. When the child discovers, through experience, that there are many situations in which he can choose and live comfortably with his choice, then he feels good about himself. He can decide whether to sit on grandpa's lap or not, and whether to play with a friend or not. He gets the feeling that "What I do is all right" and "There are many things I can do or not do." A child should be encouraged to express his opinions without fear of reprisal.

He also needs restrictions that are clear and firm, in order to prevent him from making choices that are too difficult for him. Frustration and consequent anger are frequent even in older infants who are guided with skill and understanding. Temper outbursts increase in the latter part of infancy, as the child tests himself to find out what he can do and tests his parents and his world to find out what they will let him do. Each successful encounter and choice adds to his sense of autonomy. Shame and doubt arise when disaster follows choice making and also when the child is not allowed to make enough choices. Shame, doubt, and inadequacy (lack of autonomy) lead to extremes of behavior—rebellion or oversubmissiveness, hurling or hanging on tight.*

"Me do" is the keynote phrase of the age from 18 months to 2½ years. Two-year-olds are determined to do things in their own ways at their own times. The doing and the choosing are the means of growth, for these are the ways in which toddlers test themselves, other people, and the world in order to establish themselves as creatures who function independently and adequately.

No-No

Somewhere in the second year of life, however, the child will go through a period of saying "no" to everything. Many mothers mistakenly take this to mean that the child is "stubborn" or "wayward" and needs to be taught to obey or he will grow up out of control. It is very easy to misinterpret this stage of development. But the "no-no" period is actually a time when the child himself is struggling to master certain controls over his own bodily functions and assessing the requirements of his environment. When he says "no," he is really saying, "I have to do it my way, not yours." He may also grasp everything in sight and say "mine." He is beginning to understand his identity and claim his territory. Also, at this stage the child is learning self-identity versus social conformity. (He will also go through this stage as a teenager.) Negative self-identity is part of the struggle for positive self-identity. At the same time, however, he must learn to conform to what society (primarily parents) expect of him. Although seeking independence, he sometimes reverts back to babyish dependence on mother.

---

*The period of development of trust is the *oral stage* in psychoanalytic theory. The mouth is the site of the most important experiences; feeding and the love relationship associated with feeding. Pain from teething is associated with biting and cruel, harsh experiences. In many psychoanalytic writings the skin senses and other senses, too, are greatly overshadowed by the significance of the mouth.

The period of autonomy is the *anal stage* in psychoanalytic theory. The central problem is dramatized by the ideal of the anal sphincters, which open or shut, hanging on or letting go. Depending on the child's experiences with bowel control and control by other people, his personality takes on characteristics like suspicion or confidence, stinginess or generosity, doubt and shame, or autonomy and adequacy.

The danger of this period is that mother and child can get involved in direct struggles over bedtime routines, toilet training, or eating habits. Instead, the parents may be wiser to find alternatives and substitutions that will avoid making an issue of every matter. Tactful parents find ways to present matters so that the young child thinks he is making the decisions and thus remains generally cooperative. In addition, the child's motor development at this age is more active, and there are certain times of frustration at not being able to do certain tasks.

Problems and Suggestions

Parents can make too many demands for control and conformity, and the child can become overcontrolled. This could lead to timid, unaggressive behavior, and as an adult he will be afraid to venture into the world. The child experiencing overcontrol may appear outwardly to conform, but he is actually containing his hostility and anger. He will insidiously break or destroy something, pinch his baby brother, or engage in some hostile or destructive act. Such a child may mature to be a self-righteous, narrow-minded moralist hiding his inner hostility.

On the other hand, parents who set limits, but then relax or reverse these limits, may find a confused, disrespectful teenager in trouble who is looking for someone to enforce the limits. As an adult he may be continuously late for work, for example, and criticize the employer's time rule, not himself. He may argue with everyone, and have a tendency to say no on all occasions. Often a pet (dog or cat) will be useful in teaching a child control and responsibility; it also means providing love, tenderness, comfort, and food. One of the greatest charms of owning a pet is that the pet offers companionship without bossiness. The child becomes boss of the animal, and reprimands are a common outlet, without the loss of the animal's love for him. Parents, however, must survive the relationship and help the child gain control over possible aggressions and cruelty to the pet.

Positive Self-Image and Limits

As previously stated, one of the major objectives in early childhood education is to help the child have a good image and feeling about himself. Shortly after the walking stage (around 1 year of age), the child finds himself enthused about prospective experimentation, testing, and adventures, while simultaneously being confronted with a new set of limits and boundaries. The "no-no" and "don't be a bad boy" syndrome, unless balanced by positive reinforcement when appropriate, can help initiate a child's poor image about himself. In refusing to accept this negative role, many children insist that they are not bad and instead project and transfer the bad image: their "brother or sister is bad," "the dolls are bad," "the cat is bad"; they may refer to a host of other animate or inanimate objects. In addition, the guilt feelings are inextricably linked to fear, and children may feel that they should be punished for their misdeeds and therefore are afraid of the dark, monsters, and the unknown. This can immobilize a child for long periods of time, and possibly extend into his adult life.

Limits, however, play an important part in the child's developing self-esteem and self-confidence. Establishing controls helps the child to meet new experiences successfully, gain security and confidence, and formulate his own rules. It is interesting and important to note that children playing a group game will quickly make up their own rules if none have been presented to them. Rules, therefore, help in giving the child respect for his individual rights and the rights of others.

One way to reduce guilt in early childhood is to prevent the child from doing wrong rather then letting him do the naughty thing and then shaming him. A 2-year-old has very little respect for authority and is developing a strong urge to assert his independence. His inclination, therefore, is to defy his mother. Removing temptations, distracting him, and continuously verbalizing the prohibition are helpful. As the child grows older, positive suggestions are most useful. Rather than say, "You are rude, selfish, and mean, and no one will like you because you don't wash your hands," we explain that "We wash our hands to keep clean and healthy." Negative statements can convince a child that he is unattractive and has an evil personality. A negative attitude also reflects the parents' lack of confidence in their own upbringing. Parents and teachers must continually help children cope with their negative images of themselves. The missing teeth at age 6, the glasses at age 7, being too short, too tall, unpopular, too thin, too fat—these are all difficult things for children to cope with. We must continually reinforce positive aspects of growth and development at each stage.

Gerontology

In the United States today, there are over 20 million people who are over 65 years of age. This represents over 10 per cent of the total population, and the figure is increasing as the average life expectancy increases and birth rates decline. The vast majority of these 20 million people face major social, economic, and health-related problems. Oriental and African cultures venerate the aged and the process of aging. Parents and grandparents in these cultures are considered to speak with the voice of time and to limit impetuosity with wisdom. Other nations, such as the Scandinavian countries, provide excellent medical care for their aged.

In our mobile, youth-oriented society, however, few old people can be cared for by members of their own family or have adequate resources to purchase needed care. Instead of the dignity that the older citizen has earned, there is more often desperation born of economic and psychological insecurity. The warmth of familial love and companionship is too often replaced with the chill of social and institutional segregation.

In order to counteract these problems, many communities have established multiservice community centers which provide senior citizens with a permanent fixed location in which they are able to develop physical and emotional security. Many communities also offer senior citizens various financial discounts (for transportation, movies, restaurants, television repair), as well as opportunities for a variety of social functions. The senior citizen once again finds himself in a valuable social and perhaps occupational position. A multiservice center provides older people with opportunities to take themselves out of the status placed on them by society and to raise their level of self esteem and independence. It can provide them with the respect, self-confidence, and happy lives that they really deserve.

Growing older is a tender, emotional process. It is a time in which a person can use his years of experience, wisdom, and understanding, to become an active, alive, and enjoyable person. Any action that enhances the dignity of older Americans enhances the dignity of all Americans, for unless the American Dream comes true for our older generation, it cannot be complete for any generation. One generation must care for the next.

Homemaker Service

There are millions of totally disabled persons who are unable to care for themselves and are dependent upon help from others. Yet, for these aged and disabled, maintaining a home of their own is perhaps the primary factor in maintaining personal dignity, self-assurance, and contentment. The Social Security Amendments of 1962 and the Older Americans Act of 1965 provided new means with which to help the aged and disabled toward self-care and independency. Many states have implemented a program of in-home supportive services to help aged, blind, and disabled adults remain in or return to their own homes.

The appropriate social service staff of a welfare agency establishes with applicants their need for the service, develops a suitable plan to meet the need, assigns and supervises the homemaker or chore service providers, and periodically evaluates whether the help given meets the needs of its recipients. Homemaker services generally include the physically or mentally handicapped person. The homemaker is trained to go into the client's home and help him learn to effectively manage his home environment, given his particular needs. For some, this may mean rearranging furniture to accommodate a wheelchair; for others, it may involve teaching how to shop for and prepare foods according to special dietary requirements.

Preventive Care

Although Medicare takes care of the elderly once they are ill, it does not encourage them to have the kinds of health checkups suggested for good preventive medical care. A community hospital in a small town in the state of Washington has instituted an "Eldercare" program, which provides for monthly health examinations for senior citizens at only six dollars each. The examinations are offered during the facility's nonpeak periods, in order to take the best advantage of the time and talents of the hospital staff. Each month a different kind of examination is scheduled, for example: March—Pap smears and prostate examinations; April—chest x-rays; May—blood tests and urinalysis; June—eye examinations; and so on for a 12-month cycle which begins again the following January. For full information about Eldercare, write to Administrator, Prosser Memorial Hospital, Prosser, Washington 99350.

Psychogeriatrics

In dealing with the aged, a number of issues repeatedly emerge and deserve special focus for maximum effectiveness:

1. To be old is not synonymous with illness and pain. The therapist has an opportunity to discredit this mythology of aging, since it is clear that many elderly persons will act old if that is the expectation communicated by families, friends, and physicians.

2. When using medication, especially psychoactive drugs, there is a possibility of paradoxic and idiosyncratic reactions to very small amounts of chemical agents. There is also a tendency for elderly persons to hoard medications, developing their own private pharmacy, with the risk of polypharmacy and all of its potential hazards of drug interactions and overdose.

3. The therapist must be able to recognize in himself feelings of anxiety which arise from his own identification with the elderly person. If he has not adequately dealt with his own problems of aging and death, his discomfort may hinder his effort to provide an optimal therapeutic relationship.

4. Much of the stress in old age results from conflicts that have remained inadequately resolved throughout the person's life. The same rigorous problem-solving techniques of diagnosis must be applied in evaluating the elderly person as are applied in evaluating any other person.

5. Elderly patients may present themselves as helpless. But the aged are not children. Care should be taken to avoid the temptation to take over, make their decisions for them, and create dependence, with consequent loss of self-esteem and depression.

6. The focus should not be limited to illness but should include support of the individual's strengths and belief in his own internal resources.

BODY CHANGES IN AGING*

Body System	Some of the Changes in "Normal Aging"
Skin and subcutaneous tissues	The skin becomes lax, inelastic, dry, and wrinkled; there is graying or whitening with progressive loss or thinning of hair; old people sweat less than younger ones.
Musculo-skeletal system	Changes in appearance and limitations in mobility occur with the stooped posture, stiffened joints and porous bone structure characteristic of advancing age.
Nervous system	Reflexes are slower with a concomitant decrease of responses to various stimuli; there may be tremors; with alterations in facial expression and mental reactions.
Special senses	The senses—hearing, sight, taste, smell, touch, balance—become less sharp with age.
Cardiovascular system	There is a decline in cardiac output at rest; there is a progressive increase in peripheral resistance to the flow of blood, and a tendency for increased systolic blood pressure.
Respiratory system	The following components of the respiratory system may show age-related impairments: ventilation (breathing), diffusion (exchange of oxygen and carbon dioxide between lungs and blood), and pulmonary circulation.
Gastro-intestinal tract	The stomach shows a reduction in gastric motility, with an increased tendency towards achlorohydria (loss of digestive acid) and a reduction in gastric volume; there is diminished peristalsis, which may be responsible for the constipation that is common in old people; hemorrhoids may develop.

Urinary tract	Filtration rate in the kidney and renal blood flow are diminished; polyuria (excessive urination) and nocturia (nighttime urination) are common.
Reproductive organs	With advancing years, the capacity for reproduction ebbs—earlier in the female than in the male; however, sexual needs and desires do not undergo an abrupt change, and sexual activity may continue long after reproductive powers have diminished.
Endocrine system	Structural changes occur in the endocrine glands, which indicates there may be a central endocrine deficit.
Hemopoietic system	There appears to be a diminished leucocytic response to infection; responses of the lymphoid system appear to diminish with age.
Nutrition and Metabolism	Digestive processes slow down, and food habits change.

*United States Department of Health, Education, and Welfare: *Working with Older People. Vol. 1: The Practitioner and the Elderly.* Washington, D.C.: Government Printing Office, PHS Pub: 1459, March, 1971, pp. 12–21.

SENIOR CITIZEN'S CHARTER

1. The right to be useful.
2. The right to obtain employment, based on merit.
3. The right to freedom from want in old age.
4. The right to a fair share of the community's recreational, educational, and medical resources.
5. The right to obtain decent housing suited to needs of later years.
6. The right to the moral and financial support of one's family, in keeping with the best interest of the family.
7. The right to live independently as one chooses.
8. The right to live and die with dignity.
9. The right to access to all the knowledge that is available on how to improve the later years of life.

RESOURCES COMPILED BY BERKELEY GROUP

A good example of grass-roots production for the benefit of the elderly is Resources for Growing Old in Berkeley. The Senior Citizen's Committee of the Berkeley League of Women Voters has produced a 12-page digest of 13 voluminous reports that their members put together after an in-depth study of the problems of aging. The digest includes listings of resources as well as narratives on such subjects as mental health, loneliness, income, transportation, death and dying, and safety. It was produced by members of the league, who are admittedly amateurs but who have done a better job than many governmental professionals, according to some reviews.

The Berkeley League of Women Voters does not have funds for free posting, but they will send you a single copy if you will enclose a 10 cent stamp with your order; additional copies of the Directory of Resources cost 20 cents each, plus postage. Send your inquiry—and money—to the League of Women Voters of Berkeley, 1836 University Avenue, Suite B, Berkeley, California 94703.

DRUG ABUSE

The problem of drug abuse is serious and immensely complex. Strenuous governmental efforts to control the supply of dangerous substances have not produced the necessary results. Stringent laws and severe penalties have failed to prevent the promotion of the use of dangerous substances and the sale of dangerous substances to youth, even on school grounds. Adult society, through its widespread acceptance of self-administered drugs and its wholesale use of various chemical euphoriants, is setting a bad example for children and youth. Advertising is all too often a purveyor of the idea that pills are the best answer to many of man's problems. The press and other mass media of communication all too often sensationalize drug abuse and, in so doing, make it appear attractive. It is obvious, then, that the problem of drug abuse has not been solved by legislation and that society is not only failing to check the spread of drug abuse but in some ways may even be promoting such abuse. Increasingly, therefore, governmental officials, professional people, and other citizens are looking forward to education as the best hope for stamping out the uniquely modern affliction of drug abuse among youth.[8]

Education for Drug Abuse

Education begins in the home at a *very early age.* This means that parents must understand and practice the guiding principles involved in child growth and development. We must give parents the opportunities to listen and be informed, to be heard, and to become actively involved.

This might involve community child growth and development seminars or classes where such topics are discussed:

1. Stages of growth and development (physiological and emotional)
2. Changing values and implications
3. How to communicate with your child
4. How to listen to your child
5. Discipline
6. Responsibility
7. Behavior modification techniques (simplified)
8. Experimentation and peer group participation
9. The meaning of maturity
10. Angry acts versus angry feelings

In any case, emphasis *must* be placed upon truth, trust, consistency, and love.

This also means we must continually examine, evaluate and change our educational framework and curriculum, at all levels. We are striving to raise children who are well informed with factual information, who have been exposed to many experiences and to all sides of many issues, who have the opportunity to freely and openly discuss these issues, and who adopt a strong set of values based on these experiences. Then, and only then, will we be confident that most children will make the right decisions most of the time.

Values, however, are changing very rapidly in our society today. Unfortunately, the transition from one set of "old family" values that were good enough in the "good old days" to the new set of values necessary to cope with the "now society" leaves many individuals with a sense of frustration and guilt feelings that cause other problems. Many students and younger persons are emotionally confused by their current beliefs and actions on the one hand, and their complete abandonment of their parents' values and attitudes. To further confuse the issue, "middle-class advertisements" are not consistent with ideals and values espoused by many in that group: Cigarette ads linked to springtime, freshness, and sex; beer ads that remind us we only go around once – grab all the gusto you can get; pills to put you to sleep, and pills to wake you up.

In any case, most persons agree that "love" helps you attain inner strength and peace. Two psychiatrists, who report that they have undertaken the first scientific study of love, say people in love have sharpened senses, expanded interests, and gain new dimensions to their thinking, feelings, and behavior. Other changes included: new directions, new enterprises, new social relationships, more friendly attitudes and a sharpened sense of humor. Can anyone in any generation deny that love is a most positive experience in our lives?[9]

Legislation for Drug Abuse

Controls over the abuse of chemicals are necessary, but simply passing laws is rarely a final solution. The abuse of alcohol was not solved by the Volstead Prohibition Act; indeed, it bred crime and provoked disrespect for the law. More successful, but hardly curative, was the Harrison Narcotics Act, which reduced the number of cocaine and opiate users but created a criminal hierarchy supported by those locked into heroin. The Pure Food and Drug laws successfully swept unstandardized, mislabeled, and falsely advertised nostrums from the shelves of the grocer and druggist. Why the varying degrees of success of the three laws? The amount of public support is one part of the answer. Whether the substance is culture-alien or culturally accepted is another. The third part of the answer involved a major task of our day. It is to teach the young how to live in a changing world and how to establish new goals when the old ones become threadbare and irrelevant.

We perennially forget the cyclic nature of a man's development. A young person is more curious, less cautious, more impulsive, more willing to take a chance, and certainly more idealistic. Many youths are fascinated by mind-changing drugs, especially the new ones. Their elders are appalled by the dangerous exploration of insufficiently studied chemicals. As the young grow and mature, they tend to withdraw from the chemical roulette. When they become parents, they are dismayed in turn by the goings-on of their children. The generation gap is the distance between the parents' forgetting and their children's not knowing.[10]

Methadone Programs

Drs. Dole and Nyswander in New York pioneered a new concept in the treatment of heroin addiction—that if heroin addicts cannot function without the drug, they might function well with a synthetic substitute. Methadone, a synthetic narcotic, is a long-acting medicine that is taken only once a day by mouth. When administered properly, it does not produce the "high" that heroin causes when injected into the vein, but it relieves the addict's hunger or craving. After the dose of methadone is stabilized, the addict simply feels normal. Even an injection of heroin no longer gives the usual euphoria, since the individual's body is tolerant to the effects of the daily medication. Methadone "blocks" the action of heroin. A promising substitute for methadone is propoxyphene napsylate (PN) known by the trade name Darvon N.

Preliminary reports from New York, Chicago, Minneapolis, New Orleans, and San Francisco have been favorable (although not unanimous). In Washington, D.C., for example, heroin arrests and property index crimes recently decreased for the first time since 1966. This happens to coincide with the time the local methadone program was instituted. Many clinics have been established in conjunction with local health departments. To be eligible, the person must have hard-core heroin addiction with one or more failures to remain off the drug after treatment; be 18 years of age or older, and be a resident of the county. The results of three consecutive daily urinalyses must show positive for narcotics, and the patient must take part in the treatment voluntarily. The long-term success of any methadone program, however, involves more than stopping the usage of heroin. It also involves a program of successful rehabilitation, within which problems involving employment, family relationships, and so forth can be solved. Help with these problems is offered in each methadone clinic.

Drug Abuse in the Western World[11]

The entire Western world is experiencing a major epidemic of drug abuse. Drug abuse is best defined as the use of drugs in a manner which may be calculated to produce harm. This definition purposefully excludes any elements of basic law or medical practice. In all of recorded history, there always has been drug abuse and a hard core of drug abusers. There is no reason to believe that this will not always be true.

The reasons for the current epidemic include the following:

1. The number of drugs and their availability has increased. Improved means of transportation, communication, supply, and purchasing power are compounded by the increased variety of drugs synthesized by modern chemistry laboratories.

2. Our society includes the largest number of anxious, lonely, bored, and purposeless people ever. These settings, with lack of goal commitment, often precede drug abuse.

3. The "pious pushers" of the medical pharmaceutical, advertising, and mass media industries have created a "cradle to the grave," drug-based society and have nurtured all of us with the concept of "better living through chemistry" and "take Sominex (scopolamine aminoxide hydrobromide, methapyrilene hydrochloride, and salicylamide) tonight and sleep, safe and restful, sleep, sleep, sleep." From the first moments of life until the last breath, we all are daily bombarded with the dictum and the example: "You got a problem? We got a pill gonna solve it for you."

4. Young people are protesting current values of society in numerous ways, both violent and nonviolent. For some, the use of drugs forms a method of silent social protest.

5. The age-old desire for experimentation persists, only the agents change.

6. Peer pressure continues to be an important force.

Most drug abusers are adults and most of the abused drugs are legal. In general, adult's drugs are legal and kid's drugs are illegal—yet, they may be the same drugs. This is especially true of the barbiturates and amphetamines. When Dad approaches Junior with a martini in one hand and a cigarette in the other and says: "Boy, don't

Ever wonder
why your kid doesn't
take you seriously when
you lecture him
about drugs?

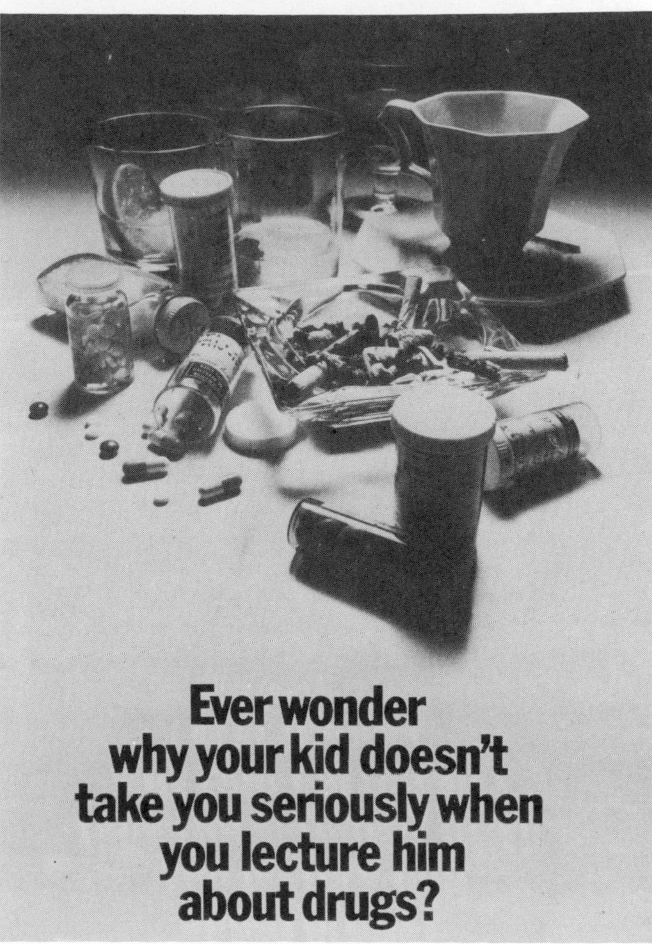

Figure 9–3 (Courtesy of the National Institute of Mental Health, Washington, D.C.)

smoke that joint, it'll hurt you," Junior knows that the martini and cigarette are more likely to hurt his father than is the "grass" (marihuana) to hurt him. Alcohol, tobacco, and sleeping pills kill every day in Los Angeles, usually legally, but there appears never to have been an authenticated case of marihuana killing anyone. Yet, look at which drugs the laws are directed and against whom they are enforced. Ignorance, hypocrisy, and greed are everywhere.

It is obvious that vast change in many areas must precede any real hope for slowing the drug abuse epidemic. What should be done?

First, by research, the scientific community ought rapidly to establish facts that are based on hard data, in perspective. The medical community should then proceed to care for individual patients, without hypocrisy and hang-ups, but with honesty, patience, and understanding. Then, both communities should make major efforts to influence public opinion in order to change the law so that it will reflect the truth.

Second, the efforts of the legal and governing community should be to produce as rapidly as possible good laws based on this data. In order for a law to be effective as a deterrent to crime, it must be accepted by the people as just. Penalties for breaking the law must be in proportion to the harm brought to the criminal, another person, or society as a whole. In almost no instance are existing laws on drugs realistic, valid, or useful.

Third, the prime efforts of law enforcement agencies should be directed against major dealers of truly harmful drugs. They should ignore the user, since his is a medical problem which requires prevention, therapy, or rehabilitation, and is not a criminal act.

Fourth, an immediate major effort should be made by educational institutions to develop young people who are willing and able to face reality without mind- and mood-altering chemicals. They should produce drug education programs aimed at teaching students to "know your poison" so that if drugs are used, they are used with knowledge that minimizes the risk.

Fifth, the primary goal of religious and sociologic organizations should be to change the world so that drug use becomes less necessary. They must attempt to develop mentally healthy people who are individually able to cope with reality.

To treat individual drug abusers, methods must be as varied as the individuals themselves.

Thus, many excellent organizations with widely differing theories and methods recently have arisen and are effective with many people. But, the problem is so massive and the inroads so few. It appears that despite all such efforts, this society, which has failed so miserably in its social, medical and legal handling of alcohol, tobacco, opiates, barbiturates, marihuana, tranquilizers, vapors, amphetamines, and hallucinogens, for the foreseeable future also will fail dismally in its handling of the new agents upon the horizon.

The Community Health Abuse Council

The Community Health Abuse Council (CHAC)* is a unique joint effort by schools and communities to achieve a positive effect on the problems that underly the misuse of chemicals. CHAC has been designed to serve as a coordinating mechanism for community and school programs dealing with the prevention and treatment of health abuse. Within this framework, the Community Health Abuse Council is dedicated to the development and implementation of:

1. *Educational Programs* in the school, the home, and the community.
2. *Counseling and Referral* services for groups, individuals, and families.
3. *Crisis Intervention* assistance to persons who are experiencing acute discomfort resulting from misuse of chemicals or other forms of stress.
4. *Preventive Alternatives* to health abuse and self-destructive behavior.

Some of the Things They Do

Information. Up-to-date information—both printed and verbal—is provided on drugs and alcohol.

Speakers' Bureau. Trained speakers from a variety of disciplines are available for presentations on youth, drugs, and patterns of abuse, new trends in health education, and the Community Health Abuse Council program.

Library Screening and Resource Center. Film and literature evaluation is provided for schools and other agencies. The CHAC resource center offers books, pamphlets, catalogues, and audiovisual materials for use by students, teachers, parents, and others who may be interested.

Educational Programs. CHAC offers parent education programs; workshops and seminars for teachers, counselors, social workers, medics, and law enforcement personnel; symposiums for businesses, industries, civic groups, and service organizations.

Counseling. The Council provides two group counseling sessions weekly (one for juveniles, one for adults); an on-campus counseling service for schools; and individual and family counseling by appointment.

Consultation. CHAC staff are available to schools and other agencies to assist with program planning, curriculum development, case conferences, and staff recruitment and training.

*Similar organizations may be known by different names in different communities.

ALCOHOLISM

Alcohol misuse and alcoholism is a health and social problem of epidemic proportions in the United States, costing the nation $25 billion annually. Following are some of the major findings reported by the National Institute on Alcohol Abuse and Alcoholism:

1. Moderate consumption of alcohol by nonalcoholic persons is generally not harmful. In some cases, such as among the elderly, it may even have beneficial physical, social, or psychological effects.
2. The proportion of American youth who drink has been increasing, and currently it is almost universal. The highest scores on an index of possible problem-drinking behaviors were recorded in the youngest age group for which data are available, the 18- to 20-year-olds.
3. Excessive use of alcohol, especially when combined with tobacco, has been implicated in the development of certain cancers, with nonwhite males appearing to be especially susceptible.
4. Heavy drinking during pregnancy can adversely affect the offspring of alcoholic mothers, but the significance of heredity on alcoholism is as yet unresolved.
5. The public suffers from much ignorance concerning alcohol and ambivalent feelings toward it. Heavier drinkers apparently know less about alcohol than do lighter drinkers or abstainers.
6. The nonexcessive use of alcohol does not appear to affect adversely the overall mortality rate or the mortality from a specific major cause of death, coronary heart disease. There is some evidence that the mortality of drinkers from this cause is lower than that of abstainers and ex-drinkers, but this is not conclusive by any means.

Alcoholism is a treatable illness, but different treatments are required by different persons. Increasingly, individual treatment needs are being determined on the basis of valid studies or clinical experience. Recommendations made by the National Institute on Alcohol Abuse and Alcoholism include the following:

1. Develop new and revised national policies

and guidelines governing the distribution and sale of alcoholic beverages.

2. Extend quality and comprehensive care to alcoholic people through coverage under health and disability benefits and the establishment of standards for care.

3. Demonstrate the values of early identification and treatment programs in business and industry on a national scale.

4. Redouble efforts to decriminalize alcoholism and public intoxication.

Criteria for the Diagnosis of Alcoholism

The American Medical Association, the American College of Physicians, the American Psychiatric Association, and other bodies have long accepted the concept of alcoholism as disease. Now the National Council on Alcoholism has issued a statement listing the criteria for diagnosis of alcoholism. No treatment can be started nor can any preventive or corrective action be initiated unless the problem itself has been confirmed, both in existence and in degree. There is no rigid uniformity in the progress of alcoholism, but since early diagnosis seems to be helpful in treatment and recovery, the disease states have been classified into three diagnostic levels—late, middle, and early. "Late" describes a patient who is definitely alcoholic; "middle" indicates a strong suspicion of probable alcoholism; and "early" points to the potential, possible, or incidental overuse of alcohol.

The criteria have also been separated into major and minor categories. The major criteria have been subdivided into physiological and clinical, behavioral-psychological, and attitudinal symptoms.

Included in the physiological criteria are physiological dependence as evidenced by the withdrawal syndrome, gross tremor, hallucinosis, delirium tremens, evidence of tolerance of the effects of alcohol, alcoholic blackout periods, and finding of a high alcohol level in the blood. Major clinical symptoms associated with alcoholism include alcoholic liver disorders, pancreatitis in the absence of cholelithiasis, chronic gastritis, hematological disorders, Wernicke-Korsakoff syndrome, alcoholic cerebellar degeneration, toxic amblyopia, beriberi, and many others.

The behavioral-psychological category of alcoholism is mainly based on the finding of drinking despite strong medical contraindication known to the patient, and the patient's subjective complaint of loss of control of alcohol consumption.

The list of minor criteria includes such symptoms as the odor of alcohol on the breath at the time of medical appointment, alcoholic extremities, hyper-reflexia, surreptitious or morning drinking, repeated conscious attempts at abstinence, medical excuses from work for a variety of reasons, preference for drinking companions, and character disorders.

The criteria for diagnosis of alcoholism also include a description of methods for diagnosing recovered, arrested alcoholism or alcoholism in remission. Suggestions include evaluation of cross-dependence between drugs and alcohol, and identification of the high-risk individual. Every physician and interested person should become acquainted with this description of symptoms of this common disorder. Reprints of the criteria may be obtained by writing the National Council on Alcoholism, 2 Park Avenue, Suite 1720, New York, New York 10016.

Sociological Aspects of Alcoholism

There are many complex aspects involved in making a person susceptible to alcohol abuse. Genetics plays a part, as do biochemical, psychological, and sociological factors. In the United States, liquor is often regarded as a sign of affluence, masculinity, and good times. Children who drink are often simply following the examples set by their parents. In Italy and Israel, on the other hand, where drinking is an accepted social custom, there is little alcoholism. The reason, perhaps, is that alcohol is considered a companion to a happy occasion. Many other countries, however, have a much worse problem with alcohol than the United States. France, for instance, has the highest rate of alcoholism in the world (an estimated 10 to 12 per cent of the population), and the Soviet Union may not be far behind.

Some experts believe that alcoholism may be encouraged by the destruction of traditional values. Supporting this notion is the experience of the American Eskimos, whose culture has been disrupted more than that of any other ethnic group on the continent. "The major problem may be one of social disintegration," says Dr. Charles Hudson, chief of psychiatric services at the

United States Public Health Service's Alaska Native Medical Center. The original social structure in many places in rural Alaska has been destroyed, much as it has been in central cities, the ghettos, and Appalachia. The things that were important to people have been taken away, and when there's nothing to do, they lose their self-esteem and stay drunk all the time. Also, perhaps once one has an alcoholic label, it becomes more difficult to lose it.

Since 1970, when Congress demonstrated Washington's changed attitude by passing an alcohol abuse and alcoholism act, a score of states have enacted laws that remove drunkenness (though not drunken driving) from the criminal statutes. Thus drunks are no longer put in jail, but are sent instead to a Local Alcoholism Reception Center (or LARC), where they are detoxified. They graduate to "halfway" houses for outpatient treatment. Because LARC makes a strenuous effort to reach alcohol abusers early, the centers can usually help improve the physical condition, earning ability, and family situation for their patients.

Treatment

The American Medical Association has waged a vigorous campaign in recent years to get practicing physicians and general hospitals to treat alcoholism as "an illness that can and should be treated." Although progress has been made in this direction, too many communities and physicians still look upon drunks as having a character problem rather than a health problem. A recent survey revealed that only one-third of the nation's general hospitals will admit patients for treatment of alcoholism. General hospital involvement is crucial because it must appeal to and be accessible for people who already fear the stigma of being institutionalized. Treatment must come from the mainstream of medicine because the problem affects the mainstream of our society.

Once an alcoholic has decided to try to conquer his problem, what kind of treatment programs are available to him and his family? A promising form of treatment gaining increasing acceptance is family therapy, in which both the alcoholic and the other members of the family are seen and counseled. This approach helps the family members solve any problems that arise from the alcoholic person's effect on them, and helps them to create or restore the kind of family atmosphere in which the alcoholic will be strengthened in his efforts to give up his dependency on drink.

Other kinds of treatment (some of them questionable) include electric shocks, drugs, aversion conditioning, individual psychotherapy, group therapy, music therapy, and anti-drinking or limited drinking seminars. Despite lay leadership, Alcoholics Anonymous has apparently achieved a success rate that surpasses those of professional therapies.

FACTS ABOUT ALCOHOLISM

*For every heroin addict in the United States today, there are 15 hard-core alcoholics.

*Alcohol plays a major part in half our highway deaths—about 28,000 each year.

*Drunkenness accounts for one-third of all United States arrests.

*People who abuse alcohol shorten their lives by an average of 10 to 12 years.

*Each year, alcohol drains the national economy of $25 billion in property damage, lost working time, medical bills, and so on.

Do you know someone who needs help with an alcohol problem? Alcoholics Anonymous—perhaps the single most successful weapon in the battle against alcoholism—maintains counseling groups and answering services throughout the country. If you wish to contact a group, or to have an Alcoholics Anonymous member call on you, consult your local telephone directory. If you live in a rural area or small town where there is no AA listing, write for information to AA World Services, Box 459, Grand Central Station, New York, New York 10017. Or phone 212–686–1100.

An Illness

The precept that alcoholism is an illness and should be treated as such is the basis for a joint statement drafted by the American Medical and American Bar Associations. The statement declares alcoholism to be a major health problem . . . says it is due to multiple causes beyond the control of an individual . . . and asserts that alcoholics should receive the same privileges in law and the same opportunities for medical treatment as are accorded to persons with other diseases.

Among other things, the AMA-ABA statement says:

* Alcoholism should be regarded as an illness in medical and hospital care insurance contracts, and should be subject to benefits comparable to those which apply to other chronic illnesses.

* Both public and private general hospitals should accept, on a non-discriminatory basis, patients diagnosed as alcoholics.

*Courses in the prevention, causes, diagnosis and treatment of alcoholism should be developed at medical schools and in hospital training programs.

* State governments should adopt comprehensive legislation covering the problems of alcoholism, including provisions for adequate rehabilitation services and for civil, rather than criminal, commitment for treatment.

* Legislation should provide for civil commitment in cases where the defendant is acquitted of a crime on the grounds of alcoholism.

* Statutes labeling public intoxication a crime should be eliminated.

This statement urges all medical and bar groups to appoint committees to study the problem of alcoholism in their respective areas, with a view to making recommendations to the AMA and ABA.[12]

The eventual eradication of alcoholism as a societal disease presents a problem of far larger dimension and must depend upon what is termed primary prevention. Primary prevention involves a revision of attitudes and environment. If effective barriers against this disease are to be erected, the status of alcohol will have to be altered so that its excessive use will no longer be tolerated. The elimination of alcoholism as the destructive disease it is would necessitate a full measure of public concern and determination, at every level of society, to distinguish between controlled drinking and pathological drinking and to tolerate only the former type. Were such a new social climate to be developed, the only persons to drink excessively would be those unable to control their drinking. Detection then would be a simple, routine matter; the alcoholic would be easily identified and recommended for treatment. The normal use of alcohol need never be condemned, but rejection of its abuse would of necessity be a matter of public responsibility. If this attitude were to prevail in our society, drinking problems would be far more amenable to correction.

Thus society's goal must be to discourage harmful types of drinking and to correct damaging attitudes born of ignorance. A substantial effort must be made to effect a change of social setting. Laws and regulations may be of some assistance in the creation of a more wholesome atmosphere, but obviously their usefulness will be minimal unless they are supported by substantial changes in public attitude. The educational approach, with widespread discussion of drinking patterns, is therefore of primary importance in the pursuit of these objectives.[13]

After having devoted years of comprehensive research to this national problem, the Cooperative Commission on the Study of Alcoholism has offered four important guidelines for the pursuit of changes in American drinking patterns:

1. Reduce the emotionalism associated with alcoholic beverages.
2. Clarify and emphasize the distinctions between acceptable and unacceptable drinking.
3. Discourage drinking for its own sake and encourage the integration of drinking and other activities.
4. Assist young people to adapt themselves realistically to a predominantly "drinking society."

As the report points out, the emotionalism is a product of numerous elements, including (a) continuing disagreement between "drys" and "wets," (b) residues of the Prohibition experience, (c) differences in attitudes toward alcohol between generations, and (d) various symbolic meanings assigned to drinking and abstinence.[14]

Prevention

The director of the National Institute on Alcohol Abuse and Alcoholism (NIAAA), cites the following seven considerations as important in the prevention of alcohol abuse and alcoholism:

1. The decision to drink or not to drink is a personal and private decision.
2. Those who drink should respect the decision of other individuals who choose to abstain.
3. Those who serve alcoholic beverages have a responsibility not to "push" drinks on their guests or customers.
4. The general public should understand the facts concerning alcohol and its effects on the human body.
5. Those who use alcoholic beverages should avoid drunkenness both in public and in private.
6. Adults should be aware of their responsibilities to youth and realize that their example and attitude on drinking greatly shape the drinking habits of youth.
7. The public must begin to understand that the line between alcohol abuse and alcoholism cannot be clearly drawn.[15]

The scope of activities of the Community Prevention Branch of NIAAA is directed to the entire community population. Its goal is to carry out programs that promote the responsible use of alcohol within a community. The emphasis is upon modes of primary prevention contained within all facets of community organization. One mode of community strategy for primary prevention deals with altering the environment in order to eliminate external forces, conditions, or events that encourage the abuse of alcohol. This might include control over advertising, limitation of alcohol content, and restriction on the distribution of alcoholic beverages. It has been suggested that there be a greater tax on alcoholic beverages, since a small percentage of the population purchases a large percentage of the liquor.

NIAAA suggests that community strategy for primary prevention might also deal with strengthening community or individual crisis-meeting resources, for example, by assisting professionals and businesses to assume a more active role in the early identification of mild disorders, the identification of crisis-prone individuals, and the mobilization of services for such people through the transmission of alcohol information via the mass media—newspapers, magazines, radio, television, and motion pictures.

A preventive campaign, presenting both positive and negative aspects of alcohol, should have these primary goals:

1. Encouragement of responsible attitudes toward alcohol use and responsible drinking behavior among those who choose to drink.
2. Identification and broad dissemination of information about alcohol, alcoholism, and patterns of problem drinking.
3. Promotion of self-awareness among drinkers and non-drinkers.
4. Understanding of peer and social pressures and how to deal with them.

Some guidelines for responsible use of alcohol can be offered:

1. Alcohol can serve a positive purpose only when it improves social relationships and does not impair or destroy them.
2. Alcohol should be taken only as an adjunct to an activity, not as the primary focus of action.
3. Everyone who drinks alcohol should be acutely aware of the danger of combining alcohol with other drugs.
4. Human dignity should be enhanced, not destroyed, by the use of alcohol.

For educators who intend to become involved in the teaching and guidance of youth on the subject of alcohol and its use and misuse, the following suggestions are offered:

1. Recognize the fact that, historically, alcohol is the most common drug man has taken to alter his reality. Be aware of the attitudes and assumptions you may exhibit and express. Attempt

to rid yourself of ambivalent attitudes about taking alcohol, or at least be conscious of such feelings. Prepare yourself with facts.

2. Share with youth the positive and negative facts about alcohol so that they will be able to make intelligent decisions. Respect the rights of those who choose not to drink and maintain empathy for those who develop the illness of alcoholism. Communicate by word and example.

3. Discussion of facts is useful, to a point, but young people's decisions concerning alcohol will be determined largely by the values, habits, and attitudes toward responsible behavior and decision-making transmitted by parents and other adults. Young people are seeking answers and searching out adult roles which they can comfortably and safely adopt.[16]

One of the approaches to reaching the individual and helping him solve problems that may result in abusive drinking is known as "values clarification." Values clarification is an education process that focuses on decision-making skills, based on an exploration of personal values and the development of a positive self-concept. It is not a means of changing individuals, but a process for developing their skills to assess goals, work through conflicts, and deal with what is important to them. Using values clarification techniques, people can examine their behavior—which may or may not include drinking behavior—and evaluate it in light of other goals which are important to them.

Since a person's ability to make responsible decisions about alcohol use depends directly on his general decision-making competence, prevention programs are dependent upon a general upgrading of decision-making abilities.

"Twelve Steps"

The "Twelve Steps" are the core of the Alcoholics Anonymous (AA) program of personal recovery from alcoholism. They are presented as suggestions only, based on the trial-and-error experience of early members of Alcoholics Anonymous. They describe the attitude and activities that these early members believe were important in helping them to achieve sobriety. Acceptance of the "Twelve Steps" is not mandatory in any sense. Experience suggests, however, that members who make an earnest effort to follow these steps and to apply them in daily living seem to get far more out of AA than do those members who seem to regard the steps casually. It has been said that it is virtually impossible to follow all the steps literally, day in and day out. While this may be true, in the sense that the Twelve Steps represent an approach to living that is totally new for most alcoholics, many AA members feel that the steps are a practical necessity if they are to maintain their sobriety. Following is the text of the Twelve Steps, which first appeared in "Alcoholics Anonymous," the AA book of experience:

1. We admitted we were powerless over alcohol—that our lives had become unmanageable.
2. Came to believe that a power greater than ourselves could restore us to sanity.
3. Made a decision to turn our will and our lives over to the care of God as we understood Him.
4. Made a searching and fearless moral inventory of ourselves.
5. Admitted to God, to ourselves, and to another human being the exact nature of our wrongs.
6. Were entirely ready to have God remove all these defects of character.
7. Humbly asked Him to remove our shortcomings.
8. Made a list of all persons we had harmed and became willing to make amends to them all.
9. Made direct amends to such people wherever possible, except when to do so would injure them or others.
10. Continued to take personal inventory and when we were wrong promptly admitted it.
11. Sought through prayer and meditation to improve our conscious contact with God as we understood Him, praying only for knowledge of His will for us and the power to carry that out.
12. Having had a spiritual awakening as the result of these steps, we tried to carry this message to alcoholics, and to practice these principles in all our affairs.

RESOURCES FOR LITERATURE ON ALCOHOLISM AND DRUG ABUSE

Alcoholics Anonymous
P. O. Box 459
Grand Central Station
New York, New York 10017

Community Mental Health Centers
National Institute of Mental Health
5600 Fishers Lane
Rockville, Maryland 20852

National Institute on Alcohol Abuse and Al-

coholism (NIAAA)
5600 Fishers Lane
Rockville, Maryland 20852

National Council on Alcoholism (NCA)
2 Park Avenue
New York, New York 10016

American Indian Commission on Alcohol and Drugs
2285 South Main Street
Salt Lake City, Utah 84115

North American Association of Alcoholism Programs
1130 17th Street, N.W.
Washington, D.C. 20036

Office of Economic Opportunity
1200 19th Street, N.W.
Washington, D.C. 20506

Center of Alcohol Studies
Rutgers University
New Brunswick, New Jersey 08903

Utah School of Alcohol Studies
Director, University of Utah School of Alcohol Studies
Salt Lake City, Utah 84112

National Institute on Drug Abuse
Rockwell Building, Room 628
1400 Rockville Pike
Rockville, Maryland 20862

National Congress of Parents and Teachers
Smoking and Alcohol Education Project
700 North Rush Street
Chicago, Illinois 60611

Public Affairs Council: Pamphlets on Drug Abuse
381 Park Avenue South
New York, New York 10016

Bureau of Narcotics and Dangerous Drugs
U.S. Department of Justice
1405 I Street, N.W.
Washington, D.C. 20537

American Medical Association
Department of Health Education
535 North Dearborn Street
Chicago, Illinois, 60610

Kiwanis International
101 E. Erie Street
Chicago, Illinois 60611

Resource Book for Drug Abuse Education
Public Health Service Publication #1964
U.S. Government Printing Office
Washington, D.C.

Committee on Drug Addiction and Narcotics
National Academy of Sciences
National Research Council
Division of Medical Sciences
Washington, D.C.

Institute for Study of Drug Addiction
680 West End Avenue
New York, New York 10025

National Coordinating Council on Drug Abuse Education and Information
P.O. Box 19400
Washington, D.C. 20036

QUESTIONS FOR DISCUSSION

1. Define:
   (a) health
   (b) mental health
   (c) psychoses
   (d) neuroses
   (e) schizophrenia
2. Discuss the merits of the following statement: "Mental health programs must place more emphasis upon treating and caring for the great number of mentally ill persons rather than providing mass prevention programs."
3. In what ways can we promote mental health and prevent mental illness?
4. What are some of the misconceptions about human emotions?
5. What agencies and organizations in your community are helping to promote mental health and prevent mental illness?
6. What are some of the various causes of mental illness?
7. Briefly discuss three new techniques and approaches in the prevention of mental illness that have proved successful in the community or school.
8. What are the purposes and function of a community mental health association?
9. How can the teacher help prevent mental illness?
10. "There was more mental illness in 1900 than there is today." Discuss this statement.
11. What sort of measures can be taken to prevent mental illness?
12. Is the World Health Organization interested in mental health? What principles did they agree on in mental health?
13. List the organizations in your community interested in the mental health of individuals. Which organizations are the most active?
14. Describe the Menninger Clinic in Topeka, Kansas. What is its role in mental health?
15. Describe the mental hospitals in your state. Are they operating effectively?
16. Describe the mental health clinics in your community. Are there other resources for the mentally disturbed?

17. What is the professional training of a psychiatrist? Psychologist? Psychiatric nurse?
18. What career opportunities are there in the field of mental health?
19. What are colleges and universities doing in helping students with mental illness? What is your institution's status in this area?
20. What are some of the most important problems that affect the emotional health of college students?
21. Develop a philosophy to encourage good mental health in an individual.
22. Discuss the new drugs used in the treatment for mental illness. What other modern techniques of treatment are in use?
23. How can one overcome worry?

QUESTIONS FOR REVIEW

1. What is the general definition of mental illness?
2. What are the two main categories of mental disease, and what are the chief characteristics of each?
3. What are three of the first five major causes of death in the 15- to 25-year age group? Which are psychogenic in origin?
4. List three factors that contribute to the increase in mental illness today.
5. Name three of the major methods of treatment of mental illness that have resulted in a more optimistic attitude toward it.
6. What are the five basic services that any community mental health center must offer (as required by the federal program)?
7. List nine of the treatment services of community mental health services.
8. What are two preventive services of mental illness?
9. List two professional organizations that are trying to meet the problem of nervous and mental disease.
10. What is the alternative for those mentally retarded persons who do not need hospitalization?
11. What are the general initial procedures in dealing with the risk of a person committing suicide?
12. List the seven guidelines that the Cooperative Commission on the Study of Alcoholism has offered for changes in American drinking patterns.

REFERENCES

1. A start at quantifying stress in life. Medical News. JAMA, *232*(7):699, May 19, 1975.
2. Smith, W. G., Hansell, N., and English, J. T.: Psychiatric disorder in a college population. Arch. Gen. Psychiat., *9*:351, 1963.
3. Allen, N. H., et al.: *Suicide in Young People.* Prepared by the American Association of Suicidology, in cooperation with MSD Health Information Services.
4. Roberts, A. R., and Gran, J. J.: Procedures used in crisis intervention by suicide prevention agencies. Publ. Health Rep., *85*:694, 1970.
5. *A Long Range Plan for Mental Health Services in California.* California State Department of Mental Hygiene, 1962, pp. N–1–N–3.
6. Nelson, W. E., Vaughan, V. C., and McKay, R. J.: *Textbook of Pediatrics.* 9th ed. Philadelphia, W. B. Saunders Co., 1969, p. 74.
7. Ibid., p. 75.
8. Kitzinger, A., and Hill, P. J.: *Drug Abuse, a Source Book and Guide for Teachers.* Published by the California State Department of Education, Sacramento, 1967, p. v (preface).
9. Weingarten, R., and Almond, R.: You're not sick, you're just in love. Associated Press.
10. Cohen, S.: *The Drug Dilemma.* New York, McGraw-Hill, 1969, p. 5.
11. Lundberg, G. D.: Drug abuse in the Western World. JAMA, *213*:2082, 1970.
12. Alcoholic "ill," AMA, ABA agree. Amer. Med. News, October 27, 1969, pp. 3–4.
13. Block, M. A.: *Alcohol and Alcoholism.* Belmont, Calif., Wadsworth, 1970, p. 46.
14. Plant, T. F. A.: *Alcohol Problems—a Report to the Nation, a Study for the Cooperative Commission on the Study of Alcoholism.* New York, Oxford University Press, 1967, p. 138.
15. *Prevention of Alcoholism* (pamphlet). NIAAA, 1974.
16. Katz, J.: Responsible decision-making. Health Education, *6*(2):5, March–April, 1975.

SUGGESTED READING

Almond, R.: *The Healing Community: Dynamics of the Therapeutic Milieu.* New York, Jason Aronson, 1974.

American Public Health Association: *Mental Health: The Public Health Challenge.* Washington, D.C., 1975.

American School Health Association: *Mental Health in the Classrooms.* Kent, Ohio, ASHA Publications, 1975.

Anderson, C. C., and Cresswell, W. H.: *School Health Practice.* St. Louis, C. V. Mosby Co., 1976.

Anderson, D. B., and McClean, L.J.(eds.): *Identifying Suicide Potential.* New York, Behavioral Publications, 1971.

Asuni, T.: Suicide in Western Nigeria. Brit. Med. J., *2*:1091–1097, October 27, 1962.

Barnes, M., and Berke, J.: *Mary Barnes: Two Accounts of a Journey Through Madness.* New York, Ballantine Books, 1975.

Bloom, B. L.: *Changing Patterns of Psychiatric Care.* New York, Behavioral Publications, 1975.

Bloom, B. L. (ed.): *Psychological Stress in the Campus Community.* New York, Behavioral Publications, 1975.

Bourne, P. G.: *Addiction.* New York, Academic Press, 1974.

Brill, L., and Harms, E. (eds.): *The Yearbook of Drug Abuse.* New York, Behavioral Publications, 1973.

Bryon, D. S.: *School Nursing in Transition.* St. Louis, C. V. Mosby Co., 1973.

Cadoret, R. J., and King, L.J.: *Psychiatry in Primary Care.* St. Louis, C.V. Mosby Co., 1974.

Cancro, R., et al. (eds.): *Strategic Intervention in Schi-*

zophrenia: Current Developments in Treatment. New York, Behavioral Publications, 1974.

Caplan, G.: *Support Systems and Community Mental Health.* New York, Behavioral Publications, 1973.

Conley, R. W.: *The Economics of Mental Retardation.* Baltimore, Johns Hopkins University Press, 1972.

Cooper, D.: *Psychiatry and Anti-Psychology.* New York, Ballantine Books, 1975.

Cowen, E. L., et al.: *New Ways in School Mental Health: Early Detection and Prevention of School Maladaptation.* New York, Behavioral Publications, 1975.

Cox, R. H., and Esau, T. G.: *Regressive Therapy: Therapeutic Regression of Schizophrenic Children, Adolescents, and Young Adults.* New York, Brunner/Mazel, 1974.

Cromwell, P. E. (ed.): *Woman and Mental Health: A Bibliography.* Rockville, Md., Division of Scientific and Technical Information, National Institute of Mental Health, 1974.

Cull, J. G., and Hardy, R. E. (eds.): *Types of Drug Abusers and Their Abuses.* Springfield, Ill., Charles C Thomas, 1974.

Davis, A. E., et al.: *Schizophrenics in the New Custodial Community: Five Years After the Experiment.* Columbus, Ohio State University Press, 1974.

DiScipio, W. (ed.): *The Behavioral Treatment of Psychotic Illness.* New York, Behavioral Publications, 1974.

Dohrenwend, B. S., and Dohrenwend, B. P. (eds.): *Stressful Life Events: Their Nature and Effects.* New York, Wiley-Interscience, 1974.

Driver, E. D.: *The Sociology and Anthropology of Mental Illness: A Reference Guide.* Amherst, University of Massachusetts Press, 1972.

Dunham, H. W.: *Social Realities and Community Psychiatry.* New York, Behavioral Publications, 1975.

Dunnette, M. (ed.): *Handbook of Industrial and Organizational Psychology.* Chicago, Rand McNally, 1975.

Enright, J. B., and Jackle, W. B.: Psychiatric symptoms and diagnosis in two subcultures. Int. J. Soc. Psychiat., *9*:12–17, 1963.

Foley, A. R. (ed.): *Challenge to Community Psychiatry.* New York, Behavioral Publications, 1973.

Golann, S. E., and Baker, J. (eds.): *Current and Future Trends in Community Psychology.* New York, Behavioral Publications, 1974.

Greenwald, H. (ed.): *Great Cases in Psychoanalysis.* New York, Ballantine Books, 1975.

Gunderson, E. K. E., and Tahe, R. H. (eds.): *Life Stress and Illness.* Springfield, Ill., Charles C Thomas, 1974.

Guttentag, M., et al.: *The Reevaluation of Training in Mental Health.* New York, Behavioral Publications, 1975.

Haim, A.: *Adolescent Suicide.* New York, International Universities Press, 1975.

Hudgens, R. W.: *Psychiatric Disorders in Adolescents.* Baltimore, Williams & Wilkins, 1974.

Hughes, C.: Psychocultural dimensions of social change. *In* Finney, J. C. (ed.): *Culture, Change, Mental Health and Poverty.* Lexington, University of Kentucky Press, 1969.

Josephson, E., and Carroll, E. E. (eds.): *Drug Use: Epidemiological and Sociological Approaches.* Washington, D. C. Hemisphere, 1974.

Kaplan, B., and Johnson, D.: The social meaning of Navaho psychopathology and psychotherapy. *In* Kiev, A. (ed.): *Magic, Faith, and Healing: Studies in Primitive Psychiatry Today.* New York, Free Press, 1964.

Kaplan, S. P., and Roman, M.: *The Organization and Delivery of Mental Health Services in the Ghetto.* New York, Praeger, 1973.

Katz, R. C., and Zlutnick, S. (eds.): *Behavior Therapy and Health Care: Principles and Applications.* New York, Pergamon Press, 1975.

Kessel, N., et al. (eds.): *Alcoholism: A Medical Profile.* London, B. Edsall, 1974.

Kiev, A.: *Transcultural Psychiatry.* New York, Free Press, 1972.

Kubler, E.: *On Death and Dying.* New York, Macmillan, 1969.

Lambo, T. A.: Malignant anxiety: a syndrome associated with criminal conduct in Africans. J. Mental Sci., *108*:256–264, 1964.

Larkin, E. J.: *The Treatment of Alcoholism: Theory, Practice, and Evaluation.* Toronto, Addiction Research Foundation, 1974.

Leighton, A., et al.: *Psychiatric Disorder Among the Yoruba.* Ithaca, N. Y., Cornell University Press, 1963.

Margolis, P.: *Patient Power.* Springfield, Ill., Charles C Thomas, 1973.

Masserman, J. H. (ed.): *Current Psychiatric Therapies.* Vol. 14. New York, Grune & Stratton, 1974.

Masserman, J. H., and Schwab, J. J.: *The Psychiatric Examination.* New York, Intercontinental Medical Book Corp., 1974.

McQuade, W., and Aikman, A.: *Stress.* New York, E. P. Dutton, 1974.

Meadow, A., and Stoker, D.: Symptomatic behavior of hospitalized patients. A study of Mexican-American and Anglo-American patients. Arch. Gen. Psychiat., *12*:267–277, 1965.

Menkes, J. H.: *Textbook of Child Neurology.* Philadelphia, Lea & Febiger, 1974.

Merskey, H., and Tonge, W. L.: *Psychiatric Illness: Diagnosis, Management and Treatment for General Practitioners and Students.* Baltimore, Williams & Wilkins, 1974.

Mico, P., and Ross, H.: *Health Education and the Behavioral Sciences.* Third Party Association, P. O. Box 13042, Montclair Station E, Oakland, Calif. 94611.

Montagu, A.: Culture and mental illness. Amer. J. Psychiat., *118*:15–23, 1961.

Moser, J.: *Problems and Programs Related to Alcoholic and Drug Dependence in Thirty-Three Countries.* Geneva, WHO Offset Publication No. 6, 1974.

Motto, J., et al.: Standards for Suicide Prevention and Crisis Centers. New York, Behavioral Publications, 1974.

Murphy, J. M., and Leighton, A. H. (eds.): *Approaches to Cross Cultural Psychiatry.* Ithaca, N. Y., Cornell University Press, 1965.

National Institute for Drug Programs: *Bibliography on Drug Abuse: Prevention, Treatment, Research.* New York, Behavioral Publications, 1973.

Newman, M., and Berkowitz, B.: *How to Be Your Own Best Friend.* New York, Ballantine Books, 1975.

Pamphlets from Public Affairs Committee, New York.

Parker, B.: *My Language Is Me.* New York, Ballantine Books, 1975.

Parker, S.: Eskimo psychopathology in the context of Eskimo personality and culture. American Anthropologist, *64*:76, 1962.

Perlin, S.: *A Handbook for the Study of Suicide.* New York, Oxford University Press, 1975.

Rogan, E. N. (ed.): *International Directory of Psychiatrists and Mental Hospitals.* New York, Behavioral Publications, 1975.

Rogler, L. H., and Hollingshead, A. B.: The Puerto

Rican spiritualist as psychiatrist. Amer. J. Sociol., 67:17–21, 1961.

Roman, P. M., and Trice, H. M. (eds.): *Explorations in Psychiatric Sociology.* Philadelphia, F. A. Davis, 1974.

Roman, P. M., and Trice, H. M. (eds.): *Sociological Perspectives on Community Mental Health.* Philadelphia, F. A. Davis, 1974.

Scheff, T. J. (ed.): *Mental Illness and Social Process.* New York, Harper & Row, 1967.

Schulberg, H. C., and Baker, F.: *The Mental Hospital and Human Services.* New York, Behavioral Publications, 1975.

Schultz, L. G.: *Rape Victimology.* Springfield, Ill., Charles C Thomas, 1975.

Sells, S. B.: *Studies of the Effectiveness of Treatments for Drug Abuse.* Vols. 1 and 2. Cambridge, Mass., Ballinger, 1974.

Shneidman, E. S. (ed.): Suicide: A Quarterly Journal of Life-Threatening Behavior. Vol. 5. 1975.

Siegler, M., and Osmond, H.: *Models of Madness, Models of Medicine.* New York, Macmillan, 1974.

Singh, J. M., and Lal, H. (eds.): *Drug Addiction.* Vol. 3: *Neurobiology and Influences on Behavior.* Vol. 4: *New Aspects of Analytical and Clinical Toxicology.* New York, Stratton Intercontinental Medical Book Corp., 1974.

Smolensky, J.: *A Guide to Child Growth and Development.* Dubuque, Iowa, Kendall/Hunt, 1974.

Steiner, C.: *Games Alcoholics Play.* New York, Ballantine Books, 1975.

Stimmel, B.: *Heroin Dependency: Medical, Economic and Social Aspects.* New York, Stratton Intercontinental Medical Book Corp., 1975.

Swazey, J. P.: *Chlorpromazine in Psychiatry: A Study of Therapeutic Innovation.* Cambridge, Mass., M.I.T. Press, 1974.

Szasz, T. S.: *The Myth of Mental Illness: Foundations of a Theory of Personal Conduct.* New York, Harper & Row, 1974.

Troup, S. B., and Greene, W. A. (eds.): *The Patient, Death, and the Family.* New York, Scribner's, 1974.

Weber, G. H., and Haberlein, B. J. (eds.): *Residential Treatment of Emotionally Disturbed Children.* New York, Behavioral Publications, 1972.

Welford, A. T. (ed.): *Man Under Stress.* New York, Halsted Press, 1974.

Williams, G. J., and Gordon, S. (eds.): *Clinical Child Psychology: Current Practices and Future Perspectives.* New York, Behavioral Publications, 1974.

Yap, P. M.: Mental illness peculiar to certain cultures: a survey of comparative psychiatry. J. Mental Sci., 97:313–327, 1951.

CHAPTER 10

Maternal and Child Health

Maternal and Child Health (MCH) has five broad aspects: maternal health; child health, which encompasses health supervision of children below school age as well as the general run of illnesses of children of all ages; school health; care for handicapped children (the term MCH is used generically to include crippled children services); and health implications of child welfare. In functional terms, the comprehensive MCH program covers (1) the promotional, preventive, and treatment services required by families in order that mothers (during and between maternity cycles) and their children may be kept well, or, if acutely or chronically ill or handicapped or crippled by social, emotional, physical, or mental conditions, may be restored to the greatest possible extent to good health, and (2) the organization and administration of programs to make available such services under public or voluntary auspices or through private practitioners.

SERVICES

Specific services include the following: physician-led family spacing interviews to counsel and aid those who would benefit by longer spacing between children or by limiting the size of their family; prenatal and postpartum clinics for women who have financial or transportation difficulties and cannot avail themselves of hospital clinics (through Social Service referral); child health conferences for physician examinations and behavioral guidance where needed; immunizations for diphtheria, tetanus, pertussus, poliomyelitis and smallpox; tuberculin and phenylketonuria tests; and growth and development counseling to parents in the care of well infants and children to age six, when there is no private physician or when referred by a private physician. These child health conferences are designed to do the following: (1) to prevent disease and reduce mortality by adequate immunizations and by teaching the principles of hygiene and good nutrition; (2) to allow observation of the growth and development of the child during the preschool period by routine physical examinations, and by psychological screening tests on selected cases with possible retardation or emotional problems; (3) to make referrals to the family physician of all cases needing medical care; (4) to help the parents understand the normal changes which occur in growing up, by anticipatory guidance and developing parental insight and wholesome attitudes toward children (this mental health education is given individually or in parent groups); and (5) to allow detection of needy parents with emotional or financial problems which hinder the normal growth and development of their children, and to arrange for home visits and agency referrals as indicated.

An immune globulin, Rh_0 (D) immune globulin (human), is now available and may save the lives of many infants. The globulin prevents Rh disease (erythroblastosis fetalis), a hemolytic disease of the newborn caused by incompatibility of the mother's blood with that of the fetus. Many health departments are including this information as part of the MCH program.

Pediatric services are provided at clinics called "child-health conferences" or "well-baby clinics" for those who are referred by their private physician. The conference includes a health examination of the well child under six as well as parent counseling. It must be pointed out here that faithful volunteers offer their time and assistance to help make these clinics successful. Arrangements are also made for home visits for demonstration of such procedures as bathing the baby or making a formula. It must be realized, however, that regular medical supervision by the family's own physician is the best basis of care for children and adults. The family physician, knowing the child in health, will be better able to care for him in illness.

Expectant-parent classes are conducted to teach the elements of good maternal health and care of the new born infant. Prenatal visits are made by the public health nurse to assist the expectant mother in making preparations for the prenatal care of the child, to interpret and implement the physician's instructions, and to keep the physician informed of any apparent abnormality.

The health department is also responsible for the promotion, implementation, and enforcement of legislation dealing with premarital and prenatal examination requirements. These may include serologic tests for syphilis, tuberculin skin tests, and chest x-rays.

CURRENT PROBLEMS

The great increase in the number of children in our population today has increased the demand for maternal and child care tremendously. The earlier age of marriage, increase in numbers of working mothers, high rate of broken homes, and rising illegitimate birth rates are but a few of the factors that change the character and volume of demands for maternal and child health services.

Because of the general emphasis in other areas in public health, the maternal and child health program has sometimes been neglected by administrators of public health. The MCH workers have been partially responsible for the lack of attention to the program, however, because they

> ... have not given leadership in producing new methods and in letting go of traditional practices. For example, too much of nursing time in maternal and child health has become a deeply felt but vague effort at giving counseling and guidance to mothers, with too little help to the nurses to make such counseling specifically pointed to meet patient needs. The public health nurse is welcomed with open arms by the young mother when she visits within 24 or 48 hours after the mother has come home with her first baby. The nurse aims at giving this insecure, young mother support, and usually does so, but may not even wake up or undress the newborn baby because she has not recently been instructed on her possible contribution to physical inspection and assessment of the health status of the infant.[1]

Another major and widespread weakness within the MCH field is the

> ... lack of the "M" in MCH. Obstetricians in public health are few and far between. Pediatricians are more numerous. The emphasis, especially recently, has been more on children than on mothers. The consequence in inadequacy of antepartum health supervision for example is clear. Why did it take so many years for MCH workers to think of the idea that antepartum health supervision, important as it is, is not enough, but that the woman who suffers an unfavorable outcome of pregnancy should be followed after the postpartum visit into the subsequent nonpregnant interval, rather than waiting for the next pregnancy before trying to correct her health imbalances.[2]

Infant and Maternal Mortality

Despite recent advances in medical science, women still die needlessly in the reproductive process. The most common single cause of maternal death is illegal abortion. The key will be education and fully accessible, safe abortions. There will always be some women who will seek clandestine or unsafe abortions because of their own feeling about the process, or because of certain circumstances, but through education and an enlightened public, these numbers will be reduced.

Girls who become pregnant before they are 17 years old run great risk for both themselves and their babies. Because they are growing most girls under 17 have greater nutritional requirements in relation to body size than those of adult women. The additional nutrient demands of pregnancy may compromise their growth potential and increase their risk in pregnancy. Complications during pregnancy frequently involve premature labor, iron-deficiency anemia, prolonged labor, and toxemia.

Pregnancy, with its psychological effects, adds to the emotional burden of the adolescent. Society's primitive attitude toward early pregnancy, particularly out of wedlock, makes the psychological adjustment harder. It is difficult for the pregnant girl to obtain medical care. She is often forced to quit school, and many states prevent her marriage. The young girl who is pregnant is forced to cope with her own psychological immaturity, the often frightening physical changes of pregnancy, and a society that rejects her.

Recommendations to alleviate the risks in adolescent pregnancy include positive community attitudes, practices, and regulations that encourage teenagers to use existing medical services and to obtain information and advice about pregnancy; increased emphasis must be given to sound family-life education, health, and nutrition in elementary and secondary schools. In Cincinnati and San Jose, for example, centers have been organized to provide help for the unwed teenage mother. The emphasis of the program is centered on encouraging girls to remain in school. The girl goes to school and receives good prenatal care and counseling in a school setting. The provision of good prenatal care is followed with postnatal visits to see that recommendations are being followed.

Infant mortality is not just a problem for the baby born out of wedlock. Our high infant mortality rate is one of our most widely discussed public health problems. Who hasn't heard that the United States ranks thirteenth among nations of the world in respect to infant mortality? The wide, shocking variation in infant mortality rates within this country is itself enough to mark our high infant mortality rate as a major and urgent problem. The worst infant mortality rates are found consistently in the central cities and in the impoverished rural areas.

A careful analysis of the problem shows that the major factor associated with infant mortality is prematurity. And prematurity, in turn, is associated with a number of other factors, including low socioeconomic class, poor maternal nutrition (especially anemia), high multiparity, short spacing of pregnancies, and no prenatal care. Perhaps the most single effective measure we can employ to reduce infant mortality would be the widespread provision of effective family planning services.

Suggestions

Many persons involved in studying child growth and development list the following suggestions: high school training for parenthood, greater responsibility for children of all ages, development of institutions and projects where teenagers would constructively work with and help small children, and development of communities where adults become involved in the lives of our children. Regarding the last point, Bronfenbrenner remarked:

> American children, however, are relatively cut off from the adult world, and the family, primarily because of changes in the larger social order, is no longer in a position to exercise its responsibilities. The role of the church in moral education has withered in most cases to a pallid Sunday school session. The school – in which the child spends most of his day – has been debarred by tradition, lack of experience and preoccupation with subject matter from concerning itself in any major way with the child's development as a person. The vacuum, moral and emotional, is then filled – by default – on the one hand by the television screen with its daily message of commercialism and violence, and on other by the socially isolated, age graded peer group, with its limited capacities as a humanizing agent.
>
> If the current trend persists, we can anticipate increased alienation, indifference, antagonism and violence on the part of the younger generation in all segments of our society – middle-class children as well as the disadvantaged. From this perspective, the emergence of the hippie cult appears as the least harmful manifestation of a process that sees its far more destructive and widespread expression in the sharp rise recently in juvenile delinquency.
>
> Why should age segregation bring social disruption in its wake? It is obvious that such qualities as mutual trust, kindness, cooperation and social responsibility are learned from other human beings who in some measure exhibit these qualities, value them, and strive to develop them in their children. It is a matter of social rather than biological inheritance. Transmission cannot take place without the active participation of the older generation. If children have contact only with their own age-mates, there is no possibility for learning culturally established patterns of cooperation and mutual concern.
>
> We are experiencing a breakdown in the process of making human beings human. What is needed is a change in our ways of living that will once again bring adults back into the lives of children and children back into the lives of adults.[3]

In spite of weakness, there is hardly any aspect of public health that does not influence and improve the health of mothers and children. Maternal and Child Health services usually constitute a major part of local public health programs and at present are often the

WOMEN, INFANTS, AND CHILDREN PROGRAM

Better health and improved life prospects for hundreds of women and children are possible because of special federal funds to support nutrition programs in the United States. A total of 40 million dollars has been granted for the special supplemental food program for women, infants, and children (WIC). The program is designed to provide potentially undernourished persons with highly nutritious food.

The WIC program, federally established in 1972, makes nutritionally desirable foods available to designated persons through local public or private non-profit health clinics or agencies selected by the Food and Nutrition Service, for as long as funds are available. These foods are intended to *supplement* the regular diet of participants—they are *not* a complete diet in themselves. The food is especially high in nutrients known to be often lacking in the diets of people who are eligible for the program.

Pregnant or nursing women, infants, and children under age 4 can receive food supplements if they (1) live in approved low-income areas served by an approved health clinic; (2) are eligible for reduced-cost medical treatment from that clinic; and (3) are determined by professionals at the clinic to need the supplemental foods. Children under 4 and mothers will receive cheese, milk, eggs, cereals high in iron, and juices high in vitamin C. Infants will receive baby cereal fortified with iron, formulas fortified with iron, and juices high in vitamin C.

The local agencies provide special food vouchers to eligible women and will follow up with clinical examinations (blood and urine tests) to assess the effects of the added nutritional elements. Food vouchers may be obtained only at the clinics and will be used to purchase designated foods at grocery stores. Gains from the program may include reductions in complications of pregnancy, the incidence of premature births, various forms of anemia, and improvement in maternal and infant health.

A major objective of the national program is the collection and evaluation of data that will identify the benefits of special nutritional supplements. Data collection and laboratory studies will be funded and carried out by an independent agency under direct federal contract from the Food and Nutrition Service.

major segment of personal health services provided under public health auspices. Founded on the medical specialties of pediatrics and obstetrics, MCH has expanded to embrace the care of handicapped children, drawing on the relevant clinical specialties, and in all of its programs emphasizes the need for public health nursing. The striking relationship between good health and the social situation of families has also brought the social worker into the maternal and child health team.

ADVANCES AND CHANGES IN MATERNAL AND CHILD HEALTH

Obstetrics—that branch of medicine dealing with pregnacy, labor, and the period after delivery—has changed greatly during the past decade. First of all, parents can decide whether they want to play any part at all in the production of future generations. The pill, vasectomy, and abortion have gained acceptance as an adjunct to responsible parenthood. Also, new medical techniques allow parents to choose the sex of their baby (there being 80 per cent accuracy with the Shettle method) and to have babies by appointment.

Society's attitudes toward childbearing have been transformed within our lifetime. Large families are a thing of the past. A nuclear family today consists of one or two children at the most. Pregnancy today is accepted as a normal condition. Expectant mothers may work and play, continuing to be active and productive. The women's liberation movement has "freed" many women. A woman is no longer considered merely the chattel of her husband and the mother of his offspring. The movement has also led to the creation of women's health clinics and self-help medical techniques. The liberated woman has revealed another facet of her personality. Some now want to experience the sensations of having their baby while unanesthetized, having their husband serve as labor coach in "natural childbirth" or the

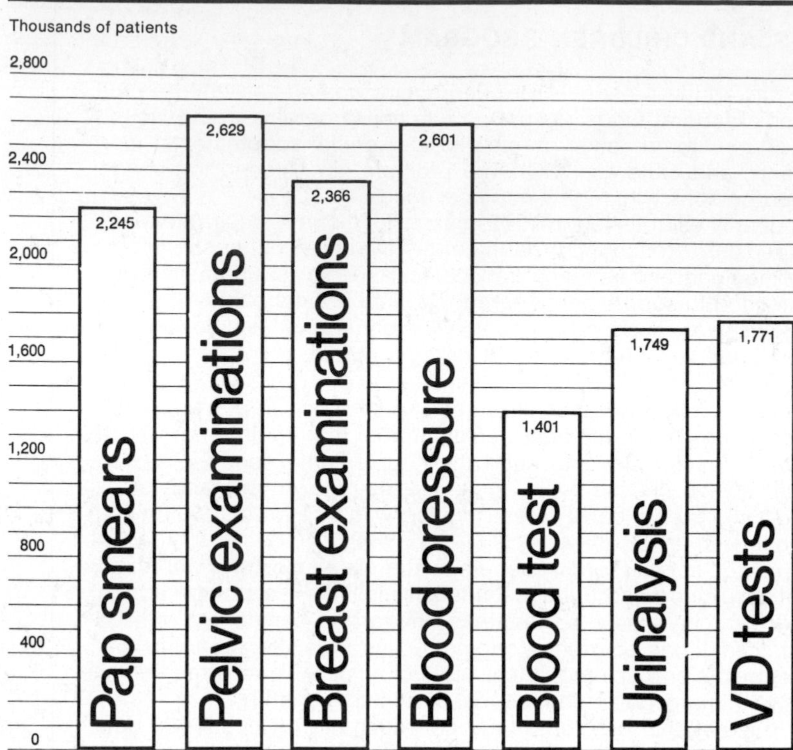

Figure 10–1 Estimated number of patients of organized programs receiving specified health services at initial and annual visits, fiscal year 1973. (From Family Planning Perspectives, 6(1):22, Winter 1974.)

Lamaze method. Many women, with the blessings of their obstetricians, are experiencing life's most dramatic moment with delight. The expectant mother plays an active, participating role in the event, with a minimum of discomfort and a maximum of safety. For the first time, the husband is an essential part of the birth process. Also, many parents and obstetricians are interested in Dr. Frederick LeBoyer's technique* for easing the birth trauma and helping the new human being to start life without pain, confusion, and fear.

In line with their yearning for a more natural life style, more and more people, particularly well-educated young people, are having their babies outside hospitals. Childbirth, they reason, is a happy event, and many find that the unlimited, cheerful, emotional support from neighbors and professionals, the lack of alarm about the pending occasion, the comfort of familiar surrounding, and best of all, the support of a loving husband, all contribute to an easier and more satisfying experience. Although some obstetricians are opposed to the movement because they consider it dangerous, many physicians around the country are willing to perform home deliveries.*

*LeBoyer, F.: *Birth Without Violence.* New York, Knopf, 1974.

*It is interesting to note that new programs are being developed that reflect these changing attitudes. For example, Mount Zion Hospital and Medical Center in San Francisco illustrates the new atmosphere with two new programs: Family-Centered Childbirth in the Maternity wing, and Care-With-Parent in the Pediatrics section. Acceptance rate by patients is high.

Medical Advances

An infant born in 1900 had a life expectancy of approximately 50 years. Today, because of the tremendous strides made in public health and medicine, an infant has before him a possible life span of more than 70 years. When the early state boards of health were created, epidemics of typhoid fever, smallpox, diphtheria, and bubonic plague threatened the country. Tuberculosis and typhoid fever were leading causes of death at that time. Today, smallpox has disappeared from the country, plague is an extremely rare disease, and significant reductions have been made in the incidence of and deaths from typhoid fever, diphtheria, whooping cough, measles, scarlet fever, tuberculosis, the dysenteries, and the tick-borne diseases. The period from 1900 to the present has revealed a steady decline in the communicable disease morbidity and mortality rates. Maternal mortality has been reduced to a great extent, and infant deaths have been lowered from almost 100 per 1000 in 1915 to less than 20 per 1000 as of 1976.

Medical advances in this area have been rapid and remarkable. For example, genetic counseling is emerging after the superstition and ignorance of centuries. Also, Rh negative problems can now be eliminated; with good prenatal care, blood typing, and an injection of immune globulin at delivery, the hazards related to this condition should soon disappear. Improvements in sedation, anesthesia, drugs, and antibiotics have helped save many mothers and babies. Adequate and regular prenatal care, including improved diet, has been very important in promoting the health of the child's mother.

On the other hand, infant mortality rates influence the rate of population increase. Infant mortality rates (deaths under 1 year of age per 1000 live births) range from a low of 12.6 in Sweden and 13.4 in the Netherlands to highs of 25.9 in Zambia and 22.9 in Gabon. Although the infant mortality rate in the United States has been reduced through the years, reaching a new low of 17.2 in 1976, most officials agree that it is still too high for this country. High infant mortality rates reflect poor nutritional status and high prevalence of disease in a nation more effectively than does any other single index. The wide range in general health status among the nations of the world, as indicated by infant mortality rates, is a real cause for concern.

Maternal Mortality

The primary vital statistic that public health has traditionally used to follow the degree of health of pregnant women has been the maternal mortality rate. This rate is defined as follows:

$$\frac{\text{All mothers dying while pregnant} + \text{All women dying within 90 days of having delivered an infant}}{\text{All live births}} \times 10{,}000$$

The numerator is considered to include all women who die from causes related to the pregnant state. While the denominator is actually a measure of birth, it will, at least in theory, include most women who have been pregnant. The resulting fraction is multiplied by 10,000 because in recent years in the United States, the maternal mortality rate has fallen to less than 1 per 1000, and it is desirable to have the statistic expressed in a whole number.

It is now felt by many that a maternal mortality of 2 deaths per 10,000 live births is not an unreasonable goal for all population groups throughout the nation. The most emia of pregnancy (a poorly understood condition which includes swelling, elevated blood pressure, and protein in the urine), hemorrhage, abortion, death due to anesthesia, and sepsis (infection of the blood stream). Approximately three quarters of these deaths are judged to have been avoidable and thus can be considered to be the result of inadequate quality of maternal care. It is important to keep in mind that while developmental periods are convenient descriptive devices, they are artificial. Growth and development are continuous processes which proceed at all times, rather than in a series of arbitrary periods.

Neo-Natal Care Units

In the United States approximately 14 infants in every 1000 die during the first week of life. Fifty per cent of these infant deaths occur within the first 24 hours following birth. Most of these fatalities occur among a group of babies considered "high-risk." A major problem is, however, that doctors can anticipate only about 60 per cent of high-risk babies from reviewing the mother's medical record. Included in this group are babies weighting less than 5½ pounds, those born prematurely (in less than the normal 37 weeks' gestation period), and those with birth defects.

High-risk babies are likely to have more difficulty than normal babies with breathing, feeding, and other vital functions. In many cases these infants are in need of immediate

MEASUREMENTS AND INDICES COMMONLY USED IN EPIDEMIOLOGY

Measure	Formula	Multiplier
Age-specific death rate	Number of persons of a given age dying during the year / Population in specified age group at midyear	× 1000
Case-fatality rate	Number of deaths from a specified disease / Number of cases of that disease	× 100
Crude birth rate	Number of live births during the year / Population at midyear	× 1000
Crude death rate	Number of deaths occurring during the year / Population at midyear	× 1000
Infant death rate	Number of deaths of children under 1 year of age during the year / Number of live births during that year	× 1000
Maternal (puerperal) death rate	Number of deaths from puerperal causes during the year / Number of live births during that year	× 10000
Neonatal death rate	Number of deaths of children under 28 days of age during the year / Number of live births during that year	× 1000
Perinatal death rate	Number of fetal deaths and infant deaths under 7 days of age during the year / Number of live births and fetal deaths during that year	× 1000

and extremely skilled medical attention if they are to live. To improve their chances for survival, hospitals are beginning to set up special nurseries called newborn special-care units, or neo-natal care units. In these units, specially trained doctors and nurses are on duty 24 hours a day. Laboratory test facilities are directly connected to these units, and sophisticated monitoring equipment, which can gauge blood pressure and heartbeat, is available. Because the infants are under constant surveillance, emergencies can be quickly met.

The baby is placed in a portable incubator, with portholes on each side through which staff members can perform blood transfusions, administer oxygen, and give other emergency services. Many of the premature babies are insufficiently developed to carry out such vital tasks as maintaining body heat, breathing regularly, and accepting nourishment. A set of electronic devices in the "isolette" guard against any vital failure. In the isolette, the baby is kept warm and special breathing bags give him the oxygen he needs when his own lung action temporarily fails. This is extremely important, because asphyxia and lung problems account for many infant deaths. A tiny plastic tube can bring nourishment through the throat into the stomach. At the age of 6 weeks, many babies receive mini-blood transfusions. In hospitals where intensive care units for newborn babies are provided, there has been a marked reduction in the rates of infant mortality and stillbirths. It has been estimated that a fully developed statewide program could reduce a state's infant mortality rate by two-thirds.

New Popularity of Midwives

The midwife was an accepted member of the social structure of ancient Greece and Rome, and once held the exclusive right to assist women at childbirth. Even today, professional midwives deal with the majority of normal births in such technologically advanced countries as Sweden, Germany, and the Netherlands. In England, which has one of the world's most advanced health care systems, 80 per cent of all births are administered by midwives. In fact, midwives deliver 80 per cent of the world's babies. In the United States, midwives dominated obstetrics as late as the nineteenth century, when their role was taken over by doctors, many of whom considered the midwives unqualified and supported efforts to legislate them into obscurity. Urbanization and medical progress also contributed to the decrease in demand for midwives' services.

Today, however, with the advent of new professional requirements and certification, high birth rate, more home deliveries, more people choosing alternate birth methods, and scarcity of doctors, midwifery is on the increase in this country. At least a dozen hospitals and medical centers offer midwife training programs for graduate nurses. The United States Air Force has plans to offer a course for nurses who wish to be midwives in Air Force hospitals. There are several reasons for the resurgence. One is the relative scarcity of women doctors and the preference of some women for a female obstetrician. Another reason is the gradual acceptance of home delivery outside of remote rural areas, where it is often a necessity. Still another reason for the midwife's growing popularity is the quality of care she is able to provide her patients. Some obstetricians feel it unnecessary to remain with their patients from the beginning of labor to its conclusion; midwives stay with their patients throughout the entire process. She also provides individual prenatal and postnatal care, gives helpful information and practical techniques to parents in working with the newborn, and helps families deal with their problems. In any case it offers women, and couples, a *choice*.

Perhaps the most pressing argument for the use of nurse-midwives is the fact that there just aren't enough obstetricians to go around and they are distributed unevenly among the population. Further, a number of general practitioners are no longer delivering babies, because of malpractice insurance problems. Hundreds of thousands of American women never even see a doctor during pregnancy and are delivered by policemen, husbands, or relatives. This is particularly true of women in the lower socioeconomic groups who receive little or no care. The shortage is worst in the inner cities and in rural areas.

Laws on midwifery vary markedly from state to state, but generally a nurse trained in the profession may deliver a baby unaided, as well as give local anesthetics, perform minor obstetric surgery, and fit contraceptives. The midwife's goal is to care for normal mothers during pregnancy and delivery under medical supervision. This gives the physician an opportunity to look after more complicated cases, emergencies, and sick patients. The midwife is not a substitute for either the physician or his nurse. In this way the quality of medical care is improved. Most physicians agree that midwives are urgently needed health care professionals, but legislation is needed in almost all states to enhance and protect their status. Many states have modern nurse-midwives who care for mothers in the prenatal and postnatal stages but may not deliver babies. New Mexico, at this writing, is the only state with special legislation to license nurse-midwives. If other states enact nurse-midwife legislation, obstetrical care may be brought to a group of women who have no care at all.

Fetal Electronic Monitoring

In recent years medicine has made great gains in many areas relating to the care of mothers and their babies, but the number of children born with brain damage has not materially decreased. Doctors now believe that in certain of these babies the brain damage probably occurred during labor or delivery, either by direct injury or because of a temporary lack of oxygen. Unfortunately, these injuries were often difficult or impossible to detect at the time. In order to avoid such tragedies, many specialized methods have been developed that can be used during labor to allow the doctor to know what is going on with both the mother and her baby. At the Yale–New Haven and Stanford Medical Centers, as well as many others, physicians are using a unique system that electronically monitors the entire birth process from labor to delivery. At present, it is desirable to use fetal monitoring only when there is high risk involved, either to the mother or to the baby. Dr. Edward Hon, originator of the world's first fetal intensive care unit, spent 13 years perfecting the system.

Through the use of these monitors, two major types of measurements can be obtained. The first of these involves the actual work of labor as it is being carried out by the uterus. It is possible now to determine and record uterine contractions—how often they occur and how strong they are. This information is then analyzed and printed on a permanent record, so that the results are continually available to those caring for the patient.

The second measurements are aimed at monitoring the baby. Previously the baby's condition could be followed only listening to its heart. As long as it beat between 120 and 180 times a minute and remained regular, the doctor had to assume that all was well. If there was a substantial change in the heartbeat, it was sometimes considered an indication that the delivery should be accomplished rapidly. Unfortunately, there was not always an exact correlation between the change in heart rate and an abnormal condition of the baby, and attempts at immediate delivery were not always without some damage to the mother or her baby.

If the fetus experiences a problem, such as compressed umbilical cord or head, or a shortage of oxygen, the heart reflects a drastic fall on the graph. Fortunately, 90 per cent of all fetal distress is caused by umbilical cord compression, which, once detected, can usually be relieved by simply changing the mother's position. Using electronic monitoring, it is possible to receive information, put it through a computer, analyze it, and make instantly available the assessment of the baby's well-being. Changes that are important and require immediate intervention can be separated from those that are not. Along with this direct electronic monitoring, it is also possible to withdraw blood from both the mother and the baby and analyse it for diagnostic purposes.

When the unit, which can monitor four babies simultaneously, was tried on 400 mothers with histories of difficult labor, the results were impressive. None of the babies died, and the number of caesarian sections for fetal distress was reduced by 50 per cent. At the present time, work is progressing to develop much more simple electronic monitoring devices that would be capable of following the fetal heart rate and the uterine contractions simultaneously. It may be possible in the future to follow all women in labor using these techniques. Continued progress will allow the delivery of more healthy, normal babies than ever before. Hopefully, Dr. Hon's new system could save as many as 20,000 babies a year.

Child Health and Disability Prevention Program

CHDP—Child Health and Disability Prevention—is a program in California to help provide *ongoing, quality* medical care to all children through:

1. Early and periodic health check-ups, and
2. Referral to medical and dental services for diagnosis, treatment, and follow-up.

The long range goal is to provide more and better health services for children, as needs for services are recognized and documented.

CHDP is a state mandated, locally administered legislative extension of the national Medi-Screen program, also known as EPSDT (Early and Periodic Screening, Diagnosis, and Treatment)—Amendment to Title 19, Social Security Act. Financing and program standards are established at the state level; health services are established at the county level.

Each community program is required to establish an advisory board, whose membership includes physicians and other health care providers, parents of children eligible for state services, school personnel, Social Services Division staff, and representatives from other groups and agencies who are interested in the health of children. The intent is to involve members of the community in their own health planning and implementation of services.

As of September, 1976, *all* first grade entrants in California are required by law to present to the school a signed certificate that states either:

1. The child has received, within the prior 12 months, the appropriate health assessment, or
2. The family chooses not to have the child receive the health assessment. (For example, the child has already had the examination, or the family declines the service for religious or personal reasons.)

School certificates and waivers are available from the providers (doctors and clinics). A child who has been receiving ongoing health care may be certified by his or her personal physician without a formal examination, if that child has received, as a minimum, all applicable procedures of the health assessment.

The CHDP program provides the following services:

1. A health and developmental history from parent or guardian.
2. An unclothed, complete physical examination.
3. Hearing, vision, and tuberculin screening tests.
4. Lab screening tests of blood and urine.
5. Evaluation of nutritional, dental, and developmental status.

6. Immunizations for diphtheria, tetanus, whooping cough, polio, mumps, rubella, and measles, if indicated.

7. Additional tests where indicated, such as sickle cell testing, and serum lead levels.

Other services are offered in the field of outreach and health education. In cooperation with schools and other health related services, parents are learning:

1. The purposes and benefits of regular and periodic health evaluation services.

2. The exact components of the "well child" examination.

3. Where examinations are provided.

4. Procedures for obtaining services.

CHDP provides for low-income, eligible families the same periodic pediatric check-up or well-child assessment as is provided in private medical practice. In place of the all-too-frequent emergency, crisis-oriented, fragmented, and episodic sick child care, this legislation provides the opportunity for *all* children, regardless of cultural, legal, or socio-economic status, to seek and receive *ongoing, periodic, high quality, preventive* health care services. It encourages families to adopt *positive health practices* through health education, and personal contact with interested physicians and health care personnel.

Two Major Medical Problems of Infants

Hyaline Membrane Disease

An infant who has difficulty breathing may not be obtaining sufficient oxygen in the brain. In such cases, permanent brain damage can result. Oxygen insufficiency can also occur because of an obstruction in an infant's airway. Or, it may be caused by *hyaline membrane disease*, when lungs become lined with a glass-like substance that makes it impossible for the baby to breathe. Each year, over 25,000 American babies choke to death within 24 hours after birth because of this disease. Probably the most widely publicized victim of this disease was Patrick Bouvier Kennedy, the short-lived infant son of President and Mrs. John F. Kennedy. Despite dramatic efforts by superior physicians, the baby died.

Today, the prognosis is somewhat more hopeful. Medical scientists have pinpointed the cause of the disease: a substance called fibrin that accumulates in the lungs of those infants who lack the specific enzyme to destroy it. The infant's immature lung is unable to produce the compounds necessary to keep its elasticity. By testing for these compounds in the amniotic fluid of the mother before birth, it is possible to predict (with 100 per cent accuracy in 700 cases) which babies will be in grave risk of being unable to breathe properly if delivered at that time. If, with this knowledge, a caesarean section or the inducement of labor can be delayed for as little as four to five days, it may well save the infant's life. If the birth cannot be delayed, the medical staff is alerted to the necessity for immediate intervention with intensive care for the premature newborn. A promising new treatment based upon enzyme therapy is available but is costly and experimental. With equipment and neonatal care now available, a baby's breathing can be monitored by tiny electrodes applied to the chest. If breathing stops, an alarm sounds, a red light flashes, and resuscitation can be initiated in seconds.

Sudden Infant Death Syndrome (SIDS)

In the United States, 15,000 times each year, previously healthy, well-cared-for infants are found dead in their cribs. The cause of these tragedies is a silent, mysterious killer known as the Sudden Infant Death Syndrome (SIDS), also called crib death. It is the leading cause of death for babies between 1 week and 7 months of age.

On autopsy, there seems to be no cause for the death. Infectious diseases had long been suspected to be a major contribution factor. A recent study indicated that death may be caused by a threshold phenomenon surrounding a minor infection. In an infant the body's reaction to the virus may cause the larynx to constrict, thus closing the air passage so the infant cannot breathe. The vocal cords are also constricted and rendered useless, so that the baby cannot cry out. An investigation into SIDS, emphasizing its correlation with upper respiratory oral infection, was conducted. The findings indicated that, of infants who died of causes unexplained by autopsy, better than half had one or more viruses or bacteria present, and high incidence of upper respiratory oral infection was found in them and in their families. However, these findings are inconsistent and inconclusive. SIDS is more common among boys than girls. There are twice as many cases in winter as in summer. Many of the victims are born prematurely or are unusually small at birth.

A growing body of evidence seems to point to apnea (cessation of breathing) as a developmental-physiological defect in SIDS babies. The problem may be an immature nervous system, which, in effect, "short circuits" during sleep, causing the part of the brain that involuntarily controls respiration to fail. When the baby's "neuro-switch" does not go on, breathing stops.

As a result, high-risk babies have electrodes fastened to their bodies 24 hours a day. When sleeping, the children are connected to electronic infant monitors that sound alarms if heart or respiration rates drop below normal for more than 10 seconds.

SIDS is now considered a legal cause of death in many states, and additional legislation in some states requires county coroners to perform autopsies. The County Health Department is required to inform the parents about the nature of the condition in order to help prevent guilt and stress. Research is advancing at the National Institute of Health, at Stanford Hospital's Sleep Disorder Clinic, and at many other centers throughout the country. Further information may be obtained by writing SIDS, P.O. Box 545, Richmond, California 84898.

Recommendations For Improved Primary Health Care

The California Nurses' Association believes that primary health care services to children and their families can be improved. It recommends the following measures:

1. The development of an effective overall health system which could still retain the features of local and institutional autonomy.
2. Improved collaboration between the various disciplines serving children and their families.
3. A better utilization of health personnel, which can bring improvement in primary health care services to children and their families.
4. More registered nurses employed in this highly responsible role in health services which help low-income groups–neighborhood health centers, Head Start programs, maternity and other clinics, and other school programs. But services of registered nurses in this role should not be limited to low-income groups.
5. Registered nurses must become more actively involved with the high priority health problems which mothers and their children face: accidents, infectious diseases, allergic disorders, early identification of hearing and visual defects, dental care, immunization, mental health, infant mortality, mental retardation, nutrition, family planning, and high-risk pregnancies. Registered nurses should also deal with the personal and social factors which affect health care.
6. Health workers, legislators, and health service consumers need to examine the California Medical Practice and Nursing Practice Arts and related laws to find ways in which health workers can have greater legal support and assistance in the development of these needed health services.
7. Finally, schools should consider the development of more curriculum in baccalaureate nursing and masters' programs, to prepare nurses for the role described here. Schools of medicine and of public health can be increasingly effective collaborators in such educational programs.

BIRTH DEFECTS

More than 1600 human diseases caused by defects in the content or the expression of the genetic information in DNA have been identified. It has been estimated that at least 25 per cent of all institutions for the handicapped in this country are occupied by persons suffering from some degree of genetic disease. Two to 5 per cent of the babies born each year are either impaired when they arrive or reveal inherited or partially inherited abnormalities by the time they are 5 years old. Most of the major birth defects have their beginnings in the first 90 days of pregnancy; many begin earlier in defective germ cells. Birth defects have many causes: faulty genes, biochemical or metabolic errors, diseases contracted by the pregnant woman (German measles, syphilis, influenza*), difficulty at birth, excessive radiation during prenatal stages, ingestion of harmful drugs (such as thalidomide or DES [synthetic estrogen hormones]), excessive smoking or inadequate nutrition during pregnancy.

Fortunately, the large majority of babies are born without serious abnormalities. It has been said that everybody is born with some kind of birth defect, and this is probably true. Some people are color-blind; some are slightly pigeon-toed. Others don't have very good coordination. Nearly everybody has a mole or small birthmark of some kind. These minor or nondisabling defects are not discussed in this book. A serious birth defect is one that either causes disfigurement, results in a physical or mental handicap, shortens life, or is fatal. Some of the more numerous and serious birth defects are listed in Figures 10–3 and 10–4. Treatment of these disorders is a highly individualized matter. Emphasis is upon early detection and prompt therapy.

---

* A recent study of malformations recorded on United States birth certificates suggested that left hip and limb deficiencies might be especially common among children born after all influenza epidemics.

Fetal Outcome After Certain Maternal Infections During Pregnancy

Agent	Increased Risk of: Abortion	Stillbirth	Congenital Malformation	Low Birth Weight	Comment Chronic Fetal Infections
Rubella virus	++	++	Eye, ear, heart, other less frequent	++	Broad spectrums of abnormality from very severe to mild, hepatosplenomegaly, meningoencephalitis, thrombocytopenia, bone lesions, deafness, mental retardation, diarrhea, failure to thrive, growth retardation, viral excretion for weeks, months after birth, babies are infectious. Rubella antibody persist after 6 mo.
Cytomegalovirus (CMV)	Unknown		Cataract microcephaly	++	Hepatosplenomegaly, thrombocytopenia, bone lesions, deafness, mental retardation. Prolonged viral excretion. CMV antibody persist after 6 mo.
Influenza A	+	+	?After first trimester	After first trimester	Available information suggests some increase in malformation following first trimester illness.
Measles	+	+	?	No	
Mumps		++ 2nd trimester	?	No	Questionable relationship between maternal mumps and cardiac fibroelastosis.
Variçella (chickenpox)	?	?	?	?	Neonatal chickenpox following maternal infection near delivery.
Variola (smallpox)	++	++	?	?	Fetal smallpox.
Vaccinia	No	?	No	No	Fetal vaccinia, elective vaccination contraindicated.
Hepatitis	?	?	No	?	Hepatosplenomegaly—jaundice, ascites.
Herpes simplex (genital)	No	No	No	No	Hepatosplenomegaly—jaundice—meningoencephalitis—occasionally generalized herpes—mental retardation.
Poliomyelitis	No	No	No	+	Paralytic polio where maternal disease near term.
Virus pneumonia	No	No	No	No	Respiratory distress, pneumonitis where maternal disease occurs at term.
Coxsackie type B	?	?	No	?	Myocarditis and pneumonitis during neonatal period—viral isolation, specific antibody persisting after 6 mo.
Toxoplasma	?	+	No	+!	Chronic congenital infection with hepatosplenomegaly, jaundice, encephalitis, retinopathy, mental retardation.

Figure 10–2 (From Hardy, J. B.: Fetal consequences of maternal viral infection in pregnancy. Arch. Otolaryngol., *98*:218–227, 1973.)

What Can Be Done

Prospective parents, to help insure a healthy, happy baby, can do some practical things: First, they should bear in mind that it is dangerous to marry a close relative. To do so increases the risk of compounding the errors in heredity.

Second, the newly married couple should select a family physician. It is important for both parents to realize that in the event of pregnancy, prenatal care is extremely important. If there is a family history of defects or if there are possible complications such as Rh incompatibility, the doctor would then be alerted. Parents should know their Rh blood group. In addition, since premature babies are more prone to defects, medical help should be readily available to avoid most premature births.

Third, every mother should be sure to tell her doctor if she thinks she is pregnant, and she should take only the medicines he prescribes. "Pep-pills," tranquilizers, sleeping pills, and painkillers are all medicines. Their effect on an embryo early in pregnancy might be disastrous. In fact, since it is not known what might be the effects of taking drugs over a long period, the rule against self-medication is an excellent one for anyone of either sex at any age.

Fourth, since there is a correlation between certain virus diseases, including German measles (rubella), and birth defects, the pregnant mother should make a special effort to avoid contact with such diseases. It would be safer for future children if all girls 12 years of age and under had German measles, a relatively light illness of short duration. One attack gives lifetime immunity.

Fifth, abdominal x-rays should be avoided during early weeks of pregnancy, except in an emergency. For this reason, any doctor consulted should be informed if the patient is pregnant. Physicians usually prescribe x-rays of the abdomen only in the first 10 days after the menstrual period.

Sixth, excessive smoking during pregnancy should be avoided, for the practice is associated with subnormal birth weight. To date, studies show that the more cigarettes a mother smokes during her pregnancy, the less her baby will weigh. The average weight loss is half a pound. For a big baby, this is not important, but for the baby under five pounds this half pound is very important, for it is related to survival.

Seventh, age should be considered. There is a high correlation between birth defects and the age of the mother, and in some cases of the father. Statistics show that mothers under 18 and over 40 have more

Estimated incidence and prevalence of selected birth defects, U.S.A., 1974

Defect	Newly Affected	Under age 20 with Condition Currently
Anencephaly	3,100	*
Spina bifida and/or hydrocephalus	6,200	53,000
Cleft lip and/or cleft palate	4,300	71,000
Congenital heart disease	24,800	248,000
Clubfoot	9,300	149,000
Congenital dislocation of hip	3,100	50,000
Polydactyly	9,300	184,000
Syndactyly	1,000	21,000
Cystic fibrosis	2,000	10,000
Hemophilia	1,200	12,400
Phenylketonuria	310	3,100
Sickle-cell anemia	1,200	16,000
Tay-Sachs disease	30	100
Thalassemia (Cooley's anemia)	70	1,000
Diabetes	+	90,000
Down's syndrome	5,100	44,000
Other mental retardation of prenatal or perinatal origin	44,000	800,000

+ Late-appearing birth defect * Fatal soon after birth

Note: Some children have more than one kind of birth defect; hence the total number with one or more of the specific defects cited is smaller than the sum of the numbers for each condition.

Birth Defects Annual Death Toll

Cause of death		Number of Deaths
Diabetes mellitus		38,256
Other hereditary metabolic diseases		598
Structural defects:		
Heart and other circulatory defects	7,624	
Genitourinary defects	1,102	
Anencephaly	933	
Spina bifida	781	
Hydrocephalus	860	
Other nervous system defects	800	
Digestive system defects	967	
Respiratory system defects	546	
Musculoskeletal defects	466	
Multiple structural defects	1,531	
Other structural defects	334	
Total structural defects		15,944
Hereditary diseases of blood		1,864
Hereditary neuromuscular diseases		1,184
Certain abdominal hernias		870
Hemolytic diseases of newborn (including Rh disease)		623
Cystic fibrosis		516
Hemorrhagic disease of newborn		402
Gout		295
Diseases of newborn due to maternal infections		180
Hemangioma and lymphangioma		87
	Total	60,819

Source: Vital Statistics of the United States, 1971

Figure 10–3 (From National Foundation–March of Dimes: *Facts 1975*, p. 12.)

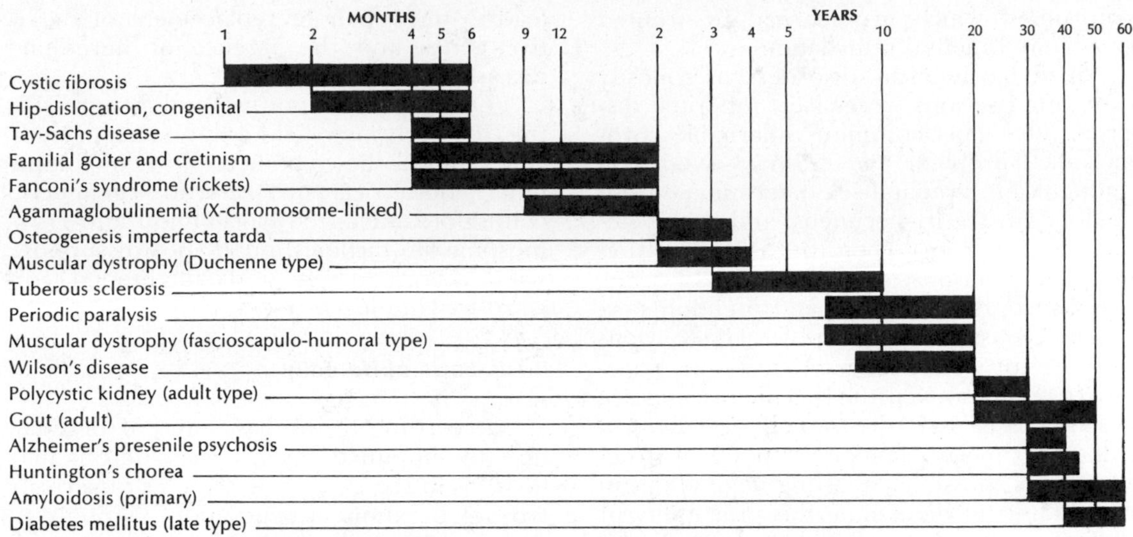

Figure 10–4 (From National Foundation–March of Dimes: *Facts 1975*, p. 10.)

children with defects than do those who give birth between the ages of 18 and 40.

Eighth, since diet affects growth, often in ways not yet fully understood, it is important for girls to acquire proper eating habits early in life. These are conducive not only to their own good health but to that of their children.

Genetic Counseling

Genetic counseling centers in hospitals and clinics are helping many parents. Trained counselors help the parents of a defective child decide whether to have more children or not and advise couples with family histories of genetic diseases before marriage. Blood and urine tests (and others) show promise in detecting more than 100 genetic diseases, including diabetes, cystic fibrosis, Tay-Sachs disease, hemophilia, sickle cell anemia, and some forms of muscular dystrophy.

By study of the amniotic fluid, through a process called amniocentesis, it is now possible to detect over 30 biochemical genetic disorders and a variety of chromosomal aberrations. Fluid usually is collected by amniocentesis sometime between the twelfth and sixteenth week of pregnancy. If amniocentesis is conducted by an experienced physician, there is very little risk of maternal or fetal complications. This test is usually performed in high-risk pregnant women who have already borne children with one of these specific disorders. Many different metabolic errors have been reliably diagnosed by amniocentesis early enough for pregnancies to be terminated. Among these are Tay-Sachs disease and Lesch-Nyhan syndrome, two serious neurological conditions; Pompe's disease, which causes infant victims to die of a weakened heart; and Hurler's and Hunter's

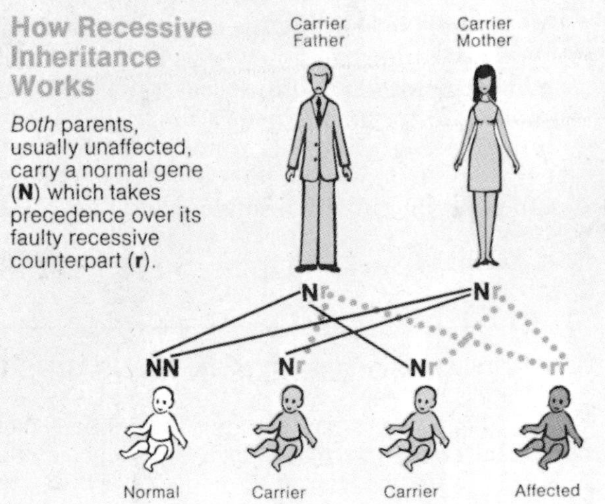

Figure 10–5 How recessive inheritance works in transmission of Tay-Sachs disease. (From National Foundation – March of Dimes: *Genetic Counseling*, p. 15.)

syndromes, which are marked by stunted growth and mental retardation.

The biochemical disorders are mostly rare, often serious, recessively inherited diseases. The most common inheritable chromosome problem is Down's syndrome (mongolism). Prenatal sex determination can be done on fresh specimens, and this sometimes is used to sharpen the risk calculation for certain serious, sex-linked recessive diseases, such as hemophilia and pseudohypertrophic muscular dystrophy. The obvious purpose for such prenatal detection is to reassure families when the specific diseases are absent and to alert them to abnormalities in sufficient time so that interruption of pregnancies is possible. Existing legislation in each state will determine the practicality of such diagnostic procedures. Successful community screening programs have helped educate the populace, screen for the defective gene, and counsel parents. Target areas include high-risk populations, for example, Jewish communities for detection of Tay-Sachs disease and black communities for detection of sickle cell anemia. Both screening tests are simple (blood test) and effective.

Dr. George Beadle, Nobel Prize winner and geneticist, claims that the most significant scientific accomplishment of the century was the understanding of the structure of the DNA molecule by Watson and Crick. He warns, however, that "Our hope, in improving man, is in guiding his cultural evolution. We can improve our government, our schools, and all of our social contacts. Why should we try to engineer a more intelligent human being when we cannot yet realize our existing intellectual potential?" (Now that we can experiment with a single gene, this could lead to the repair or replacement of defective genes and the absence of hereditary diseases.)

Optimal utilization of and progress in this relatively new field of preventive medicine requires the combined efforts of competent obstetricians, clinical geneticist-counselors, advanced biochemical and chromosome lab facilities, public health support, scientific researchers, and enlightened, forward-looking legislation.*

Basic Laws of Heredity

According to the basic laws of heredity (greatly simplified here), genetic defects may be transmitted in varying degrees of severity from generation to generation, through either dominant or recessive inheritance.

Dominant Inheritance. This means that an affected child must have one parent with the same disorder. A rare exception would be a new mutation, or change, in one parent's germ cells. In such a family, there is a 50 per cent risk that each child will manifest the defect, though it may not be evident at birth. There is an equal likelihood that a child will not receive the abnormal gene; thus, both he and his children should be free of the defect. Currently, some 943 dominantly inherited disorders have been catalogued. Examples include:

*achondroplasia – a form of dwarfism

*chronic simple glaucoma (some forms)

* Parents or prospective parents who want genetic counseling should consult their family doctors and/or write to the National Foundation--March of Dimes, 800 2nd Ave., New York, N.Y. 10017, for a list of counseling units in the United States and Canada.

AMNIOCENTESIS IN TAY-SACHS DISEASE

Tay-Sachs disease is an inborn metabolic disorder, essentially peculiar to Jews, consisting of deficiency or absence of the enzyme hexosaminidase A. The disease is invariably fatal, usually before 2 or 3 years of age. The carrier or heterozygous state occurs in approximately 1 in 30 Ashkenazi Jews, and is a harmless condition. If two carriers marry, the statistical probability is that one-quarter of the offspring will have the fatal disease, one-half will be carriers like the parents, and one-quarter will be totally free of the Tay-Sachs gene, according to simple Mendelian genetics.

Widespread screening for the carrier state has been undertaken in the United States and the United Kingdom. Many laboratories are now offering to carry out tests for the prenatal diagnosis of Tay-Sachs disease by the application of amniocentesis. If the fetus is determined to have Tay-Sachs disease, an abortion is then recommended.

—a major cause of blindness if untreated
*Huntington's disease—progressive nervous system degeneration
*hypercholesterolemia—high blood cholesterol levels, propensity to heart disease
*polydactyly—extra fingers or toes

Recessive Inheritance. In recessive inheritance, both parents of an affected child appear essentially normal, but by chance, both carry the same harmful gene, although neither may be aware of it. Unfortunately, the child who receives the defective gene from both parents may have a significant birth defect. As a rule, recessive abnormalities tend to be more severe than dominant ones, but they are also less likely to occur. When both parents are carriers of a harmful recessive trait, each of their children will run a 25 per cent (1 in 4) risk of manifesting that genetic disease. Each child will also have a 25 per cent chance of not inheriting the gene from either parent; and each has a 50/50 chance of receiving only a single defective gene and becoming a carrier of the genetic trait like both parents. Should the carrier-child ultimately marry another carrier, he or she runs the same risk.

Among 783 recessively inherited disorders catalogued are:
*cystic fibrosis—disorder affecting function of mucus and sweat glands
*galactosemia—inability to metabolize milk sugar
*phenylketonuria—essential liver enzyme deficiency
*sickle cell disease—blood disorder primarily affecting blacks
*thalassemia—blood disorder primarily affecting persons of Mediterranean ancestry

Phenylketonuria (PKU)

Phenylketonuria, called PKU for short, is an inherited condition some children have that makes it impossible for their bodies to properly use phenylalanine, an amino acid found in most foods. If this condition is not treated, the brain does not develop normally. It is easier to understand phenylketonuria if you can think of it in terms of food. Foods such as meat, fish, milk, eggs, cheese, dried beans, peas, and most breads and cereals have proteins that are necessary for growth and development. When a person eats these foods, the proteins are broken down into amino acids which the body uses with the help of body chemicals called enzymes. In phenylketonuria, a particular liver enzyme is lacking. As a result, the amino acid phenylalanine is not all used by the body and collects in large amounts in the blood, preventing the brain from developing normally and causing other harm to the body. Treatment of this condition was discovered very recently. Medical scientists are now trying to control the condition through a diet restricted in phenylalanine. If the diet is started early enough, the child's brain development will be normal in most cases. But even at a later age, a phenylalanine-restricted diet often results in noticeable improvement, especially in behavior.

Inheritance

Phenylketonuria is found in about 1 out of every 10,000 births. It is inherited, although it is not a strong enough trait to be inherited unless both the mother and father carry this tendency. Even then, not all the children of these parents will have phenylketonuria. Usually only 1 out of 4 children of such parents will have this condition, but this is not always true. When one child with phenylketonuria is found in a family, all the other children should be checked, especially infants. When the child with PKU becomes an adult, and if he or she marries and has children, the chances are small that the children will have PKU. This is because of the slight chance of marrying another adult with PKU or a carrier of the tendency.

Diagnosis

The diagnosis is not always simple, especially in the newborn period. Most states now have laws requiring that all infants have their blood tested for phenylalanine soon after birth. If the results indicate that the child might have PKU, the child will be tested more completely to determine if he has the condition. With older children a urine test is often used for this purpose. Since the disease is rare, many physicians refer to these cases to medical centers where experts are available to assist in making the diagnosis and starting the dietary treatment.

Symptoms

A child with PKU whose condition has not been found soon enough, and who therefore has not had the advantage of the phenylalanine-restricted diet, may have severe mental retardation, occasional eczema, excessive uncontrolled body movements, and convulsions. Many of these children are irritable and seem to be unhappy. When such a child is found to have PKU and is placed on the proper diet, his behavior and itching or eczema, if present, usually show the first signs of improvement. When an infant or young child with PKU is already retarded at the time the diet is started, some improvement in mentality (I.Q.) may be expected, but usually there remains some amount of permanent retardation. This is why it is so important that phenylketonuria be discovered early and the child kept on the phenylalanine-restricted diet. It is still not known how long the child needs to remain on the diet.

Management

Every child with PKU under treatment should have blood tests very frequently or whenever his doctor feels that it is important. From these tests, his doctor knows how much phenylalanine is in the child's blood. Some phenylalanine is necessary for a child to grow normally, as the body cannot manufacture it. From the blood tests, the doctor will decide how much phenylalanine can be allowed in the diet. With this amount of phenylalanine, a diet plan suitable for the age of the child will be planned with the parents. A low-phenylalanine product has been developed for children with PKU to substitute for protein foods such as milk, meat, eggs, and fish. This product, called Lofenalac, is low in phenylalanine but is otherwise similar to milk in food value. The product is expensive because the manufacturing process is complex and its use is limited. Diets containing Lofenalac, along with foods that have very little phenylalanine, such as fruits and most vegetables, must be carefully planned for each child with PKU. With proper dietary management, the child should gain weight, or lose if overweight, and grow normally. The parents are responsible for the diet, but they will have many understanding people to help them—doctors, nutritionists, nurses, and other professional people.

Prevention

Although PKU is rare in the general population (our current rate is about 1 case per 10,000 births), it is an important cause of mental retardation, constituting 1 per cent of our institutionalized population. The humanitarian benefits to the child and his family are obvious, but the preventive program has proven to be a boon to the taxpayers. The costs of state administration of this program on an annual basis have averaged \$50,000 to detect approximately 20 cases, or \$2500 per case. Treatment for 10 years would cost \$8000 from CCS* funds, totaling a lifetime cost of \$10,500 per case for the state. Alternately, the cost of institutional care for 1 case for 1 year averages \$5400. Estimated costs for even a 30-year life expectancy would be \$162,000, more than 3 times the cost of the preventive program. Based on a conservatively estimated savings of \$112,000 per case, the cases detected so far represent a potential saving of \$6,720,000.

Sickle Cell Anemia

Sickle cell anemia is an inherited blood disease that is transmitted from parent to child. It is not contagious. The disease affects blacks *almost* exclusively and is seen in two forms: (1) patients with the active disease, who are very sick, and (2) carriers of the "trait," who are usually healthy. A child born with the active disease is often chronically anemic; he may have chronic ulcers on his legs, ankles, or both; and he may suffer from yellow jaundice, intermittent pain in his arms, legs, and remainder of his body, and loss of appetite. At present the disease is incurable; victims rarely live more than 20 years and have less than 50 per cent chance of survival during the first year of life.

Normal red blood cells are shaped like a doughnut. In sickle cell anemia, the red blood cells tend to twist into the shape of a sickle or crescent. This impairs their ability to carry oxygen, and the sickle-shaped cells pile up and block blood vessels, thus producing pain and other symptoms. Sickle cell anemia is transmitted from generation to generation by carriers who have the trait. A person with sickle cell trait is usually in good health but carries the gene for sickle cell

*Crippled Children's Services

trait, which may be passed on to his children. About 1 in 10 black Americans is a carrier of sickle cell trait; 1 of every 500 black babies is affected. Both sexes are equally affected. A simple blood test can determine whether the sickle cell trait is present.

The two forms of sickle cell disease, sickle cell anemia and the carrier trait, are transmitted by blacks and persons whose parents stem from Africa, the Caribbean, Central America, and South America and has helped protect these people from contracting malaria by changing the shape of the red blood cell. When both a mother and father are carriers of the sickle cell trait, then with each child born there is a 25 per cent chance of the child's having the "full-blown" sickle cell anemia. Half the children will be born with the trait, and 25 per cent will be completely normal. In about 1 family in 150, both parents carry the trait. Both are usually perfectly healthy and unaware that they are carriers. The sickle cell anemia trait has been transmitted from black parents to their children for many centuries.

Sickle cell anemia is one of the most common chronic illnesses among black children. It occurs in about 1 out of every 500 births. Every black person in the community must be informed of this problem. Every black person may be an unknown carrier of the sickle cell trait; he must know where to go for tests and, if necessary, medical treatment and counseling. It is particularly crucial that black parents learn to anticipate the possibility of the disease occurring in their own children by seeking a blood test for sickle cell disease as part of a routine medical examination. Women with the sickle cell trait have increased difficulty with pregnancy. There is an increased death rate of babies born to such mothers. Greater awareness should lead to better detection, more counseling, improved care, and the stimulation of more research to combat the disease.

Psychological problems are common, as in other chronic handicapping illness. They may arise from (1) frequent absence from school with retarded educational progress, (2) feelings of inferiority because of inability to compete physically with peers, and (3) parental overconcern and overprotection. Some points for the parent and teacher to keep in mind are:

1. Sickle cell anemia is a chronic hereditary handicapping disease;

2. Colds and other infections may precipitate crises;

3. Crises cause frequent absence from school, especially in younger children;

4. Between crises, a child with sickle cell anemia may carry on the usual activities of his peer group, with the exception of strenuous sports.

Mass Screening Programs for Sickle Cell Anemia

With the enactment of Public Law 92–294, the National Sickle Cell Anemia Control Act, by the 92nd Congress in 1972, a new era of detection, treatment, and prevention of genetic disease on a national scale was established. The only precedent was the emergence of mass screening laws for phenylketonuria in the early 1960's. Unlike the Sickle Cell Act, however, these screening laws were passed by state legislatures in a time of relative unconcern for social aspects of health care delivery. The Sickle Cell Act made genetics a household word and resulted in a national dialogue of unprecedented proportion. Not only did 34 states commence statewide screening services (by means of a simple blood test), within one year after the federal law was passed, but over 250 screening programs offered diagnostic tests for hemoglobin S (Hb S).

Toxoplasmosis

Toxoplasmosis is a parasitic disease most likely to damage the eyes, brain, and spinal column of the fetus when the mother is infected during pregnancy. The parasites are found in two common sources that a pregnant woman is in danger of contacting every day: raw or undercooked meat, and cats. After the organisms enter the cells of the developing fetus, they multiply with such force that they burst the cell membranes, move into new cells, and the destructive cycle continues. If the mother was infected before pregnancy and built adequate antibodies to the disease, her baby is protected. If she has not had the disease before pregnancy, the parasites are capable of crossing the placenta and entering vital organs of her baby.

The question arises why so many children, although infected during pregnancy, show no ill effects of the disease when they are born. A study conducted by Cornell New York Hospital Medical Center in New York City reports that only one-third of the babies infected during intrauterine life showed evidence of the disease. Scientists now have discovered a "time bomb" factor. Sometimes the parasites stay dormant for as long as 20 years after the child is born and then strike without warning, often causing degrees of blindness and mental retardation. The symptoms can be so mild that a person is unaware of the infection. Before recent studies, doctors often confused toxoplasmosis with mononucleosis because of the similarity of symptoms: low-grade fever, lethargy, and swollen lymph glands. Laymen sometimes confuse it with the flu.

Dr. Georges Desmonts, a French scientist, linked the disease to raw or undercooked meat. He studied the reactions of hundreds of children being cared for in a tuberculosis sanitarium. Part of the treatment there involved eating large amounts of raw mutton and horse meat. His investigations convinced him that the more undercooked meat they ate, the greater the infection rate of toxoplasmosis. Similar studies were done in Japan among slaughterhouse workers. Nearly 90 per cent were found to have toxoplasmosis at some time.

These probings confirmed that raw or undercooked meat is definitely a source of infection. The parasites succumb quickly to temperature changes and cannot live in meat that has been well cooked. Since undercooked meat could not account for all cases of toxoplasmosis, there had to be another source of infection. Toxoplasmosis scientists hold the cat equally responsible. Cats are unique among animals as incubators for toxoplasmosis. The parasites harbor in feline intestines and form infectious bodies called oocysts which reach the outside world in cat feces. Toxoplasmosis oocysts survive for years and can be uprooted and spread by another cat, rodent, or gardner. At least two-thirds of all cats are believed to carry the disease. How the infection is transmitted to humans is not known. The Cornell team urges all pregnant women to avoid raw or undercooked meat and to stay away from cats, unless blood tests reveal that the mother is immune to toxoplasmosis.

Toxoplasmosis can be diagnosed in pregnancy, but the knowledge of the disease is still so new that many doctors understandably are not looking for it in their examinations of pregnant women. Studies have been conducted since 1908, but cohesive, related findings are only recent. A blood test for laboratory analysis shows if a patient has had the disease. Faster and less expensive means of testing are being explored. The Cornell team hopes that all pregnant women will now be given routine tests for susceptibility to toxoplasmosis. Data suggest that the fetus is in less danger if the mother contracts the disease during the first three months of pregnancy. Studies indicate that no woman can take the risk of ignoring medical warnings about avoiding cats and not eating raw or undercooked meat during her pregnancy. There is no vaccine against toxoplasmosis at this time.

To protect against possible infection from the cat, which has been shown to harbor the organisms, a woman who has cats as pets should have them checked as soon as she learns she is pregnant. By studying a cat's feces, a licensed veterinarian can determine whether the pet is free of infection. Once it is established that it is, the disease can be avoided by preventing the pet from playing with other cats or hunting mice, and by not feeding it raw or undercooked meats. Other safeguards against contracting feline infection during pregnancy are:

1. Do not introduce a newly acquired cat into the house during pregnancy without having a vet examine the animal. There's no way of knowing about his prior diet or history of infection.

2. Have someone other than the expectant mother empty the cat's litter box. This should be done daily, because the parasites are harmful for about two days after excretion. For added protection, use two litter boxes. When one is in use, the other can be washed clean of possible contaminants and given time to dry thoroughly. Finally, make sure that litter is incinerated or disposed of carefully, so that others will not come into contact with it.

3. Feed the cat canned or commercially dried cat foods. Unlike table scraps, which may harbor parasites, these packaged foods are germ-free.

4. Avoid digging in the garden if there is a chance that cat feces are buried there.

5. Avoid holding or fondling cats when visiting another home.

BREAST-FEEDING

There has been a dramatic decline in maternal nursing in recent years. The decline is in some ways surprising, since breast-feeding is the traditional and ideal form of infant nutrition, usually providing all of a child's complex nutritional needs for the first 4 to 6 months of life. For most infants in low-income countries, prolonged breast-feeding may be the key to survival, affording the only ready source of high-quality protein containing all the essential amino acids. By contrast, the use of expensive and less healthful substitutes for human milk has often resulted in human and economic suffering. Breast milk meets most of the metabolic needs of the baby during the months essential to normal brain development. Furthermore, the unbalanced or inadequate diets that often replace mother's milk tend to contribute to illness later in life. Although breast milk alone is inadequate after about six months, it can, when supplemented by solid foods, continue to be of great value for many more months.

Natural milk provides a host of protective factors. Breast-fed babies are more resistant to malaria and to infection caused by bacteria or viruses (including the polio virus). They are less likely to suffer from rickets or iron-deficiency anemia. The role of colostrum, the yellowish fluid that comes from the breast after childbirth and before the beginning of milk flow, is becoming clearer—and more obviously crucial. It appears that colostrum protects the child against infections, particularly those of the intestinal tract, and against food allergies. This explains why allergies are more common in artificially fed babies. In addition,

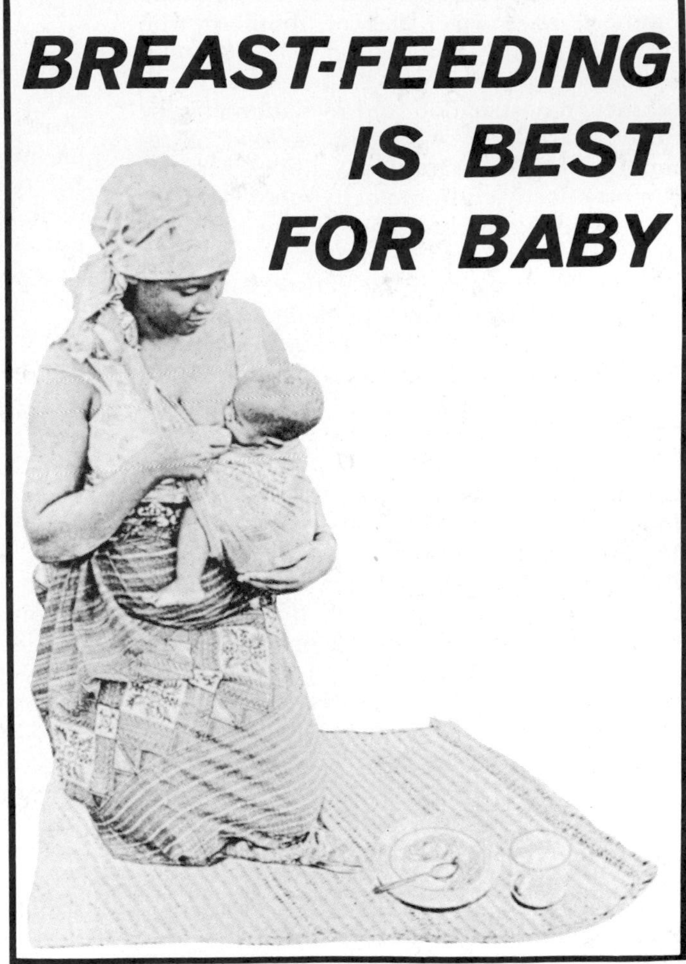

The decline in breast-feeding has prompted the Zambian government to issue this advertisement.

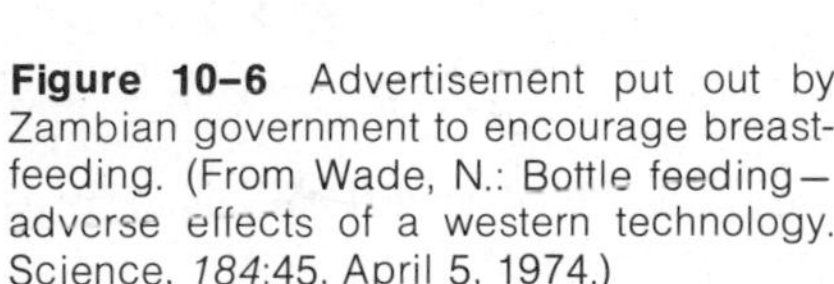
Figure 10–6 Advertisement put out by Zambian government to encourage breast-feeding. (From Wade, N.: Bottle feeding—adverse effects of a western technology. Science, *184*:45, April 5, 1974.)

the milk is easily digestible and requires no preparation.

New social values, spread through urbanization and faster communications, make breast-feeding in many places seem an old-fashioned or even vulgar peasant practice. Indeed, anthropologists in some countries even measure the level of acculturation by the incidence of artificial nursing—the less nursing, the higher the sophistication level. In most developing countries the bottle has become a status symbol. This trend in the poorer countries is apparently a reflection of behavior in the wealthier ones. A continuing nationwide study in the United States found that in only 10 years the number of mothers breast-feeding when they left the hospital had declined by half. This drop is most pronounced in the poorer states.

One recent study reported that the incidence of pregnancy in the first nine months after childbirth among non-nursing mothers was twice that of mothers who breast-fed, including those who simultaneously used other foods. In the lactating mother, menstruation and ovulation may be delayed from 10 weeks to as long as 26 months. The contraceptive value of lactation is most effective if in the early months the infant receives only human milk, for the sucking stimulus appears to inhibit ovulation. In Taiwan, for example, scientists have estimated that lactation has prevented as much as 20 per cent of the births that would have occurred otherwise. In India the same ratio would mean prevention of approximately 5,000,000 births each year.

Countries that should be concerned with the decline in breast-feeding—many of them unaware of the economic losses they are suffering—are acting slowly, if at all, and often in the wrong direction. Free milk programs, for example, especially those that offer dry skim milk, tend to discourage breast-feeding. The Chilean government during the last 10 years has increased twelvefold the free milk available to infants; during this time breast-feeding has declined markedly, and infant mortality in urban areas has risen. Like governments, educational authorities generally neglect the importance of nursing, often emphasizing instead the importance of artificial feeding. Of the 1600 pages in a major United States textbook on pediatrics, only one and one-half pages concern breast-feeding. For the vulnerable infant and young child a reversal of the current trend could be of greater significance than any other form of nutrition intervention.*

CHILDHOOD SAFETY

Safety education begins in the home; only parents can protect their children from accidents. Accidents remain the foremost cause of death among schoolage children and account for many more fatalities than are attributed to any single disease. Parents must protect infants from burns, drowning, poisoning, falls, and machinery. When the child begins school, the parents must depend upon the child's knowledge, attitude, skill, habits, and behavior to protect him. Therefore, parents must be effective teachers and must set good examples for their children.

Children must be motivated to develop and practice protective skills and acquire the habit of conscientiously observing general as well as specific safety principles. Education should engender in every child the desire and the ability to shield himself from potential danger in all circumstances, including those that are new to him and that involve hazards he has not previously encountered. Safety education must be extended to all students in the school and be given proper emphasis in the school curriculum. First aid, swimming instruction, driver training, and bicycle training should be included in the safety education program.

Accidental Poisoning in Children

One of the most important and increasingly common causes of childhood accidents is poisoning. Drugs and medications cause most poisonings in children, and the drug most often involved is aspirin. Deodorants, barbiturates, household preparations such as detergents, insecticides, stimulants, and analgesics contribute to the magnitude of the problem. More than 300 products, many containing a variety of ingredients, are the causative agents. Internally taken drugs cause nearly 50 per cent of all poisonings.

Around 55 per cent of all poisoning occurs in persons under 20 years of age. Household materials such as cleaning, sanitizing, and polishing agents, solvents, and pesticides are the main offenders. Parents

*For further discussion, refer to *The Nutrition Factor*, published by the Brookings Institute, 1973.

Children will try anything once.
Keep all household cleaners
drugs and medicine out of children's reach.
The Health Education Council

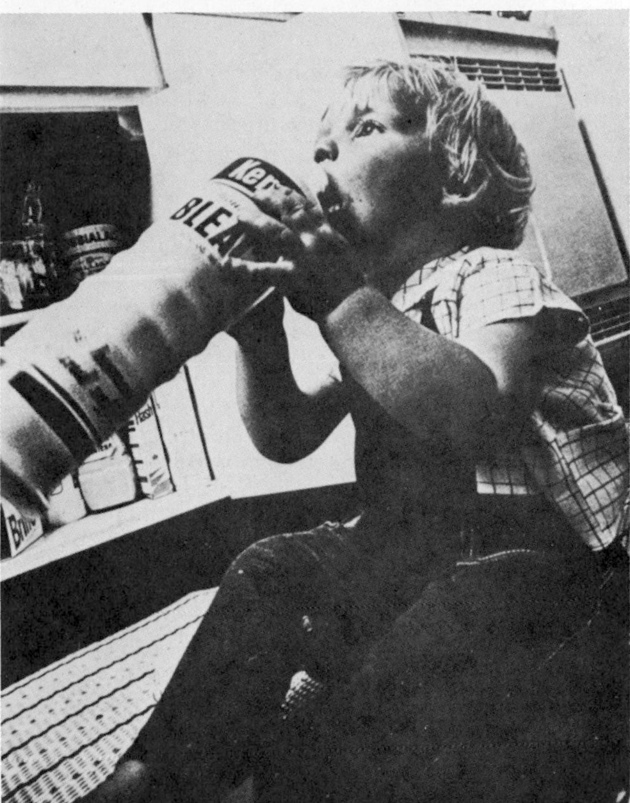

Figure 10–7 A Health Education Council warning on the hazards of accidental child poisoning. (From Calnan, M. W.: Health education policy of accidental child poisoning. The Health Education Journal, *34*(1):31, 1975. Health Education Council, 78 New Oxford St., London, England.)

should be alerted to the harmful effects of ingested paint containing lead, and they should avoid its use for indoor painting.

Flavored baby aspirin is a frequent cause of salicylate poisoning. Poisoning of children occurs most frequently in the kitchen. The bedroom and the bathroom also contain possible hazards. In an effort to protect small children against potential harmful substances, many manufacturers, especially of aspirin, are experimenting with and have in operation hard-to-open safety containers and bottles. "Palm-n-Turn" safety caps, which require pressure and turning to open, cannot be removed by children under four years old. Manufacturers also limit the number of aspirin in each container.

The prevention of poisoning revolves around education, legislation, poison control centers (usually located in large cities in the United States, where doctors can get information quickly on antidotes of specific poisons), and educational programs conducted by the public health departments in each community. Public schools, as well as colleges and universities, should also include a teaching unit in their health classes in this area. A safety and accident prevention program is predicated on the assumption that education is the most potent weapon in the control and prevention of accidents. All media, including press, radio, and television, should be effectively utilized. Health education should be widely promoted through schools, clinics, drugstores, P.T.A.'s, and health and welfare agencies.

A few precautions necessary to prevent poisoning are:

1. Keep all drugs, poisonous substances, and household chemicals out of the reach of children.
2. Do not store nonedible products on shelves used for storing food.
3. Do not transfer poisonous substances to unlabeled containers.
4. Never re-use containers of chemical substances.

5. Do not leave discarded medicine where children or pets can get it.

6. Read labels before using chemical products.

7. Never give medicines in the dark.

Hazards of Children's Vitamin Preparations Containing Iron

Ingestion of iron preparations and vitamin preparations containing iron are the fourth most common cause of poisoning in children under five years of age. [Overdose of aspirin is still first.] Unless treated promptly, mortality from acute iron poisoning has been reported to be approximately 50 per cent in these young children. Iron compounds, commonly given to mothers during or immediately after pregnancy, have most frequently been associated with accidental poisoning of children. The iron compound frequently used is ferrous sulfate, and the usual formulation is a tablet containing 300 mg. The tablets are often attractively packaged and sugar coated. Six or seven of these tablets are equivalent to 400 mg. of elemental iron, a dose that is potentially fatal to a young child.

The Committee on Nutrition of the American Academy of Pediatrics has recommended that all infants be given an iron-fortified formula until they are 1 year old. Iron-fortified cereals and other food products are being marketed with increasing frequency. Thus, the availability of iron and possible accidental poisoning is increasing. In addition, iron is being incorporated into the formulas of several pediatric vitamin preparations, and some of these products are fruit-flavored and animal-shaped and are chewable. These preparations are marketed in bottles containing as many as 250 tablets. They are particularly hazardous, since a bottle contains sufficient iron to provide 5 to 10 times the lethal dose for a child. These vitamins are available without prescription and most parents consider them safe. None of the bottles contains a warning of the danger, and labels often do not clearly indicate the iron content.

An article from the poison information center of the Ottawa (Ontario) Civic Hospital indicates that the incidence of iron poisoning in children caused by children's chewable vitamins is increasing. A similar increase in the United States is probable unless the public becomes aware of the hazards of iron-containing compounds. As a first step, labels should be standardized and all iron-containing products should be labeled as potentially hazardous if large amounts are ingested accidentally.

Safety Education

The death rate for children between the ages of five and 14 has shown a remarkable reduction since safety education was introduced into school programs. The decreasing number of pedestrian accidents and the continuing low rate of bicycle accidents almost certainly reflect the school's efforts to promote safety in these areas, particularly the increasing use of student traffic patrols.

Although the death rate for young people between the ages of 15 and 24 has shown little change during the last 30 years, more

LEAD POISONING

In 1971, the Surgeon General announced guidelines for a nationwide campaign against lead poisoning, which he said may affect as many as 400,000 children and may cause mental retardation or death. Lead poisoning occurs mainly in city slums where dwellings are old and children eat the paint peeling from walls, doors, and window frames. Lead poisoning can come from other sources as well, such as glazed earthenware pottery used for drinking.

Lead-based paints were commonly used for house interiors many years ago. They are still used for exteriors of dwellings. The Surgeon General indicated that it was urgent that more cities establish programs to locate and treat children suffering from lead poisoning and to remove lead-based paint. The Public Health Service recommends that screening programs for the prevention and treatment of lead poisoning include all children aged one to six who live in old, poorly maintained houses.

It is estimated that 6000 children suffer severe and permanent brain damage each year from lead poisoning, and another 200 die from it. Children in slum housing should be given blood tests. Those with 40 μg. or more of lead in 100 ml. whole blood have too much lead. Children with 80 μg. or more of lead should be hospitalized immediately. In some cities, lead poisoning may be so widespread that an overwhelming number of children screened will be found to have 40 μg. or more.

than 50 per cent of all fatalities in this group are due to automobile accidents, with drowning and firearm accidents responsible for most of the rest. If driver education courses become more widespread, and more students elect to take them, the death rate for adolescents and young adults should be reduced. At present, over 4,000,000 students are enrolled in these courses, which are offered by 15,000 high schools. Statistics show that both the accident rate and the incidence of traffic violations are lower among these students than other drivers of the same age.[5] On a proportionate basis, five times more infractions are committed by the untrained group than by the trained group.

In stressing the relationship of safety education to the community, Dr. Florio and Dr. Stafford, safety educators, noted:

> If safety education is to meet its challenge, it must be extended not only to more and more students, but to their parents as well—in fact to all members of the community. The school's program functions best when it is supported by outside agencies; the effectiveness of classroom instruction is weakened when parents do not support the program, e.g., permitting a child to ride a bicycle in the street before he has acquired sufficient skill and knowledge. When a student brings home a checklist of home hazards, it is important that his parents pay attention, for any indifference or opposition on their part may negate the value of what he has learned. The training students receive at school must be strengthened by their outside experiences; otherwise they may take the proper precautions only when they are closely supervised. It is far easier to induce children to behave safely at all times if adults set a good example.[6]

BATTERED CHILD SYNDROME

No concern is more important to a community than the health, welfare, and protection of its children. In the days of our ancestors, however, it was common practice to "beat the devil" out of children. Physical punishment is part of our cultural heritage. Many children are considered as private property by their parents and are helpless in the face of their punitive whims. The Society for the Prevention of Cruelty to Children was instituted in New York City in 1875 by an incensed group of church workers. It was not until this decade, however, that various state legislatures reacted to the public's demand for strong punitive measures for parents who inflicted such injuries on their children.* All persons who are involved in maternal and child health are faced with new responsibilities that involve a complex socio-legal-medical syndrome.

Because the statutes in all states were based on model laws suggested by the Children's Bureau and the American Humane Society, they have great similarity in outline and intent, although in procedures and implementation there are many differences. The objective in most of the statutes is to identify children who have been abused so that they may be protected. Most of the state laws make a legal distinction between "abuse" and "neglect," defining abuse as nonaccidental physical attack or injury inflicted on a child by a person caring for him. By this definition, accidental neglectful causes of injury are ruled out. The *nature* and *intent* of an overt act,rather than its severity, is usually the crucial factor. All the state laws focus on the child who is hurt and the care-taking person who hurts him. In legal terms, in order for a child to be physically injured by his parents or guardian several factors must come together in a very special way. First, a parent (or parents) must have the potential to abuse. This potential is acquired over the years and is made up of at least four factors:

1. The way the parents themselves were reared, i.e., did they receive the "mothering imprint"?

2. Have the parents become very isolated individuals who cannot trust or use others?

3. Is one parent so passive that he or she cannot give?

4. Do the parents have very unrealistic expectations from their child (or children)?

Second, the child must be a very special one, who is seen differently by his parents—one who fails to respond in the expected way, or possibly one who really is different (retarded, too smart, hyperactive, or suffering from a birth defect). Most families in which there are several children can readily point out which child would have "gotten it" if the parents had the potential to abuse. Often the perfectly normal child is viewed by his parents as being, bad, willful, stubborn, demanding, spoiled, or slow.

---

*One definition of the battered child (Drs. Kempe and Helfer) is: "Any child who received nonaccidental physical injury (or injuries) as a result of acts (or omissions) on the part of his parents or guardians."

Finally, there must be some form of crisis that sets the abusive act into motion. The crisis can be a minor or a major one; the precipitating factor could be almost anything—faulty plumbing, persistent crying of an infant, a collection of bills to pay, in-law problems, and so on. It would seem most unlikely for the crisis to be the cause of the abuse, as some would like to believe; rather, it is the precipitating factor. The simplistic lay view that child abuse is caused by parents who "don't know their strength" while disciplining their child has been shown to be false. It is this combination of events, occurring in the right order and at the right point in time, that leads to physical abuse.

Parents who physically abuse their children come from all walks of life and all socioeconomic levels. They do share, however, a common pattern of parent-child relationships characterized by a high demand for the child to perform so as to gratify the parents, and by the use of severe physical punishment to ensure the child's proper behavior. Abusive parents also show an unusually high vulnerability to criticism, disinterest or abandonment by the spouse or other important person, and overreaction to anything that lowers their already inadequate self-esteem. Such events create a crisis of unmet needs in the parent, who then turns to the child with exaggerated demands for gratification. The child is often unable to meet these parental expectations and is then punished excessively for his failure. This pattern of demanding, aggressive behavior toward the child and the crises of emotional deprivation which trigger the pattern of abuse both stem directly from the parent's own childhood experiences and learning.

These childhood experiences are profound, and provide lasting imprints which are revealed in the way the adults feel about themselves and their children. Abusive parents have no basic, firm cushion of self-esteem or awareness of being loved and valuable to carry them through periods of stress. Instead, they are in constant need of reassurance. They are inwardly shattered by anything resulting in disapproval from their spouse, relatives, employer, or any other person significant in their lives. In such a crisis of insecurity, they repeat what they learned in childhood about how parents behave, and they turn to their own infant or child for the nurturing and reassurance they so badly need to restore this sense of self-esteem.

Indicators of a Child's Need for Protection

The Child's Behavior

1. Is the child aggressive, disruptive, destructive? Such a child may be acting out of a need to secure attention. He may be shouting for help. His behavior may reflect on a hostile or emotionally destructive climate at home, or he may be imitating destructive parental behavior.

2. Is the child shy, withdrawn, passive, or overly compliant? This child may be as emotionally damaged as the aggressive child. He has internalized his problem; his cry for help is a whisper instead of a shout. He may be inattentive; he may daydream; he may be out of touch with reality.

3. Is the child a habitual truant—chronically late or tardy? Is he frequently absent from school, giving flimsy reasons and lame excuses? This behavior points to problems of adjustment—problems at home, in school, within the child, or a combination of these.

4. Does the child come to school much too early? Does he loiter and hang around after school is dismissed? This child may be seeking to escape from home—he may lack love and attention at home, or he may even be "pushed out" in the morning and have no place to go after school because there is no one to supervise or care for him.

The Child's Appearance

1. Is the child inadequately dressed for the weather? Is his clothing torn, tattered, or unwashed? Is the child unbathed? Do other children refuse to sit next to him because he smells? These are all signs of physical neglect, a condition not necessarily related to poverty. It reflects a breakdown in household management and in concern for the child.

2. Is the child undernourished? Is he coming to school without breakfast and does he go without lunch? Again, this is often a problem unrelated to poverty.

3. Is the child always tired? Does he sleep in class? Is he lethargic or listless? Such conditions are symptomatic of parental failure to regulate the child's routines, or of family problems which disrupt family routines.

4. Is the child in need of medical attention? Does he need glasses or dental work?

5. Does the child bear bruises, welts, and contusions? Is he injured frequently? Does he complain of beatings or other mal-

treatment? Is there reason to suspect physical or sexual abuse?

Parental Attitudes

1. Are the parents aggressive or abusive when approached about problems concerning their child?

2. Are they apathetic or unresponsive?

3. Is parental behavior, as observed by school personnel, or as related by the child, bizarre and strange?

4. Do the parents show little concern about the child? Do they fail to participate in school activities or to permit the child to participate?

There appear to be four major categories that may assist in the early identification of those who may injure their small children:

1. Parents who physically abuse their children have almost invariably been reared in a similar manner.

2. Lack of family unity, structure, and relationship is seen in these cases.

3. The family may have built a wall of isolation around them which could keep them from turning to others for help.

4. The parents have unrealistic expectations of their children. There is a feeling that the children must provide them with emotional support when they are upset.

Efforts have been made to design and validate a questionnaire with the goal of uncovering parents who have the potential to abuse their small children. The crucial areas that must be examined involving attitudes of abusers and nonabusers are: (a) feelings of loneliness and isolation, (b) expectations for performance of their children, (c) relationships with their own parents and spouses, and (d) feelings of anxiety in response to children's behavior. Following is an excerpt from a questionnaire in which parents are asked to respond to statements in each of the crucial areas.

Sample Items From Clusters[8]

Cluster 1 — Isolation and Loneliness

I like myself.

People are always criticizing me (reflected).*

I am close to others.

I am a warm person.

Cluster 2 — Expectations of Children

Children are ready to be toilet trained at 1 year of age.

I expect too much of my children (reflected).

If parents don't expect a lot of their children, they won't be successful.

Cluster 3 — Relationship to Their Parents and Children

Most women remain close to their mother after marriage.

I would describe my relationship to my mother as very close.

At least one of my children reminds me of someone I don't like (reflected).

People say one should automatically feel love for their children but it's not that easy (reflected).

Cluster 4 — Upset and Angry

When my baby cries, I often feel like crying.

People become very upset and angry when they are fed up with their children.

Children are easily spoiled by others and then give trouble to their parents.

I am afraid of many things.

The typical parent who abuses a child is very young, emotionally immature, lonely, and rejected. One such mother studied by case workers was unloved, rejected by her parents, and probably physically abused. Child care and development was learned only through her hostile environment. She married young in a desperate search to find someone who would love her, help her gain self-respect, and overcome her feelings of inadequacy, failure, and isolation. (Many times child abusers are unwed mothers who openly resent their child.) For some women, pregnancy can be a way to escape from unresolved conflicts, to achieve instant identity, to strengthen a poor self-image, or to gratify a need for love and attention they feel they never had as children.

When perfection and love are found lacking in their mates, a mother may turn to her baby to fulfill these expectations. When the 2-month-old baby lies in his crib and cries endlessly, the mother feels that her child, like everyone else, is rejecting her, criticizing her efforts, illuminating her inadequacies. In frustration, she then strikes out. The immature mother expects perfection in her

*The term "reflected" indicates that a person agreeing with the other items in this cluster will disagree with the reflected item.

child, but has no knowledge of child development. When she tries to toilet train her 6-month-old child and fails, she feels inadequate and rejected, and abuses the child. It is interesting and important to note that, for some, the earliest months of life are the hardest to cope with because the child is so much more demanding and much less rewarding.

Additional factors involved in the child abuse syndrome include the following:

1. Parents usually select a certain child—usually the oldest—as a scapegoat, and they tend to abuse this child while leaving the others alone. Often this child resembles the mother herself, and has certain qualities the mother objects to in herself, her husband, or other members of the family. The same is true in cases where the husband perpetrates the attack. The majority of abused children are under 22 months, with the largest group under 1 year of age. Most parents are under 25 years of age; often the mothers are still in their teens.

2. A crisis, or frustration caused by social pressures, usually precedes the attack. Illness, moving, or loss of a job are examples of the kinds of things that cause strain leading to child abuse.

3. A battered child may grow up to be a battering parent. This is a learned response and is passed on from one generation to the next ("I turned out O.K.; therefore my parents must have raised me correctly"). Rejected by their own parents, convinced of their own inadequacies, child abusing parents have difficulties in establishing normal relationships with other people and expect a great deal of their children. Those expectations are never fulfilled, because no normal child can be the perfect being that these parents want. And so the child is beaten, and the cycle starts all over again. Some parents feel that by battering their child they are "getting even" with their own parents.

4. Many parents are simply not knowledgeable and are unprepared for the stresses of parenthood. Many young girls have no idea of the time and energy involved in raising a child. Some parents expect children to act like adults, and when their child fails to perform properly, they attribute this behavior to deliberate stubbornness, willful disobedience, or a malicious desire to thwart their wishes. The parents, of course, feel justified in their actions. Some parents have little knowledge as to ages and stages of development in children; some don't realize the difference between hitting a child on the bottom and hitting him on the head.

5. Feelings of jealousy.

6. There are those who, perhaps because of certain religious beliefs, adhere to the ways of our Puritan ancestors in their belief that physical punishment will effect a positive change in behavior.

Recent studies have indicated that there is a definite link between maternal deprivation and feelings of rejection in the mother. One recent study explored the feasibility of bringing mothers into premature nurseries early and allowing them to touch their very sick infants. This would be expected to assist normal maternal-child bonding and lessen the usual isolation experienced by the mother of a small premature infant. It appears likely that the enforced separation so commonly practiced in premature units contributes to abnormal maternal-child relationships, including rejection, neglect, and finally battering.[9, 10]

Legislation in many states now requires teachers, administrators, and physicians to report all suspected cases of child abuse. When child abuse is suspected, all personnel concentrate on admitting the child to the hospital or Children's Shelter (depending upon severity of injury) and giving psychiatric help and counseling to the parents. To help the child, the parents must be helped first. Because the parent is filled with guilt and suppressed anger, an accusing tone would bring indignant denials and stubborn refusal to release the child. In many cases, the cure for child abuse is to give parents enough self-respect and dignity to achieve the deep friendships they lack. This may be facilitated by discussions of possible alternative ways of problem solving, relieving frustration, and coping with children. Parents must be reinforced for their efforts and be given constructive and judicious praise. Growth involves the development of a sense of value and self-esteem. These parents also need a great sense of reassurance, patient support, and sometimes direct, realistic aid. The establishment of a positive therapeutic relationship with the therapist is often the most important step in protecting the child. The parent needs help and rehabilitation, not punishment; taking the child away from the parent often does not solve the problem.

New programs include meetings with groups of parents conducted by a trained psychologist, counselor, social worker, or lay therapist, and surrogate parents who live in the home for short periods of time and offer counseling, guidance, and friendship. Parents Anonymous is an organization through which parents call each other on the phone and discuss their anger, fear, anxiety, or frustrations with someone who has been through the same ordeal. The organization's basic tenets and guidelines are expressed in its brochure, Guidelines for Achievement, and are reprinted below:

1. WE will recognize and admit to ourselves and to other Parents Anonymous (P.A.) members the child abuse problem in our home as it exists today and set about an immediate course of constructive actions to stop any further abusive actions in our homes.

2. WE want and accept help for ourselves and will follow any constructive guidance to get the strength, the courage, and the control that we must have in order that our children will grow up in a loving healthy home.

3. WE will take one step, one day, at a time to achieve our goals.

4. WE may remain anonymous if we desire, but we may identify ourselves and at anytime call upon other P.A. members or seek constructive help before, during, or after our problem of child abuse occurs.

5. WE must understand that a problem as involved as this cannot be cured immediately and takes constant acceptance of the P.A. program or other constructive guidance.

6. WE admit that our children are defenseless and that the problem is within us as a parent.

7. WE believe our children are not to be blamed or subjected to our abusive actions regardless of what the cause is.

8. WE promise to ourselves and our families that we will use, to the fullest extent, the P.A. program.

9. WE admit that we are alienating ourselves from our children and our family and through the P.A. program we will make ourselves the center of reuniting our family as a loving, healthy family unit.

10. WE admit we must learn to control ourselves and we do these things in order to achieve harmony in our home and to earn the love and respect of ourselves, our family, and our society.

In any case, community education and a multidisciplinary team approach, involving social worker, public health nurse, counselor, pediatrician, psychiatrist, and juvenile court officials, is essential. The development of child abuse centers in large metropolitan areas for the purpose of education, demonstration, and research in the area of abused and neglected children is in sight. New and practical ways must be found of helping "Wednesday's Children."

QUESTIONS FOR DISCUSSION

1. Discuss three major current problems in maternal and child health.
2. What is the importance of the WIC program?
3. What steps can be taken to *prevent* birth defects?
4. Discuss three major medical advances in maternal and child health.
5. Discuss genetic counseling, using Tay-Sachs disease as an example.
6. Briefly discuss the significance of PKU testing and breast-feeding on public health.
7. Discuss accidental poisoning in children (aspirin, vitamins, lead, etc.).
8. Why is the "battered child syndrome" within the scope of state or local health departments? What can be done to prevent this syndrome?

QUESTIONS FOR REVIEW

1. What are the five broad aspects of maternal and child health?

2. Name and describe the disease that can be prevented by the Rho immune globulin.

3. List some recommendations for the reduction of pregnancy risks in adolescents.

4. What is one of the most increasingly common causes of child accidents?

5. List the precautions necessary to prevent poisoning.

6. What are two sources of lead poisoning?

REFERENCES

1. Committee on Relationships Between Schools of Public Health and Maternal and Child Health and Crippled Children's Field Services: Report on the teaching of maternal and child health. Amer. J. Publ. Health, *52*:1932, 1962.
2. Ibid.
3. Bronfenbrenner, U.: Parents, bring up your children! Look, *35*:45, 1971.
4. California's Health, *27*(4):3, 1969.
5. Brody, L., and Stack, H. J.: *Highway Safety and Driver Education.* New York, Prentice-Hall, 1954, pp. 360–361.
6. Florio, A. E., and Stafford, C. T.: *Safety Education.* New York, McGraw-Hill, 1956, p. 15.
7. Murphy, B. F.: Hazards of children's vitamin preparations containing iron. JAMA, *229*(3):394, July 15, 1974.
8. Schneider, C., Helfer, R. E., and Pollock, C.: The predictive questionnaire: a preliminary report. *In* Kempe, C. H., and Helfer, R. E. (eds.): *Helping the Battered Child and His Family.* Philadelphia and Toronto, J. B. Lippincott Co., 1972, p. 277.
9. Barnett, C. R., et al.: Neo-natal separation: the maternal side of interactional deprivation. Pediatrics, *45*:197–205, 1970.
10. Klein, M., and Stern, L.: Low birth weight and the battered child syndrome. Amer. J. Dis. Child., *122*:15–18, July, 1971.

SUGGESTED READING

American Medical Association: *The Quality of Life.* Vol. 1: *The Early Years.* Vol. 2: *The Middle Years.* Baltimore, Publishing Sciences Group, 1974.

Anderson, B. A., et al.: *Pregnancy and Family Health: A Programmed Text.* Vol. 1: *The Child-Bearing Family.* New York, McGraw-Hill Book Co., 1974.

Anderson, C. L.: *Community Health.* 2nd ed. St. Louis, C. V. Mosby Co., 1973.

Arms, S.: Immaculate Deception: A New Look at Women and Childbirth in America. Boston, Houghton Mifflin, 1975.

Auerbach, S. (ed.): *Child Care: A Comprehensive Guide.* Vol. 1: *Rationale for Child Care—Programs vs. Politics.* New York, Behavioral Publications, 1975.

Barten, H. H., and Barten, S. S. (eds.): *Children and Their Parents in Brief Therapy.* New York, Behavioral Publications, 1973.

Baumslag, N. (ed.): *Family Care.* Baltimore, Williams & Wilkins, 1973.

Berlin, I. N.: *Bibliography of Child Psychiatry,* with a selected list of films. New York, Behavioral Publications, 1975.

Bonvechio, L. R.: *School Health Resource Guide.* Dubuque, Iowa, Kendall/Hunt, 1974.

Bryant, P.: *Perception and Understanding in Young Children: An Experimental Approach.* New York, Basic Books, 1974.

Burgess, A. W., and Lazore, A.: *Community Mental Health.* Englewood Cliffs, N.J., Prentice-Hall, 1976.

Child Care Quarterly. Vol. 4. New York, Behavioral Publications, 1975.

Cockburn, F., and Drillien, C. M. (eds.): *Neonatal Medicine.* Oxford, Blackwell Scientific Publications, 1975.

Cohn, V.: *Sister Kenny: The Woman Who Challenged the Doctors.* Minneapolis, University of Minnesota Press, 1976.

Cravioto, J., et al. (eds.): *Early Malnutrition and Mental Development.* Saltsjobaden, Sweden, Swedish Nutrition Foundation, 1974.

Davis, H. C., and Land, D.: *Out of the Mouths....* London,The Gibbs Oral Hygiene Service, 1973.

Day Care and Child Development Council of America: *Alternatives in Quality Child Care: A Guide for Thinking and Planning.* New York, Behavioral Publications, 1972.

Duffy, J. C. (ed.): Child Psychiatry and Human Development (journal). New York, Behavioral Publications, Inc.

Dummett, C. O.: *Community Dentistry: Contribution to New Directions.* Springfield, Ill., Charles C Thomas, 1974.

Elliott, K., and Knight J. (eds.): *Size at Birth.* New York, Elsevier, 1974.

Gellis, S. S. (ed.): *The Year Book of Pediatrics 1975.* Chicago, Year Book, 1975.

Grynebaum, H., et al.: *Mentally Ill Mothers and Their Children.* Chicago, University of Chicago Press, 1975.

Hartman, H.: *Let's Play and Learn.* New York, Behavioral Publications, 1975.

Helfer, R. E., and Kempe, C. H. (eds.): *The Battered Child.* Chicago and London, University of Chicago Press, 1974.

Holt, J.: *Escape from Childhood.* New York, Ballantine Books, 1975.

Hundley, J. M.: *The Small Outsider.* New York, Ballantine Books, 1975.

Hubbard, C. W.: *Family Planning Education: Parenthood and Social Disease Control.* St. Louis, C. V. Mosby Co., 1976.

Husting, E. L., et al.: *Guidelines for Self-Evaluation of Programs Serving Adolescent Parents.* Published by Maternity Care Research Unit, Graduate School of Public Health, University of Pittsburgh, Pittsburgh, Pa., 1973.

Hyatt, R., and Rolnick, N. (eds.): *Teaching the Mentally Handicapped Child.* New York, Behavioral Publications, 1974.

Illich, I.: *Medical Nemesis.* New York, Pantheon, 1976.

Jelliffe, D. B.: *Human Milk in the Modern World.* St. Louis, C. V. Mosby Co., 1976.

Jerge, C. R., et al.: *Group Practice and the Future of Dental Care.* Philadelphia, Lea & Febiger, 1974.

Kissane, J. M.: Pathology of Infancy and Childhood. 2nd ed. St. Louis, C. V. Mosby Co., 1975.

Klerman, L. V., and Jekel, J. F.: *School-Age Mothers—Problems, Programs, and Policy.* Hamden, Conn., Shoe String Press, 1973.

McCalister, D. V., et al.: *Readings in Family Planning: A Challenge to the Health Professions.* St. Louis, C. V. Mosby Co., 1976.

Melnick, A.: *Pediatrics: Some Uncommon Views on Some Common Problems.* St. Louis, Green, 1975.

Meltzer, D.: *Birth.* New York, Ballantine Books, 1975.

Mico, P., and Ross, H.: *Health Education and the Behavioral Sciences.* Third Party Associates, P.O. Box 13042, Montclair Station E, Oakland, Calif. 94611.

Milunsky, A.: *The Prenatal Diagnosis of Hereditary Disorders.* Springfield, Ill., Charles C Thomas, 1973.

Morley, D.: *Pediatrics: Priorities in the Developing World.* London, Butterworth, 1973.

Montessori, M.: *The Discovery of the Child.* New York, Ballantine Books, 1975.

Montessori, M.: *The Secret of Childhood.* New York, Ballantine Books, 1975.

Oakland, T., and Phillips, B. N. (eds.): *Assessing Minority Group Children.* (Special issue of Journal of School Psychology.) New York, Behavioral Publications, 1974.

Piaget, J.: *A Child's Conception of Movement and Speed.* New York, Ballantine Books, 1975.

Piaget, J.: *The Child's Conception of Time.* New York, Ballantine Books, 1975.

Piaget, J.: *Construction of Reality in the Child.* New York, Ballantine Books, 1975.

Pollack, M. B., and Oberteuffer, D.: *Health Science and the Young Child.* New York, Harper & Row, 1974.

Roberts, A. R. (ed.): *Childhood Deprivation.* Springfield, Ill., Charles C Thomas, 1974.

Sarason, I., and Sarason, B.: *Constructive Classroom Behavior: Guide to Modeling and Role-Playing Techniques.* New York, Behavioral Publications, 1974.

Schreiber, F. R.: *Your Child's Speech.* New York, Ballantine Books, 1975.

Shirley, H. C.: *Pediatric Therapy.* 5th ed. St. Louis, C.V. Mosby Co., 1975.

Smolensky, J.: *A Guide to Child Growth and Development.* Dubuque, Iowa, Kendall/Hunt, 2nd ed., 1977.

Stone, L. J., et al. (eds.): *The Competent Infant: Research and Commentary.* New York, Basic Books, 1974.

Taichert, L. C.: *Childhood Learning, Behavior, and the Family.* New York, Behavioral Publications, 1973.

Torrens, P. R. (ed.): *Policies and Issues in Health Care.* St. Louis, C. V. Mosby Co., 1976. (Individual series books include: Breslow, L.: *Politics of Health Care in the United States*; Jelliffe, D. B.: *Maternal and Child Health Programs*; Roemer, M. I.: *Rural Health Services*; Shonick, W.: *Area-Wide Health Planning*; Torrens, P. R.: *Health Organizations and Issues.*

Wallace, H. M., et al. (eds.): *Maternal and Child Health Practices: Problems, Resources, and Methods of Delivery.* Springfield, Ill., Charles C Thomas, 1973.

Walters, C. E.: *Mother-Infant Interaction.* New York, Behavioral Publications, 1975.

Windsor, C. F., and Hurtt, J.: *Eye Muscle Problems in Childhood: A Manual for Parents.* St Louis, C.V. Mosby Co., 1974.

CHAPTER 11

Environmental Sanitation

From his earliest beginnings, man has sought ways to manipulate and control his environment and to create favorable conditions for his work, play, and home activities. Our complex industrial, mobile public, made more aware of luxury and comfort products by increased education and mass communication, is demanding a higher living standard and a better living environment. Unfortunately, however, environmental sanitation programs in many local health departments have not changed or expanded to meet present and future needs. Many legitimate new public health activities have been indifferently lost to enthusiastic allied agencies.

Correction and control of water and air pollution require changes in industry, in living habits, in technology, and in numerous aspects of society. In turn, this means that numerous special interests are involved, and that many of these will resist change. For example, air pollution control is hindered by lack of comprehensive community and regional planning involving local, state, and federal action. Another example involves millions of dollars allocated to regional water resources development, the real purpose of which is sometimes questioned, as related in the following testimony:

> "There are a variety of motivations behind such violent shifts of water assets as the Pacific Southwest Water Plan and the Central Arizona Project," Adolph J. Ackerman, a Madison, Wisconsin, engineer, told the Senate Interior Committee a fortnight ago. For one thing, he stressed an implied yearning on the part of politicians to become pyramid builders. He mentioned also "a new type of massive speculation in real estate in arid regions, based on the idea of persuading the government to bring in water from distant sources at public expense." At the time California officials were agitating for the start of the Feather River Project, he told the Senate inquiry, "some private interests in Southern California began to acquire control of vast areas of Antelope Valley, an arid region of some 4,800,000 acres on the edge of the Mojave Desert."

PROGRESS INVOLVES DANGERS

Needless to say, ecologists, students of natural resources, physicians, and public health officers have long recognized that technological innovations cause dangers to human health. The problem is not to protect man from exposure to a few poisonous substances, but rather to consider, as a whole, the dangers to health that are created by the innumerable products and techniques of modern technology. Dr. Rene Dubos stimulates our thinking in this area:

> For the time being, we must accept as a fact that it is impossible to detect beforehand all the potential dangers of new technological developments. No legislation or administrative regulation can cope with this problem, because the scientific background is far too inadequate. It must be recognized, furthermore, that to exact a certificate of absolute safety before licensing a new process or a new product would completely paralyze technological progress.
>
> It is almost certain that any substance possessing biological activity will also prove to have some toxic properties. Each one of the drugs introduced into the practice of medicine during the past twenty years–from penicillin to cortisone or the tranquilizers–is now known to be capable of causing severe toxic reactions under certain cir-

cumstances; this is true even of acetylsalicylic acid (aspirin). Thus, the problem is not to rule out of use substances which are potentially toxic but rather to use educated judgment in weighing advantages against dangers. The case of isoniazid illustrates well the need for common sense as opposed to sweeping regulations. It has been known for many years that isoniazid causes neurological symptoms in a certain percentage of human beings, and it was reported last year that it can elicit cancers in several strains of mice.[2] On the other hand, isoniazid is an indispensable drug for the control of tuberculosis. Clearly, therefore, it must be used extensively despite its potential dangers. And a similar case could be made for many other substances which have become essential in medicine, industry, or agriculture, even though they present some danger for human health.

All technological innovations, whether concerned with industrial, agricultural, or medical practices, are bound to upset the balance of nature. In fact, to achieve mastery over nature is synonymous with disturbing the order of nature. Technological progress necessarily involves dangers, and these cannot always be foreseen. Thoughtful men are of course concerned with safety, but on the other hand, vigorous societies are always willing to take risks for the sake of technological development. In consequence, it is probably useful now and then to overstate the dangers of technological innovations lest there be no control of them. In this respect books such as Our *Synthetic Environment* and *Silent Spring* serve a necessary social role, even though they present an unbalanced picture of the problem posed by the use of chemicals in modern life. Half a century ago the popular emotion aroused by Upton Sinclair's novel *The Jungle* compelled Congress to give adequate authority to the Food and Drug Administration. It may turn out that the fictional description of a birdless midwestern town will play a similar role with regard to the problem of environmental pollution in our society. It will also spur the search for better scientific knowledge of the biological effects of chemicals and thereby help technologists control natural forces more intelligently without poisoning thereby either human beings or the birds which enliven the spring.[3]

It is now apparent that if man is to have a suitable environment, he must be concerned with the total management of the natural resources of water, food, land, air, and space. This means that state and local governments must develop organizational patterns and tools in an effort to promote the fullest possible coordination and cooperation with all agencies that have a significant influence on public health.

HISTORY OF PUBLIC SANITATION

Many important sanitation principles had their beginnings in England. Slow sand

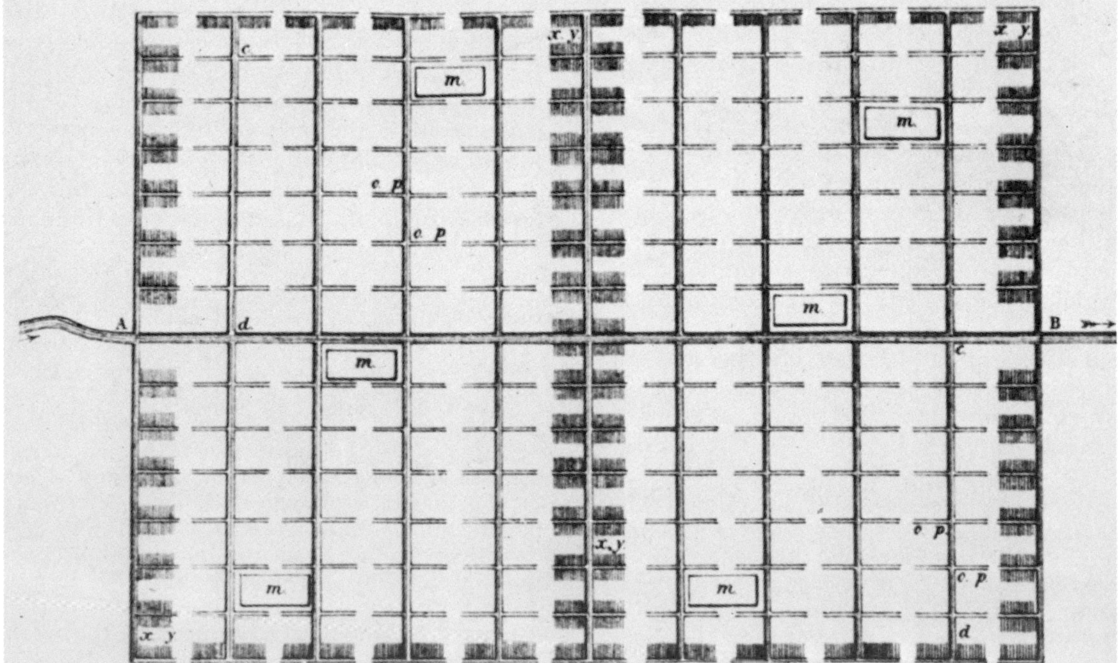

Figure 11–1 Sir Edwin Chadwick's sewage system. (From Dubos, R., and Pines, M.: *Health and Disease.* New York, Time-Life Books, 1971, p. 67.)

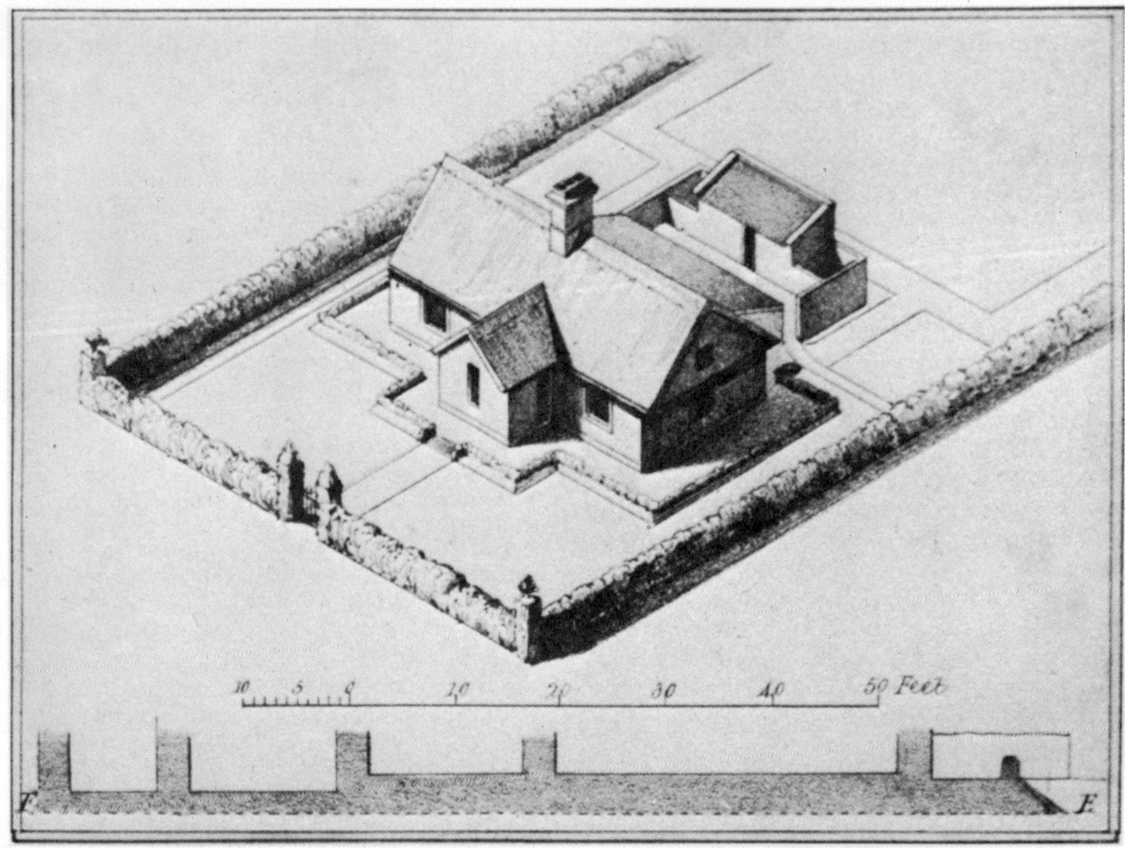

Figure 11–2 Early plan for public housing. (From Dubos, R., and Pines, M.: *Health and Disease.* New York, Time-Life Books, 1971, p. 66.)

filtration of community water supplies was initiated in England in 1829 by the Chelsea Water Company. Edwin Chadwick initiated the establishment of a board of health in 1848 to combat environmental hazards; in 1849 John Simon and John Snow demonstrated conclusively that a community water supply polluted with human wastes could be dangerous.

The foundation for public health and sanitation in America was laid in 1850 with the publication of the Report of the Sanitary Commission of Massachusetts, 1849, by the Commissioners appointed under a resolution of the Legislature of Massachusetts and commonly called the Shattuck Report.[4] In the report, Lemuel Shattuck had strongly urged the formation of a state board of health in Massachusetts; however, it was not until 1869 that this state organized the second state health department in the country. In 1872, Stephen Smith founded the American Public Health Association , and in 1874, state laws concerning food sanitation were initiated by the state of Illinois. The Rockefeller Sanitary Commission, established in 1909 to combat hookworm, aided states in the establishment and organization of full-time county health departments and advanced sanitation programs. Although many sound sanitation principles were advanced early by a few pioneers, there has always been a social lag between discovery and adoption of these principles.

Through the years, the inventions of man have created new causes of pollution in his environment. The new, more subtle, insidious contaminants are the man-made undesirable by-products of technological progress. New, ubiquitous, and rapidly increasing chemicals, drugs, and pollutants are finding their way into the air people breathe, the water they drink, and the food they eat. Although the problem is enormously complex and difficult, the gap between technology and biology must be closed quickly. In the last analysis, however, progress in this area will depend upon the attitudes and values of the people; these may be reflected by some citizens demanding reasonably clean air and water at reasonable costs, and other citizens demanding clean air and water at all costs. In either case, it is necessary for all to realize that water, air, and food respect no city or state boundary, and that cooperation, coordination, and support of local bond issues are necessary to further the growth, development, and health of the nation.

The sanitarian of today understands and practices modern sanitation principles, and his concerns include restaurant inspection, nuisance abatement, milk and food sanitation, air and water purity, garbage and rubbish disposal, and many other conditions of civilized living. In order to keep pace with the increasingly complex environment, the sanitary *engineer* has become a very important person in community health. Inspection, education, and enforcement must be supplemented by principles of sanitary engineering. A masters degree in public health sanitary engineering can be obtained at most of the approved schools of public health.

ADMINISTRATIVE GUIDE FOR ENVIRONMENTAL PROBLEMS

The Fringe Area Sanitation Practices Committee, Engineering and Sanitation Section, American Public Health Association, developed a guide to help identify basic principles and offer suggestions for good practices in the solution or prevention of environmental problems. The group explored demographic, governmental, legislative, planning, subdivision, financial, and community participation factors of environmental health problems associated with community growth. The following basic plan of action may be adopted according to the character of the local community, its problems, and its capabilities:

1. Establish and support an adequately staffed local health department with professional sanitary engineering direction of a comprehensive environmental health program to prevent, solve, and control environmental engineering problems.
2. Establish a metropolitan or county planning agency. A comprehensive plan to guide community development and improvement, supplemented by short-range detail plans, is required.
3. Authorize the preparation of regional or metropolitan area comprehensive engineering plans for public water supply and sewerage, air and water pollution control, traffic circulation, recreational, industrial expansion, residential housing, shopping centers, and so forth.
4. Adopt and enforce a modern sanitary code including control of reality subdivisions, air pollution, and ionizing radiation.
5. Adopt and enforce an up-to-date building code, plumbing code, fire prevention code, and zoning ordinance with full-time professional direction.
6. Adopt and enforce a modern minimum standards housing ordinance, and a taxing policy that encourages rather than penalizes housing conservation and rehabilitation. Retain, improve, and integrate useful parts of the community and guide desirable construction so as to strengthen and protect the character of the neighborhoods. Capitalize on good points; eliminate "foci of infection"; replan and redevelop. Professional guidance and direction are essential.
7. Provide parks and cultural and recreational facilities, and protect residential areas to promote a healthful environment.
8. Adopt a capital improvement program geared to needs and the ability of the people to pay. Step-construction programs based on long-term comprehensive engineering plans, with a balanced allocation of the available income expected each year, make possible that which appears to be impossible.
9. Provide an operating budget sufficient to meet all essential community services. Remember that in the long run, good salaries attract good people. Large sums of money stand to be misdirected when administered by incompetent people. Evaluate budgetary requests and salaries on basis of services rendered, rather than on gross amounts alone.
10. Encourage local research and continuing evaluation of local government programs. Apply new knowledge and seek out new methods and procedures.
11. Utilize available professional and technical skills in government and in the community.
12. Finance initial community improvements and services, such as roads, water supply, and sewerage, through the persons affected in proportion to the benefits received.
13. Keep the taxpayer continually informed of how his taxes and fees are being spent, of plans for future community improvements, and of the benefits and services rendered. Obtain and invite understanding and cooperation of taxpayers, business, and community organizations.

COMMUNITY PARTICIPATION

The Sanitation Practices Committee recognized the fact that legislators react to public demands for changes and additions to laws necessary for protecting public health,

Approaches to Comprehensive Environmental Protection.

	Symptomatic Approach	Environmental Systems Approach	Functional Approach
Evolving Recognized Programs Programs	Air pollution program Water pollution program Food sanitation program Occupational health program Radiological health program Community noise Housing and health Drug abuse Motor vehicle accident prevention Home accident prevention Consumer health habits	Health Aspects of The urban environment The rural environment Occupational environment Recreational environment Transportation environment Domestic environment Educational environment	Environmental monitoring and surveillance Environmental quality evaluation Environmental quality protection

Classification of Health Department Activities Relevant to a Functional Approach to Comprehensive Environmental Protection

Program	Environmental Monitoring and Surveillance	Environmental Quality Evaluation	Environmental Quality Protection
Air/Sanitation, including* cigarette smoking, environmental respiratory diseases	Statewide cooperative air monitoring network; health surveillance; special studies	Air quality criteria and standards; motor vehicle standards	Motor vehicle pollution control and other control efforts
Food and drug, including* drug abuse	Food inspection; cannery and other facility inspection; drugs, cosmetics, hazardous household substances inspection; devices, medical nutritional quackery inspection	Food standards and tolerances; food processing standards; drug standards; hazardous substances evaluation; processing requirements	Labeling control; fraud prosecution; food processing licenses; food, drug, cosmetic adulteration, labeling and advertising
Housing	Environmental monitoring; epidemiological studies of housing, related illness, and accidents	Health standards; new housing; current housing standards	(No California State Department of Health Program)
Occupational health, including* pesticides	Special studies; noise monitoring; occupational environment surveillance; occupational health surveillance	Threshold limit values; safety standards; ergonomic standards	Prevention of occupational disease; diagnosis and treatment of occupational disease
Radiological health	User registration; air, water, food monitoring and surveillance; special studies; inspection of radiation facilities	Radiation health criteria; radiation machine standards; radioactive material standards	Licensing of isotopes; radiation machine control; radioactive material control
Water sanitation	Domestic water supply sampling; recreational water monitoring; shellfish surveillance; reclaimed water surveillance; special studies	Water supply standards; waste and reclaimed water standards; water related recreational standards; shellfish standards	Domestic water supplies and permits; waste treatment and reclamation preemptory orders; shellfish quarantine
Vector Control, including* solid waste management and rat control	Vector surveillance; vector resistance surveillance (pesticides); arthropods (principally insects); small mammals (principally rodents)	Insecticide formulation and application standards; solid waste criteria	Zoonoses suppression; water-related vector control; field wilderness vector control; community area vector control; solid waste management control

***Programs included are new ones and the grouping with more established programs is based on similarities of technical staff requirements.**

Figure 11–3 Factors involved in environmental protection. (From Goldsmith, J. R., and Starr, A. C.: Environmental health monitoring. ExChange (journal published by the California State Department of Health), *1*:5, June–July, 1973, p. 31.)

and the Committee suggested the following contributing factors and indicated solutions:

Contributing Factors

1. The public is often uninformed. The need for the following services and resources is usually not recognized by the public during the early stages of community growth: water and sewerage services, refuse collection and disposal, housing controls, planning of land use, clean air, and clean water.

2. Fragmentation hinders effective participation. The existence of noncontiguous patterns of fringe area growth makes it very difficult for people to reach common objectives and take concerted action in securing necessary facilities.

3. Community support is not solicited. Many government officials fail to involve the total community to secure public acceptance of specific environmental health programs. Promoters of community projects often overlook an adequately planned public relations program, have little community understanding, and only a vague knowledge of the process by which government operates.

Indicated Solutions or Prevention

1. Improve neighborhood identity. A sense of community should be established to overcome the sense of isolation, of helplessness, and frustration that often haunt the residents of a modern community. Resources of service clubs and other civic organizations can be utilized.

2. Overcome civic apathy. Careful planning for citizen participation is necessary. Study and action committees and business and neighborhood organizations are potential groups to stimulate community interest.

3. Present the facts. Health leaders should participate in community activities so that accurate and essential information is disseminated. This makes possible informed decisions concerning environmental health programs within the total framework of community goals.

4. Keep the people informed. Community participation can be stimulated through the dissemination of information. The distribution of a monthly or quarterly newsletter to civic, professional, and business organizations is an excellent approach. Mass media should also be utilized to the maximum extent.

5. Know your subject and your people. Public officials should know the characteristics of the various segments of the population so that they can reach and motivate the people.

6. Clarify who does what. Prepare and keep current a central reference pamphlet listing all official and voluntary community agencies, their basic functions and responsibilities to the people, annual budget, and sources of funds.[5]

ECOLOGICAL BALANCE

Clear Lake, California, is a shallow, 40,000-acre body of fresh water that lies about 100 miles north of San Francisco. For centuries, it was home for a large colony of Western grebes, lovely birds that swim with the stately grace of swans and dive as skillfully as loons. But many years ago, in an environmental tragedy unwittingly perpetrated by man, large numbers of grebes began dying off, and the once-clear waters of the lake turned murky and green. Now, by introducing a new ecological cycle, scientists have saved Clear Lake's grebes and even clarified its water.

The grebe's problems began in the late 1940's when the local mosquito abatement district sprayed thousands of pounds of DDD, a chlorinated hydrocarbon pesticide, on Clear Lake to rid the area of swarms of buzzing black gnats. The chemical, a close cousin of DDT, worked so well that developers previously repelled by the gnats began building houses around the lake.

Unhappily, after an absence of several years, the gnats returned. In 1954 and again in 1957, stronger doses of DDD eliminated them. About the same time, the lake's population of grebes began to decrease, dropping from 1000 pairs to only 20 within one year. The baffling change was explained in 1962 by Rachel Carson in her book, *Silent Spring.* Grebes, she explained, feed mainly on fish. The fish, in turn, eat insect larvae and zooplankton, and these foods had become saturated with the DDD dumped into Clear Lake. Thus, over a long period, the grebes accumulated lethal amounts of the long-lasting pesticide in their tissues and died by the hundreds. Even worse, because of the DDD in their eggs, thousands of grebes never hatched. Between 1958 and 1963, only one young bird was seen at Clear Lake.

Meanwhile, the proliferation of houses around the lake was having another, equally unforeseen effect. Household wastes, laden with nutrients, seeped into the water and fertilized algae. By 1961, the lake and its beaches were covered with green slime.

What could be done to solve the problem? The mosquito abatement district switched from the persistent DDD to methyl parathion, a chemical that is effective against gnats but that deteriorates and becomes harmless in a short time. At the same time, the district hired a team of scientists from the University of California at Davis to find a way to control the gnats biologically. The team decided that a small freshwater smelt, the Mississippi silverside, might find the gnats appetizing. In 1967, they "planted" 3000 fingerlings in the lake.

The silversides have multiplied prodigiously. They not only eat the gnats, but also compete for the nutrients that stimulate algae growth. As a result, the algae are disappearing, and the lake has regained 80 per cent of its original clarity. No longer troubled by DDD, the grebes are returning. Large game fish now have to be imported to feed on the wildly proliferating silversides. An ecological balance is not easily restored.

Local Wars Against Pollution

Northern California. Stringent controls have been imposed on development of the San Francisco Bay shoreline as a result of an eight-year fight by concerned citizens. These "Save Our Bay" advocates argued that further filling of the Bay would have adverse effects on the region's climate because less water would mean less wind to disperse pollutants and the Bay's cooling influence in summer and warming influence in winter would be diminished.

Lake Tahoe. Public pressure has forced drastic limitations in plans for real estate development at Incline Village, Nevada, on the shore of Lake Tahoe.

Arizona. After smog became a problem in the desert air, citizens of Phoenix, Tucson, and other cities demanded and got tougher statewide standards on air quality. Reduced maximums were set for sulphur dioxide gas and solid particles polluting the air.

Chicago. A "pollution revolution" was triggered by a smog siege which, some officials said, might have been a contributing cause of about 50 deaths. A campaign spearheaded by *The Chicago Tribune* resulted in a sharp shakeup of the city's air pollution control department and the establishment of a city department of environmental control to work on all pollution problems.

Duluth, Minn. The Izaak Walton League of America filed suit for a permanent injunction against drilling for minerals in the "boundary-waters canoe area" of northeastern Minnesota.

Miami. One of the nation's hardest fought environmental battles ended with victory for conservationists when plans to build a huge jetport in the Florida Everglades west of Miami were scrapped. Opponents asserted that the facility would create such environmental hazards as serious air pollution from fallout of jet exhausts, noise intolerable to people and animals, impediments to water flow through the Everglades, and major problems of waste disposal and water purification arising from commercial and residential development adjacent to the airport site.

Houston. One indication of public reaction here to the pollution problem: A radio newsman appeared before the city council with a mother and her 11-month-old daughter. The newsman said pollutants from a principal industrial area of the city worsened the infant's asthmatic conditions to a point necessitating almost constant hospitalization. After the council appearance, the newsman said, he received hundreds of supporting complaints. Houston's concern with another environmental ill – water pollution – was heightened when an expert called the city's ship channel one of the 10 filthiest waterways in the U.S.–"too thick to drink and too thin to plow."

Fairport Harbor, Ohio. A group of 200 irate citizens of this Lake Erie waterfront town east of Cleveland filed suit for 1.4 million dollars for damages caused by air pollution. Two industrial firms were named as defendants. Door-to-door solicitation and a car-washing project by youngsters raised $5000 to finance the lawsuit.

Escanaba, Mich. Action by a citizens' group here is credited with forcing a paper-manufacturing company to revise its expansion plans in order to achieve a "cleaner" operation and reduce what residents described as a "rotten egg" smell.

A state official commented, "When people get involved, when they start screaming, companies become much more sensitive to their responsibilities. There's no doubt companies move faster under that kind of pressure."

Cornwall, N.Y. The long battle over plans of the Consolidated Edison Company to build the world's largest pumped-storage hydroelectric generating plant at Storm King Mountain in the Hudson River highlands is an example of what can happen when a utility undertakes a big project in a scenic area. The company was fought in the courts by a conservation group, the Scenic Hudson Preservation Conference. The conservationists have succeeded to the extent that the company has modified the project and now plans to put the plant underground. Consolidated Edison says that the Storm King generators will reduce the air pollution in New York City–which the company serves–by making it possible to shut down older and less efficient units.

Calvert Cliffs, Md. Proposals to build nuclear power installations run into opposition as soon as plans for them are announced.

Greensboro, Ga. Alarmed citizens of rural Greene County successfully opposed a move to establish a nuclear waste disposal area. Opposition developed quickly when it was learned that the Nuclear Industrial Service Corporation of Springville, N.Y., had taken an option on 7000 acres in Greene County. When public sentiment against the proposal made itself evident at a mass meeting attended by nearly 300 persons, the corporation president announced that he would give up the option. "We don't want to be located where they don't want us," he said.

COMMUNITY WATER SUPPLIES

Sources of Water

The average American uses over 147 gallons of water each day. With the increase in population and the increase of per capita use of water, it is estimated that this figure will rise to over 225 gallons per day by the year 2000. Periodic droughts have caused water shortages in many areas throughout the world. Water rationing is in effect in many cities. It is therefore most important that conservation methods be practiced by all citizens. Many large cities use the water from the rivers or lakes on whose shores they were founded (Fig. 11–4). Many communities depend on underground sources such as wells and springs for their water supplies. Some cities like New York and Los Angeles transport water from distant upland sources: e.g., water from the Colorado River is carried 400 miles through aqueducts as large as 16 feet in diameter to supply southern California. Various sources of water are discussed on the following pages.

Lakes and Reservoirs. Since lake

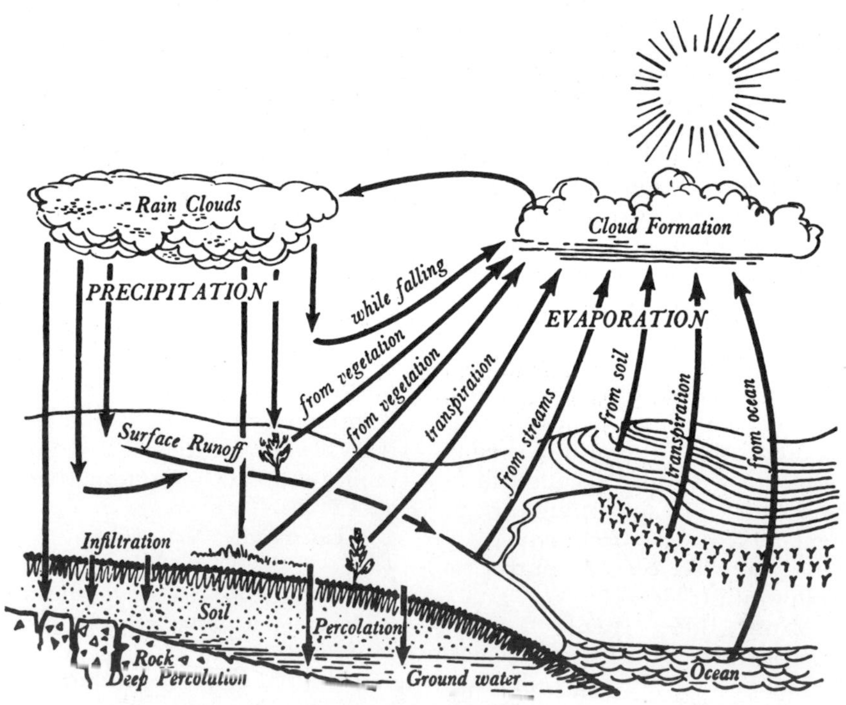

Figure 11–4 The hydrologic cycle. (From the *Yearbook of Agriculture,* 1955, United States Department of Agriculture.)

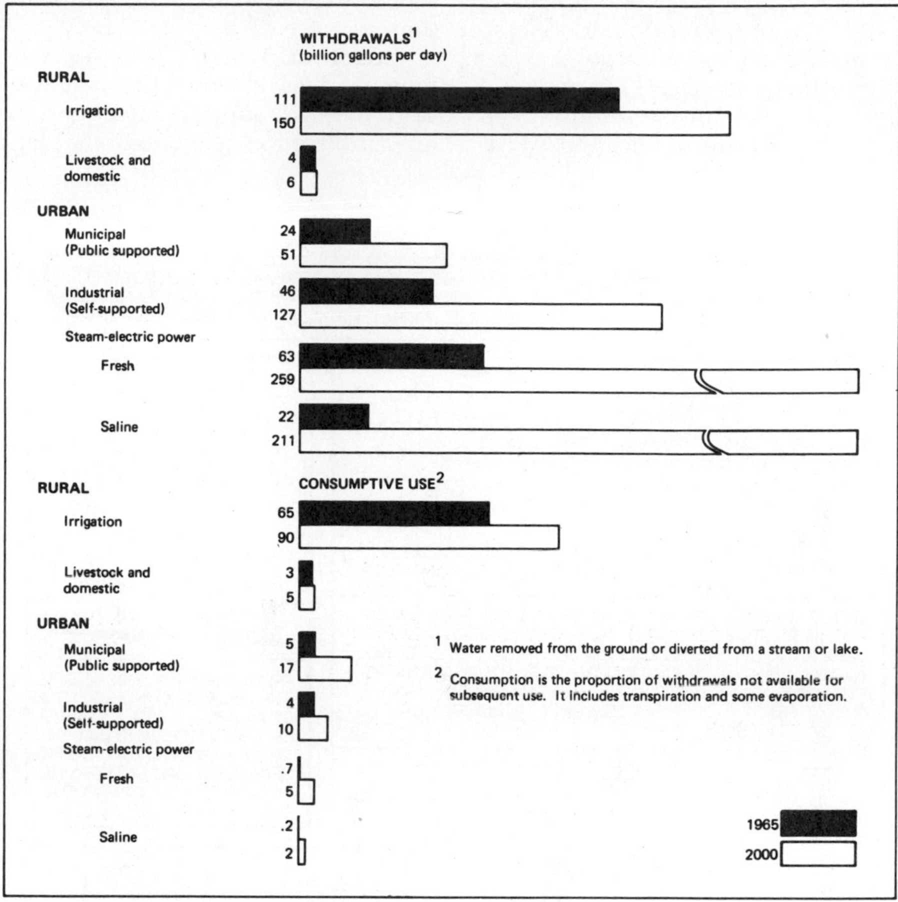

Figure 11–5 Comparison of water uses for 1965 vs. the year 2000. (From *Our Land and Water Resources.* Washington, D.C., U.S. Department of Agriculture, May, 1974, p. vii. Data from *The Nation's Water Resources Summary Report.* Washington, D.C., U.S. Water Resources Council, 1968.)

water is clearer and less polluted than water from most streams, it is the most satisfactory source of surface water. A lake, often called a reservoir, is a large body of open fresh water fed by small tributary streams or springs. Lakes may be either natural or man-made. The clarity of lake water arises from the fact that lakes used for drinking water generally have forested watersheds and are fed by short tributary streams flowing in rocky channels. Storing water in lakes permits clarification by natural sedimentation and the substantial removal of objectionable bacteria by time and sedimentation. Most lake water requires no treatment other than chlorination; a prominent example is the New York City supply. An auxiliary value of the lake may be its location at a higher elevation than the city served. The cost of pumping water is thus saved, and occasionally electric power may be generated as well.

Certain limiting factors prevent the extensive use of lakes and reservoirs as sources of supply. Frequently, suitable sites and catchment areas within an accessible distance are lacking. Lake supplies are often costly, because of the large investments in land having watersheds for sanitary protection, long aqueducts, and sometimes the cost of pumping. Slightly turbid lake waters may be more difficult to filter than more turbid stream waters. Seasonal taste and odor from plant growth are other problems.

Streams. Streams are the most common source of surface supply because more cities are accessible to an adequate stream source than to lakes and reservoirs. They are also the most common source of supply for cities above 25,000 population in this country, because adequate ground water resources are less frequently available. Stream supplies include brooks, creeks, and rivers. Many mountainside spring-fed brooks, serving small communities, compare favorably in water quality with lake and reservoir supplies, and they do not require filtration. Most creek supplies and practically all river supplies must or should be filtered and chlorinated because of turbidity, color, and pollution.

Ground Water. Ground water is obtained from below the surface of the ground. Such supplies include wells, springs, and infiltration galleries, the latter being

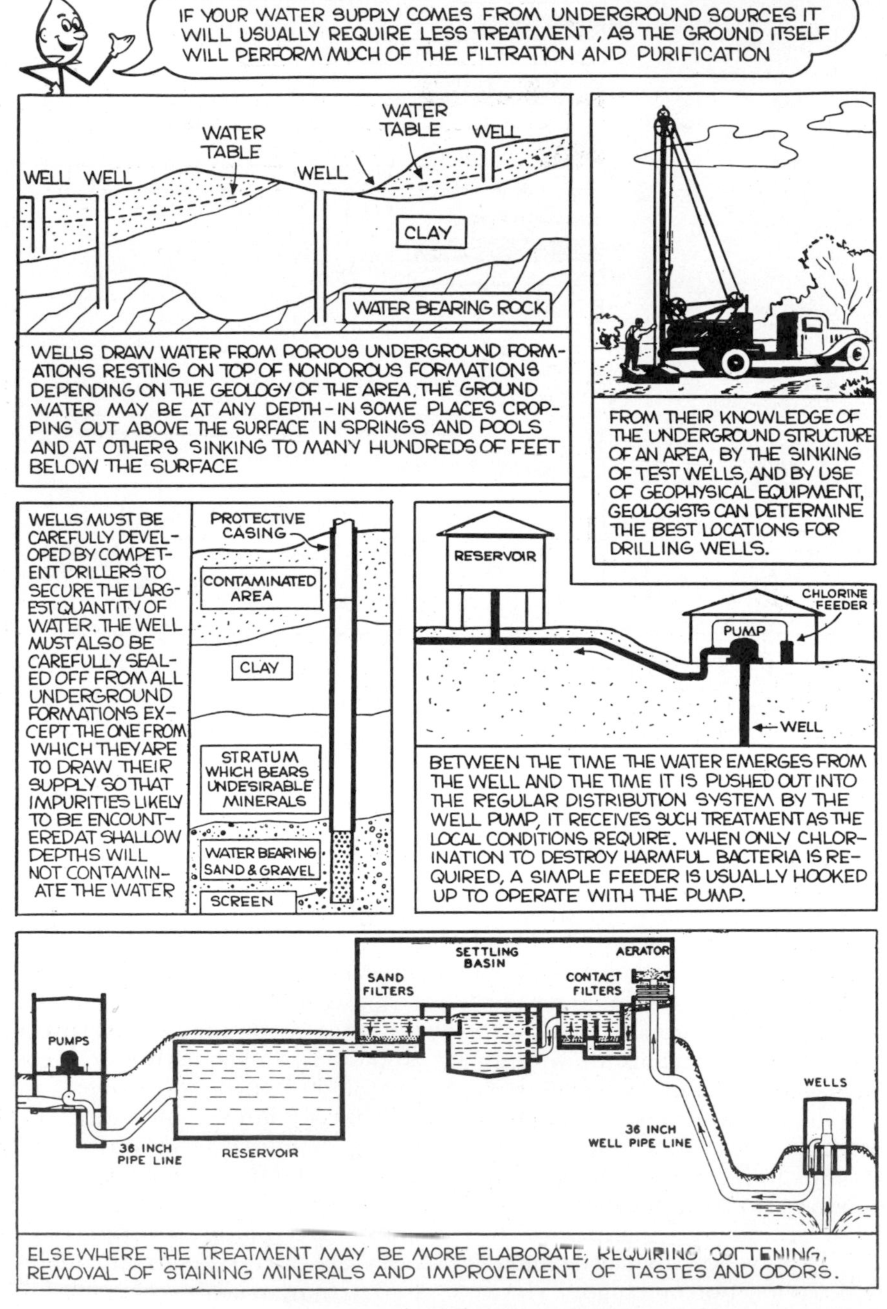

Figure 11–6 (From *The Story of Water Supply.* New York, American Water Works Association, 1957.)

rare. Wells and springs are the most common sources of supply for communities up to about 600 population (Fig. 11–6).

Water-borne Diseases

Contaminated water may carry infection from human or animal waste or may have been rendered unwholesome by poisonous chemical compounds; this contamination can be easily checked by field or laboratory analysis. The greatest danger of pollution is from the discharges from the human body; there is very little danger of infection from lower animals or from the organic matter of plant life. Organisms discharged from humans are grouped as "colon bacilli" and are called the "coliforms." These are always present in human intestines and feces and their presence indicates water contamination. A laboratory technician can test for this pollution by placing a water sample in a tube of lactose broth and then incubating it at a temperature of 37° C. for 48 hours. The coliforms will ferment lactose and their presence is indicated by gas in the tube.

The most common of the water-borne diseases from pollution are typhoid fever, paratyphoid fever, the dysenteries (amebic and bacillary), gastroenteritis, infectious hepatitis, schistosomiasis, and Asiatic cholera. Typhoid, paratyphoid, dysenteries, gastroenteritis and Asiatic cholera are transmitted by urinary and intestinal discharges of ill persons and human carriers. Gastroenteritis is a diarrheal disorder involving the alimentary tract; infectious hepatitis is caused by a virus and could be transmitted by direct personal contact or from food, water, or milk. Poliomyelitis is also a virus disease which has been found in the feces of infected persons and in sewerage; schistosomiasis organisms are parasites which have their life cycle in certain species of water snails. These organisms can leave the snail and are able to enter the skin of bathers or swimmers in the water. (See Chapter 8.)

Water Treatment Methods

Since most lakes, reservoirs, streams, and ground water are subject to pollution, many community water supplies are purified and periodically analyzed for chemical or bacteriological contamination. The most common type of water treatment is the rapid sand gravity filtration method that consists of chemical addition and mixing, flocculation and sedimentation, filtration, and chlorination. The first three steps are designed to remove turbidity and color, although flocculation and sedimentation assist in the removal of bacteria and other organisms such as algae and protozoa. Filtration removes most impurities from the water, and effective filters include sand, diatomaceous silica, and anthracite coal (Fig. 11–7).

Disinfection of water depends upon the number and nature of organisms present, temperature, time of contact, pH (potential of hydrogen), oxidation potential, and the type of disinfectant used. Chemicals that have good disinfecting qualities include potassium permanganate, copper, silver, ozone, chlorine dioxide, and the halogens.

Tracing the Origin of Polluted Water

The classic method of detecting and tracing typhoid carriers is by investigation of probable typhoid cases, followed by an analysis of individual fecal or rectal swab specimens. These procedures are complicated and time consuming and require extensive contact with large numbers of people. The newer swab technique provides a simplified and impersonal screening procedure for reducing the suspected area in which the carrier will probably be found with a minimum of community disruption. Typhoid organisms are traced to a specific sewer, then a specific area, and finally toilet swab tests are conducted in the homes in that area. A positive swab test is confirmed by analysis of stool specimens provided by individuals living in that particular home.

Polluted water may be detected by the use of dyes to help trace the movement of water underground. *Fluorescein,* also called uranin, is considered a harmless organic dye, which can be removed by the use of filtration. The solution is mixed by adding one pound of fluorescein to one pound of caustic soda in 10 gallons of water. If surface pollution of a well is suspected, some of the solution is sprinkled on the surface and the water is observed for color.

Fluorescein dye is also commonly used

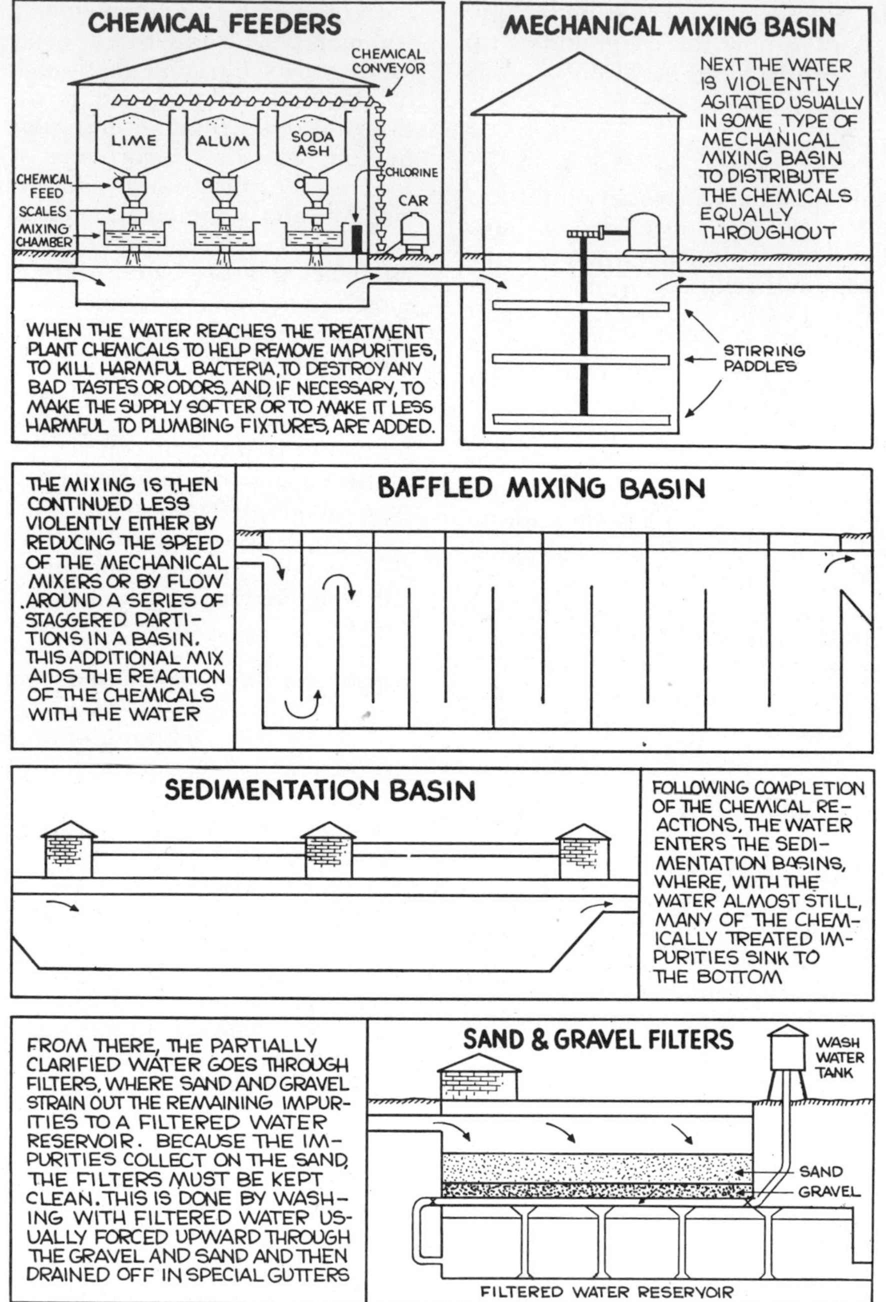

Figure 11–7 (From *The Story of Water Supply*. New York, American Water Works Association, 1957.)

as a tracing agent in sanitary field practice, for the following purposes:

1. Tracing the flow patterns and estimating rates of flow in sewers and streams.
2. Estimating the detention times in sewage settling tanks.
3. Detecting cross-connections between potable and nonpotable water supplies.
4. Detecting the surface entry of contaminated ground water into supply wells.
5. Determining the zone of influence of waste discharges in receiving waters.
6. Detecting emergent flows of waste effluents from subsurface disposal fields.

Care should be taken in the use of fluorescein and it should be avoided when the community may have contact with it in heavy concentrations. Care should also be taken to see that the dye does not enter potable water supplies of the community. Under normal sanitary uses, the dye will be low in toxicity. Water supplies should be diluted so that the dye is not detected by the naked eye. Precautions and expert handling of the dye should be followed carefully.

Rural Water Supplies

Rural water supplies are usually obtained from simple, shallow, and unprotected wells. The great increase in infectious hepatitis in the United States can be traced to shallow wells that have become polluted by inadequate disposal systems or ineffective septic tanks. Inadequate sanitary laws, and the lack of public health education, very often lead to poor sanitation conditions in the rural or suburban areas of a state.

The tops of driven wells should be carefully protected, since polluted water may run down the sides of the pipe in the well. The well should have a heavy top bolted tightly to prevent loosening of the joints. The gound should slope away from the well and the area around the well should be kept clean.

Most county or state health departments have adopted specifications for property owners to follow in constructing wells. They will gladly send a consultant to help plan the well in order to prevent pollution. Basic well construction measures include the following:

1. The well should be of considerable depth to avoid excess seepage from the ground.
2. The well should be cased, in order to prevent shallow levels of water from seeping in.
3. A concrete collar should be constructed around the upper part to prevent surface washing from seeping in.
4. There should be a covering on the top to prevent tampering, and to keep dirt from entering.
5. The water should be lifted by means of a pump instead of a rope and bucket.

Chemicals in the Water

Chlorine is added to the water to kill the harmful or pathogenic bacteria that it may

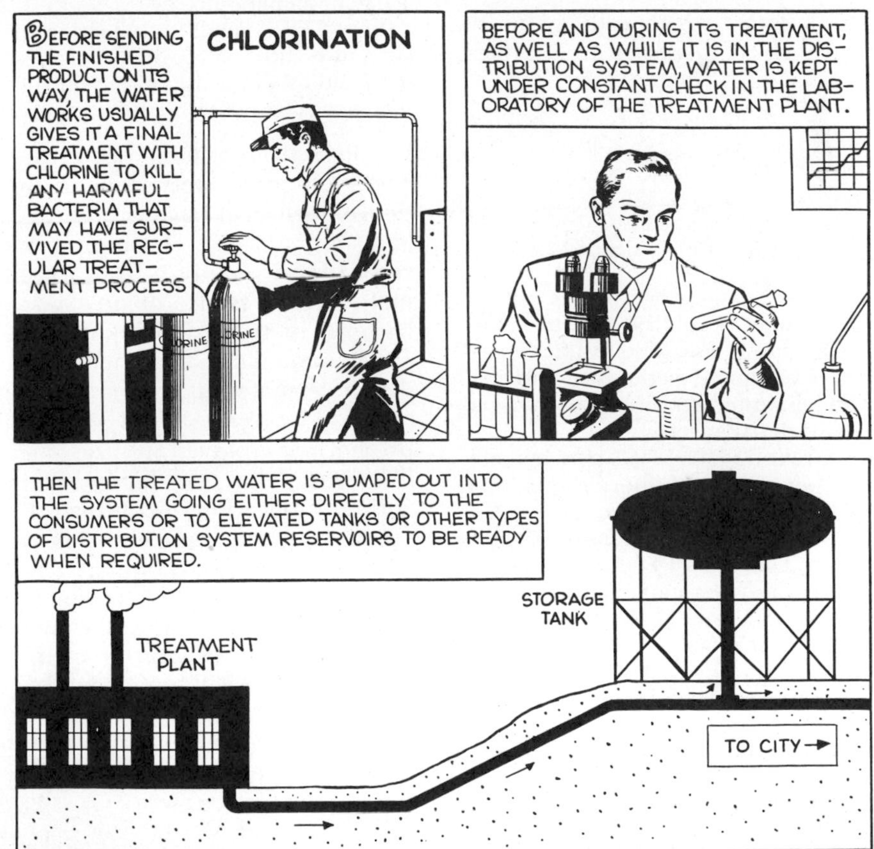

Figure 11–8 (From *The Story of Water Supply*. New York, American Water Works Association, 1957.)

contain (Fig. 11-8). Chlorine is universally used in water purification because it is reliable, inexpensive, and easy to administer. Chlorine plus water yields hypochlorous acid plus hydrochloric acid ($Cl_2 + H_2O \rightarrow HCl + HClO$). Hypochlorous acid is a very efficient disinfectant, especially at low pH values.

Copper sulfate is added to water to control the algae growth. It is applied in a proportion of 0.1 to 1.0 part per million parts of water. Some of the copper precipitates, settles to the bottom of the tank, and is then removed from the water. Copper is not an accumulative poison; it is found even in the milk that we drink.

Physicians have experienced a problem with patients for whom they must prescribe strict sodium-free diets. Because public water supplies contain this mineral in varying degrees, many states and communities are now busy determining the sodium content of most of the public water supplies. With this knowledge, a physician will be able to determine whether or not a patient on a sodium-restricted diet can drink from his usual source of water, or if distilled water must be prescribed.

Fluoridated water, which reduces tooth decay in children, was discussed in Chapter 6.

Safe Community Water Supplies

When planning a safe community water supply, the following criteria should be considered:

1. The community should be able to obtain water at nominal water rates. The water department should have adequate methods of distribution and provide minimum requirements adopted by the local health department.
2. A concentration of from 0.7 part per million to 1.5 parts per million of fluoride should be added to the water supply in order to give protection against tooth decay. Fluoridation has been approved by the American Dental Association, the American Medical Association, and the American Public Health Association. Research studies have proved that fluoridation of public water supplies in various communities has resulted in as high as a 65 per cent reduction in dental caries in children.
3. All water supplies should be chlorinated with a concentration of two parts per million to five parts per million. This procedure reduces the water-borne diseases to a minimum.
4. If surface water is used, it should be inspected and controlled at the watersheds.
5. The water supply intake should be located to reduce the possibility of pollution.
6. Plumbing codes should be designed to regulate plumbing cross-connections and prevent back siphonage.

The public health department, the city or county housing and planning commission, builders' organizations, and professional health organizations should all cooperate to provide safe water for the community.

Guideposts to Water Quality

Three key tests that may be used as guidelines when water quality is considered are:

1. Residual chlorine. This is the amount of disinfecting chlorine left in the water after treatment. The taste of chlorine in water is a major reason for public complaints.
2. Abs. The term "abs" refers to those parts of household detergents left after chemical decomposition in sewage or other treatment plants. Their presence in drinking water is considered the best way to determine if there has been sewage contamination.
3. "Differential" examination of the bacteria currently showing up in water supplies. This is designed to tell health and water officials whether the bacteria are potentially dangerous.

Present methods of testing water for bacteriological safety depend on the detection of coliform bacteria. Fecal coliform organisms may be considered indicators of recent fecal pollution by warm-blooded animals. The presence of any type of coliform bacteria in treated drinking water suggests either inadequate treatment or access of undesirable materials to the water after treatment. The most rapid of the techniques presently employed utilizes the membrane filter test. This test depends on the growth and multiplication of coliform cells until they reach sufficient numbers to be visible to the unaided eye as a colony. The other test, referred to as the fermentation tube method, depends on sufficient growth and metabolic activity of the coliform bacteria that visible gas will be formed from lactose in a fermentation tube. This may take from two to four days, whereas the membrane filter technique requires 24 hours.

A final judgment on the quality of drinking water should not be based on the

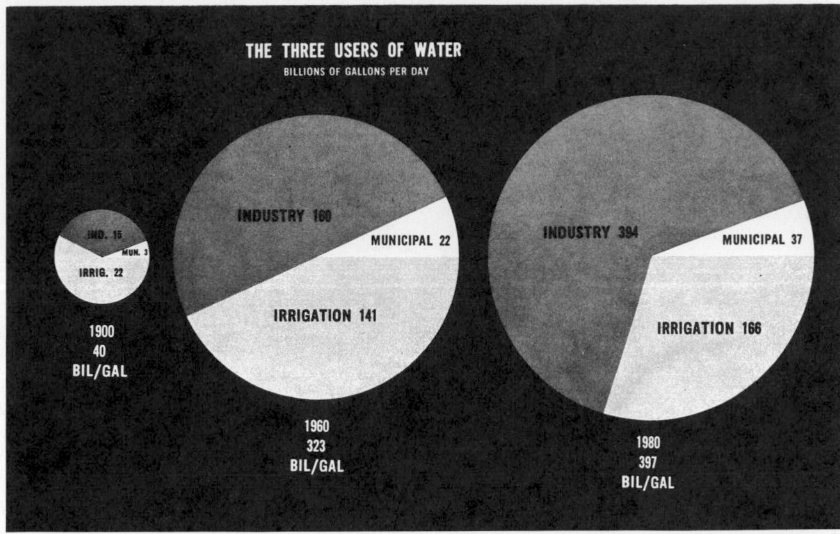

Figure 11–9 Changing demands for water. Demand for water is determined by population, technology, and standard of living. The changing character of America is shown by the changing demands for water among industry, agriculture, and municipalities.

bacteriological examination alone but should also include a sanitary survey of the area. This is why *water samples collected by trained public health personnel are of greater value than those collected by the general public.* Water samples from public water supplies are collected periodically by authorized individuals using techniques prescribed in *Standard Methods of Water Analysis,* a publication of the American Public Health Association. Regular bacteriological examination of public supplies of water by health authorities is good insurance against water-borne epidemics. Such outbreaks can quickly be recognized and the necessary remedial action taken by public health authorities.

A relatively simple method of monitoring the levels of fresh water contamination that can be used almost everywhere has been developed at the University of North Carolina School of Public Health. The method consists of measuring the cholinesterase activity in the brains of fish from waters known or suspected to contain insecticides. When cholinesterase activity is depressed to about 20 per cent of normal, death usually occurs. In some species of fish, death may occur at higher levels, depending on the insecticide used, the concentration, and other factors. Researchers at the school worked out a table of normal values for cholinesterase activity in the brains of several species of fish; then, by varying the time interval and the concentration of insecticides, they have been able to determine the extent to which fish can be exposed without lethal effects. The data obtained by this method can be used to allow insect control to go on without harm to fish and other aquatic life, to monitor the safety of water used for recreation, or to detect any possible pollution of drinking water supplies taken from a lake. Further information can be obtained from the Department of Sanitary Engineering.

WATER POLLUTION

Water pollution is a hazard to our health, a threat to our economic growth, and a menace to recreation. Millions of fish are killed in coastal waters and rivers each year by pollution. Radioactive wastes, detergents, pesticides, and other chemicals are found in many rivers and streams, and septic tanks often drain into underground waters. In many cities, drinking water is becoming less and less palatable because of pollutants in the water supply, or chemicals that have been added to overcome pollutants. In addition, demands on our municipal water supplies have increased because of increase in both the general population and the urban population, and because of a higher standard of living, growing industry, an increase in irrigation and lawn sprinkling, and the manufacture of new chemicals.

If precipitation and population were uniformly distributed throughout the country, water supply and waste disposal would be less of a problem. However, 50 per cent of our population now lives on less than 10 per cent of the land area. In 30 years, the urban population has grown from 56 per cent to 70 per cent of the total population, and this trend is accelerating. The unequal distribution of precipitation over the country and its variability in time aggravate the situation.

Virtually all of our water supply has its origin in rainfall. When society was predominantly rural, the rain was able to percolate through the soil and join underground rivers and lakes, to be drawn on when needed. Increased suburbanization with extensive areas used for bedrooms, two-car garages, drive-in movies, and shopping centers has interfered with the percolation of the rain. Now the rain hits the top of the ranch house, carport, driveway, or shopping area parking lot and runs quickly off to a storm drain and thence to a channel and stream, threatening flood rather than becoming part of the underground water resource.[7]

A Congressional study highlights the following facts. The United States now uses approximately 335 billion gallons of water each day, but by 1980 requirements will have climbed to 600 billion gallons per day. By 1980, however, the total dependable fresh water supply available will be about 515 billion gallons per day. By A.D. 2000, water requirements for the United States will be more than 1000 billion gallons per day. Furthermore, the most that the United States can ever hope to have available as a result of engineering works will be about 650 billion gallons per day. Thus, provision of sufficient water of proper quality at the right place and time for a growing population will be a major problem.

Water is not limitless; the supply is relatively fixed. The increasing use of water already has resulted in its re-use in many locations. As water is used and re-used, it becomes contaminated or polluted in many ways. Before each re-use, it must be cleaned in varying degrees, posing economic and technical problems of considerable magnitude. Water re-use is not new. At times, the water in the Ohio River is used 3.7 times before it reaches the Mississippi, and some water in almost every stream is used one or more times.

In light of the best available information on population increase, industrial and general economic expansions, surveys, and estimates of water use and good engineering judgment, it seems that the nation must do two things: complete as rapidly as possible the works necessary to capture the maxi-

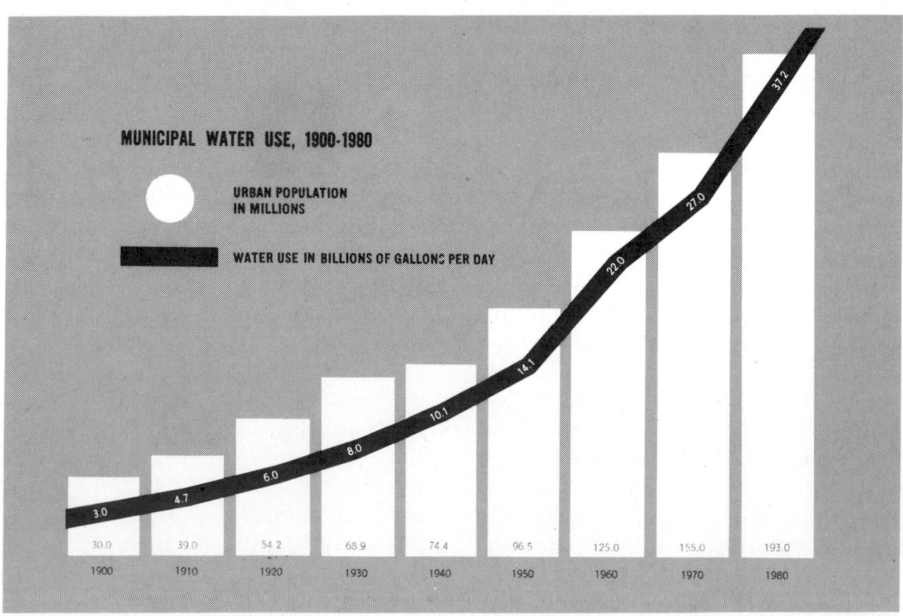

Figure 11–10 Water for cities. Municipal demands for water are presently 7 times those of 1900 and will be 12 times the 1900 level in another 20 years. This reflects in part a larger population, and in part our higher standard of living. The use of water in bathrooms, kitchens, and home laundries is far greater than it was a generation ago.

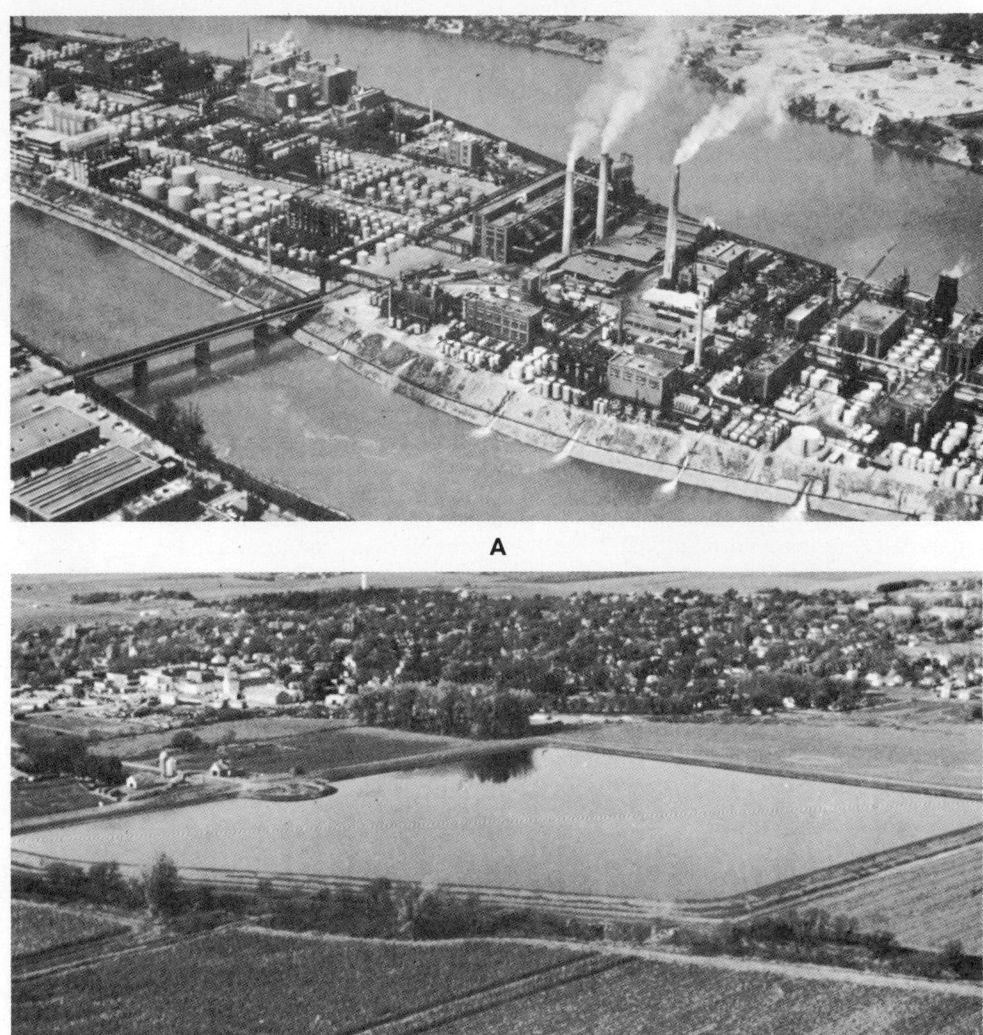

A

B

Figure 11–11 Water pollution and purification. *A*, Industrial concentrations can cause gross pollution without adequate treatment. Note sewers dumping wastes. *B*, Sunlight, algae, and oxygen work together to purify waste water in a lagoon or oxidation pond. (From *A Primer on Waste Water Treatment.* Environmental Protection Agency, March, 1971, pp. 8, 9.)

mum 650 billion gallons of water per day, and treat the water to make each gallon usable at least twice.[8]

Types of Pollution

Water pollutants are classified by the Committee on Public Works as follows:

1. Organic wastes from domestic sewage and industrial discharges of plant and animal origin that remove oxygen from the water through decomposition.

2. Infectious agents contributed by domestic sewage and by some kinds of industrial wastes that may transmit disease.

3. Plant nutrients that promote nuisance growths of aquatic plant life such as algae and water weeds.

4. Synthetic organic chemicals such as pesticides and detergents resulting from the constantly changing chemical technology, that may be toxic to aquatic life and humans.

5. Inorganic chemicals and mineral substances from mining, manufacturing processes, petroleum plants, and agricultural industry that interfere with natural stream purification, destroy fish and other aquatic life, cause excessive hardness in water supplies, produce corrosive

damage, and in general add to costs of water treatment. Mercury poisoning, caused by industrial pollution into a harbor, was fatal to 300 persons and crippled 1000 more in the area around Minamata, Japan.

6. Sediments that fill stream channels, reservoirs, and harbors; erode hydroelectric power and pumping equipment; affect fish and shellfish by blanketing fish nests, spawns, and food supplies; and increase costs of water treatment.

7. Radioactive pollution from mining and processing of radioactive ores, from use of refined radioactive material, and from fallout following nuclear testing.

8. Excessive temperatures (heat) from use of water for cooling purposes, for example, and from impoundment of water in reservoirs. This may result in harmful effects on fish and aquatic life and may reduce the capacity of the receiving water to assimilate wastes.

WHAT IS A POLLUTANT?

It is illegal under the 1972 Federal Water Pollution Control Act to discharge pollutants into the nation's waters except under a National Pollutant Discharge Elimination System permit. Pollutants covered by this permit requirement are: solid waste, incinerator residue, sewage, garbage, sewage sludge, munitions, chemical wastes, biological materials, radioactive materials, heat, wrecked or discarded equipment, rock, sand, cellar dirt, and industrial, municipal, and agricultural wastes discharged into water.

Excluded from the National Pollutant Discharge Elimination System permit program are: discharges of sewage from vessels; pollutants from vessels or other floating craft in coastal or ocean waters; discharges from properly functioning marine engines; water, gas, or other material injected into oil or gas wells, or disposed of in wells during oil or gas production if the state determines that ground or surface water resources will not be degraded; aquaculture projects; separate storm sewer discharges; and dredged or fill material. Discharges excluded from the National Pollutant Discharge Elimination System permit system are covered by other pollution control requirements.

Unfortunately, a municipality, institution, industry, public agency, or other group seldom is faced with a simple or single class of pollutant. Wastes are mixed, the organic with inorganic, organic with bacterial, industrial with domestic, and so on. problems of identification frequently have not been solved, and only general characterization is possible. It is not usually feasible to separate pollutants from the water medium or from each other for independent study for disposal.

Another principal problem involves the type of water affected. Waters generally are classified as surface waters or ground waters. Surface waters are lakes, reservoirs, streams, and coastal waters. Generally, treating polluted surface waters is somewhat simpler than is the elimination of pollution from ground waters, where the pollution can travel rapidly or slowly, depending on the nature of the ground strata through which the supply moves and on the nature of the pollution itself. Pollution of ground waters by septic-tank effluents in suburban and rural areas is frequent. Ground waters also may be polluted from waste lagoons or oxidation ponds, oil field brines, and in some coastal areas, by salt water intrusion.[8]

Because we do not have enough "new" water to meet all water needs, we must use water that has been used before in the water system of upstream cities and industries. To make this water suitable for re-use, we must treat the wastes going into the water upstream. This means sewage treatment plants, the most efficient of which utilize two processes—a physical separation and screening of the waste water, and bacterial treatment of this water. The processes are known as primary and secondary treatment. In addition, the resulting water is often purified by adding chlorine.

Mussel Poisoning

The first report of shellfish poisoning was recorded over 175 years ago when the Russian Baranoff expedition in 1790 lost some 100 men from what they called "mussel poisoning" in Sitka, Alaska. In 1793, an outbreak took place in the exploring party of Captain Vancouver near the island that bears his name.

Since that time, outbreaks have been reported from Juneau, Alaska to the Gulf of California, Mexico. But shellfish poisoning is by no means limited to the Pacific Coast of North America. Outbreaks have been reported from the Bay of Fundy, Nova Scotia, New Brunswick, and many areas in coastal waters of northern Europe. An outbreak affecting 78 persons was reported in 1968 from the Northumbrian Coast of England.

MUSSEL QUARANTINE ORDER

A quarantine is hereby established of all species of mussels from the ocean shore of California, extending from the California-Oregon boundary south to the California-Mexico boundary, and including the Bay of San Francisco and all other bays, inlets, and harbors. During the period of this quarantine, mussels may concentrate a toxic material that is highly poisonous to man. This quarantine prohibits the taking, sale, or offering for sale of the mussels in or from these designated areas, except for use as fish bait. Mussels for use as bait shall be broken open at the time of taking, or prior to sale, and shall be placed and sold in containers adequately labeled in boldfaced Gothic type letters at least one-half inch in height as follows:

MUSSELS MAY CONTAIN POISON
UNFIT FOR HUMAN FOOD

The quarantine order applies only to mussels. In addition, clams should be cleaned and washed thoroughly before cooking. All dark parts of clams should be discarded, because a poison present during May through October would be concentrated in the dark parts. Only the white meat should be prepared for human consumption. In addition, clams should be taken only from areas free from sewage contamination.

This long experience has led to the imposition of an annual mussel quarantine which is usually in effect from May 1 to October 31. The shellfish toxin is produced by plantlike dinoflagellates of the genus *Gonyaulax*. These plankton are ingested by mussels, clams, oysters, and other bivalves, which store the neurotoxin in their muscle and digestive tissue. The strychnine-like poison is extremely potent and heat resistant. It is found in shellfish broth as well as tissues. As several subspecies of toxin-producing *Gonyaulax* are colorless, increased toxin production is not necessarily correlated with the often described "red tide."

Several other misconceptions also exist: that shellfish are not safe in "R" months, that the toxin may be detected by the discoloration of a clove of garlic, a silver spoon, or a coin, or that home cooking will destroy the toxin.

The symptoms of shellfish poisoning are characteristic. Gastrointestinal symptoms in man are quite variable and subordinate to the paresthesias and paralysis that may appear within 10 minutes of eating the offending shellfish or broth prepared from them. Tingling numbness around the lips is followed by prickly feelings in the fingertips. The victim may be giddy and may have trouble walking. The staggering and drowsiness have been likened to the early stages of drunkenness. Dryness and gripping sensations in the throat are among the complaints. Incoherence of speech is common and may lead to complete inability to speak. In severe poisoning, muscle paralysis, coma, cessation of respiration, and death may follow.

There is no specific antidote or treatment for shellfish poisoning. Induction of vomiting with syrup of ipecac or apomorphine is helpful in evacuating stomach contents. A tracheotomy set and a mechanical respirator should be kept available should breathing stop. Prognosis is generally favorable when the patient has survived for 12 hours beyond the onset of symptoms.

Surveillance activities for shellfish toxin have been increased along the coast. Suspect shellfish or gastric contents from suspect cases preserved in one-tenth normal hydrochloric acid should be submitted to the local health department. All suspected cases must be reported immediately to the local health department.

Zero Discharge

"Zero discharge" of wastes into all waterways by 1985 is the target set by Congress. The enforcement of pollution controls, whether by direct setting of standards on emissions or by effluent charges, will require growth in the technical capabilities of regulatory agencies in government, not only at the federal level but also at the state and local levels. One of the principal lessons of the last few years is the political and economic difficulties that occur when we are forced to establish standards of air and water quality on the basis of wholly inadequate scientific evidence as to their effects, especially on human health. The implementation of standards entails large economic costs which are difficult to justify without strong evidence of the need for such standards, and scientific uncertainties provide leverage for agitation against their enforcement. The need for continual changes of standards in the light of new information is also economically and politically costly; great effort is warranted in obtaining the necessary information and understanding in advance of the establishment of regulations.

Increasingly stringent court interpretations of producers' liability for product safety and environmental protection will also provide a strong incentive for "defensive" research in industry, aimed at avoiding the risk of unexpected damage suits involving very large penalties.

Legislation

The first significant national legislation on water was the Water Pollution Control Act of 1956. It authorized the United States Public Health Service to intervene where interstate waters were contaminated to such an extent that they jeopardized the health or welfare of residents of adjoining states. This was done through the so-called "conference procedure," a series of hearings at which the problems were examined and corrective programs could lead to federal court action and citations for contempt. Recognizing that much pollution is due to the inadequacy of community sewage treatment, the act also instituted a program of federal grants to help communities improve their facilities. A major addition to the legislation was made in the Clean Waters Act of 1966, which called for the states to establish federally approved standards of water quality for their waterways, as a step toward imposing controls on pollution sources.

Congress enacted the Water Pollution Control Act of 1972, designed as comprehensive legislation to supersede all other measures. Covering municipal, industrial, and agricultural pollution, the law calls for zero discharge by 1985, with the intermediate steps of "best available" treatment facilities by 1983 and "most practicable" facilities by 1977 (the two terms to be defined technologically by the Environmental Protection Agency). Secondary treatment or the equivalent is the minimum treatment acceptable under the law. Since secondary treatment relates basically to community sewage, "equivalent" treatment (for such things as chemically complex industrial discharges) was left for the Environmental Protection Agency to define. The heart of the law is a new permit program for the three categories of pollution sources. Permits are to be granted to individual dischargers only after they show that their effluents, individually and collectively, will not contaminate a waterway in excess of federal–state quality standards, or lower its existing quality. The law allows polluters time to install new facilities, but provides that corrective programs must meet the 1977- and 1983-phased requirements.

In place of the cumbersome "conference procedure" of enforcement, the new law sets penalties ranging from $2500 to $25,000 a day, plus a year in prison, for willful or negligent violations of pollution abatement requirements, and up to double the penalty for repeated offenses. Unintentional violations entail civil penalties of fines of up to $10,000 a day. The law gives citizens an active role in the abatement program. It stipulates that states must give public notice of pending permit applications and make all pertinent data available for public inspection; that interested citizens and governmental agencies can request public hearings on the granting of permits; and that, if requested by a state, federal hearings must be held regarding discharges into interstate waters. The law also gives individuals and groups the right to sue violators or state or federal agencies in federal courts to compel enforcement of the law's provisions.

Another significant provision of the law was that state water pollution boards—which in most states administer and enforce water pollution regulations—should be purged of members with financial connections with polluters. Such implicit conflicts of interest had been considered a possible factor in the slow pace of pollution abatement in many areas. Unfortunately, the program as of this writing has not produced the dramatic results promised, because of reduced funds, a proliferating and changing array of guidelines, and changing directives from the Environmental Protection Agency.

1974 EPA Inventory Report on Water Quality in Rivers

The 1974 Water Quality Inventory report from the Environmental Protection Agency (EPA) points out that the two water pollutants receiving the most widespread controls—coliform bacteria and oxygen-demanding organic materials—showed general improvement in 22 major U.S. waterways during the past 10 years. However, the levels of nitrogen and phosphorus, the two nutrients most often associated with eutrophication, are reported to be rising.

The 1974 report states that between 1963 and 1967 and between 1968 and 1972, the dissolved oxygen and oxygen-demand levels improved in up to 74 per cent of the regions that were studied in the 22 waterways. Coliform bacteria levels improved in up to 78 per cent of the reaches. In contrast, nitrogen levels increased in up to 76 per cent and exceeded reference levels (0.8 milligrams per liter) in one-half of them.

Other pollutants present at high levels are phenols (industrial compounds that can affect the taste of fish) and suspended solids (which interfere with some aquatic life processes). The data on phenols and suspended solids are not as disturbing as the nutrient data, according to the report, since those waters for which detailed information was available had shown a general improvement in both phenols and suspended solids in the preceding five years.

The 1974 report is the first systematic analysis of the quantitative impact of water pollution on a national scale. It is based on data obtained by EPA, by other federal agencies, and by the individual states. In addition to the 22 major waterways, it focuses on 5000 major problem areas in 56 states and territories. It reflects the beginning of new activities in 1973 by the Environmental Protection Agency and the states to collect the data on stream quality and effluents needed to implement the 1972 Water Act. More comprehensive data will be available for future reports as these new activities get into full operation.

Copies of the National Water Quality Inventory Report are available from the Environmental Protection Agency, Office of Water Programs, Monitoring and Data Support Division (WH-453), Waterside Mall, Washington, D.C. 20460.

International Action

Extending the water pollution abatement effort beyond the nation's shoreline, Congress in 1972 also passed the Marine Protection, Research, and Sanctuaries Act. It prohibits ocean dumping of highly radioactive wastes and of chemical, biological, or radiological warfare compounds within 12 miles of the coast, and requires federal permits for other specified sorts of dumping. At the United Nations environmental conference in Stockholm in June 1972, representatives agreed in principle that nations have a mutual responsibility for care of the oceans, as well as for the earth's atmosphere; and an array of measures to protect ocean quality were included in the program of international action adopted by the conference. Five months later, at a conference in London, representatives of 92 nations, including the United States, agreed on a global convention (subject to ratification) to end the dumping of poisonous and noxious waste materials at sea.

Sewage Treatment

Today, disposal of sewage into the waterways is considered a privilege rather than a right. Nevertheless, raw sewage is drained into many rivers and bays throughout the country, and many sewage treatment plants are inadequate and ineffective in coping with the increase of sewage, chemicals, and detergents. Sewage treatment plants should at least provide primary and secondary treatment in larger communities (Fig. 11–12).

Primary Treatment. Primary sewage treatment consists of screening and sedimentation. Screens may be coarse or fine and help remove large objects that may damage

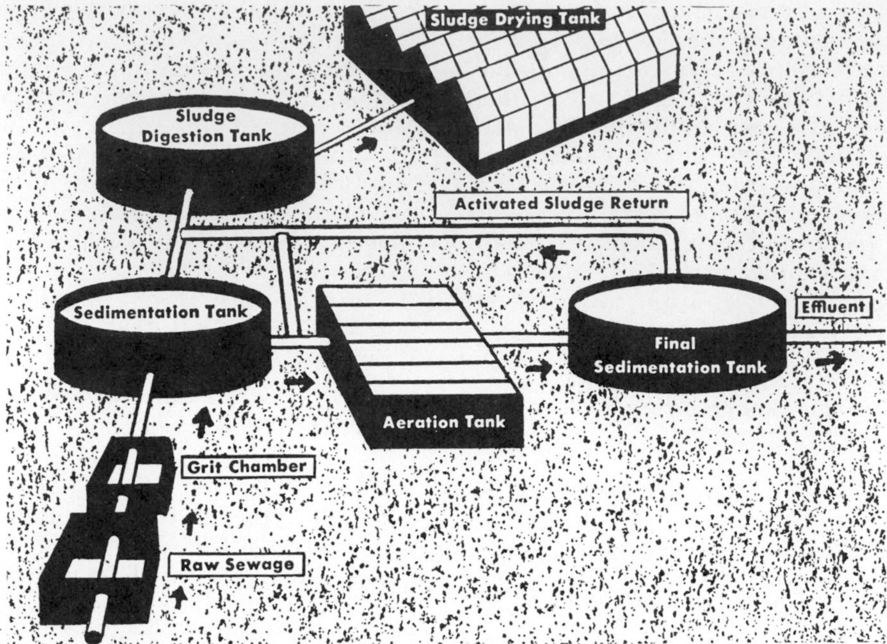

Figure 11–12 This activated sludge type of sewage treatment is used by many large cities. Solid matter is broken down by action of bacteria and air after it settles. (From Rosenblum, M.: *Public Health.* Merit Badge Series, Boy Scouts of America, 1956.)

pumps. Sedimentation, which takes place in settling tanks, allows the solids to settle when the velocity or flow of the turbid liquid is reduced or stopped. The solid portion of the settling tank, called sludge, is then transported to the digestion tank, where sludge particles support a colony of anaerobic bacteria, initiate biochemical oxidation of the sludge, and release carbon dioxide and methane. These gases supply energy to operate the pumps. The sewage is transported to open-air drying beds, and is then buried, burned, dumped, or sold for fertilizer.

To complete the primary treatment, the effluent from the sedimentation tank is chlorinated before being discharged into a stream or river. Chlorine gas is fed into the water to kill and reduce the number of disease-causing bacteria. Chlorination also helps to reduce objectionable odors. Although 30 per cent of the municipalities in the United States give only primary treatment to their sewage, this process by itself is considered entirely inadequate for most needs.

Secondary Treatment. Secondary treatment removes up to 80 per cent of the organic matter in sewage by making use of the bacteria in it. The two principal types of secondary treatment are trickling filters and the activated sludge process. After the effluent leaves the sedimentation tank in the primary stage of treatment, it flows or is pumped to a facility using one or the other of these processes. A trickling filter is simply a bed of stones from 3 to 10 feet deep through which the sewage passes. This system utilizes aerobic bacteria, air, water, and sunlight, all of which help oxidize and purify the liquid portion of the sewage. Bacteria gather and multiply on these stones until they can consume most of the organic matter in the sewage. The cleaner water trickles out through pipes in the bottom of the filter for further treatment.

The sewage is applied to the bed of stones in one of two ways. One method consists of distributing the effluent intermittently through a network of pipes laid on or beneath the surface of the stones. Attached to these pipes are smaller, vertical pipes that spray the sewage over the stones. Another much-used method consists of a vertical pipe in the center of the filter, connected to rotating horizontal pipes which spray the sewage continuously upon the stones. Currently, the activated sludge process is favored over trickling filters. This process speeds up the work of the bacteria by bringing air and sludge heavily laden with bacteria into close contact with the sewage. After the sewage leaves the settling tank in primary treatment, it is pumped to an aeration tank, where it is mixed with air and sludge loaded with bacteria and allowed to remain for several hours. During this time, the bacteria break down the organic matter.

From the aeration tank, the sewage, flows to another sedimentation tank to remove the solids. Chlorination of the effluent completes the basic secondary treatment. The sludge, now activated with additional millions of bacteria and other tiny organisms, can be used again by returning it to an aeration tank for mixing with new sewage and ample amounts of air. The activated sludge process, like most other techniques, has advantages and limitations. The size of the units necessary for this treatment is small, thereby requiring less land space, and the process is free of flies and odors. But it is more costly to operate than the trickling filter, and the activated sludge process sometimes is not completely effective in eliminating difficult industrial wastes. An adequate supply of oxygen is necessary for the activated sludge process to be effective. Air is mixed with sewage and biologically active sludge in the aeration tanks by three different methods.

The first, mechanical aeration, is accomplished by drawing the sewage from the bottom of the tank and spraying it over the surface, thus causing the sewage to absorb large amounts of oxygen from the atmosphere. In the second method, large amounts of air under pressure are piped down into the sewage and forced out through openings in the pipe. The third method is a combination of mechanical aeration and the forced air method. The final phase of the secondary treatment consists of the addition of chlorine, as the most common method of disinfection, to the effluent coming from the trickling filter or the activated sludge process. Chlorine is usually purchased in liquid form, converted to a gas, and injected into the effluent 15 to 30 minutes before the treated water is discharged into a watercourse. If done properly, chlorination will kill more than 99 per cent of the harmful bacteria in an effluent.

Tertiary Treatment. To eliminate troublesome contaminants remaining after the two-stage treatment, scientists in recent years have developed "advanced waste treatment," a three-stage process sometimes called tertiary treatment. It consists essentially or filtrating secondary-treatment effluent through some medium such as carbon granules, sometimes with the addition of chemicals. The product of tertiary treatment is so pure that it is even drinkable, after precautionary chlorination. This process costs about 50 per cent more than secondary treatment, which typically costs one cent a day per person. A number of advanced waste treatment plants are in operation, the best known of which is at Lake Tahoe, California. Because the lake provides an abundant supply of drinking water, the tertiary effluent is piped over the rim of the Tahoe Basin to arid country on the opposite slope in the Sierras, where it serves as a water supply for agriculture and man-made recreational lakes.

Problems

In considering waste treatment plants, there are three basic problems. First, there are not enough of them. One-fourth of our municipalities still discharge their wastes into the most convenient stream without treating them. Another 31 per cent of our communities provide only primary treatment. Approximately 7500 municipal sewage treatment plants are now operating in this country. If our water sources are to be improved, authorities state that we must build, enlarge, or modernize almost 6000 more.

Second, our waste treatment plants are not efficient enough. Primary treatment at best removed 35 per cent of organic wastes and secondary treatment removes up to 90 per cent. (In terms of total wastes, organic plus inorganic, they remove much less than this.) It is obvious that there is still an enormous amount of pollution being discharged into rivers and streams. The pollution load in our rivers is already six times as much as it was 60 years ago.

Third, because the procedures of waste treatment plants are based mainly on bacterial action, they have difficulty in removing many of the new pollutants found in waste water today. Even common salt cannot be removed by existing waste treatment processes. A great effort is being made to find an economical means of water desalinization, so that arid areas of the world near the sea can begin to convert ocean water to drinkable water.

Also, treatment plants have difficulty in removing wastes resulting from the use or manufacture of such new substances as plastics, detergents, nylon and similar fibers, pesticides, herbicides, and medicines. The plants are ineffective against other mineral and chemical substances, such as acids produced by mine drainage, against radioactive substances, and against heat, which harms aquatic life by affecting the metabolism of fish and by lowering the water's ability to hold oxygen.[10]

Even if provision of secondary treatment by conventional methods is greatly accelerated for all sewage by 1985, the amount of municipal pollution reaching watercourses then will be substantially the same as today. If the present rate of municipal treatment-plant construction is not accelerated, considering the projected urban growth for 1985, the municipal sewage discharge in that year will be the equivalent of untreated waste produced by a population of 114 million, or 52 per cent greater than the pollutant load from the same source in 1960.

Advanced Methods of Treating Wastes

To return water of more usable quality to receiving lakes and streams, new methods for removing pollutants are being developed. The advanced waste treatment techniques under investigation range from extensions of biological treatment capable of removing nitrogen and phosphorus nutrients to physical-chemical separation techniques such as carbon adsorption, distillation, reverse osmosis, and ozonation. These new processes can achieve any degree of pollution control desired and, as waste effluents are purified to higher and higher degrees by such treatments, the point is reached where effluents become "too good to throw away." Such water can be deliberately and directly reused for agricultural, industrial, recreational, or even drinking water supplies. This complete water renovation will mean complete pollution control and at the same time more water for the nation.

Coagulation–Sedimentation Technique

The process known as coagulation–sedimentation may be used to increase the removal of solids from effluent after primary and secondary treatment. Besides removing essentially all of the settleable solids, this method can, with proper control and sufficient addition of chemicals, reduce the concentration of phosphate by over 95 per cent. In this process, alum, lime, or iron salts are added to effluent as it comes from the secondary treatment. The flow then passes through flocculation tanks where the chemicals cause the smaller particles to "floc," or bunch together, into large masses.

The larger masses of particles or lumps will settle faster when the effluent reaches the next step—the sedimentation tank. Although used for years in the treatment of industrial wastes and in water treatment, coagulation–sedimentation is classified as an advanced process because it is not usually applied to the treatment of municipal wastes. In many cases, the process is a necessary pretreatment for some of the other advanced techniques.

Adsorption Technique

Technology has also been developed to effect the removal of refractory organic material. These materials are the stubborn organic matter that persists in water and resists normal treatment. Adsorption consists of passing the effluent through a bed of activated carbon granules which will remove more than 98 per cent of the organics. To cut down the cost of the procedure, the extremely hard carbon granules can be cleaned by heat and used again. Carbon also has a huge surface area to weight—each pound of carbon represents from 100 to 125 acres of surface area.

An alternative system utilizing powdered carbon is under study. Rather than pass the effluent through a bed of granules, the powdered carbon is put directly into the stream. The organics stick to the carbon and then the carbon is removed from the effluent by using coagulation chemicals and allowing the coagulated carbon particles to settle in a tank. The use of this finely ground carbon will improve the rate at which the refractory organics are removed. The potential widespread use of powdered carbon adsorption depends largely on the effectiveness of regenerating the carbon for use again. Except for the salts added during the use of water, municipal waste water that has gone through the previous advanced processes will be restored to a chemical quality almost the same as before it was used.

Electrodialysis

Electrodialysis is a rather complicated process by which electricity and membranes are used to remove salts from an effluent.

The Tahoe Water Reclamation Process

The Tahoe process of purification and nutrient removal begins where conventional waste treatment systems end. Effluent from the secondary clarifier receives chemical clarification by the addition of lime as a coagulant. This removes the suspended matter and most of the phophates. The high pH (11.5–12) effluent from the chemical clarifier is pumped to a lath-packed stripping tower which removes the ammonia-nitrogen. As it leaves the tower, the water is recarbonated to reduce the pH, using carbon dioxide recovered from furnace stack gases. Filtration on mixed media separation beds filters out remaining turbidity, phosphates, and calcium carbonate. Final polishing is provided by granular activated carbon, which removes color, odor, and almost all of the remaining organic material.

Costs are reduced by facilities for reclaiming materials for reuse. Spent carbon is regenerated in a six-hearth furnace, developing temperatures up to 1700 degrees. Lime sludge is thickened in a centrifuge and recalcined in a similar furnace, and carbon dioxide from the stacks is used for recarbonation. Disposal of the biological sludge from the primary and secondary treatment units is accomplished by burning it in multiple-stage smokeless incinerators.

Lagoons and Septic Tanks

There are many well-populated areas in the United States that are not served by any sewer systems or waste treatment plants. Lagoons and septic tanks may act as less than satisfactory alternatives at such locations. A septic tank is simply a tank buried in the ground to treat the sewage from an individual home. Waste water from the home flows into the tank where bacteria in the sewage may break down the organic matter, and the cleaner water flows out of the tank into the ground through subsurface drains. Periodically the sludge or solid matter in the bottom of the tank must be removed and disposed of. In a rural setting, with the right kind of soil and the proper location, the septic tank may be a reasonable and temporary means of disposing strictly domestic wastes. Septic tanks should always be located so that none of the effluent can seep into sources used for drinking.

Lagoons, or, as they are sometimes called, stabilization or oxidation ponds, also have several advantages when used correctly. They can give sewage primary and secondary treatment or they can be used to supplement other processes. A lagoon is a scientifically constructed pond, usually 3 to 5 feet deep, in which sunlight, algae, and oxygen interact to restore water to a quality that is often equal to or better than effluent from secondary treatment. Changes in the weather may change the effectiveness of lagoons.

When used with other waste treatment processes, lagoons can be very effective. A good example of this is the Santee, California, water reclamation project. After conventional primary and secondary treatment by activated sludge, the town's waste is kept in a lagoon for 30 days. Then the effluent, after chlorination, is pumped to land immediately above a series of lakes and allowed to trickle down through sandy soil into the lakes. The resulting water is of such good quality that residents of the area can swim, boat, and fish in the lake water. Competent engineering is required to determine whether or not a lagoon is the best answer to a community's sewage problems.

A Program to Abate Water Pollution

Controlling water pollution is a complex problem involving the conservation of water, its distribution, and its uses. The key to the successful development of any water plan involves water management, which includes initial collection and impoundment, controlled use and re-use of water, and disposal or reclamation of immense volumes of water that have become overmineralized or otherwise degraded to such an extent that further use is not feasible. A program to abate water pollution must include construction, law enforcement, research, and cooperation. Citizens must unite and promote the construction of sewage treatment plants in order to protect their health, and to restore the pu-

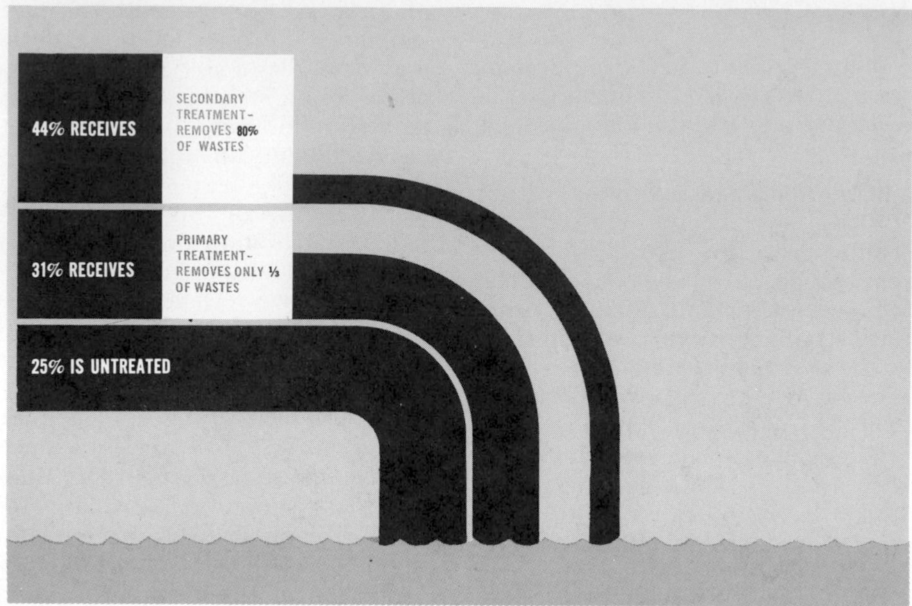

Figure 11–13 Municipal wastes. Fortunately, water is a resource that can be cleaned and used again. Many cities have sewage treatment plants and clean their wastes before returning them to watercourses. Unfortunately, this is not true in all cases; 25 per cent of municipal wastes are still dumped into our rivers and streams as raw sewage, and another 31 per cent are given only primary treatment, which only removes solids that settle.

rity and beauty of their lakes, rivers, and streams.

The Ohio River Valley offers an excellent example of what can be done. In 1950, the basin's 17 million residents had few sewage treatment plants, and raw sewage from 5 million persons went directly into the river system. A small group of interested citizens organized the Ohio River Valley Water Sanitation Commission and initiated an educational program, followed by a fund raising campaign. The Junior Chamber of Commerce, Boy Scouts, newspapers, and other civic-minded organizations supported local bond issue campaigns. River testing stations gained active cooperation from industry. The Commission gained the support of 1000 basin towns and cities to build modern sewage treatment plants that cost up to $150 per capita. Today, treatment plants serve over 12 million residents, and new plants are being added rapidly. The results are already measurable in terms of clean, new beaches, fishing, boating, and water skiing.

As suburbs continue to grow, contagious disease hazards increase because of poor and inadequate sanitary facilities. Because no public sewer system exists in many suburban areas, many people are using septic tanks for sewage disposal. Where soil has poor drainage, effective absorption of septic tanks effluent is impossible, and the effluent may find its way into wells or main drainage ways. The logical solution to this problem in suburbs is annexation to the nearest city and installation of public sewer systems. People should be educated to realize that an increase in taxes may be small compared to hospital bills.

Public Cooperation. Progress in the struggle for clean water depends on public understanding, support, and cooperation. Many states have joined to form interstate compacts, enabling them to discuss and meet the problems that affect them all. These compacts cover important areas. A typical one is the Interstate Commission on the Potomac River, which enables Maryland, Virginia, Pennsylvania, West Virginia, and the District of Columbia to develop and carry out joint programs for controlling pollution of this river. Cooperation is also the basis for the several comprehensive river basin studies that are now under way and that involve industries, municipalities, state and federal agencies, and research institutions. One such plan involves the Arkansas-Red River Basin, 180,000 square miles of land lying principally in Kansas, Oklahoma and Texas. A cooperative study has been undertaken involving these three states, their municipalities and industries, and a number of federal agencies, including the United States Geological Survey and the United States Army Corps of Engineers. Somewhat similar studies involve the Colorado River Basin, the Columbia River Basin, the Great Lakes-Illinois Waterway area, the Delaware Estuary, and Chesapeake Bay. These studies require from two to six years and cost two million to 12 million dollars. However, they result in systematic plans for maximum water use for all purposes over the longest possible period.[11]

Industries are becoming more aware of their significant contribution to the desecration of the land, but they still need more effective methods to control the waste materials they discard. Today about 125,000 individual industries are cooperating with their nearby communities, but about 25,000 of all major types of industry are still discharging untreated wastes directly into community streams. One way industries can help improve the water supply is to build their own treatment plants or to help communities build them. They can also recover valuable natural resources from wastes rather than

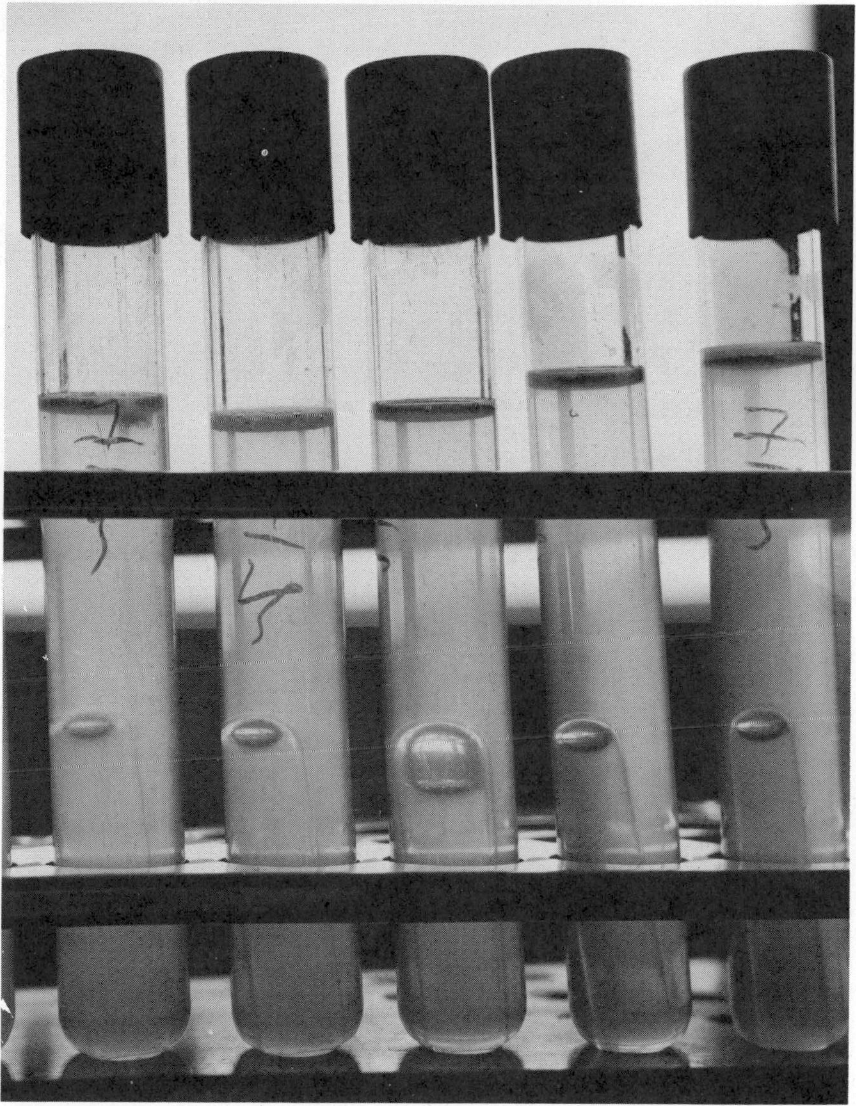

Figure 11–14 The *presumptive test* is the first test that water undergoes. Gas bubbles are plainly visible in the small inverted glass vials inserted in the larger test tubes. Bubbles are the product of fermentation brought about by the action of coliform group of intestinal bacteria with a liquid food source that contains lactose. If the water sample contains these intestinal organisms, they will ferment the sugar. The gas produced will be trapped in the small inverted vial. These bubbles indicate a positive presumptive test and the possibility that the water is contaminated. (From Water analysis. Oregon Health Bull., *41*:2, 1963.)

dispose of them in the waterways. The steel industry pioneered in development of a process for the recovery of valuable chemicals from waste liquids.

POLLUTION IN THE GREAT LAKES

People began to worry about pollution in the Great Lakes as early as 1912. Nobody did anything about it, however, until 1965, when Congress passed the Water Quality Act, which set standards for all states. Then, in 1970, the International Joint Commission completed a major study of pollution and, in effect, urged both the United States and Canada to stop using the Great Lakes as a sewer. This led, two years later, to the signing of an agreement by the two countries to clean up the lakes. The same year, Congress implemented the agreement with rigid Water Pollution Control Amendments, which at last gave the Environmental Protection Agency both the money and legislation to do the job. Since 1972, more than 2 billion dollars has been spent by the United States and Canada on the world's largest area of fresh water. Progress has been steady, at times even spectacular, even though much remains to be done.

In general, Great Lakes pollution has three sources. Sixty per cent comes from municipal sewage, 30 per cent from industry, and 10 per cent from agricultural runoff and other sources. This breakdown is based on volume and does not reflect toxicity; damage by industry (mercury) or by agriculture (pesticides) can often be more dangerous than the smaller amounts suggest. The primary job in 1972 was dealing with municipal waste; all municipalities had to be equipped with adequate (i.e., secondary) sewage systems. To this end, the federal government agreed to put up 75 per cent of the funds, with local governments providing the rest. There are 974 municipal sewer plants on the United States side of the Great Lakes. In 1972, a mere 5 per cent of the population was adequately served by them. By 1982 the figure will rise to 98 per cent.

Meanwhile, water pollution is being attacked on other fronts. DDT has been banned, and mercury discharges have been largely eliminated. Phosphorus, perhaps the worst offender of all because of its role in

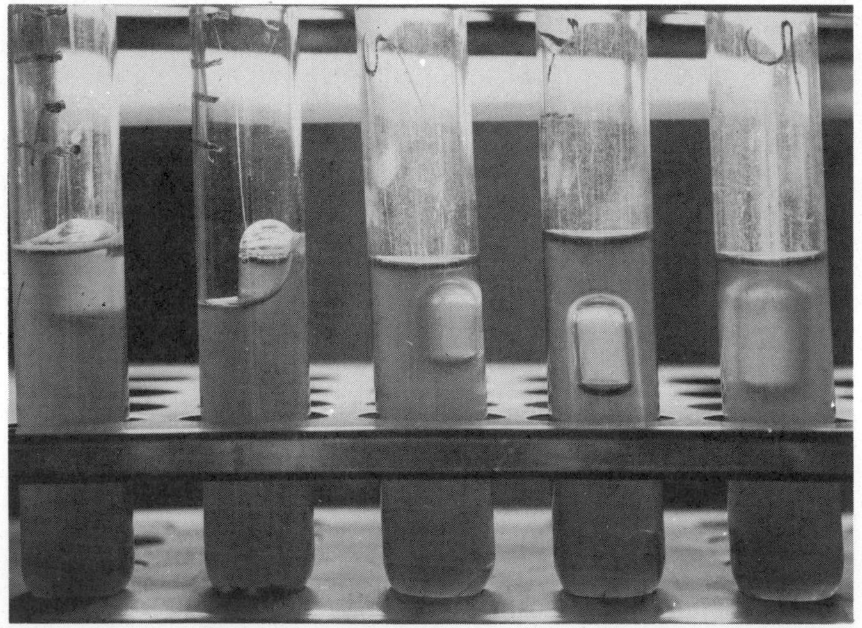

Figure 11–15 Samples producing bubbles shown in Figure 11–14 are subjected to a second confirming test. The Oregon Public Health Laboratory uses a special liquid medium, or source of food, that will encourage the growth of only the coliform group of bacteria. Known as brilliant green lactose bile broth, the dye and chemical inhibit the growth of other bacteria and yeast, which could give a false positive presumptive test by bacteria that are not indicators of sewage pollution. The appearance of bubbles in this second test indicates that the water sample has been contaminated by sewage, and therefore the water from this source is unfit for human consumption. (From Water analysis. Oregon Health Bull., *41*:3, 1963.)

promoting algae and contributing to the depletion of a lake's oxygen, has been handled in several ways. Canada reduced its content in detergents, as did three American states. Most states, fearful that phosphate substitutes might be worse than the original detergents, requested removal at municipal plants. All new systems have this capacity.

Perhaps the most dramatic improvements have occurred in industry. The heart of the industrial cleanup campaign is a system of permits issued by both the Environmental Protection Agency and the states. Individually tailored to each plant, a permit specifies the amount and type of waste that may be discharged, and a timetable for reducing the total. When a company violates this permit, a suit can be initiated. The law allows a reasonable amount of time to install new and usually expensive facilities to curb pollution. (The steel industry, for example, has already spent over 1 billion dollars on them.) All programs must be completed with the "best practical technology" by 1977, and with the "best available technology" by 1983.

What Can Citizens Do To Help?

Concerned citizens, especially those organized in voluntary citizen organizations to work for a cleaner environment, can contribute greatly to the campaign against water pollution. Among other things, they can work to insure that water pollution control agencies—at the community, state and federal levels—have adequate funds and staff to implement water pollution control laws and regulations. They can support, encourage, and stimulate control agencies and polluters to move steadily and speedily toward compliance with water pollution control laws and regulations. They can keep the public informed, on a continuing basis, on the success or failure of water pollution control programs, including the permit system.

Citizen groups can play a direct role in the national permit program. They can monitor permit applications and proposed permits. They can obtain and analyze draft permits and fact sheets. They can request and take part in public hearings and the formal adjudicatory hearings when deemed necessary. They can learn the terms and conditions of permits, obtain monitoring and compliance reports, and check to see if compliance schedules are being met on time. They can report supposed violations of permits to control agencies. If all else fails, they can use their right to take court action to compel compliance. In brief, concerned citizen organizations can serve as public ombudsmen—watchdogs of the national program "to restore and maintain the chemical, physical, and biological integrity of the Nation's waters" under the Federal Water Pollution Control Act.

WHAT YOU CAN DO

1. Get the facts about causes and effects of pollution in your community.
2. Join an organized citizens group working on pollution problems. If none exists, organize one.
3. Promote a cleanup campaign in your company. Tell your customers and community about it. It's good business.
4. Find out the water quality standards established for your local rivers and lakes.
5. Publicize your community's clean water goals and programs. Get your local newspaper editor interested. Get him photographs. They tell a story. Send copies to your mayor, your state agency, and your local news media.
6. Vote for the candidates who support clean water.
7. Vote yes for local and state bond issues to support improved pollution control programs.
8. Don't be a polluter yourself. Don't throw your trash on beaches, parks, stream banks, and highways. Don't throw your wastes and garbage overboard. Prevent oil and fuel spills.

Organizations

The Environmental Protection Agency, Washington, D.C. 20460, and its 10 regional offices have many publications on water pollution, summaries of legislation, and manuals on citizen action. The Izaak Walton League of America, 1800 North Kent, Rosslyn, Virginia 22209, has a pamphlet on citizen action entitled "Clean Water – It's Up To You." The pamphlet includes a list of other organizations and public officials concerned with pollution. The League of Women Voters, 1730 M Street, N.W., Washington, D.C. 20036, also has helpful background literature.

Other conservation organizations with local chapters in many parts of the country are the National Wildlife Federation, 1412 16th Street, N.W., Washington, D.C. 20036; the National Audubon Society, 950 Third Avenue, New York, New York 10022; and the Sierra Club, 220 Bush Street, San Francisco, California 94104. The National Wildlife Federation publishes an annual Conservation Directory listing state and national environmental officials and organizations throughout the country.

Among the most active organizations in environmental litigation have been the Sierra Club; Friends of the Earth, 620 C Street, S.E., Washington, D.C. 20003; the Environmental Defense Fund, 162 Old Town Road, East Setauket, New York 11733; and the Natural Resources Defense Council, 15 West 44th Street, New York, New York 10036. Public affairs pamphlets include "The Campaign for Cleaner Air," by Marvin Zeldin, No. 494; "An Environment Fit for People," by Raymond F. Dasmann, No. 421; "Noise – the Third Pollution," by Theodore Berland, No. 449; "Cleansing our Waters," by Gladwin Hill, No. 497.

Private Organizations Interested in Pollution Control

The following organiztations may be contacted for further information on pollution control:

American Fisheries Society
1040 Washington Building,
15th Street and New York Avenue, N.W.,
Washington, D.C. 20005

American Littoral Society,
Sandy Hook,
Highlands, New Jersey 07732

Conservation Foundation,
1717 Massachusetts Avenue, N.W.,
Washington, D.C. 20036

Garden Club of America,
598 Madison Avenue,
New York, New York 10022

General Federation of Women's Clubs,
1734 North Street, N.W.,
Washington, D.C. 20036

Izaak Walton League of America,
1326 Waukegan Road,
Glenview, Illinois 60025

League of Women Voters,
1730 M Street, N.W.
Washington, D.C. 20036

National Association of Counties,
1001 Connecticut Avenue,
Washington, D.C. 20036

National Association of Soil
and Water Conservation,
1025 Vermont Avenue, N.W.,
Washington, D.C. 20005

National Audubon Society,
1130 5th Avenue,
New York, New York 10028

National Council of State Garden Clubs, Inc.
4401 Magnolia Avenue,
St. Louis, Missouri 63110

Sierra Club,
1050 Mills Tower,
San Francisco, California 94104

Sport Fishing Institute,
Suite 503
719 13th Street, N.W.
Washington, D.C. 20005

Trout Unlimited,
5850 E. Jewell Avenue,
Denver, Colorado 80222

UAW-CIO Department of Conservation
and Resource Development,
8000 E. Jefferson Street,
Detroit, Michigan 48214

Wildlife Management Institute,
709 Wire Building,
Washington, D.C. 20005

Wildlife Society,
Suite S–176
3900 Wisconsin Avenue, N.W.,
Washington, D.C. 20016

AIR POLLUTION

Smog and other forms of contaminated air, previously considered a local annoyance, are now recognized as a national problem and a menace to the future health of this country. Evidence from disastrous occurrences elsewhere, and from available data, though limited, indicates that air pollution poses a significant public health problem. Further investigation reveals that air pollution is injurious to agricultural crops and livestock and is hazardous to air and ground transportation.

At present, over 10,000 communities in the United States have some kind of air pollution problem. Each year additional communities find it more difficult to keep the air supply fresh and healthful for people to breathe. This should be a major consideration, since each of us breathes in about 15,000 quarts of air per day. But the tendency to associate the smoking industrial stack with prosperity has consistently allayed community rebellion. This popular concept is now waning; people all over the industrialized world are awakening to the air pollution hazard.

Air and Health

There is no conclusive evidence that concentrations of community air pollution are producing severe harmful effects on the average person. However, studies reveal that air pollution may cause reduced visibility, eye irritation, respiratory irritation, damage

TABLE 11–1 Established Pathogens Found in Motor Vehicle Exhausts (Partial List)*

POLLUTANT	POTENTIAL EFFECTS
Aldehydes	Respiratory stress in infants; extreme dermal hypersensitivity; eye irritation.
Carbon Monoxide	Anoxia; chronic optic neuritis; hearing impairment; vestibular disturbances.
Chrysene Benz (a) anthracene Benzo (a) pyrene Benzo (e) pyrene Benzo (j) fluoranthene 1,1 H-Benzo (b) fluoranthene Dibenzo (a,h) anthracene Dibenzo (a,e) pyrene Dibenzo (a,l) pyrene	Carcinogenic.
Nitrogen Oxides	Anoxia; central nervous system depression; asphyxial convulsions; central paralysis; respiratory irritation; pulmonary edema; bronchopneumonia; bronchiolitis; pneumonitis.
Ozone	Eye irritation; decreased cold resistance; partial paralysis of respiratory organs; chest pains; headaches.
Sulfates	(Associated with air pollution disasters in London, New York City, Meuse Valley, Germany, and Donora, Pennsylvania.) Alters rate and depth of breathing; chest pains; coughing; bronchial restriction; pulmonary flow resistance; aggravates bronchial asthma
Lead	Body burden significantly increases with exposure to vehicular traffic.

*Adapted from a report of the Surgeon General, U.S.P.H.S., to the U.S. Congress, June, 1962. *In* Hilleboe, H. E., and Larimore, G. W. (eds.): *Preventive Medicine.* 2nd ed. Philadelphia, W. B. Saunders Co., 1965.

TABLE 11-2 Comparison Among Three Major Air Pollution Crises*

	MEUSE VALLEY, 1930	DONORA, 1948	LONDON, 1952
Weather	Anticyclonic, inversion, and fog	Anticyclonic, inversion, and fog	Anticyclonic, inversion, and fog
Topography	River valley	River valley	River plain
Most probable source of pollutants	Industry (including steel and zinc plants)	Industry (including steel and zinc plants)	Household coal-burning
Nature of the illnesses	Chemical irritation of exposed membranous surfaces	Chemical irritation of exposed membranous surfaces	Chemical irritation of exposed membranous surfaces
Deaths among those with preexisting cardiorespiratory disease	Yes	Yes	Yes
Time of deaths	Began after second day of episode	Began after second day of episode	Began on first day of episode
Ratio of illnesses to deaths	Not available	75 : 1 to 300 : 1	Illness rates not in expected proportion to that of deaths
Autopsy findings	Inflammatory lesions in lungs included parenchyma	Inflammatory lesions in lungs did not include parenchyma	Inflammatory lesions in lungs included parenchyma
Suspected proximate cause of irritation	Sulfur oxides with particulates	Sulfur oxides with particulates	Sulfur oxides with particulates

*From Herman, H.: Effects of air pollution on human health. *In* Barker, K., et al. (eds.): *Air Pollution.* New York, Columbia University Press, 1961, p. 180.

to certain rubber and plastic products, crop damage, and discomfort. Other medical studies link air pollution with lung cancer, emphysema, and certain other diseases. In London, for example, chronic bronchitis-emphysema, an irreversible pulmonary disorder that can cause eventual heart failure, is the third leading cause of death (behind heart diseases and cancer) of men over 45 years of age. Many British doctors attribute its rapid rise to polluted air.*

*There has been approximately a fourfold increase in the mortality rate from emphysema among Californians in the last 20 years.

Three episodes of acute air pollution have been characterized by sudden death. These tragedies occurred in Belgium's Meuse Valley in 1930, in Donora, Pennsylvania in 1940, and in London in 1952. In each case a heavy fog had settled over the area and did not lift, in each case the phenomenon was produced by a temperature inversion or a layer of warm air over a layer of cold air, and in each case there was a heavy concentration of smoke and pollutants. During these periods, 63 deaths in Meuse Valley, 20 deaths in Donora, and 3000 deaths in London were attributed to air pollution. Most of those who died, however, were elderly people already suffering from

TABLE 11–3 Symptoms Produced by Air Pollution in Donora, in Decreasing Order of Occurrence in All Ages*

Symptom	%
Cough	33.1
Non-productive	20.2
Productive	12.9
Sore throat	23.1
Constriction of the chest	21.5
Headache	17.0
Dyspnoea without orthopnoea	12.9
Smarting of the eyes	12.3
Orthopnoea	8.4
Lacrimation	8.0
Vomiting	7.4
Nausea without vomiting	7.1
Nasal discharge	6.6
Fever	2.6
Choking	2.3
Aches and pains	1.9
Weakness	1.8
Cyanosis	1.0
Diarrhoea	0.1

*From *United States Technical Conference on Air Pollution* by L. C. McCabe (ed.). Copyright 1952, McGraw-Hill Book Company, Inc. Used by permission of the publisher.

diseases of the respiratory or circulatory systems. A $500,000 study was completed in 1974 by the National Academy of Sciences (Academy of Engineering). The report estimated that air pollution is implicated in about 1 per cent of all deaths in the United States each year, and that automobiles contribute up to one-fourth of this pollution (4000 deaths).

Sources of Air Pollution

Three general types of substances are known to pollute the atmospheres of all industrial environments. These are chemical, radioactive, and biologic substances. Chemical pollutants are becoming the major concern because of expanding industrial, automotive, and domestic wastes. But we must also keep in mind the radioactive pollutants which add to the total exposure in both urban and rural air. Biologic dusts and pollens likewise may cause harmful effects, especially in persons who react to them with hay fever, asthma, and other allergies. The accidental industrial fumigation of the Mexican town, Poza Rica, during a temperature inversion in 1950 poisoned 329 persons and killed 22 in the immediate vicinity of an oil refinery. This catastrophe showed that hydrogen sulfide can diffuse through the air in concentrations sufficient to kill individuals in normal health. Other immediate lethal concentrations can occur to a degree far above tolerance levels.

Two major causes of air pollution are the steady and rapid industrialization and urbanization, and the weather. More than 40 foreign substances have been identified in the atmosphere of California coastal cities. The principal sources of some of the substances are identifiable: hydrocarbons in the atmosphere arise from motor vehicle exhausts, petroleum refinery processes, the storage and marketing of petroleum products, and from other sources; nitrogen oxides occur in exhausts from autos, household and industrial fuel, and oil and gas burners; smoke may be traced to domestic incinerators and fuel oil burners; dusts and fumes result from certain mineral and earth processes, metal industries, grain and feed processes and a wide variety of chemical industries, sulfur oxides are emitted from fuel oil burners, petroleum processes and chemical processes.

Most states have adopted and are enforcing legislation regarding the use of auto crankcase devices in order to reduce pollution; major auto companies are compelled by law to install these devices as standard equipment. Although legislation has been enacted to ensure that all new cars are completely smog-free, millions of older cars will be on the road without full smog controls. This means that it will be most difficult to maintain air quality below the standards for nitrogen dioxide, carbon monoxide, lead, hydrogen sulfide, and sulfur dioxide. Sometimes "advanced technology" leads to one giant step backward. It was found, for example, that the catalytic converters installed in some 1975 automobiles were responsible for discharging sulfuric acid into the air. Chlorine combines with certain pollutants in the water to form possibly carcinogenic compounds.

Tests made with air filters give an idea of the extent to which the atmosphere is being filled with dust, oxides, lint, chemicals, and substances that cannot be identified. For example, a study made in Louisville, Kentucky, revealed that a daily average of 440 tons of man-made substances are thrown into the air over the city's main industrial section; in Seattle, Washington, autos and

Estimated Emissions of Air Pollutants, Nationwide 1971 (in millions of tons per year)

Source	Carbon Monoxide	Partic- ulates	Sulfur Oxides	Hydro- carbons	Nitrogen Oxides	Source Total	Source Percentage
Transportation	77.5	1.0	1.0	14.7	11.2	105.4	50.6
Fuel combustion in stationary sources	1.0	6.5	26.3	.3	10.2	44.3	21.2
Industrial processes	11.4	13.6	5.1	5.6	.2	35.9	17.2
Solid waste disposal	3.8	.7	.1	1.0	.2	5.8	2.8
Miscellaneous	6.5	5.2	.1	5.0	.2	17.0	8.2
All Sources	**100.2**	**27.0**	**32.6**	**26.6**	**22.0**	**208.4**	**100.0**

Figure 11–16 (From *Air Pollution Primer.* American Lung Association, 1974. Data from Environmental Protection Agency.)

trucks alone were found to be putting 100 tons of hydrocarbons, 20 to 80 tons of nitrogen dioxide, and 4 tons of sulfur dioxide into the city's air each day; in Chicago, the Illinois Institute of Technology found that each month, dust fall, a measure of air contamination, was averaging 52.9 tons per square mile compared with 71 tons in the same period of the year when industrial activity was significantly higher.[12]

The virulence of Los Angeles' smog stems from the meteorological factors that give Southern California its superb mild climate. Warm air, trapped in the basin bounded on three sides by mountains, often hangs over the city. When it is warmer than the air at ground level (a condition known as thermal inversion), this stagnant air mass becomes a transparent lid, preventing the rise and dispersion of the contaminants. Sunlight then "cooks" the hydrocarbon byproducts of incomplete combustion, converting them into noxious polluting gases and vapors that sting eyes, hamper breathing, scorch vegetables, and embrittle rubber. Low-altitude temperature inversions, common throughout the United States, create this photo-chemical smog in at least 19 states plus the District of Columbia. Los Angeles' smog differs only in frequency rather than in severity from that of most large United States cities.

Several organizations have made estimates of the kinds and amounts of air pollution originating from urban areas in California, particularly Los Angeles. More than 12,500 tons of pollutants are discharged (80 per cent by autos) into the air each day in the Los Angeles basin. This figure would be 3300 tons higher without the city's severe industrial controls. Toxic substances include lead, acids, sulfur dioxide, oxides of nitrogen, organic substances, hydrocarbons, ozone, aldehydes, and carbon monoxide. Average carbon monoxide content in Los Angeles has risen from 5.5 parts per million in 1956 to 15 parts per million in 1975. Under the Los Angeles air pollution control system,

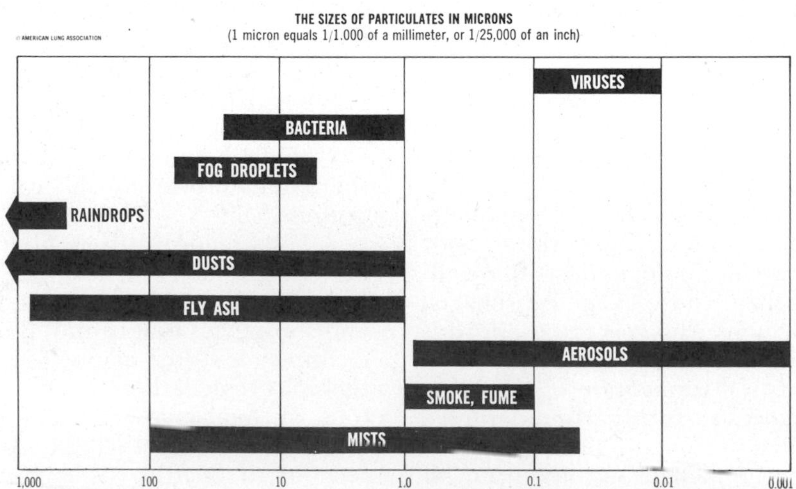

Figure 11–17 (From *Air Pollution Primer.* American Lung Association, 1974.)

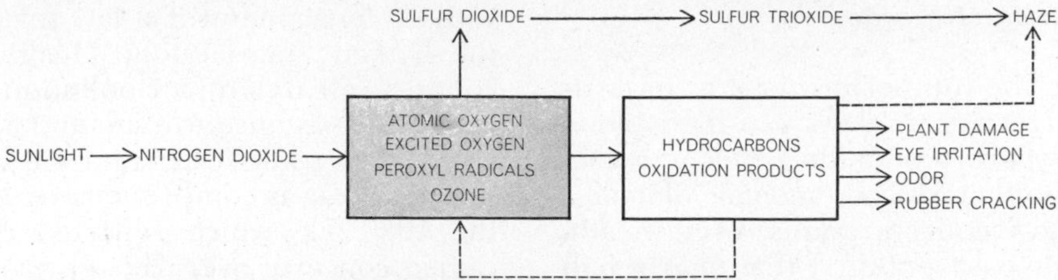

Figure 11–18 Photochemical reaction playing a major role in smog formation begins with sunlight acting on nitrogen dioxide, a product of combustion, to yield oxidants *(gray box).* They attack hydrocarbons, which come mainly from automobile exhausts, to produce irritating materials. Oxidants also attack sulfur dioxide, a product of coal and oil burning. Broken lines indicate interactions. (From Haagen-Smit, A. J.: The control of air pollution. Copyright © 1964 by Scientific American, Inc. All rights reserved.)

an alert would be called if carbon monoxide ever reached a level of 100 parts per million parts of air. It is estimated that a concentration of 200 parts per million for two hours is necessary to produce minimal effects in humans. Major contributors to air pollution include motor vehicles, oil refineries, fuel oil and fuel gas, gasoline marketing and distribution, refuse incineration and disposal, manufacturing, processing, chemical industries, exotic sources, combustion of fuels other than petroleum products and gas, locomotive and aircraft fuel combustion, and material from abrasion of rubber tires.

Many rural areas are now engulfed by air pollution. Unlike the air pollution problems in cities, however, the rural problems differ greatly in character from place to place. They reflect the nature of localized agricultural and industrial activities. Principal rural air pollution problems include dust storms, smoke and charred sawdust from sawdust burners, dust clouds in delta lands, dust from cement plants, smoke, irritating vapors from hot road mix plants, odors from faulty disposal of organic industrial wastes, toxic aerosols from the use of insecticides, hairsprays, deodorants, and smoke from orchard heating. Recently it has been found that aerosol spray products discharge fluorocarbons into the air which diminish the protective ozone layer. Many scientists believe that the ozone layer is necessary to protect against ultraviolet rays, which can cause skin cancer.

The Cost of Air Pollution

City officials and businessmen have learned how expensive air pollution can be. They count the billions of dollars' damage from smog in cleaning bills, corrosion, crop losses, and lowered property values. Economic damage alone is estimated at 11 billion dollars per year. This can be expected to increase if toxic substances in the air are allowed to rise. Devices designed to "launder" the air used in manufacturing and utility plants have doubled in the last several years at a cost of about 600 million dollars per year. Private industry is now spending about one billion dollars per year on air-pollution control work, and much more will be spent in the future.

WHAT'S YOUR AIR POLLUTION I.Q.?*

1.	Air pollution is harmful only in cities	YES	NO
2.	Air pollution is worse in big cities than small ones	YES	NO
3.	Nationwide, automobiles are the major source of air pollution	YES	NO
4.	Smog is a problem only in Los Angeles	YES	NO
5.	Inversions—in which air at ground level is trapped by warmer air above—come from air pollution	YES	NO
6.	Chronic respiratory diseases are aggravated by air pollution	YES	NO
7.	Air pollution affects only the respiratory system	YES	NO
8.	Air pollution can kill	YES	NO
9.	When the plume from a smokestack is white, no pollution is coming out	YES	NO
10.	Air pollution is expensive	YES	NO

*From the American Lung Association.

Carbon Monoxide Hazards

Among the numerous health hazards related to cigarette smokers is a high blood level of carbon monoxide, which causes blurred vision, reduced mental alertness and, in heavy concentrations, even death. American air is so polluted that nearly half of all nonsmokers as well have blood concentrations of carbon monoxide exceeding federally established safety levels. Since nonsmokers have not built up as high a tolerance to carbon monoxide, they are perhaps in more danger than smokers from the polluted air they breathe. Occupations in which exposure to carbon monoxide is especially great include taxi driver, printing, welding and processing metals, and working with chemicals, stone, or glass. Moreover, some experts claim that there is potential risk in giving a transfusion of smoker's blood with a high carbon monoxide concentration to a heart patient whose blood oxygenating system is already impaired.

Pickup trucks with campers or canopies can have high carbon monoxide (CO) levels, especially when a tailpipe is rusted or broken off and is shorter than the designed length. Idling or trolling boats develop high CO levels when rear bulkheads or canvas covers are removed and through-ventilation is absent. Catalytic heaters, although not utilizing an open flame, do produce CO, and have been responsible for several deaths in the state of Washington. Charcoal braziers or fisherman's heaters (a bucket of charcoal briquettes) should never be brought inside; burning charcoal gives off very large amounts of CO. Idling school buses parked in a long line soon have CO levels high enough to cause headaches and nausea.

Legislation

Air pollution laws of some kind have existed in many areas for a long time. Until the late 1940's, when Los Angeles began to break new ground in an effort to deal with the photochemical smog resulting principally from automobile emissions, the laws were mostly smoke ordinances, requiring large users of fuel to minimize their emissions of smoke. Fortunately, ordinances could be enforced without great difficulty once the emitter recognized that a smoking stack was wasting money. The federal government's involvement in air pollution began in 1955 with the enactment of a law that authorized the United States Public Health Service to conduct research on air pollution and to give technical assistance to state and local governments. Later laws extended the federal role, but none was as comprehensive or as strict as the 1970 act, which reflected the growing public concern over the environment and also a recognition by Congress that most of the federal, state, and local agencies concerned with air pollution had been unable to accomplish much. Congress decided that the only way to press the attack on air pollution effectively was by means of a strong law that established deadlines for accomplishing results and authorized large fines for violators.

The basic philosophy of the act is most easily discussed in terms of the concept of the threshold value. In the act, Congress assumed that for most of the major air pollutants (sulfur dioxide, carbon monoxide, nitrogen oxides, particulates, and oxidants) there is some concentration below which the pollutant has no measurable effect. That concentration is termed the threshold value. Congress based the principal set of regulations on the threshold concept. It also recognized, however, that there are or may be other pollutants that are harmful in any amount and thus have no threshold. They are the ones covered in the separate set of regulations on hazardous pollutants.

For threshold-value pollutants, Congress directed the administrator of the act to determine on the basis of medical evidence what the threshold value is for each pollutant and then to use that value, minus "an adequate margin of safety," as a basis for setting primary and secondary standards, which are called national ambient-air quality standards. The primary standards are designed to make sure that the pollutants cause no damage to human health; the secondary standards relate to human welfare and are supposed to ensure that the pollutants do not damage property, vegetation, or animals. Once the standards were set, the states were directed to prepare state implementation plans showing how they would make certain that the standards were never exceeded anywhere in any state after a certain date.

Control Efforts

Air pollution control efforts are now beginning to be based on the premise that no one has the right to use the atmosphere

10 points for each correct answer

You're well informed ...	100
Good, but try again ...	80–90
What you don't know may hurt you ...	under 80

NO		1. The air carries pollution far beyond the city. So do automobiles and out-of-city factories
	YES	2. Although special circumstances cause exceptions, pollution generally increases with population
	YES	3. Industry, power plants, space heating, and refuse disposal follow far behind, in that order
NO		4. Los Angeles–type smog forms in many places—wherever automobile exhaust is acted upon by sunlight
NO		5. Inversions occur naturally. They do keep pollution from being dispersed, however
	YES	6. Studies indicate that pollution worsens these diseases and brings more deaths from them.
NO		7. Among other things, pollution is linked to heart failure in chronic respiratory disease patients
	YES	8. In a number of famous long-lasting inversions, pollution brought death to many people
NO		9. Many polluting gases are colorless and many polluting particles are white
	YES	10. The government estimates that air pollution damage to animals, crops, paper, clothes, rubber, leather, and stone costs each man, woman, and child in the U.S. $65 a year. That's a lot to pay for something you don't even want, isn't it?

as a receptor of wastes in a manner that will adversely affect the health, comfort or property of others. It is recognized too that economic, social, and technical factors are concerned in air pollution control efforts and must be considered in the application of controls and in the appropriate modification of such controls. It is generally accepted that responsibility for administration of a program for the prevention and abatement of air pollution should be at a level of government capable of dealing with the problem in its entirety. Although this may indicate the desirability of air pollution control programs at a local or regional level, due consideration should also be given to the role of the state. It is essential that jurisdictional boundaries be established coincidental with natural geographical and topographical features that may affect air pollution conditions in any local area.

The goal of air pollution legislation should be to maintain a reasonable degree of purity of our air resources consistent with public health and welfare, protection of plant and animal life, protection of physical property, visibility requirements for safe air and ground transportation, continued economic development and growth, and maintenance of an esthetically acceptable environment. In programs at all levels of government, control can be most effectively brought about only by legislation that is reasonable and based on technically substantiated criteria, which provides adequate flexibility and yet is reasonably specific in meeting the needs of the area under consideration. Legislation should be adapted to the structure and practices of the government of the state or community. It should clearly establish its scope, specifically assign responsibility, and scrupulously avoid technical details, establishing the procedure by which such details are worked out, implemented, and revised to meet changing conditions. In this way a high degree of flexibility can be attained.

State air pollution control activity has developed traditionally from the authority of health departments to preserve public health. On the local governmental level, however, air pollution control authority has been vested in a variety of agencies, including health, building, fire, public safety, and other departments, as well as air pollution control departments. Early state statutes frequently provided an administrative approach that was largely negative—that is,

DON'T TOP OFF MY TANK!

» Here is an important way in which you can help to reduce air pollution. It won't cost you a penny but with your help it could be possible to remove up to an estimated 11 tons of pollutants from the California air each day!

» Urge your gasoline station attendant not to 'top off' your automobile gas tank. This means that the tank should not be filled to the brim and that filling should stop after the automatic hose nozzle cutoff occurs.

» PEEL OFF THE ATTACHED STICKER AND PLACE IT OVER THE CAP OF YOUR GASOLINE TANK OR PLACE IT INSIDE THE GAS TANK DOOR. This will let people know that you are concerned with air pollution and will remind your gasoline station attendant not to "top off" your tank.

A message from your LUNG ASSOCIATION — the Christmas Seal people.
Dennison Eastman Corp. Oakland, Calif.

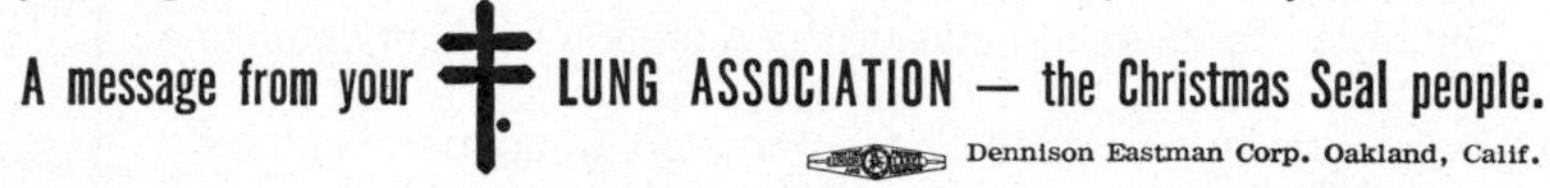

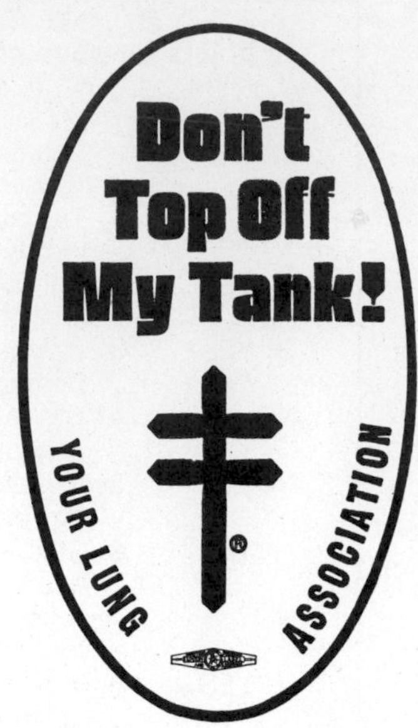

Figure 11–19 Automobile sticker for combating pollution.

when a particular activity was found to cause air pollution, the administrative agency was authorized to take steps to abate such pollution. Newer legislation shows a shift in emphasis from the abatement of existing air pollution to control through prevention.[13]

POLLUTION POINTERS

Most people today have experienced mild effects of air pollution, particularly in densely populated areas and on crowded highways. Symptoms include coughing, headache, shortness of breath, nausea, and burning of the eyes. Suggestions offered by medical authorities for protection against these symptoms include the following:

1. When walking in a city, keep away from curbs as much as possible. Hold your breath while you walk through clouds of exhaust.
2. If you reside in a heavily polluted area, remain indoors whenever possible during the hours of the day when the sun is hottest; keep windows and doors closed. Avoid dust and aerosol sprays.
3. Use an air conditioner that combines an absolute filter with activated carbon, and set the unit to circulate inside only. Electrostatic air conditioners do not remove hazardous chemicals from the air.
4. When exposed to heavy pollution, reduce physical activity to a minimum.
5. When driving, avoid heavily traveled highways and tunnels as much as possible.

Problems

When Congress passed the Clean Air Act of 1970, its aims were laudable: to keep the nation's air clean and to protect the public from noxious fumes. The trouble was that the act's provisions, if strictly enforced, could also end construction of new factories, power plants, and smelters that might emit fumes in areas that now have clean air. Sufficient alternative forms of transportation could not be developed within the time allotted in some areas. Many persons felt that the Act, if fully implemented, would cause disastrous social and economic disruption in certain states and cause an improper intrusion on the land use authority of state and local government. Although many states are attempting to achieve a balance between levels of health protection and economic stability, some officials object to "clean air at the expense of unreasonable economic or social hardship." To further complicate matters, catalytic converters required on 1975 autos were later found to be responsible for forming sulfuric acid in the atmosphere.

The most potent threat to the Clean Air Act is coming from utilities and heavy industries such as steel, copper, and chemicals. They complain about the unavailability of clean fuel and assert that current abatement technology is unwieldy, unreliable, energy-wasting, and expensive. These enterprises are pushing for intermittent control strategies, otherwise known as "pollution by dilution," which would involve building tall stacks to disseminate pollutants, switching back and forth between clean and dirty fuels (depending on what the atmosphere can stand), and using other methods to hold effluents under prevailing limits. On the other hand, according to congressional staff members, state agencies responsible for promulgation and enforcement of air quality standards find the basic act workable and oppose any attempts to weaken it. In fact, some states like the primary standards so much that they are moving ahead to set deadlines for secondary standards, which are designed to protect property, vegetation, and esthetic things such as visibility.

Environmental restrictions have served the nation well. One prime example is the requirement in the National Environmental Policy Act that federal agencies describe the probable environmental effect of new projects. This requirement has caused, through advance planning, better routing of highways, safer nuclear plants, and the development of new techniques of extracting oil from Gulf of Mexico reserves without oil spills. The law also delayed the Alaska pipeline for years, but perhaps this was a good thing. We can conserve, explore other sources, and be independent of foreign suppliers. Environmental groups report that they are steadily gaining new support from citizens who never showed much interest before, especially in regions where new energy developments are being proposed. In many cases, immediate economic arguments are replacing the old environmental cry that pristine nature must be protected. Midwestern farmers often oppose proposed nuclear plants, partly because they fear radioactive accidents and partly because the power companies take good farm land for power-plant sites by eminent domain. For example, the majority of residents polled in Durham, New Hampshire, opposed construction of a refinery. Their main reason was that coastline is too valuable an economic resource (for recreation and shellfishing) to be replaced by oil.

Thoughtful environmentalists see the current energy crisis as a potential blessing. They feel that any resolution of the energy problem will go hand-in-hand with a solution to environmental problems. For example, if car pooling becomes popular, it will not only conserve gasoline but will also reduce smog. The energy shortage shows that resources are finite and must be conserved. The crisis, environmentalists say, has thus accomplished what they could not. For one thing, Americans have started thinking much more about gas mileage before they buy cars. For another, industries are checking into ways of fueling their boilers with garbage and other combustible wastes.

In any case, the Environmental Protection Agency has agreed to allow industries more time to achieve particular air quality standards in some areas and to delay deadlines related to vehicle emission standards. Meanwhile, more research, greater fuel economy, leadfree gas, and more efficient (and smaller) engines and cars may conserve energy *and* preserve the environment.

AIR POLLUTION IN NEW GUINEA

Cause of Chronic Pulmonary Disease Among Stone-Age Natives in the Highlands

Inhabitants of villages in the Highlands of New Guinea wear scant clothing. To keep warm during cold nights they burn smoky fires in small closed huts, where they inhale extremely high levels of particulate matter and aldehydes. Pulmonary disease, mainly obstructive but also restrictive, appears at an early age and was present in 78 per cent of subjects over age 40 years. Severely affected subjects have diminished breath sounds, coarse rales, and decreased chest cage movement. Pathologic specimens from affected subjects demonstrated centrilobular emphysema, thickened pleura, pulmonary fibrosis, mucous gland hypertrophy, and deposition of anthracotic pigment. Other factors probably responsible for the high prevalence of pulmonary disease include smoking of home grown tobacco, protein malnutrition, poor sanitation, and various endemic diseases.[14]

THE AIR DOESN'T HAVE TO BE POLLUTED

* Better control devices can be installed on automobiles. Other kinds of power—electricity or steam—can be used to make them go. Buses, subways, and trains can replace the automobile to a great extent.

* Trash and garbage can be disposed of in modern efficient incinerators, or used for sanitary landfill or heating. (Part can be salvaged for re-use.)

* Sometimes pollutants coming from fuel can be removed before the fuel is burned.

* Excess packaging can be stopped. So can the use of nonreturnable containers and virtually indestructible plastics.

* Some manufacturing processes can be altered so that a pollutant is not produced.

* New sources of energy—such as natural gas or nuclear fission—can be used instead of coal and oil.

* Many unwanted gases can be washed out of industrial emissions by machines called scrubbers, or they can be absorbed by substances such as charcoal, or burned off.

* Most unwanted particles can be filtered out or removed by machines such as centrifuges or electrostatic precipitators. Automobiles create more dirty air than any other source—they are responsible for more than half of all air pollution in this country. You can reduce auto pollution by taking the following measures:

* Walk when you can. Use buses and trains. Shop with others. Join a car pool. Ride a bike.

* Buy gasoline with the least amount of lead and the lowest octane level your car can take. Ask your service station or car dealer what it must have.

* See that the pollution controls on your car are doing their job. Give your engine regular tune-ups.

* Switch off the motor when you park, even if it's only for a few minutes. Work with others for a good public transit system so you won't need your car so much. Campaign for the development of cars that won't pollute.

Air Sampling Network

The Public Health Service's National Air Sampling Network, which gathers scientific data on air pollution throughout the country, presently has 275 air sampling stations, located in every state, the District of Columbia, and Puerto Rico. The network samples suspended particulates—smoke, dust, and other solid contaminants emitted into the atmosphere from a variety of sources to remain suspended for varying periods. The pollutant samples are collected biweekly by a high-volume air sampler, which draws air through a glass-fiber filter for 24 hours. The filter is later analyzed at the laboratories of the Public Health Service's Robert A. Taft Sanitary Engineering Center, Cincinnati, Ohio. Thirty-five of the network stations also sample for two gaseous pollutants—sulfur dioxide and nitrogen dioxide. The data collected provide state and local air pollution officials with basic information for control programs.

Forecasting Air Pollution Potential Coast to Coast

Since August 1960, the Weather Bureau Research Station at the Robert A. Taft Sanitary Engineering Center of the Public Health Service at Cincinnati has conducted a special program of forecasting air pollution potential for all portions of the United States east of the 105th meridian (Rocky Mountains). On October 1, 1963, the program was expanded to include all of the contiguous United States. Observations over the United States have indicated that when certain meteorological conditions are met in the vicinity of a source or sources of air pollution, the pollutants tend to accumulate in the atmosphere instead of being dissipated by diffusion or transport. The stagnation and intensified pollution usually continue until meteorological conditions change so as to provide better ventilation for the affected area. Air pollution potential, therefore, may be defined from the meteorological standpoint as a set of weather conditions conducive to accumulation of air pollutants in the atmosphere.

To be notified of these advisories, air pollution control or research units must initiate arrangements with the nearest Weather Bureau station. The advisories from Cincinnati are transmitted daily at 12:07 Eastern Standard Time over the Weather Bureau's Service C teletype circuit, and they are available through the stations on that circuit. Once arrangements have been made, the local weather station notifies the participating units of the beginning and ending of each period of high air pollution potential.

Air pollution potential forecasts provide an exceptional opportunity for air pollution control and research units to conduct special observations of air pollution problems in their own localities, and particularly to study the influence of meteorological factors on the pollution conditions observed. In addition, the advisories may be regarded as an alert to air pollution control officials to be on the watch for heavier or more troublesome accumulation of pollution than is likely at other times.

Because the forecasts are issued for a given area only when meteorological conditions warrant, it is possible that some affiliates of the program will not receive any notifications at all, and many will receive them only rarely. Because the forecasts are for special purposes, it is suggested that they should be disseminated through local air pollution agency channels. Any public announcements should be given in terms of expected pollution conditions rather than as weather news, and should relate to the issuing agency rather than to the Weather Bureau office.

Questions or comments about the advisory service may be directed to: The Meteorologist in Charge, Weather Bureau Research Station, Robert A. Taft Sanitary Engineering Center, Cincinnati, Ohio 45226.

Prevention and Control

Present control programs are aimed at reducing the quantity of waste materials disposed into the air because no other method of improving air quality has yet been developed. Before a community can intelligently plan an air pollution control program, it must have an understanding of the quantity of air available, a knowledge of the kind and amount of pollutants, and an understanding of the reactions that take place in the atmosphere.

To narrow the gap between the known and unknown factors in the air pollution problem, investigations are being carried on by many groups. Effective control of smog is not now possible because of a lack of fundamental information. No simple, inexpensive solution is at hand, but all groups involved in air pollution are working toward a solution and realize that they must:

1. Identify the compounds that cause typical smog conditions.
2. Extend scientific studies to determine the nature of reactions taking place in the atmosphere, the substances entering into these reactions, and the compounds formed.
3. Learn more about the adverse effects of air pollution on humans and identify the specific substances responsible.
4. Develop additional knowledge so that standards for air quality can be established and hazards to health and damage to vegetation can be prevented.
5. Devise reliable and practical means for continuously measuring air quality.
6. Develop practical and effective means of controlling certain emissions (particularly hydrocarbons from motor vehicles).[15]

Long-term sacrifices in life style will have to be made if people want cleaner air to breathe. Once higher air quality is achieved, it will require much sacrifice and effort to keep the quality high for a significant period of time. The public must be aware of this and must realize that clean air is worth the price.

Smoke Control in Pittsburgh. Initiated by the health department and backed by law, control measures reduced smoke in Pittsburgh by more than 90 per cent between 1946 and 1955, but control efforts continue. A 1962 agreement between the health department and the steel industry established a schedule for future smoke and dust control activities calling for elimination of 95 per cent of the air pollution from the steel industry. They have enjoyed superior results.

Smoke Control in London. London has effectively combatted its age-old air pollution problem. In 1956, a Clean Air Act aimed at industrial and domestic air polluters was passed by Parliament. Most important, the traditional burning of soft coal in hearth grates was prohibited in large areas across Britain. To comply with the new regulations, British industry has spent nearly a billion dollars in the past decade to clean up the emissions from its smokestacks.

London has led the way in smoke control. The 156,000 tons of sooty grime it once dispelled into the air annually have been cut by 80 per cent, and about three-quarters of the city is actually smokeless. It is estimated that London now gets 50 per cent more sunlight in the winter than before the act. Also, many of Britain's public buildings have been scrubbed down, and look brighter than they have in decades, if not centuries.

Perhaps the most pleasing result, for London bird watchers at least, is that the songbirds missing from the city for almost a century are returning. The first house martins in nearly 80 years have been found nesting, and rare birds such as the snow bunting, the hoopoe, the great northern diver, and the bearded tit have reappeared. It may be only a matter of time before nightingales return to sing once again in Berkeley Square.

Engineering

The solution of a community's air pollution problems will depend in part on the successful application of these engineering principles:

1. Control air pollution emissions at the source. For example, by use of devices on internal combustion engines, electrostatic precipitators on smoke stacks, auto exhaust filters.
2. Substitution of materials and methods. For example, sanitary land fill in place of backyard incineration.
3. Zoning in locating new industrial plants.
4. Improving ventilation of communities by thermal, catalytic, or mechanical methods.
5. Neutralizing the pollutants in the atmosphere.
6. Governing emissions according to meteorologic conditions, relayed in advance perhaps, by a weather detector photographic satellite.[16]

NOISE POLLUTION

Noise has physiological, psychological, and social effects on people. Prolonged exposure to very loud noise in an occupational setting will result in hearing loss. Noise causes physiological stress by activating the nervous system, creating changes in heart rate, respiratory rate, gastric activity, pupil size, and sweat gland activity. Experimental study has revealed that artificial noise (90 decibels) will produce dilation of the pupils,

Possible Effects of Noise on Health

Symptoms of aggravation or disease:	Headache Muscle tension Anxiety Insomnia Fatigue Drug consumption Other reactions
Impairment of functions:	Impairment of hearing, including temporary threshold shift and presbycusis
Interference with activities:	Interference with relaxation and rest, communication, (conversation, listening to radio, telephone and TV)
Feelings of annoyance:	Fear Resentment Distraction Need to concentrate
Individual actions to modify the environment:	Installation of air conditioning so that windows can be closed. Installation of acoustic insulation materials to reduce noise in the home. Shutting windows. The use of masking noises, such as turning on the radio and TV or fan. Departure from environment.
Social effects:	Concentration of lower income families in noise polluted residential areas. Spending less time at home because of the noise problem. Withdrawal from communication. Family disorganization.

Figure 11–20 (From Goldsmith, J. R., and Jonsson, E.: Health effects of community noise. Amer. J. Publ. Health, 63(9):784, 1973.)

reduced blood volume in the skin, and general vascular constriction. In some people, diastolic blood pressure increases. There is some research that suggests that noise may produce mental illness or maladjustment. One study, for example, revealed that steelworkers who worked in the noisiest parts of the plant had a greater frequency of social conflicts both at home and at work.

The most important known effects of general noise on psychological states include:

1. *Effects on sensory and perceptual processes.* These are the temporary threshold shifts—temporary losses in hearing and sensitivity.

2. *Effects on action and thought.* These are the changes in quality of work performance when noise is over 90 decibels, especially when the noise is random and intermittent rather than continuous. But rhythmic sound, such as music, may help pace work, or may improve morale in dull, repetitive work.

3. *Effects on attitudes and feelings.* These are the negative feelings which grow with loudness or intensity, with high frequency sounds, with intermittent sounds, and with sounds which convey unpleasant meaning, such as sirens or airplanes flying too low.

4. *Effects on needs and motivation.* These are the intrusions on privacy, relaxation, rest and sleep, but here we have the least solid evidence of effect.

Researchers emphasize that we need more realistic social research. But we also need to begin establishing noise controls now.

Although we are adapting to noise, and perhaps speaking a little louder, many of the more affluent are already willing to pay for silence. But the noise problem can only be solved when the public *demands* noise reduction and is willing to pay the cost. Some of the things we can do to reduce noise include: (1) passing legislation which limits the amount of noise which can be produced in residential areas, but this legislation must be more easily enforceable than at present; (2) specifying noise standards for appliances; (3) inspecting for noise emission and smog emission necessary for car licensing; (4) demanding screening walls for freeways and a limit to the number of night flights over residential areas; and (5) demanding better shield-

Santa Cruz City Noise Survey

"A healthy and pleasing sound level should be maintained through the City through regulation of noise emitters and acoustical design."

The foregoing statement is an adopted policy of the City of Santa Cruz. The Santa Cruz City Planning Department is working toward the realization of that policy and the first step is the completion of a Noise Element to our General Plan. In order that it be a truly responsive and representative document, the Planning Staff is seeking every citizen's input. By returning the completed questionnaire to the Planning Department, City Hall, 809 Center Street, the impact of noise in our community can be evaluated, problem areas can be pinpointed, problem sources can be identified, and community attitudes can be analyzed.

Noise pollution in the nation as a whole has been doubling every ten years. It won't double during the next ten years if we all act now. Please help the Planning Department in curbing noise pollution in Santa Cruz by taking a moment to complete this short questionnaire. Only through the help of our residents can the best interests of the community be served.

The completed questionnaire can either be returned by mail or in person to the Planning Department, Room 206, City Hall Annex, 809 Center Street. Thank you.

The Santa Cruz City Planning Department

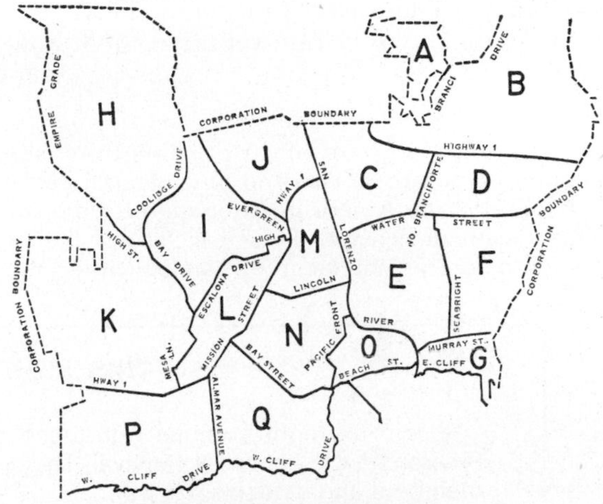

NOISE ELEMENT QUESTIONNAIRE

(1) Do you believe noise to be a significant pollution problem in the City of Santa Cruz?
YES ______
NO______

(2) Please rank the following pollution problems in their order of significance (1 through 5), in the City of Santa Cruz.
AIR______
LITTER______
NOISE______
VISUAL ______
WATER ______

(3) Please indicate those noise sources affecting only your neighborhood by ranking them in order from most irritating to least irritating.
AMPLIFIED MUSIC ______
ANIMALS ______
AUTOMOBILE TRAFFIC ______
CHURCH BELLS AND CHIMES ______
EMERGENCY VEHICLES ______
FREEWAY ______
GARBAGE TRUCKS ______
INDUSTRIAL NOISE ______
MOTORCYCLE TRAFFIC ______
POWER TOOLS ______
RECREATION NOISE ______
SCHOOLS AND DAY-CARE CENTERS ______
SPORTING EVENTS ______
TRAIN TRAFFIC ______
TRUCK TRAFFIC ______
OTHER ______

(4) What times of day does the most irritating noise normally occur?
MIDNIGHT to 6:00 A.M. ______
6:00 A.M. to 9:00 A.M. ______
9:00 A.M. to NOON ______
NOON to 4:00 P.M. ______
4:00 P.M. to 7:00 P.M. ______
7:00 P.M. to 10:00 P.M. ______
10:00 P.M. to MIDNIGHT ______

(5) Have you ever complained to the City about noise?
YES ______
NO______

(6) If yes, what was the nature of your complaint? ______

(7) Based on the neighborhood map above, please circle the letter that represents your neighborhood.
A B C D E F G H I J K L M N O P Q

(8) If you'd like to give us your address, it will also help us pinpoint noise problems: ______

Figure 11–21 Noise survey and questionnaire by the Santa Cruz City Planning Department. (From *Santa Cruz Sentinel*, October 20, 1974, p. 37.)

ing of aircraft engines, including those small planes used for private purposes. Some states have enacted legislation requiring that an office of noise control be established within the state health department.

Effects of Noise Pollution on the Circulatory System

An article in the Journal of the American Medical Association reported the following:

Recently a group of 30 panelists from nine countries met to discuss the physiological effects of sound at the American Association for the Advancement of Science. Their conclusions are expressed in the statement of one panelist: "You may forgive the noise around you, but your circulatory system never will."

Dr. A. E. Arguelles, senior lecturer at the Buenos Aires State Medical School in Argentina, reported on studies involving 36 patients, including 12 coronary victims, 12 cases of hypertension (high blood pressure), and 12 psychotic patients. All were exposed to the same noise level for 30 minutes (2000 cycles per second at 90 decibels).

Coronary patients are known to have an elevated cholesterol level. Following exposure to noise, blood cholesterol rose in eight of the 12 coronary subjects tested. Of the 12 hypertensive patients in the study, blood pressure increased in eight following noise stress.

Results were similar with most of the 12 psychotic patients, even though they had been given anti-psychotic drugs prior to testing. According to Dr. Arguelles, the aggressive outbursts of these patients might be precipitated by noise stimulation, and without drug treatment their responses may have been much greater.[17]

THIS MONTH'S ECOTIP*

Join the fight for quiet with these suggestions for individual action from ENACT, Environmental Action for Survival. They were compiled by University of Michigan faculty members and students.

- Support existing local noise pollution ordinances and campaign to get them strengthened.
- Check your own car muffler, radios, air conditioners, TV, etc. Be sure they don't add to the noise problem.
- Be sure that boats, motorcycles, model airplanes, construction equipment, etc., have adequate noise control devices.
- Support efforts to ban sonic booms.
- Tape record objectionable and unnecessary noise in your local environment and play it back at city council meetings to support demands for noise control.
- Petition for noise-free bubbles or cubicles to be provided in city parks.
- Demand that airports be developed and zoned away from population centers; deter flight patterns.
- Encourage the Federal Aviation Agency to set noise abatement standards for airlines.

* Today's Health, July, 1970, p. 18. Published by the American Medical Association.

FOOD SANITATION

The local health department is responsible for protecting the public's health against food contamination. This includes epidemiological investigations, regulation and enforcement of minimum sanitary food standards, supervision of food establishments, and health education. Sanitarians must keep pace with the rapidly changing technology of quick freezing, radiation, and the use of antibiotics in perishable foods.

Salmonella and staphylococci germs are very prevalent and multiply rapidly in food, and thus gastroenteritis and "food poisoning" are the predominant infections transmitted by food. Other diseases transmitted by food include the common cold, typhoid fever, amebic dysentery, and bacillary dysentery. Tapeworms and other parasites occasionally contaminate the food supply. However, many other germs may be carried by utensils; the drinking glass is the most important vehicle of transmission, and the poorly operated and managed bar, soda fountain, and luncheonette are the worst offenders among food handling establishments.

Food poisoning symptoms include cramps, diarrhea, and vomiting within three hours to two days after eating contaminated food. Foods that are intimately handled, stored, and mixed after cooking have the highest frequency of food-borne infection. These include salads, sauces, creamed foods, and cream-filled pastries and pies. If food is kept longer than one hour at room temperature before it is eaten, food poisoning may contaminate it.

The broad objective of a food-service sanitation program is the protection of the health of the consumer. More specifically, however, such a program is designed to accomplish the following:

1. Protect food against bacterial infection. Sanitation standards are used to reduce to a minimum the opportunity for microorganisms to gain entrance to and multiply in food. Organisms that may cause communicable disease and food-borne illness merit primary consideration.

2. Ensure the wholesomeness of food. Basically, a food is wholesome when it is in sound condition, clean, free from adulteration, and otherwise suitable for human consumption. If sound and healthful, it may be considered wholesome. Consumer acceptability may also be a factor, although it is readily recognized that this shows wide variability when dietary habits and cultural patterns are considered. Wholesomeness is frequently thought of in terms of purity. However, to be wholesome, a food need not be a "natural food." It may be a mixture of wholesome ingredients.

Food should be free of any substance deleterious to the health of the consumer. The addition of toxic chemicals, either by accident or otherwise, may render food unsafe. Chemical additives should be used only if officially approved, and if the amount present is within the limits of established official tolerances. This applies to pesticides, veterinary drugs, and the migration of substances from packaging material or from food equipment surfaces into the food itself.

3. Meet consumer expectations. A food service establishment may take many precautions to prepare and serve a safe food product and yet fail to provide an appealing, pleasant atmosphere, or otherwise to meet consumer expectations. People expect to be served wholesome, appetizing food prepared and handled in a sanitary manner and in a clean environment. That food prepared in an unsanitary environment might be clean or that an unclean food might be safe to eat does not make it acceptable to the consumer.[19]

In order to meet these objectives, sanitarians observe and supervise the following criteria:

1. The food and drink served should be safe.

2. The personal hygiene and food handling practices of the food handlers should be satisfactory.

3. The water supply should be safe.

4. Sewage, other liquid wastes, garbage, and other solid wastes should be disposed of in a sanitary manner.

5. Food should be protected from contamination during production, processing, display and storage.

6. Utensils and equipment should be washed, sanitized and stored in a sanitary manner.

7. The general sanitary maintenance of an establishment should be satisfactory. This includes exclusion of rodents, vermin and flies; refrigeration, handwashing and toilet facilities should be clean; good housekeeping, adequate light, ventilation and satisfactory arrangement of facilities should be provided.

Education and guidance have replaced threats and legal suits in restaurant sanitation; education activities are directed toward the public, management and food handlers. The most significant development in this area has been the establishment of short training courses for food handlers by many health departments. Education of food handlers may be supplemented by periodic physical examinations in order to detect tuberculosis, typhoid fever, and other diseases that may be transmitted by carriers. Large food companies are now employing trained, experienced public health engineers and sanitarians to supervise food production and promote education. Trained specialists in food sanitation are also employed by restaurant associations and chains in an effort to educate and self-police members and units.

Case Studies[20]

A person who prepares and serves food can be the cause of a food poisoning outbreak, whether the person is a chef, waitress, dishwashing machine operator, homeowner or other person who handles food or food equipment. The following examples are but a few of thousands of recently reported cases.

Case 1. Seventeen persons aboard a ship became ill within eight hours after eating a noon meal. Nausea, vomiting, cramps, and diarrhea were the symptoms. Macaroni had been cooked prior to the meal, and chopped pimientos, lettuce, boiled eggs, mayonnaise, and mustard were hand mixed by two mess cooks. One of the cooks had several minor cuts on two fingers. These finger cuts yielded *Staphylococcus aureus*, the same kind of bacteria found in the salad.

Prevention. Hands should never be used to mix foods when clean sanitized utensils can be used. Food should never be worked with when infected cuts are present because the germs causing the infection may be a source of food-borne illness.

Case 2. After drinking punch served in a coffee shop, 14 of 25 persons drinking the beverage became ill with cramps, and diarrhea. The punch had been prepared in a galvanized iron container, then stored in a refrigerator. On investigation, it was shown that the container had been corroded by the action of the acid in the punch. Chemical analysis of the remaining punch showed that a considerable amount of zinc had been dissolved from the container lining.

Prevention. Utensils containing toxic materials should never be used in the preparation or storage of foods. Food containers made with metals such as antimony, zinc, cadmium, and lead have been sources of food-borne illnesses. All containers used for storing, transporting, preparing, and serving food should be made of smooth, easily cleanable, nontoxic materials.

Case 3. Approximately one hour after supper, four persons vomited, became nauseated and dizzy, and had difficulty in swallowing, talking, and seeing. During supper they had eaten what they thought were collard greens. Actually, these "greens" were the leaves of a wild tobacco plant.

Prevention. Care must be taken to identify foods picked for personal use. Some plants may look alike, yet actually be quite different.

Case 4. Two persons became ill about 15 minutes after eating mushrooms. Symptoms included nausea, dizziness, numbness, and vomiting. The mushrooms had been picked fresh, refrigerated, peeled, cleaned, boiled, and fried. Examination of similar types of mushrooms showed that they were poisonous.

Prevention. Mushrooms should never be picked unless they can be identified as nonpoisonous varieties. In most cases, only an expert can tell the difference.

Case 5. Sixteen persons experienced acute upset stomachs within five hours after their evening meal. Egg salad was the food suspected. The eggs were boiled and shelled early the same afternoon. One of the cooks then added mayonnaise and relish to the chopped eggs. After preparation, the salad was not refrigerated. The cook who prepared the salad had tonsillitis.

Prevention. Food service workers should not work when they are ill. Potentially hazardous (readily perishable) food should be refrigerated at temperature of 45° F. or below, or kept at 140° F. or above until serving.

Case 6. A group of 145 persons became ill with severe diarrhea and stomach pains. The suspected meal of roast beef and gravy had been prepared the day before and allowed to cool in open trays without refrigeration for 22 hours. *Clostridium perfringens* organisms were found in the beef and gravy.

Prevention. Potentially hazardous (readily perishable) foods should be thoroughly cooked and then kept either hot (140° F. or above), or cold (refrigerated to 45° F. or below) until serving.

Case 7. At a church dinner, over half those who had eaten barbecued chicken became ill within six hours. The chickens had been cooked the day before, immediately refrigerated overnight, then reheated the next morning. After reheating, the chickens were cut into quarters with the butcher's meat saw. The chickens were without refrigeration from 10:00 A.M. until being reheated again around 5:00 P.M. Large numbers of staphylococci were recovered from the chickens. These bacteria could have come from the meat saw or from the cook's hands, which contained numerous small cuts and abrasions.

Prevention. Food service workers should never use a utensil or work surface in food preparation unless it has been cleaned and sanitized. The worker should not work with food if he has open, infected cuts or abrasions. As an added precaution, potentially hazardous (readily perishable) food should be kept hot (140° F. or above) or cold (45° F. or below) except when being prepared or served.

Case 8. Eleven cases of trichinosis occurred in a small community among seven families who had eaten raw smoked sausage prepared from the same hog. Symptoms were high fever, muscle pain, stomach cramps, chills, and general weakness. This illness was caused by *Trichinella spiralis*, a small parasite present in the uncooked pork.

Prevention. Pork should never be eaten unless it has been thoroughly cooked. All pork, unless otherwise treated to destroy trichina, should be cooked sufficiently to reach an internal temperature of at least 150° F. This destroys the parasite.

Case 9. Four cases of botulism, including one death, occurred as a result of the consumption of home-canned chili. Symptoms were vomiting, dizziness, difficulty in breathing and speaking, and blurring of vision. There was paralysis for a time. The chili had been home-canned with insufficient temperature and pressure. This permitted a toxin to be formed in the chili.

Prevention. A pressure cooker should be used to can all meats or low-acid foods. The high temperature and pressure used will destroy the spores that produce toxin. The smell of foods that contain the toxin often is no different from that of safe foods, but even a taste, if the toxin is present, may be sufficient to cause illness or death. Commercially canned foods are [usually] safe to use because temperatures and pressures used in their preparation are high enough to destroy the bacterial spores.

Salmonellosis

Salmonellosis is a major public health problem in the United States. It has been estimated that 2,000,000 human cases occur each year at a cost of up to $200 million to the American economy. Many of these cases occur among patrons of restaurants and food catering establishments. Six factors seem to be involved in today's salmonellosis problem:

1. Americans are eating in restaurants more frequently than ever before and, even at home, are more likely to consume mass-produced foods. Thus, much of the average diet contains ingredients from a variety of subsidiary suppliers. Each additional supplier is another potential source of *Salmonella* organisms.

2. Pets are fed scraps from the table much less frequently. Their food tends to be mass-produced, and sometimes "fortified with highly *Salmonella*-containing material from rendering plants."

3. Rapid, inexpensive transportation means that foods—including any that may become *Salmonella*-contaminated—can be conveyed great distances. And whenever such contamination occurs, it's like "biological warfare in practice."

4. Food-processing equipment is not always properly designed for sanitary maintenance.

5. More *Salmonella* serotypes are being identified, but 50 to 57 serotypes of the approximately 1400 now known account for 94 to 96 per cent of organisms sent to the Federal Center for Disease Control in Atlanta for identification. There is no satisfactory antibody test for identifying the serotype involved.

6. There is no *Salmonella* vaccine for humans except S. typhi, paratyphoid A and B.

Contamination of food by *Salmonella* poses a significant public health problem. There are more than 1400 known serotypes of this organism, all capable of causing infection in man. These bacteria are found throughout the environment. Outbreaks of salmonellosis (*Salmonella* infection) have been reported in increasing numbers in recent years.

Salmonella microorganisms, when taken into the body, multiply in the gastrointestinal tract and produce gastrointestinal irritation with resulting nausea, vomiting, abdominal cramps and pain, diarrhea, and fever. Symptoms of infection range from mild nausea to life-endangering general infections.

Susceptibility to salmonellosis and the severity of the infection depend a great deal on the age and physical condition of the individual. Infants and the elderly tend to be more severely affected than other age groups. Infections generally are treated with drugs which relieve the symptoms. Antibiotic treatment may be used in severe cases.

Where Contamination Occurs

Contamination of food by *Salmonella* may occur during production, handling, and storage in manufacturing plants. It also can occur while food is prepared and handled in the home. Since food animals may harbor the organism, raw poultry, meats, eggs, and dairy products are among the foods most frequently found to carry *Salmonella*. Insects, rodents, and pets—especially some types of small pets such as turtles, birds, dogs, and cats—are the main carriers. Humans get salmonellosis mainly through eating contaminated food or through contact with an animal or human carrier.

Prevention

All foodstuffs made from animal and poultry sources should be *thoroughly cooked*. Turkey and egg dishes are particularly susceptible. Other important measures include the following:

Refrigerate all prepared food before use, as well as all leftovers. This also aids in prevention of rodent and insect contamination.

Food service workers and housewives should always *wash their hands* before and after food preparation.

Kitchen utensils and working surfaces or tables should be *cleaned carefully* and *frequently*.

If the purity of drinking water is questionable, it should be chlorinated or boiled before use.

After handling or playing with animals, find time to *wash hands*.

Do not change the water from a pet turtle tank in the kitchen sink.

Protection Provided Consumers

Because of the rapid advances in food processing and packaging techniques in this country, all consumers, in a sense, are served from the same great communal kitchens—the processing plants of national manufacturers. When one of these "kitchens" becomes contaminated, thousands of families across the nation may be affected.

The Food and Drug Administration is

responsible for assuring consumers that foods destined for their table are free from *Salmonella* and other contamination. FDA accomplishes this by making food plant inspections and laboratory examinations of food products collected from locations throughout the United States.

FDA cooperates with and receives excellent assistance from state and local health officials in carrying out a mutual mandate for protecting consumers. Whenever a problem occurs at one of the great communal kitchens, FDA relies extensively upon the assistance of state and local health investigators to prevent continued sale and shipment of contaminated products.

Housewives and others who follow good sanitation practices in preparing and handling food in the home contribute to this protection.

SALMONELLA GASTROENTERITIS FROM RESTAURANT FOOD

Contaminated meats served to patrons of a large restaurant over a two-week period resulted in 250 cases of salmonella gastroenteritis. Sixty-two of 134 (46 per cent) restaurant food-handling employees were also infected. Sanitation and food-handling procedures within the restaurant were generally adequate and widespread contamination of the enviornment was not found. A meat slicer contaminated with *Salmonella enteritidis* was the most important factor in dissemination. The outbreak illustrates the strategic role of slicing equipment as a reservoir of contamination and underscores the need for improvements in the design of slicing machines. Currently available slicers are difficult to clean thoroughly because of the hazard and inconvenience to personnel.[18]

BOTULISM

With the rapid increase in food prices has come an increase in home canning, as families buy foods in bulk at their peak seasons to save on the grocery bill. And with the increase in home canning has come a serious health hazard—botulism—a form of food poisoning that produces critical illness and is fatal in 25 per cent of all cases.

Botulism bacteria grow only in airless places—for example, in the vacuum-sealed containers used in home canning. The bacterium and its toxins can be destroyed by exposure for 10 minutes or more to a temperature of 212° F., the temperature reached in water-bath canning. However, the spores of botulism are not destroyed at this temperature and can produce more of the deadly bacteria. Water-bath canning should be used, therefore, only for foods that do not harbor spores of the bacteria (high-acid foods such as citrus fruits and tomatoes). Low-acid foods such as meat, string beans, and corn must be processed in pressure cookers, which reach temperatures above 249° F. for 15 minutes.

Canned food that is in any way suspect must not be tasted until it has been thoroughly cooked. There is no easily recognizable, characteristic odor to foods infected with botulin, and cans do not necessarily bulge, as in other kinds of spoilage.

Education of the home canner and the consumer is the most pressing need in respect to prevention and control of botulism. Public health agencies should provide information to the home canner about proper techniques and common errors involved in the preservation of foods.

Botulism is the least common and the most highly lethal of bacterial food poisons in the United States. In Germany and France, the mortality rate is less than 25 per cent. Some experts feel that there is some difference in the type and amount of toxin that must be present in the organisms at various geographic locations. Though the disease is relatively rare, the importance of outbreaks lies in the fact that they have resulted from ingestion of commercially processed products that had widespread distribution. Prior to 1960, there had been only one reported instance of botulism from food commercially processed or canned in this country since 1925. There have always been a number of small epidemics yearly, but these have resulted primarily from home-prepared foods with limited distribution. Then, mysteriously, in 1963 the total number of botulism cases and deaths increased markedly, and included 20 cases and

Food Products Causing Botulism Outbreaks, 1970-1973					
	Botulinal Toxin Type				
Source	**A**	**B**	**E**	**Unknown**	**Total**
Vegetables	6	4	0	3	**13**
Fish and fish products	2	1	3	0	**6**
Other source*	3	1	0	0	**4**
Undetermined	3	0	0	4	**7**
Total	**14**	**6**	**3**	**7**	**30**

*Includes meatballs and spaghetti sauce, vichyssoise soup, antipasto, and blackberries.

Commercial Food Contaminated With Botulinal Toxin or *Clostridium botulinum*, 1970-1973			
Date	**Food**	**Type**	**Cases**
4/70	Mushrooms	B	0
8/70	Meatballs and spaghetti sauce*	A	4
6/71	Vichyssoise	A	2
8/71	Chicken vegetable soup	A†, B†	0
2/73	Mushrooms	B	0
3/73	Mushrooms	B†	0
4/73	Mushrooms	B	0
5/73	Peppers	B	7
7/73	Mushrooms	B	1‡
9/73	Mushrooms	B	0
12/73	Mushrooms§	B	0
12/73	Mushrooms§	B†	0

*Food epidemiologically incriminated; laboratory confirmation not obtained.
†Only *C botulinum* organisms detected.
‡Canadian case.
§Contamination detected late 1973; products recalled early January 1974

Figure 11–22 Statistics on botulism. (From Merson, M. H., et al.: Current trends in botulism in the United States. JAMA, *229*(10):1305, September 2, 1974.)

nine deaths which were attributed to commercially packed food. In addition, an outbreak of type B toxin from a liver paste canned in Canada and distributed in the United States demonstrates that the problem lies not only with new sources of infection but with easy and rapid dissemination of the toxin made possible by modern transportation.

The well publicized occurrence of cases resulting from canned tuna in Detroit, from soup, and from whitefish originating in the Great Lakes region has serious implications. While types A and B *Clostridium botulinum* have accounted for most of the cases in this country, both of the outbreaks caused by fish appear to have been due to the rare type E toxin. This toxin type has been associated primarily with marine products, and has been reported most often in Japan in connection with the consumption of izushi, a fermented raw fish preparation. A number of outbreaks in Labrador and Alaska, due to ingestion of whale and seal flesh, have been reported. Salmon eggs have been implicated previously in botulism only in Alaska, British Columbia, and Yukon Territory. More recent occurrences seem, therefore, to indicate a new endemic infection of marine wildlife with type E *Clostridium botulinum.* Scandinavian and Russian scientists have found type E spores in the soil, shore sand, and sea bottom. Ocean currents can carry these spores for thousands of miles. Certain American scientists suggest that expelling industrial wastes into the lakes may have changed the bottom in a way that has favored growth of type E. Tough type E spores are resistant to smoking, drying, vinegar, spice pickling, and low energy nuclear radiation, and exposure to many preservative processes will not significantly destroy preformed toxin.

New and more stringent public health regulations relating to commercial packaging and processing are necessary. No defect in the technique of canning has yet been identified in relation to the canned tuna. The whitefish was prepared by a method in use commercially for many years without previous difficulty. The Food and Drug Administration recommended the destruction of all products that were made from the Great Lakes fish or processed in the Great Lakes region, except in instances in which the techniques of processing and distribution were such that no development of toxin was possible. Suggestions for safer processing include chemical additives, cooking smoked fish at a temperature of 180° F. for 30 minutes and then freezing until sold, and quick-freezing the fish immediately after smoking, Studies on the susceptibility of *Clostridium botulinum* spores to radiation have shown that as much as 4 million rads is necessary in some cases to inactivate the spores. The vegetative cells of the organism can be killed with about 50,000 rads. The FDA has approved the use of radiation in processing bacon. Although laboratory studies indicate that 2.5 rads is sufficient to destroy the spores, a minimum level of 4.5 rads is required by FDA to ensure complete safety in the product.

Information on the efficacy of antitoxins and supportive therapy is required, as well as new methods for quickly evaluating the specific types of *Clostridium botulinum* poisoning. The mouse tests currently used are of little value because they require up to 72 hours to obtain satisfactory evaluation. In addition, the commercial availability of antitoxin that will include protection against type E toxin is also desirable. The Communicable Disease Center in Atlanta procured from the Danish State Serum Institute a limited supply of antitoxin for emergency use by qualified medical practitioners against type E botulism. Prompt recognition of the syndrome and treatment with the appropriate type of antitoxin is extremely important. In any case, the United States Public Health Service and the Food and Drug Administration, in cooperation with appropriate state agencies, have displayed a high level of professional competence in protecting the health of the public in recent outbreaks. Each year a number of cases of botulism occurs. Sadly, this danger lurks in an old and honored American practice—putting up one's own fresh fruits and vegetables, home canning "as Grandma used to do." The following case serves as an example.

Case Study

Botulism in West Virginia. A 25-year-old West Virginia man died of botulism within 24 hours after eating home canned green beans. Six hours after ingestion, the patient experienced severe abdominal cramping and vomiting, which caused his admission to a hospital. At that time, his pupils were dilated and fixed. In the hospital, his vomiting continued; he went into shock and expired early the next morning. At autopsy, the stomach and small bowel were dilated, but otherwise there was no evidence of gastrointestinal pathology. The lungs were markedly edematous and congested. The brain was mildly edematous.

The victim's wife had prepared six quarts of cold pack green beans, obtained from the family garden, in early July 1963. Five of these quarts were consumed by all members of the family (including the victim) at varying intervals during the month of July. No member of the family experienced any illness from these. The remaining quart, opened approximately one month after it was cold packed, was noted to have both a milky appearance and a bad odor. The patient disregarded advice from other members of his family and consumed approximately half the can of beans. No other member of the family tasted the beans from this particular can. *Clostridium botulinum* was cultured from the remaining green beans.[21]

PROTECTING THE PUBLIC FOOD SUPPLY

Influence of Sinclair's The Jungle

The Jungle, published in 1906, was the most popular and most influential of all of Upton Sinclair's numerous novels. This savage indictment of labor and sanitary conditions in the Chicago stockyards first appeared serially in *The Appeal to Reason*, a Socialist weekly, when the author was a mere 27. The times were ripe for *The Jungle*. Still fresh in the public's memory was the "embalmed beef" scandal of the Spanish-American War. Theodore Roosevelt, hero of the battle of San Juan Hill, had testified before a Senate investigating committee that he would just as soon have eaten his old hat as the canned food that, under a government contract, had been shipped to the soldiers in Cuba. Languishing in Congress as Sinclair was composing his celebrated exposé was a bill prepared by Dr. Harvey W. Wiley, "Father of the Pure Food and Drugs Act," to tighten the laws and to protect consumers against unscrupulous manufacturing and business practices.

. . . After bitter debate, both the Pure Food and Drug Act and the Beef Inspection Act were passed in modified form and became laws of the land—less than six months from the appearance in book form of *The Jungle*.[22]

Federal Action to Protect the Public Food Supply

A series of dramatic disclosures over a period of years, essentially involving harmful food adulterants and fake medical preparations, led to the enactment in 1906 of the Federal Food and Drug Act. For 25 years before 1906, attempts by Dr. Harvey W. Wiley and his associates to obtain passage of similar legislation had failed. It is unfortunate, yet true, that most of the major changes and improvements in the nation's food and drug laws have been made following dramatic, and often tragic, circumstances.

For example, it took more than 30 years to get a much-needed major revision of the 1906 statute. The spark in this case was the so-called "Elixir of Sulfanilamide" tragedy in 1937. More than 100 Americans, many of them children, died because a new sulfanilamide preparation contained diethylene glycol, a highly toxic solvent. This episode was promptly followed by enactment of the Federal Food, Drug, and Cosmetic Act of 1938—the law that to this day remains the foundation stone of American consumer protection.

The mission of the Food and Drug Administration is to protect consumers by ensuring that foods are safe, pure, and wholesome; drugs and therapeutic devices are safe and effective; cosmetics are safe; all the foregoing are honestly and informatively labeled and packaged; and that certain hazardous household chemical aids (e.g., cleaning agents, paint removers and thinners, polishes and waxes) carry adequate warning labels. This is done through enforcement of the Federal Food, Drug, and Cosmetic Act and other consumer protection laws.

The laws on which the authority of the FDA rests are primarily regulatory in nature and consequently make FDA a law enforcement agency. The laws that FDA enforces also have the potential of profoundly affecting the rate of progress this nation can make in food, drug, and cosmetic science and technology. These laws have fundamental impact on the industry and commerce of our nation. Not only is this true in the case of new drugs, but it also applies to the development and use of new food additives, color additives, agricultural chemicals, and therapeutic devices. These statutes affect manufacturing, processing, and distribution techniques. They apply to research and testing procedures and to a host of other factors profoundly related to the progress this nation can make in providing better health and improved standards of living.

In the past, FDA has been severely hampered because salaries, number of staff members (16,500 employees today), and budgets did not keep pace with certain trends, which include:

1. Population increase. In addition to sheer numbers, most of the technological developments for the preservation, packing, and distribution of food, for example, have been stimulated by the industry's need to provide for a fast growing urban population. Further, the increase in the older age groups is related to an increase in medical and nutritional quackery.

2. A growing economy and a more affluent population. These have led to a large number and variety of products to please an even greater diversity of tastes and demands.

3. Technological advances. These have led to new methods of production and distribution, and new and complex products, including pesticides, animal feeds, food additives, and drugs.

The trouble with the FDA, claims Dr. Jacqueline Verrett, FDA biochemist, is the same as that in all regulating agencies: too many of its personnel are recruited from the industries it is supposed to control. Furthermore, there was evidence suggesting political dictation from the White House via the Secretary of Health, Education and Welfare.*

Food Additives

For many reasons, laboratory technicians and manufacturers have had to infuse foods with an infinite variety of chemicals. Two vital questions now face both consumers and pure-food authorities: (1) Are these additives necessary or even desirable? and (2) Are they safe? In virtually no case is a simple declarative answer possible. See Feingold, B. F.: *Why Your Child Is Hyperactive* (New York, Random House, 1975), for a discussion on the relationship between food additives, dyes, sugar, and hyperactivity.

In crude or dilute form, nature supplies some of the substances that have recently gained notoriety as additives. The first additives, aside from salt and seaweed, were spices. Some contained natural preservatives. Benzoic acid, used as a preservative for almost a century, occurs naturally in berries and in some fruits, such as plums.

The first U.S. Pure Food and Drug Law, passed in 1906, gave the enforcing authority

---

*See Verrett, J.: *Eating May Be Hazardous to Your Health.* New York, Simon & Schuster, 1974.

(now the Food and Drug Administration) no power to rule on the safety of any substance that a food processor proposed to put in his packages. Not until 1958 did Congress give the FDA the power to pass on additives before they went on the market, but by then it had delayed so long that hundreds of additives had been in wide use for many years. So the new law contained a grandfather clause, exempting substances already employed and "generally recognized as safe for their intended use" (GRAS).

The FDA's list of GRAS items classifies hundreds of additives by their principal purposes. Among them are anti-caking agents, which keep such things as salt, sugar, and milk powder from clumping; preservatives (31 listed); emulsifying agents, used to help homogenize substances that do not normally mix (like fat in milk); and sequestrants, which keep trace minerals from turning fats and oils rancid and are also used to prevent some soft drinks from turning cloudy. In addition, the FDA has 80 "miscellaneous" GRAS substances, from alfalfa to zedoary (an aromatic East Indian herb), from pipsissewa leaves to ylang-ylang, used as flavoring.

In all, there are thousands of permitted additives, dyes, and substitutes, and few have ever been tested thoroughly for possible long-term harmful effects in man. No one can be really certain that any particular substance may not induce cancer over a 50-year period, or cause thalidomide-like deformities in the unborn. Although there is only the remotest chance that even a minority might be hazardous, further testing of many additives by chromatographic techniques, which did not exist when the substances were first introduced, is clearly indicated. The FDA has arranged with the National Academy of Sciences' National Research Council to supervise such studies of saccharin and monosodium glutamate.

It has become clear that far too many additives were used and allowed on the GRAS list without sufficient testing. Moreover, an automatic guillotine such as that applied to cyclamates is too crude an instrument for determining acceptability. The food industry obviously has to use some additives to keep its products from spoiling and—in the case of such staples as bread, milk, and iodized salt—to give them maximum nutritive and health-protective values. Some scientists claim, however, that the benefit of adding nitrite to bacon to protect against botulism, for example, is outweighed by the possible carcinogenic chemical risk involved in the frying process. Just as clearly, the public demands low-calorie sweeteners as well as precooked heat-and-serve meals. It is well within the competence of chemists and manufacturers to meet society's demands safely. At the same time, the FDA needs the unquestioned authority and financial resources to ensure that the world's greatest consuming society can be far better informed and protected.

Committee on Meat and Poultry Inspection

The Committee on Meat and Poultry Inspection is of the opinion that there is an urgent need for the reevaluation of all governmental food hygiene activities and programs, including programs operated by the Public Health Service, the Food and Drug Administration, the Department of Agriculture, and other federal agencies. The examination of present programs and procedures could lead to better utilization of laboratory facilities and personnel among these agencies. New approaches to surveillance and sampling could lead to increased safety for the consumer and more efficient utilization of resources. A full-scale examination of programs might result in considerable savings while releasing scarce professional personnel such as chemists, food technologists, and veterinarians for other critical activities in food protection programs. The Committee recommends that a research and evaluation program should be initiated to explore the more extensive application of microbiological and other scientific and technical methodologies to meat, poultry, and food hygiene. In addition to the use of sampling and surveillance, methodologies should be studied with respect to modifying the present wasteful and inefficient systems of carcass by carcass inspection of meat and poultry.

Recommendations

1. The American Public Health Association should convene a committee to explore the total system of food inspection in the United States, in order to guide funds now expended in food protection. There is a need for the reevaluation of all governmental food protection programs.

2. Meat and poultry products are a main source of *Salmonella* organisms incriminated in food-borne disease outbreaks. However, a food hygiene program must take into account the total infection cycle for *Salmonella.* Control activities for *Salmonella* should not be limited to a specific point or product, but should be directed to the total problem.

3. A group of experts should evaluate the effectiveness of on-line carcass by carcass inspection procedures in meat and poultry inspection. These experts should be brought together by an organization such as the National Academy of Sciences.

4. Inspection legends should be designed to

fully inform the public of the actual meaning and extent of protection that is implied in the statement to the public. The food industries should further develop informational material and educational programs to indicate to the consumer the meaning of the legend.[23]

Milk Sanitation

Milk is an excellent food but it is also a favorable culture medium for many diseases. Milk-borne diseases include streptococcal infections, diphtheria, dysentery, tuberculosis, brucellosis, typhoid, and paratyphoid fever.

Opportunities for milk infection are numerous; the first source of infection is the cow. Diseases indigenous to the cow include brucellosis and bovine tuberculosis. Brucellosis and tuberculin testing of cows is standard procedure today. In addition, infected udders are a source of human streptococcal infection, but this perhaps should be considered an exotic disease of the cow since it is generally contracted by the cow as a localized infection from a human milk handler. The usual form of bovine mastitis is caused by other streptococci which are non-pathogenic to man. Opportunity for infection arises with the milk handler who may contaminate the milk through carelessness, lack of personal hygiene, or disease. Other opportunities for milk infection involve unsanitary utensils, equipment, and barn, and impure water used in cleaning the utensils and equipment. Nevertheless, milk samitation programs emphasize education rather than compulsion to achieve results.

TIPS FOR CONSUMERS

In the supermarket:

1. Buy only federally inspected and graded meat. You can tell it by the purple "roll stamp" that appears on all large pieces. Usually the grocer will aid you by adding his own label reading "USDA Prime," "USDA Choice," or some other indication that the meat comes from federally approved plants. All the experts we consulted agreed that you are better off with USDA-inspected meat, in spite of the system's failings.
2. Never buy meat that is distinctly "two-toned"—the darker portion is likely to be too old, or spoiled.
3. Never buy meat if the packages are torn or broken.
4. If you want the best possible ground beef, grind it yourself, or have it ground to order by your butcher.
5. If you see anything wrong with the meat, let your butcher know about it. If you don't see the cut you want with a federal stamp, ask for it. Let your butcher know that it makes a difference to you.

In the community:

1. Since inspection of retail outlets is uneven at best, and often even nonexistent, find out what the inspection practices are in your area by calling local health officials. If you are not satisfied with what is being done, tell them so. Write letters to local legislators and to newspapers. Nothing encourages fair dealing like public scrutiny.
2. If you are concerned about meat inspection and additives in meat, write your congressman and let him know about it. Tell him you want to be kept up to date on the government's control of the safety of meat, and let him know when you're not satisfied—and when you are.
3. Take a tour through a meat plant in your area. It will be interesting in itself, and packers are more likely to be on their toes if consumers show an interest.

Pasteurization

Pasteurization is a bactericidal process which applies heat to milk for a sufficient time-temperature period to kill all milk-borne pathogens without impairing the flavor or nutritive quality of milk. Cooling of milk before and after pasteurization is an important supplemental safeguard. The tubercle bacillus and the Q fever organism seem to be the most resistant germs under most time-temperature combinations. Pasteurization may best be performed in a neutral time-temperature zone.

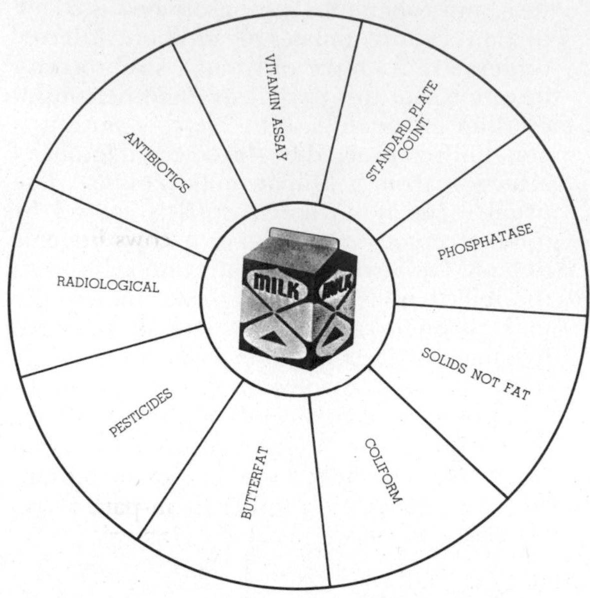

Figure 11–23 Factors affecting the production of safe milk. (From Health has a place in the sun. Annual Report, Maricopa County Health Department, Phoenix, Arizona, 1963.)

The present United States Public Health Service recommended standards for pasteurization are as follows:

1. The vat process, which is defined as continuously heating every particle of milk to not less than 145° F. for not less than 30 minutes, and immediately cooling to 50° F. or less.
   a. When milk or milk products contain high fats or added sugar, the recommended temperature is 150° F. for 30 minutes.
2. The high temperature process for short-time pasteurization, which is defined as heating every particle of milk continuously to at least 161° F. for not less than 15 seconds, and immediately cooling to 50° F. or less.
   a. When milk or milk products contain high fats or added sugar, the recommended temperature is 166° F. for 15 seconds.
3. The vacreator process of pasteurization, which is defined as heating milk or milk products by steam in vacuo to not less than 194° F. in approved equipment (Series No. 600 or more), and immediately cooling to 50° F. or less.[24]

Pasteurization should not be considered a substitute for proper sanitation, but rather an essential supplementary safeguard for all fluid fresh milk. To the milk sanitarian and other public health workers, properly pasteurized milk is safer than certified raw milk. The necessity for pasteurizing raw milk, even when produced under spotlessly sanitary conditions, is highlighted by the fact that no practical system of inspection has been developed that can ensure the noninfectiousness of the cow and the milk handler at all times. Cows may contract brucellosis and human streptococcal organisms between frequently performed veterinary inspections; milk handlers may become harborers of streptococcal and salmonella organisms without evidence of illness, and typhoid carriers are not always detected by single or random stool examination. When milk is produced and handled under other than virtually aseptic conditions, as is generally the case, the argument for effective pasteurization is strengthened.

Sanitary milk tests include:

1. Direct microscopic counts for total bacteria.
2. Direct microscopic examination for specific organisms, especially streptococci.
3. Plate counts for total bacteria.
4. Phosphatase test to determine the effectiveness of the pasteurization process (this enzyme is present in raw milk, but is thermosensitive at pasteurization temperature).
5. Coliform test (pasteurization kills all coliform organisms).
6. Reductase test to determine the bacterial condition of milk.
7. Sediment test to indicate the cleanliness of the milk.

Effective control programs are administered by trained city and county sanitarians with the support of state health and agriculture departments and private dairies. Most of their work is guided by basic state laws and supplemented by local ordinances. Individual states have vested authority over milk sanitation in either the health department or the agriculture department. In an effort to standardize milk sanitation and pasteurization regulations, the Public Health Service published a code interpreting the standard milk ordinance. This code has been accepted by many states as the basic regulation for an interstate certification program and an industry-wide education program. In addition, the Public Health Service initiated the interstate Milk Certification Program, which provides for milk shipments to be inspected and rated by state health officials and certified by the Public Health Service. Milk from a certified shipper may then be accepted in other states and municipalities without further inspection.

Q Fever

Raw milk, untreated and unpasteurized, contains a variety of organisms which may cause serious illness in humans. One of them is Q fever, which was first recognized in Queensland, Australia in 1935. The parasitic microorganism which causes the fever (*Rickettsia burnetii*) may occur in animal reservoirs, may be transmitted to man by arthropod vectors, and may even be transmitted from man to man. The most common method of contracting the disease is via the respiratory tract, but consuming raw milk or raw milk products can also result in the disease.

The disease is found all over the world. During World War II, Q fever caused widespread sickness among members of the allied forces in the Mediterranean area. It is characterized by high temperatures, ranging from 101 to 105 degrees and lasting from five to seven days, associated with shivering, backache, sore throat, headache, chest pains, stiff neck and sweating. In many cases, patients have an irritating cough and occasionally a rash on the trunk. Sometimes, chest x-rays show pneumonic solidification of the lungs which may take many weeks to clear. Chronic heart disease due to Q fever organisms has also been reported. Treatment of the fever is usually isolation, bed rest, and aspirin or antibiotics.

There has been at least one report of a fatal case of endocarditis (inflammation of the lining of the heart) occurring as an aftermath of Q fever. *Rickettsia burnetii* has also been implicated as a cause of subacute endocarditis; if a patient has had Q fever and later in life develops an unexplained low-grade fever, the possibility of rickettsial endocarditis should be considered.

In a recent Q fever epidemic in Great Britain, in which the patients had consumed unpasteurized milk, examination of the cows showed that they were actively excreting Q fever organisms in their milk.

Enforcement of Sanitary Standards

It is interesting to note the activities of the Baltimore City Health Department, Milk Control Division in maintaining standards of sanitary control:

Dairy Farm Inspection. The Bureau of Milk Control sanitarians made at least two inspections of each dairy farm shipping milk into Baltimore City during the year, and at least two samples of milk from each dairy farm were tested by the City Health Department's Bureau of Laboratories for the presence of bacteria, added water, and antibiotics. In addition, approved industry field men made similar sanitary inspections on each farm. Samples of milk from these farms were also tested each month by certified industry laboratories and the results were submitted to the bureau. Because of the enormous amount of data collected as a result of this vigorous milk control program, beginning in January 1963, all laboratory test results and the sanitary inspections of each dairy farm holding a City Health Department dairy farm permit were recorded for computer processing. This system enabled the bureau for the first time to establish a complete and readily available record of each dairy farm permittee and aided in attaining an enforcement compliance rating of 94.88 per cent in a United States Public Health Service interstate milk shippers' survey conducted early in the fall. The monthly program of obtaining samples of milk from each producer's milk shipment and testing them for the presence of added water and antibiotics, begun in 1960, was continued. Seven milk producers were suspended for seven days because of the presence of added water, and three milk producers because of the presence of antibiotics, in their milk shipments. This program has been instrumental in helping to maintain a pure milk supply.

Milk Plant Inspection. During the year, members of the bureau's milk plant inspection staff in cooperation with the United States Public Health Service and the Maryland State Department of Health, obtained samples of milk from the local milk plants once a week for testing for strontium-90 and iodine-131 in milk. At no time during the year were levels reached that required the taking of action to protect the public health. More than 34,000 samples of pasteurized milk and cream were phosphatase tested by City Health Department's Bureau of Laboratories and by certified industry laboratories. For the eighth consecutive year not a single instance of improper pasteurization was reported.[25]

REFUSE DISPOSAL

The average per capita production of refuse in the United States is four pounds per day. Disposal of this ever-increasing amount of refuse is a task our civilization must solve if it is to remain healthy. It is not a problem confined to big cities alone, for a small city of 10,000 would have to dispose of 40,000 pounds of refuse, or 20 tons each day.

Major Components of Waste Handling

The major components of a good waste handling program are divided into three parts: refuse storage at the home or point of origin, collection of the refuse, and the ultimate disposal of the refuse.

Home Storage. At the point of origin, it is recommended that a water-tight container with a close-fitting lid be used to prevent rodents and other animals from getting into the garbage and tipping over the can. The breeding of flies can be reduced if garbage cans are kept clean and if the garbage is wrapped. Garbage cans should not be larger than the 30 gallon size. They should be light enough that a man can lift them when they are full. Adding a second garbage can is preferable to overloading a large one, which cannot be dumped.

Collection. The life cycle of the domestic fly is a factor in fly control. Flies require from four to six days to develop from egg to adult. If fly larvae are hauled away before this amount of time has elapsed, they never have a chance to emerge as flies because they will be buried at the landfill. During warm weather, therefore, collection twice a week is desirable.

Garbage Trucks. The tops of garbage trucks should be covered so that papers will not blow off when the truck is driven. The bottoms of trucks should be leakproof to prevent the spreading of smelly liquids as the truck makes its rounds. Some trucks are known as "paper trucks" because of a hydraulic arrangement used to compress their loads. Added efficiency is gained because each truck can thereby haul more garbage per trip. Length of haul is a factor to consider. If the trucks haul their loads more than 20 miles, it might be more economical to build an adequate incinerator. Trucks should be washed out at least at the end of each day's operation. The fluid washed from the trucks should drain into a sewer or some other facility that would prevent flies from breeding in the organic material present.

Ultimate Disposal. Choice of the type of disposal depends on many factors, including availability of land, accessibility and distance to site, size and type of city or county organization, and air pollution. Sanitary landfills have been increasing in number throughout many states in recent years and this method continues to grow in acceptance by communities. As landfill sites disappear, and the prospects of sanitary landfills grow more and more remote, however, incineration becomes more economical and feasible. The incinerator burns the refuse at a high temperature. Though the figure varies from city to city, in Los Angeles it is more economical to use incineration if the distance to the landfill site exceeds 50 miles, even when transfer operations are conducted. Los Angeles turned to the use of relatively remote landfill sites in recent years only after costly smoke-control edicts forced it to close down most of its incinerators.

Other big cities are in a considerably worse situation, when it comes to landfill sites. New York City, which generates enough refuse daily to fill a freight train seven miles long, expects to run out of all its feasible landfill sites by approximately 1985. The city is now in the process of completing 11 incinerators at a cost of more than 90 million dollars.

Chicago, which constructed its first incinerator in 1930 and did not build another for 25 years, after operating costs proved higher than anticipated, has aimed at incinerating practically all its refuse. Though there have been a number of innovations in incinerator operations since 1930 that make incinerators more economical to operate—automatic stoking and filling, for instance—Chicago's move from landfill to incineration is being dictated by the disappearance of landfill sites.

Incinerators do not eliminate the need for dump space, however, because ash and noncombustibles, such as tin cans and glass, still remain. Noncombustibles account for about 15 per cent of the total refuse and ash for about 10 per cent, which means that about one-fourth of the original volume needs to be disposed of after incineration. When New York City proposed to use the remaining trash to fill in marshes along the shore of Jamaica Bay in Long Island, it promptly stirred the ire of every duck hunter and nature lover for miles around. Chicago, which had hoped to use exhausted rock quaries for the purpose, was faced with the costly task of hauling dirt from considerable distances for cover.

The following are some present experiments in finding ways of handling trash: (1) pipeline techniques for collection and removal of household solid waste, (2) recycling and reuse, (3) composting of garbage on a commercial scale for sale as fertilizer, (4) total recycling in which nothing would be thrown away, (5) a combustion power unit which would burn trash at high pressures to produce hot gases to power a turbine, therefore driving an electrical generator, and (6) plates, bottles, glasses, cans, and other items made of collagen (a water-soluble protein) that will dissolve instantly in boiling water.

Another method of disposal is reduction, in which refuse is cooked under steam pressure with recovery of the melted fats and dry solid residue. The fats are used for soap-making, and the residue is used as a fertilizer. Biological digestion consists of placing the refuse into tightly sealed vaults, allowing it to decompose. After approximately 25 days, the residue can be used as fertilizer. This method is not a popular procedure in the United States, although some European countries still use it.

Sanitary landfills are becoming more popular as a satisfactory method of refuse disposal. Generally, they can be operated inexpensively in many different types of terrain. The term *sanitary landfill* denotes an operation in which refuse is deposited in or on the ground in an orderly manner, compacted, covered daily with 6 inches of earth, and again compacted.*

Before a sanitary landfill is used, the following steps should be taken:

1. An accessible site of sufficient size should be selected as near as possible to the areas served. (It is generally estimated that one to 1½ acres of land excavated or developed to a depth of about 6 feet is required for disposal of refuse per year for a population of 10,000 people.)
2. A topographic map of the proposed landfill site should be prepared and the final elevations of the filled areas should be based on the future use of the reclaimed land.
3. An all-weather access road should be provided to the landfill site.
4. Provisions should be made to prevent the obstruction of natural drainage channels and pollution of surface or underground water in excess of limits set by the State Sanitary Authority.
5. An adequate water supply should be provided for fire protection, dust, paper control, and the cleaning of trucks and equipment.
6. An appropriate structure should be provided at the disposal site for tools and the storage and maintenance of equipment.

The collection and disposal of refuse is a proper and important community function and should be controlled by officials of the public health department. In some communities, the refuse is collected by a private concern under contract. In either case, refuse collection and disposal should be controlled and regulated by the health department to meet the necessary standards in order to protect the health of the community.

Solid Waste

Today, a new concept of solid waste management is evolving; it assumes that man can devise a sociotechnological system that will wisely control the quantity and characteristics of wastes, efficiently collect those that must be removed, creatively recycle those that can be reused, and properly dispose of those that have no further use. The Solid Waste Disposal Act of 1965 marked the first significant interest by the federal government in management of solid wastes. The act provided for assistance to state and local governments, and others involved in managing solid wastes, by financial grants to demonstrate new technology, provide technical assistance through research and training, and encourage proper planning for state and local solid waste management programs.

The Resource Recovery Act of 1970 amended the legislation to provide a new focus on recycling and recovery of valuable waste materials. Under current legislation,

*A modified landfill, however, is not necessarily covered daily with 6 inches of earth.

the Environmental Protection Agency has the following functions:

1. Carrying out research to find improved methods in all aspects of solid waste management and providing technical assistance to speed the application of new knowledge. Special emphasis is given to studies to determine means of recovering materials and energy from solid waste; methods of accelerating the reclamation of such materials (by economic incentives, subsidies, depletion allowances, federal procurement to develop market demand, and so on); and the feasibility of reducing the amount of solid wastes by changes in product characteristics, production, or packaging practices.

2. Making financial grants for the construction and operation of plants or processes for demonstrating new technology. In the city of Franklin, Ohio, for example, an advanced system for recovery of municipal wastes has been demonstrated. It features a hydropulper, by which solid wastes are processed into slurry form. Heavy materials are ejected and ferrous metals removed for salvage by an electromagnet. Paper fiber is recovered for re-use. An additional step planned involves extraction of glass, with separation into various colors by an optical sorting device. The residue has a relatively high percentage of aluminum, which also may be reclaimed.

3. Development of a comprehensive plan for a system of national disposal sites for storage and disposal of hazardous wastes.

4. Providing financial assistance to state and local governments and interstate agencies for the development of resource recovery and solid waste disposal systems and for solid waste management planning.

5. Providing training to develop the highly skilled engineers and technicians needed to design, operate, and maintain complex new regional systems.

Recovery of Solid Waste. Environmental concern has drawn attention to means for recovering material and energy resources from urban solid waste, particularly from the household portion. Metals, for instance, can easily be recycled to make new products. Combustible refuse can be sold to power companies or factories as a supplementary fuel (trash when burned releases about 50 per cent of the heat value of coal); oxygen-free furnaces can convert organic trash into oil or gas (pyrolysis); cellulose in wastepaper and grass clippings combined with sludge may trigger a natural sequence of soil enrichment and turn a desert into a vast garden (Odessa, Texas.

Recovery from solid waste is essentially a two-phase process, involving first, materials recovery (glass, metals, and some paper) and second, recovery of the organic portion and re-use through conversion, probably as a source of energy.

One scheme for recovering materials and energy from solid waste is shown in Figure 11–24. "Front end" refers to materials recovery with disposal of the organic portion by conventional means – for example, by landfill or incineration. This is a suboptional system because it is incomplete. "Back end" refers to the recovery of the organic portion and its re-use as fuel or as raw material for a product.

OCCUPATIONAL HEALTH

History

Medical history reveals that the health of the individual was often influenced by his occupation. Many match sellers and glass blowers were afflicted with eye trouble, miners developed lung disease, hat cleaners contracted psychic disturbances, musicians developed hernia, and flute players had lung edema. Hippocrates described diseases in the metal workers in the year 460 B.C. and Pliny the Elder is said to have invented the first gas mask, but it remained for farsighted Bernardo Ramazzini to give a comprehensive description of the many diseases associated with occupation. His book, *A Treatise on the Disease of Workers,* is still an authoritative classic, although it was first published in the year 1700.

Modern occupational health is an outcome of the industrial revolution in England in the nineteenth century. At the time numerous laws were passed for the protection of workers as a result of the increasing deplorable work conditions, and the exploitation of women and children in industry. Dr. Alice Hamilton, author of *Industrial Poisons in the United States,* published in 1925, is considered the founder of industrial toxicology in the United States and is recognized as having opened the era for the modern practice of industrial medicine. Medical care for employed groups had its beginnings in 1887, when the Homestake Mining Company of

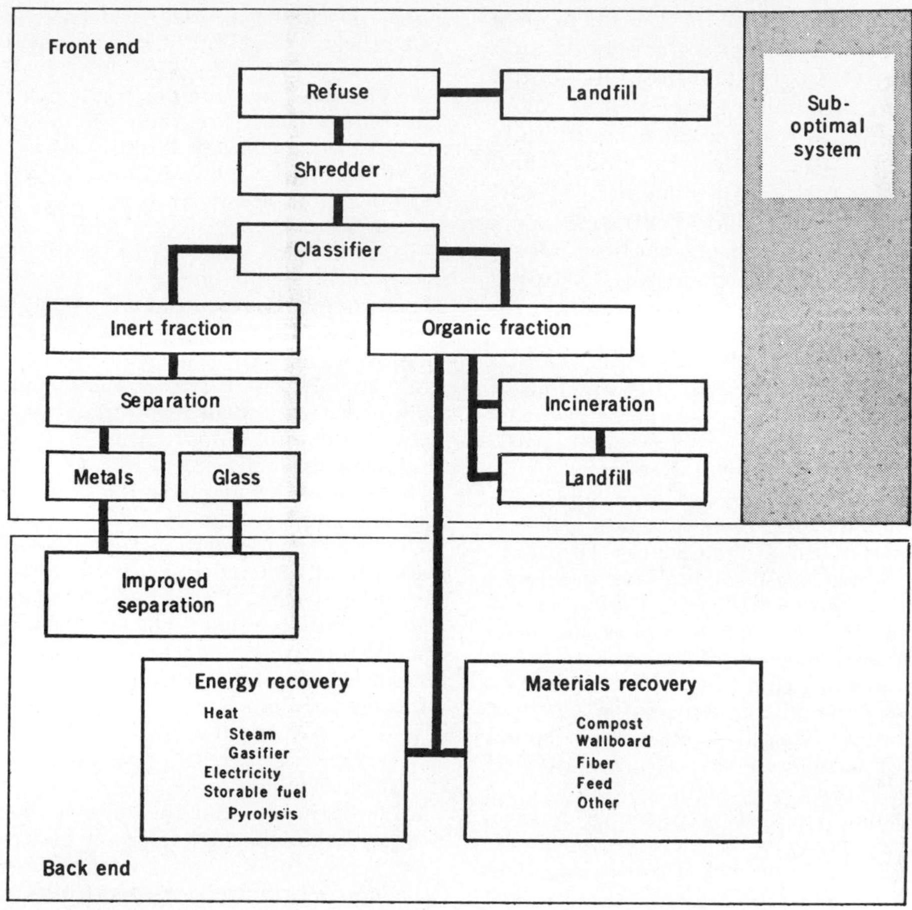

Figure 11–24 A modular approach to resource recovery. Front end refers to materials recovery. Back end refers to direct utilization, or conversion, of the organic portion of the waste. (From Abert, J. S., et al.: The economics of resource recovery from municipal solid waste. Science, *183*:1053, March, 1974. Copyright 1974 by the American Association for the Advancement of Science.)

South Dakota established a medical department with a full-time staff providing complete medical services to employees and their families.

The theory of workmen's compensation as a social answer to legal problems and failure of existing laws originated in England and gradually spread throughout the world. The first workmen's compensation law in the United States was enacted in 1908 and covered certain injuries and diseases of federal employees. New York, Maryland, California, and Wisconsin were the first states to enact workmen's compensation laws. The slow progress in this area, however, is illustrated by the fact that today, 19 states have only partial coverage, two states have no provisions, and about half the states limit medical benefits in occupational disease cases.

With changing times and the dynamic growth of industrial, political, economic, and social life, industrial hygiene needs have become very complex and have evolved into matters of grave responsibility for anyone who has created employment. Today, thousands of people work together in concentrated areas; machinery and materials of production are complex and everchanging. A multitude of laws and rulings regulate employer and employee, and the whole atmosphere of industrial activity is under the constant scrutiny of government and public alike. The need for an industrial hygiene program becomes even more evident in the light of demands made by industry's new environment, the medically enlightened but apprehensive public, the broadened compensation rulings for medical disorders and their effect on the employer, and increased union and governmental activities in occupational medicine and hygiene, the need for a well planned program, and the benefits that can be achieved. Every such program should have realistic, attainable goals spelled out in terms of better employee and community relationships, actual savings in dollars and cents, and the proper fulfillment by a corporation of its role as a good citizen.[26]

The following editorial, entitled "Occupational Health—Talk or Action," emphasizes the need for occupational health programs:[27]

Occupational health is just the opposite of the weather. Almost nobody talks about it, except we specialists who talk to ourselves, while everybody does something about it. Not many of this "everybody" know that they are doing something about occupational health, yet practically all employed persons in the United States take part in workmen's compensation medical care programs. Often they demand more, better or different services, thereby shaping the future of occupational health. A small proportion of the working public is involved in more comprehensive, occupationally centered, preventive and health services, and a handful, under special environmental conditions, receive complete medical care as well as preventive services.

Thus, some kind of occupational medical health services seems to be almost universal. Yet this universality coexists with a certain separateness. Each preventively oriented occupational health service continues because someone in management wants it. The "someone" may be in a private industry, a government bureau, a hospital, a health department, a union headquarters, or any organization one may name. This "someone" looks at his budget and decides how much he will devote to medical and health services. The amount is based on the expected needs of the *particular* organization. This logical train of events has helped generate the myth that an occupational health service is the sole concern of the organization providing it. Actually, it is a general concern. We, in occupational health, often find ourselves pointing out that an employee cannot park his heart, lungs, or anxieties at the gate before starting his day's work. Therefore, the employer needs periodic evaluation of each worker's health. Despite our acceptance of the "whole man" theory, neither we inside the specialty nor medical and health specialists in other areas seem much concerned about our *joint* responsibilities for the health of the worker as a *member of the adult public.* One state's "Guiding Principles for Occupational Medicine"[28] says in part "the physician considers himself a deputy health officer in practice if not in fact." How many occupational physicians currently believe this? How many other physicians? How many public health specialists? Of those who believe that existing occupational physicians are a logical extension of the public health forces of the community, how many act on this belief?

The lost opportunities for better preventive and public health programs are most glaring in the area of small plant health services. Thirty or forty years ago, Geier, McCord, Selby, and other men of vision pioneered in providing high quality, preventively oriented health services for workers in small plants. Now we find the United States little farther along the road than it was then, while other countries are passing us. Britain has demonstrated a viable pilot model of comprehensive services for small industries in its Slough Industrial Health Service.[29] With joint financing by a private foundation and the industries themselves, and with support from the public health authorities in such areas as rehabilitation, the program has steadily increased the health benefits for persons employed in the area. It now provides health services to workers in many establishments with less than ten employees and covers about seventy per cent of all establishments on the so-called Trading Estate. The only essential ingredient which we have lacked in this country is an emotional one. One reaction has been "No give away of tax money to profit making industries! Let them pay for their own services." On the opposite side one may hear "No government interference!" We have lacked emotional commitment to joint private and public efforts, despite their logic. Part of the logic of joint effort relates to cost. Successful small plant health programs must be adequately financed. Support must come from outside the struggling, competitive small industries themselves, if occupational health services are to be extended beyond the two per cent (a generous estimate) of all establishments now providing preventively oriented occupational health programs. When we accept the necessity for a vigorous partnership of private and public health efforts we can begin to progress at speeds commensurate with our capacities.

The Occupational Safety and Health Act

The Occupational Safety and Health Act of 1970 gives specific responsibilities to the Department of Health, Education and Welfare (HEW). The principal HEW responsibilities under the Act, which became effective on April 28, 1971, include research on occupational safety and health problems, hazard evaluation, toxicity determinations, manpower development and training, and the establishment of a National Institute for Occupational Safety and Health (NIOSH). Other responsibilities include special industry-wide studies of chronic or low-level exposure to hazardous substances and research on psychological, motivational, and behavioral factors as they relate to occupational safety and health. This legislation is designed to assure safe and healthful working conditions for the nation's working men and women and as such it provides broad authority to the Department of Labor and the Department of Health, Education and Welfare. Safe and healthful working conditions, resulting in better health for the worker, are the objective.

When Congress created the Occupational Safety and Health Administration (OSHA) it acted out of justifiable concern about the shocking high rate of United Sates job-caused injuries and illnesses. Unfortunately, in operation, OSHA has pleased very few. Labor leaders complain, correctly, that job-accident rates have not dropped, and charge that OSHA lacks the money and manpower to begin to do its job adequately. Many businessmen protest that OSHA inspectors often arbitrarily enforce regulations that are too strict and prohibitively expensive to obey. Others insist that the agency's 700 inspectors are enough and contend that few businessmen want advice on how to remedy unsafe conditions.

For information about the NIOSH Hazard Evaluation Service program and related services, write: NIOSH, Division of Technical Services, Post Office Bldg., Cincinnati, Ohio 45202.

For information about NIOSH training programs, write: NIOSH, Division of Training, 1014 Broadway, Cincinnati, Ohio 45202.

Current Status

Current staffs of industrial hygiene agencies are totally inadequate to cope with a fast-growing industrial labor force. Occupational health as an activity of local health departments has grown at a snail's pace. State and local programs continue to vary in scope, depending on size of staff, administration, and industrial economy. The best developed phases of programs deal with engineering services. Emphasis in other programs is dependent on state conditions.[30]

One authority in this area claims that occupational health has been neglected in the official agency public health planning because:

1. There has been a failure to realize the importance of occupation in the immediate and anticipated health needs of modern industrial society.
2. Health agencies often have a philosophy inappropriate to modern industrial society and inconsistent with the health needs of the gainfully employed.
3. Too often public health planners do not conduct accurate and imaginative community research into the scope and problems of occupational health within their communities.
4. Frequently, there has been a defeatist attitude regarding available or providable funds, rather than intelligent planning that would provide a firm basis for obtaining funds and personnel.
5. Public health planners have not taken leadership roles in identifying occupational health programs as vital public health programs and thus increasing their community acceptance.
6. Occupational health plans already formulated are often those designed "for the books" and for lip service.
7. There has been a failure of imaginative leadership in realizing the potential of a good occupational health program as a means of improving, strengthening, and focusing a community's attention on its general public health problems.[31]

Present Concepts

Occupational health is primarily preventive, aimed at the protection and promotion of health of employed workers. The objectives of the occupational health program as advanced by the American Medical Association Council on Occupational Health are:

1. To protect employees against health hazards in their work environment.
2. To facilitate the placement and ensure the suitability of individuals according to their physical capacities, mental abilities, and emotional makeup in work they can perform with an acceptable degree of efficiency without endangering their own health and safety or that of their fellow employees.
3. To assure adequate medical care and rehabilitation of the occupationally ill and injured.
4. To encourage personal health maintenance.[32]

Such programs have been found to help improve employees' health, morale and good will, and they have also resulted in savings from decreased workmen's compensation costs, lower insurance premiums, increased efficiency, fewer infections and disease, better placement and less turnover, improved working conditions, better health education, and diminished absenteeism. For example, the National Association of Manufacturers reported that health costs in the average company with ordinary risks of accident and disease are as follows:

> A 500 man plant has an expectancy of 335 days of disability due to industrial accident and disease, and 4,500 days due to nonoccupational injury and illness. Translated into money, this represents an average wage loss of $48,350 to employees, based on a daily wage of $10. Proportionately, in a 200 man plant the wage loss is $20,000 per year; in a 100 man plant, $10,000 per year.[33]

Industrial health programs are increasing in large industries that can afford facilities and personnel for such a program. Industrial medicine is a growing specialty, and there are over 2000 physicians working in this field. A good industrial health program may include preemployment and periodic physical examination for employees, counseling and guidance, prevention of industrial health hazards and disease, health education, and immunization and rehabilitation programs. This program usually involves the services of a physician, nurse, and industrial hygiene or safety engineer.

Official Agency Programs

Official agency programs were initiated because occupational diseases and deaths were increasing throughout the nation and most of these were preventable. Funds for occupational health programs were allocated to state and local health departments as a result of the Social Security Act in 1935. Renewed interest in this field developed after certain industrial tragedies occurred that could have been prevented by such a program. The continued existence of these programs is related to rapid industrial expansion and the daily introduction of complex health hazards in the form of chemicals or processes.

The first state occupational health programs were initiated by New York and Ohio in 1913. The following year the Office of Industrial Hygiene and Sanitation was created as a branch of the United States Public Health Service. An occupational health division may include a physician, nurse, industrial hygiene engineer, industrial hygiene chemist, and public health educator who work as a team in an effort to protect and promote the health of the workers in the community. Today, most state health departments and a few local health departments have occupational health divisions. In some states, occupational health matters are the joint concern of the Department of Public Health and The Division of Industrial Relations. However, the state occupational health divisions generally are hampered by lack of funds and personnel, and are able to reach only about 10 per cent of the nation's workers each year.

The scope of the local health department's occupational health program is broad, since it includes all occupations, but most programs direct their major efforts toward the manufacturing segment of industry; more people are employed in this category and the number of hazards is greater. Services of the occupational health division may include periodic physical examinations of government employees, prevention of industrial health hazards and disease, consultation, and education. The Federal Environmental Health Center located at Cincinnati, Ohio, now employs hundreds of scientists and technicians, and is leading the way in environmental health research and field investigations. In general, the local health department may be divided into engineering, medical and nursing, and laboratory services.

1. Engineering services include: review of plans for new procedures or processes or for proposed changes in established operations; engineering survey of an entire plant or selected operations for job hazards; consultation on industrial waste disposal and air pollution problems; consultation and assistance in the design of engineering control measures, including industrial exhaust systems.

2. Laboratory services refer to: analytical chemistry determinations in connection with any of the engineering studies; consultation concerning chemical methods of control or concerning the development of laboratory testing procedures related to occupational health, and the analysis of materials of known or suspected toxic composition.

3. Medical and nursing services include: consultations concerning the need for, or the organization and conduct of, employee health plans; assistance in planning medical facilities and in the selection of equipment; consultation and assistance in defining causal relation of diseases noted in the working environment and in the prevention, diagnosis and management of occupational

diseases. In addition, the division actively promotes on-the-job rehabilitation beginning with the injured employee and progressing through the plant nurse and all of the agencies involved.

4. Special studies relating to possible occupational disease or hazards in certain groups is of particular concern. An example of such a study is one which has to do with radiation exposure of dentists and dental assistants.[34]

The following investigations of industrial exposures conducted by the Bureau of Industrial Hygiene, Baltimore City Health Department, are of particular interest:

1. A workman cleaning a tank trailer was overcome by carbon tetrachloride vapors and four workers attempting to rescue him suffered ill effects. As a result of the accident, the company issued a set of safety procedures and made a substitution in the solvent used by the employees.

2. An investigation was made at a chemical plant as the result of a worker's illness from parathion exposure. The employee complained of stomach trouble and had vomited after working outdoors in the liquid parathion area. Blood tests for cholinesterase determination indicated low levels in the worker's plasma and in red blood cells. The patient was treated at a local hospital by the plant physician. It was indicated that poor personal hygiene and a contaminated glove contributed to exposure.

3. A mercury vapor study was conducted in the anesthesiology research laboratory of a large hospital. There was evidence of mercury spillage in several areas. Atmospheric samples ranged from 0.12 to 0.40 mg. of mercury per cubic meter of air. An employee working in the immediate area was requested to submit a 24 hour urine sample for the determination of mercury. Recommendations were given to control exposure of mercury.

4. A small fire occurred in the radium treatment room of an eye, ear, nose, and throat clinic. Through the efforts of hospital staff personnel, a 300 mg. radium source was removed safely. A radiation survey of the area indicated no contamination.

5. Two persons working in an office were affected from carbon monoxide gas as the result of a leak caused by a clogged flue. Repairs were promptly made by the company to eliminate the hazard.

6. Investigations were made of 29 radioisotope users who were authorized by the Atomic Energy Commission to use 143 isotopes. There were 47 different isotopes in use. The isotopes were used in medical diagnosis and therapy; in the industrial field for radiography, density measurement, process control, and instrument calibration; and for research. Joint field inspections were also made with representatives of the United States Atomic Energy Commission.

7. Forty-four cases and one death of lead paint poisoning in children were reported. Altogether 950 visits were made to the homes of parents whose children had lead paint poisoning or whose children had the habit of pica but had not absorbed sufficient lead to cause poisoning. It was stressed to the parents that they should assume the responsibility for their children through adequate supervision.[35]

The public health problems in this area are increasing rapidly. A major problem is the increasing production of new compounds and chemicals, many of which may be harmful or injurious to workmen, farmers, and others. Increasing uses of radioactive materials present new and different occupational health problems. With increased numbers of working women, opportunities for health promotion and protection are being expanded. State and local health departments must continue to expand their occupational health programs in order to cope with these increasing problems, protect and promote the health of the worker, and save the taxpayers' money.*

Guidelines for Suggested Activities for Public Health Nurses in Local Health Departments in Occupational Health

A. Introduction:

The nursing director participates with the health officer and others in appraisal of need for services, health department staff involvement, and establishment of channels of communication. The nurse who will provide services in an occupational health program needs to have an opportunity to become acquainted with industries and management for the purpose of:

1. Identifying key personnel such as occupational health nurses, physician, safety engineer, personnel manager, and others, and general orientation to the plant.

2. Interpreting health department services; identifying key personnel in the health department.

3. Interpreting other community facilities.

4. Identifying resources within health and welfare provisions of the plant organization.

5. Becoming familiar with industrial laws, labor code, and other legal controls.

---

*For further reading in this area refer to Carnow, B. W., et al.: A bookshelf on occupational health and safety. Amer. J. Publ. Health, *65*(5):503–520, May, 1975.

B. Possible activities of nursing director in places of employment that do not employ a nurse:

1. Serves as a resource to plant management and to employees on community health resources and community agencies, including local, state, and federal. Requests or promotes consultation as indicated for specific problems.

2. Serves as a resource person to management and employees in such areas as: nutrition and foodhandling; establishing of policies for health programs; first aid, including equipment and supplies; safety on and off job; plant safety; plant sanitation; health education materials; local, state, and federal consultant services.

3. Serves as a resource in identifying occupational health hazards and diseases and the prevention of such.

4. Encourages and/or participates in direct service and followup:

a. Screening activities: tuberculosis, venereal diseases, multiphasic glaucoma, diabetes, audio, immunizations, physical examinations.

b. First aid: helps management in planning for the provision of adequate, safe first aid.

5. Assists and/or participates in establishing in-plant educational programs for employees pertaining to health. Examples: first aid classes, in-service education in plant (nutrition, etc.), bulletins for plant newspapers.

6. Promotes educational programs in health and safety.

7. Plans, assists, and participates in special health surveys and studies.

8. Establishes adequate records and reporting system for nursing service.

9. Recognizes the health of the employed adult as part of family health. Also recognizes and interprets to employer the interrelatedness of the health of the employed adult and his family.

C. Possible activities of nursing director in places of employment that do employ a nurse: Assumes responsibility and leadership in promoting close and effective working relationship with occupational health nurses, and serves as a resource person to the plant nurse regarding community health facilities and services as listed above. She shares current information and new knowledge in regard to health and nursing. She may participate in some direct service as listed above.[36]

Environmental Agents

One of the major objectives of an occupational health program is the prevention

OCCUPATIONAL HEALTH

Silicosis—still the No. 1 occupational disease.

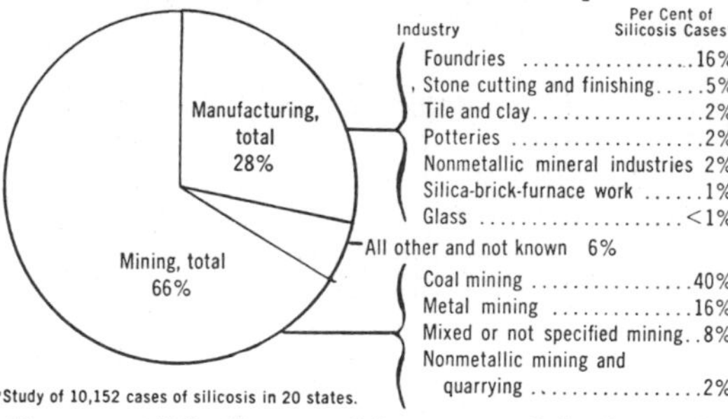

Industry	Per Cent of Silicosis Cases*
Foundries	16%
Stone cutting and finishing	5%
Tile and clay	2%
Potteries	2%
Nonmetallic mineral industries	2%
Silica-brick-furnace work	1%
Glass	<1%
All other and not known	6%
Coal mining	40%
Metal mining	16%
Mixed or not specified mining	8%
Nonmetallic mining and quarrying	2%

*Study of 10,152 cases of silicosis in 20 states.

Despite the accomplishments of dust control measures, silicosis is still the major occupational disease in the U.S. in terms of disability and compensation costs. Silicosis cases, which represent only 3% of claims, account for more than one quarter of all compensation awarded in occupational disease cases by the New York State Workmen's Compensation Board. The latest count of persons with silicosis in 26 states in the U.S. was 12,763; however, this number does not include many persons with non-disabling silicosis. At least half and probably closer to three quarters of workers disabled by silicosis are over 50 years of age.

Dermatitis is a widespread industrial problem.

Causative Agent	Per Cent of Cases*
Petroleum products and greases	19%
Alkalies and cement	12%
Solvents	8%
Plants and wood	7%
Metals and metal plating	6%
Rubber and its compounds	3%
Burns, physical and mechanical agents	3%
Chemicals, unspecified	3%
Paints, enamels, varnishes	3%
Acids and acid fumes	2%
Dyes and dye intermediates	2%
Chromates and chromic acid	2%
Biological agents	1%
Coal tar products	1%
Furs, fur dyes, hides	1%
Synthetic resins	1%
Nonmetallic elements	<1%
Oils, vegetable (oils, fats, waxes)	<1%
All other known exposures	19%
Unknown exposures	6%

Figure 11–25 The most common industrial health problem is occupational dermatitis. Dermatitis of occupational origin tends to be temporary in nature and less costly than most other occupational diseases. Average cost per case in New York is [illegible]. About 90 per cent of dermatoses are caused by contact with chemicals, four-fifths of which are primary irritants; the remainder are sensitizers. It is estimated that slightly less than half of occupational dermatitis cases in manufacturing industries are caused by petroleum products. In the case of dermatitis, 41,628 workers were studied. (From *Patterns of Disease*. Parke, Davis and Co., January, 1960.)

of adverse effects by environmental agents. Environmental agents may be divided into three categories; chemical agents, physical agents, and biological agents. Chemical agents may be the gaseous contaminants, such as carbon monoxide, or particulate matter contaminants such as dust, fumes, mist, and fog. Physical agents include high or low air pressure, temperature and humidity, illumination, radiant energy, mechanical vibration, and noise. Biological agents include many communicable diseases which often have an occupational origin, such as anthrax and brucellosis.

Injurious substances reach the body and cause damage by inhalation, skin contact, and ingestion. The nature and degree of injury are determined by the nature of the substances involved, the intensity and length of exposure, and the susceptibility of the person exposed. Despite the accomplishments of dust control measures, silicosis is still the major occupational disease in terms of disability and compensation costs. Dermatitis continues to be the most common industrial health problem (Figs. 11–25 and 11–26). It is interesting to note that the most dangerous occupations in terms of accidental death and disabling injuries include coal mining, logging, steel erection, and electric light and power work. Nevertheless, occupational diseases and hazards are decreasing, owing to expanding industrial medical services, legislation, development and use of protective engineering and safety measures and devices, and continuous health education programs.

Health hazards—from fiber glass to actinic rays.

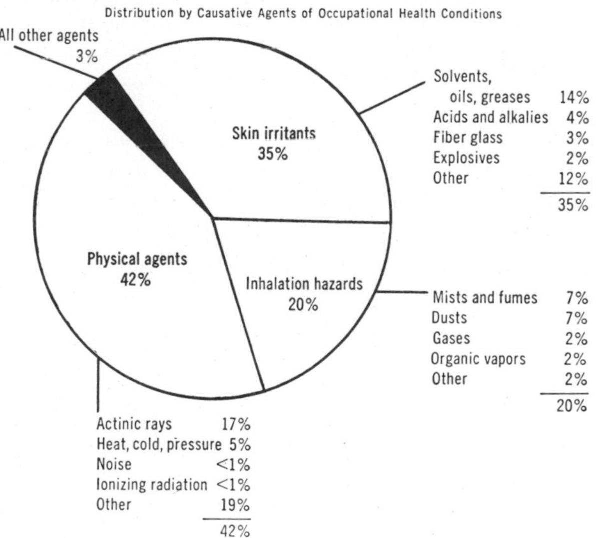

Figure 11–26 Study of 1733 occupational medical conditions occurring among 314,000 civil service employees during 1957. (From *Patterns of Disease.* Parke, Davis and Co., January, 1960.)

The proliferation in recent years of a multitude of new industrial chemicals—an estimated one every 20 minutes, the effects of which are as yet unknown in the workplace, and against which humans may have no defense because of the absence of post-exposure experience—is causing great concern. Also, it has been estimated that almost one half of all workers in this country are exposed to significant levels of known toxic substances. In addition to physical hazards, there is increasing concern for new hazards, such as lasers and microwaves.

Occupational Lung Diseases

Workers who are exposed to hazards in the air—cotton fibers, coal dust, asbestos, and other substances—can develop lung disease. Pneumoconiosis is a general term for these lung diseases. "Black lung" is a common name for coal worker's pneumoconiosis. Heavy coal dust exposure over many years can cause impaired lung fuction. More than 95,000 totally disabled miners and 75,000 widows are currently receiving federal benefits as victims of the disease. Improved ventilation in mines and wet drilling may help reduce black lung disease.

Asbestosis is a lung disease caused by inhaling asbestos fibers, which irritate lung tissues and cause thickening of the walls of the air sacs. By the time minimal changes become apparent on x-rays, the walls are already considerably thickened, thus interfering with the exchange of oxygen and carbon dioxide. Lung cancer is much more prevalent among asbestos workers—especially those who also smoke—than among the general population. Some 200,000 workers in the United States are directly involved in the production and installation of asbestos products. Fibers in the air are believed to be a factor in the deaths of more than 3000 workers each year (see p. 417).

Berylliosis is a disease of the lungs caused by inhalation of dust from the metal beryllium, used in nuclear reactors and missile systems. There may be years between the last exposure and onset of symptoms. Treatment with drugs can relieve some of the symptoms, such as breathlessness, if administered early in the course of the disease.

Silicosis is another dust disease of the lung, caused by breathing silica dust. Workers in rock, granite, and marble industries are exposed to the dust, as are metal miners, coal workers, and those who make china and pottery. Other, less common dust diseases are caused by such airborne materials as sugar cane dust or fungal spores in moldy hay. Some dusts, such as iron, do no damage.

Fungus Infections

Spores of fungi or moldlike substances are constantly present in the air we breathe. Many reach our lungs without producing disease. A few fungi, however, can cause lung diseases whose symptoms resemble tuberculosis. Histoplasmosis is triggered by spores that are tiny and light enough to float in dusty air. The spores flourish in warm, moist, dark places: old chicken houses, pigeon lofts, barns, and under trees where birds roost. When the spores are inhaled, they go into the air passages of the lungs; some may travel on to the air sacs, then multiply in the lymph nodes. If the infection remains in the lungs it is not as serious as when it spreads throughout the body. When the disease does spread, it can be fatal.

Skin tests, blood tests, and chest x-rays can help detect the infection. Drugs may be required to treat severe cases. Coccidioidomycosis is another lung disease caused by inhaling dust contaminated by spores. Perhaps 60 to 70 per cent of all people infected with cocci develop no symptoms at all. Those who have symptoms may develop a fever that goes as high as 104 degrees. Symptoms usually appear one to three weeks after the spores invade the lungs and body. There are usually aches and pains as well as a cough. A week or two after the fever rages, some patients get a rash that resembles measles. There may also be sores on the shins and pains in the joints. Usually symptoms disappear within a month or so. Tests of body fluids, blood, and skin can detect the disease. Chest x-rays can reveal abnormalities. Cough and fever can be treated. When the disease spreads throughout the body, drugs must be administered into the blood stream.

Pesticides

No one disputes the fact that by now most Americans have a significant amount of dieldrin (corn crop pesticide) and DDT in their bodies, but there is still debate about whether the levels are sufficient to cause cancer. Mice given food with levels of dieldrin similar to those in human foods have developed cancer, especially in the liver. Some scientists say there is no evidence that those results apply to humans; however, the Environmental Protection Agency insists that dieldrin has "unreasonable and adverse effects on man."

One of the main objectives of the "environmental movement" is the banning of the insecticide DDT. The drive to obtain this ban has become a crusade in which every effort is made to get public support. As a result, people frequently ask questions about the "dangers" of DDT, which has an astonishing record of safety and usefulness. Simmons, in a study on DDT, said:

> Except for the antibiotics, it is doubtful that any material has been found which protects more people against more diseases over a large area than does DDT. Most of the peoples of the globe have received some measure of benefit from this compound, either directly by protection from infectious diseases and pestiferous insects, or indirectly by better nutrition, cleaner food, and increased disease resistance.[37]

Most of DDT's benefits to health are in warm climates, where malaria and other arthropod-borne diseases are prevalent. The World Health Organization (WHO) states that more than 960 million people who used to be subject to endemic malaria are now free of this sickness.[38] DDT has also been of great use in agriculture, especially on potatoes and other vegetables, cotton, rice, and oil seed crops. WHO notes that there have been no detectable toxic effects in spraymen who have worked for years in malaria eradication. These men constantly breathe DDT spray, and more than 130,000 have been employed in the program.

In 1970, the American Medical Association councils on occupational health and on environmental and public health stated that it was an established fact that pesticide handlers who have been studied with great care during the past 30 years have DDT concentrations in fat up to 50 times that of the general population.[38] However, careful research has shown no interference with their health, despite long-continued exposure. Injuries to humans have been observed only in persons who accidentally received acute massive doses.[38]

On the other hand, DDT is fatal to many insects and quite toxic to crustaceans and fish; at high levels, it is toxic to wild birds. This has occurred following misuse, as when birds were exposed to heavy spraying. DDT has killed fish and other aquatic life when sprayed over bodies of water. This practice has been discontinued. DDT killed robins that were in elm trees during spraying for insect control, and DDT is no longer used for this purpose. In any case, there is a great deal of disagreement, bureaucratic morass, and political maneuvering. Hopefully, decisions will be made that will conserve the quality of life and lead to the prevention of disease and the promotion of health. In all controversial matters such as this, we must continually evaluate current knowledge and research and weigh *risks* versus *benefits.*

Asbestosis

In the asbestos industry alone, 200,000 workers are currently employed; another 800,000 workers have been employed. Among these 1 million workers, it is estimated that over 3000 deaths will occur each year for the next 20 or 30 years from cancer of the lungs and respiratory disease. For example, while producing insulation for the boilers and pipes of naval ships, workers in the Pittsburgh Corning Corporation (P.C.C.) in Tyler, Texas, were exposed to enormous quantities of asbestos dust, which, once inhaled, never leaves the lungs. Now, based on previous experience with asbestos-caused diseases, medical experts estimate that as many as 300 of the 869 employed at the plant since 1954 will die of asbestosis (a permanent and often progressive scarring of lung tissues from inhaled asbestos fibers), lung cancer, or cancers of the colon, rectum, or stomach.

Asbestosis and related cancers may not develop until 30 years after exposure to the particles, but once they do, they are painful and often fatal. The large number of deaths that result from these cancers should come as no surprise to either company or government officials. Doctors have long suspected that asbestos dust is hazardous; there has been ample documentation of increased incidence of lung disease and cancers among people exposed to the mineral. Pittsburgh Corning Corporation officials ordered a study of the asbestos-dust hazard at Tyler in 1963. The report seriously underestimated the hazard. A 1966 dust survey found asbestos levels to be above recommended thresholds in many areas of the plant, and a 1967 survey by the United States Public Health Service's Division of Occupational Health confirmed that the levels were high, but did not warn of the health hazard. After a Labor Department study two years later reported the same conditions, respirators were issued to workers in the plant's dustiest areas. But, according to workers, at no time did Pittsburgh Corning Corporation officials tell them that they were exposed to a health hazard.

It was not until a 1970 law created the National Institute for Occupational Safety and Health (NIOSH) and gave the Labor Department's Occupational Safety and Health Administration (OSHA) the authority to enforce compliance with asbestos standards that thorough investigation was initiated. In 1971 a NIOSH team visited Tyler, confirmed the danger of the dust levels, and emphasized the extraordinary hazard. The team pointed out many examples of poor hygiene practices: the company lunchroom was close to the production area and workers were using compressed-air hoses to blow dust off each other (thereby spreading the dust about), and the company was selling burlap bags contaminated with asbestos. NIOSH promptly notified OSHA, which inspected the plant, fined P.C.C. $210, and gave it four months to come up to standards. When a reinspection showed that the company still had not installed the necessary dust-control equipment, OSHA fined it $7990 and promised further action. Forced to make a decision, P.C.C. closed the plant, citing economic as well as environmental reasons.

One group of former employees is suing P.C.C. for $100 million in damages; some individuals are also bringing $1 million suits against the government for failing to protect them. But neither the suits nor any belated medical care that the workers may now receive is likely to alter the odds against their survival.

Occupational Environments

There is no occupation and no place of employment that is completely free of the potential for causing occupational disease. Approximately 13,000 known toxic substances are so widespread throughout our society that all employed persons come into daily contact with many of them. At present, there is little data indicating the frequency and types of occupational diseases. However, the Michigan Occupational Health Program has identified the leading occupational diseases in the state as follows:

OCCUPATIONAL DISEASE	COMMENTS
1. Dermatitis	Involves irritation or damage to the skin caused by chemicals used in industry, construction, or agriculture. More than 46% of all workmen's compensation claims are due to dermatitis.
2. Carbon monoxide poisoning	Encountered throughout society. Greatest exposure potential in manufacturing plants, warehouses, foundries, service garages, and steel-making operations.
3. Chemical intoxication	Results from inhalation of toxic vapors and fumes in foundries, metal finishing, dry cleaning, and general industries.
4. Pneumoconiosis	Caused by penetration of dust into the lungs.
Silicosis	From dust in foundries, mines, and quarries.
Asbestosis	In manufacturing and insulating trades.
5. Hearing loss	Caused by exposure to excessive noise in many industrial plants, in transportation, and in service industries.

Industrial Safety Programs

The industrial safety programs have helped reduce the national industrial accident frequency by 75 per cent. This reduction was due largely to the application of preventive medicine in industry. During this period, absenteeism was cut in half, compensation costs were reduced by two-thirds, and accident sickness costs were decreased 40 to 50 per cent. Many small plants joined medical service plans which served many companies.

Industrial accidents are caused by personal or mechanical difficulties. It has been said that 80 to 85 per cent of industrial accidents are due to faulty human actions and less than 20 per cent are due to mechanical design factors. Perhaps safety may be improved if mechanical design is more closely related to the anatomical, physiological, and psychological characteristics of workers. Personal causes include unnecessary exposure, accident proneness, improper starting or stopping of machinery, operating machinery at unsafe speed, lack of skill or knowledge, improper machine guards, hazardous arrangements, and unsafe wearing apparel. A good accident-prevention program in industrial safety includes personnel selection combined with adequate medical examination, human engineering, and job supervision.

Occupational and Community Health Safety Recommendations: Actual Cases

Ventilation in Garages. A Cincinnati Health Department survey of garages during cold weather disclosed widespread deficiencies in ventilation. Air in 48 garages with capacities of four to more than 25 cars was analyzed by using an MSA squeeze bulb sampler. Carbon monoxide concentration in 13 garages exceeded 100 ppm; it was between 25 and 100 ppm in 23 others. These readings were not taken at peak periods. A drive to improve conditions was initiated by complaints from several sources. Owners were concerned with the failure of some mechanics to use exhaust hoses. Service managers criticized owners who neglected defective mufflers and tailpipes. Mechanics reported frequent headaches, nausea, and loss of appetite.

Auto Body Shops. California studies of automobile body repair operations often poorly ventilated, with little or no suitable sanitary facilities, have pointed up several hazards: skin contact with plastic body fillers, solvents, grease, and dirt; inhalation of paint spray, solvent fumes, plastic dust (from grinding), and carbon monoxide; and exposure to flammable and explosive materials. It has been observed that right-handed workers are likely to develop boils on the left side of the body because more plastic dust is directed at that side during grinding. Multiple boils have been seen on the left forearm, under the left arm, on the left thigh, and particularly below the left knee, where dust is easily forced into the skin of the kneeling worker.

Innovation in Sewer Maintenance. Closed-circuit television is used in Pennsylvania for sewer and pipeline maintenance. A section of the sewer is first rodded from manhole to manhole; then a television camera is attached to the rod and pulled through the line. Personnel in an air-conditioned portable trailer watch the findings on the screen.

Silicosis in Sandblasting. Two patients with advanced silicosis were discovered among eight workers employed by a Massachusetts company to sandblast and clean external walls. When the first was discovered, it was learned there had been no x-ray survey of these workers. One of the patients had developed silicotuberculosis, and the other, who was clinically asymptomatic, showed evidence of pulmonary deficiency after removal of a cancerous lobe of lung.

Phosdrin-Contaminated Clothing. Investigation of repeated illness of an 8-year-old California boy revealed it occurred only when he wore his jeans. The suspect jeans, which had been purchased at a salvage depot, were found to be impregnated with Phosdrin, a potent insecticide. In the next few weeks, four other boys and two adults had similar symptoms, and one boy became critically ill. Through radio, television, and newspaper publicity, all purchasers of jeans from the same lot were urged to submit them to the local health department for laboratory testing. All recovered clothing was tested by the California Department of Agriculture, and one batch was found contaminated with up to 5 per cent pure Phosdrin. Further investigation disclosed a container of Phosdrin had been punctured in transit with a consignment of jeans, which had absorbed most of the spilled insecticide. The jeans had been stored seven months before being placed on sale.*

X-ray Exposure. The California Bureaus of Occupational Health and Radiologic Health investigated the illness of a 38 year old woman who had worked for 12 years as an x-ray technician and was believed to have an occupationally induced blood disease. In October 1961, she noticed an abrupt onset of fatigue, weakness, muscular aching, nausea, and loss of appetite. Her physician-employer did a routine white count, red count, and blood smear on at least three occasions and found she had a white count of 2500 with relative lymphocytosis of 90 per cent but with an absolute reduction in both lymphocytes and granulocytes. Results of bone marrow biopsies compared with the appearance of peripheral blood, together with her negative history of drug intake and major illness, strongly suggested excessive exposure to ionizing radiation. The x-ray equipment she used during the previous five years exposed the technician in the process of obtaining a radiogram to approximately 1000 mr./hr. When she held a patient during an exposure, she was in a field of about 20,000 mr./hr. She was frequently in the room during fluoroscopy without protection from a leaded apron. The direct beam overlapped the lead glass fluoroscopic screen by two inches on either side. The technician received most of her exposure, estimated at a monthly total of about 12,000 mr., during fluoroscopic examinations. (Maximum permissible dose recommended is 100 mr./wk. or 400 mr./mo.) At no time during the last five years did she carry a dosimeter or wear a film badge to monitor her exposure.[39]

Parathion Deaths in Florida. Ten Florida residents, most of them small children, lost their lives in 1961 from contact with the organic phosphate insecticide, parathion. Several cases and two deaths occurred in Tampa among five children who took an innocent-looking burlap bag from a trashpile. The bag had previously been placed around a sack of fertilizer taken from a watermelon field and transported to Tampa. The children filled the bag with rags and used it as a swing. Approximately eight hours after swinging from the bag, one little girl was taken to the hospital and died soon after admission. Her little brother became ill shortly thereafter and died in the hospital during the same night. Three other children who had played with the swing were taken to the hospital but recovered. The burlap bag, on chemical examination by the United States Public Health Service, was found to have been contaminated with an oil solution of parathion. A third death resulted when a child was exposed to 15 per cent parathion and chlordane dust that had been applied inside the home by an unlicensed pest control operator; he was untrained and offered his services illegally. The most recent death in Tampa occurred in a 17 year old boy who was handling empty parathion drums that had not been decontaminated before their sale to a junk dealer. Six other children died during 1961 from contact with parathion, which in most cases had been taken into the home.[40]

Cadmium Poisoning in California. Thirty to 45 minutes after drinking pink lemonade, 23 school children, aged 5 to 9, experienced abdominal cramps and vomiting in an outbreak due to cadmium contamination. All recovered within 48 hours. The severity of symptoms correlated with the amount of lemonade consumed. Nine other children, who only tasted or consumed small amounts of the lemonade, did not become ill. Each child brought a lunch from home; the lemonade was the only food common to all 32. The lemonade was prepared by adding the proper amount of city water and ice cubes to three cans of a commercially prepared concentrate. The mixture was placed in a three gallon cadmium plated war surplus container for the 3½ hour interval between preparation and serving. Laboratory analysis of a sample of the remaining lemonade revealed 21 parts per million of cadmium, a

*Occupational health notes. Publ. Health Rep., *78*:260, 1963.

dosage considered sufficient to cause the symptoms in the children.[41]

Antimony Poisoning in Illinois. A group of 35 preschool age children all experienced vomiting 30 to 45 minutes after drinking a raspberry flavored beverage at a Chicago Sunday school Halloween party. Some children also became pallid; others dizzy. Three were hospitalized for less than 24 hours. No fatalities occurred. Only this drink and potato chips were served. Because of the rapid onset of symptoms, the premises were carefully inspected for evidence of insecticides, rodenticides, and other toxic materials. None was found.

The investigators learned that the beverage had been prepared by mixing the contents of several packages of the raspberry powder with sugar and water in an old porcelain roasting pan, and then refrigerated for 40 hours prior to serving. No trace of chemical could be found in the powder concentrate or in the potato chips. Antimony was detected in the small quantity of remaining beverage and from acid washings of the pan. An insufficient quantity remained for quantitative analysis. Accordingly, the Chicago Board of Health laboratory workers repeated the entire procedure, using the same roasting pan; 2.8 mg. per cent antimony was detected.[42]

Antimony Poisoning in Virginia. Twenty persons experienced nausea, vomiting, abdominal pain, and varying degrees of prostration 15 to 45 minutes after drinking punch poured from a large gray "granite" enamelware coffee pot while attending an annual church-school meeting. Cherry juice, powdered citric acid mix, sugar, saccharin, and lemon juice concentrate were mixed in a two gallon gray enamelware coffee pot, and stored in a refrigerator for 24 hours.

Children attending Bible classes were served cookies and punch by age groups in the order of kindergarten, primary, junior, and junior high. The nursery group was not served because others were already becoming ill by the time their turn arrived. The small quantity of remaining punch, negative for the usual bacteriological pathogens, had a pH of 4.6 and a positive qualitative test for antimony. Simulated punch, made in the laboratory in the same coffee pot using the same ingredients and refrigerated for the same length of time, showed a pH of 4.6 and a concentration of antimony of 11 parts per million or 0.325 mg. per ounce. The punch was served in 3 ounce cups, and most drank only one serving.

Recovery was prompt and uneventful. It is noted that of the groups who drank the punch, only the first two groups were affected; none of the older children (junior and junior high) were ill and only one of the 11 teachers. In an effort to explain this phenomenon, consideration was given to the possibility of varying concentrations of antimony at different levels due to settling. However, samples taken at different levels in the pot of simulated punch did not show any appreciable variation. Virginia State Health authorities postulate that at this low concentration of antimony, the smaller body weight of the younger group may have been significant in the poisoning. Notably, a similar episode occurred the previous year during this annual church-school meeting.[43]

Alkyl Mercury Poisoning in Humans. Three members of a family of nine that ingested mercury-contaminated pork became ill with classic symptoms of methylmercury poisoning and rapidly progressed to coma or semicomatose states. Treatment with dimercaprol (BAL in oil) and n-acetyl-d, I-penicillamine was not associated with significant immediate clinical improvement, although both drugs appeared to increase urinary excretion of mercury. All three patients improved considerably but still remain severely impaired. A case of congenital methylmercury poisoning also resulted from the outbreak. This is the first known instance in the United States of methylmercury poisoning resulting from ingestion of mercury-contaminated meat.[44]

Other Hazards

Glazed Tableware

A new law regulates the amount of lead and cadmium in glazed tableware. Passage of this law was motivated by public concern after a family was poisoned by orange juice contaminated by lead from the glaze of a pitcher in which the juice had been stored. The acid in the juice had leached the lead out of the improperly glazed earthenware. Since improperly glazed or decaled tableware can release lead or cadmium over a long period of time, there is the additional danger of accumulating these metals in the body until a toxic quantity has been stored and illness or death results. Any manufacturer or importer who introduces glazed ceramic tableware for sale in California now needs a Certificate of Acceptability, which assures that lead and cadmium levels are below those specified in the law. Manufacturers and importers will be required to submit test results to the Department of Health before a certificate is issued for the pattern produced. The department will monitor tests to ensure that all laboratories are making accurate analyses.

Some historians have suggested that the decline of the Roman Empire was due, in part, to lead poisoning as a result of the wide use of lead-based pewter for eating utensils.

In any case, poisonings attributed to lead salts have plagued man from the time he started putting food on plates. If the glazes are properly formulated, applied, and fired, the lead salts are sealed and cannot be leached out by acidic foods such as fruit juices, soft drinks, cider, or those containing vinegar. Some manufacturers save the cost of testing by producing glazes that do not contain lead or cadmium.

Nerve Illness

The Ohio Department of Health was involved in the investigation of an outbreak of peripheral neuropathy in a wall-covering manufacturing plant. (Neuropathy is a general term denoting functional disturbances and/or pathological changes in the peripheral nervous system.) The illness caused weakness and muscle wasting in affected employees. The cause was ultimately identified as a solvent used mainly in printing inks. The solvent was removed from production processes; measures to prevent exposure of workers to chemicals were instituted. All employees most severely affected showed remarkable and encouraging improvement. Many have had complete return of muscular strength.

Vinyl Chloride

Vinyl chloride (VC) is a colorless gas that has been used as a propellant in such popular products as hair spray and disinfectant and insect sprays. It is also the principal ingredient of polyvinyl chlorides, the plastics that go into a host of familiar products, including food wrappers and containers, suitcases, detergent bottles, and garbage bags. Increasing evidence links vinyl chloride to a crippling bone disease and a rare but invariably fatal form of cancer. In 1974, B. F. Goodrich Co. reported that, since 1971, three men who worked with VC in its Louisville, Kentucky, plastics plant had died of angiosarcoma of the liver. Since then, doctors have identified nine more cases of the cancer in the United States, one in Great Britain, and another in Norway. Since such cancers may not develop for at least 15 years after initial exposure, environmental health researchers suspect that more cases will be uncovered.

In the United States alone, over 6500 workers are involved in making VC gas for converting the gas into PVC; thousands more are engaged in converting the plastic into finished products. European and Japanese films are also heavily involved in VC production. The Department of Labor's Occupational Safety and Health Administration has issued emergency regulations reducing allowable VC levels to 50 parts per million. Whether this is adequate to provide long-term protection for plastics workers remains to be seen. An industry-sponsored study has shown that when mice are exposed to those levels, they develop angiosarcoma.

Silo-Filler's Disease

Silo-filler's disease is a little-known health hazard caused by a highly toxic gas, nitrogen dioxide (NO_2), emitted by grain (particularly corn) during the first few days of storage. Whether or not corn will emit this gas in significant amounts depends on the conditions under which it is grown. Excess nitrogen in the soil and factors interfering with conversion of nitrates into plant protein can cause excess nitrate accumulation in the grain. In confirmed spaces such as bins, it takes only a small amount of the gas to reach hazardous or even lethal concentrations.

Meat-Wrapper's Asthma

Sokol et al. have reported the following:

> Three patients employed as meat wrappers developed respiratory symptoms when exposed to the fumes of a polyvinyl chloride film cut with a hot wire. The patients were middle-aged women who smoked cigarettes and demonstrated reversible airway obstruction on pulmonary function testing. The cause of their symptoms is not known, but some ingredient of the polyvinyl chloride film is suspected.[45]

Green-Tobacco Sickness

Tobacco-associated occupational illness occurs regularly in North Carolina tobacco fields. Green-tobacco sickness is a self-limited illness characterized by pallor, vomiting, and prostration. It occurs principally in young men who handle uncured tobacco leaves in the fields. A survey among 53 harvesters who had had green-tobacco sickness and 49 control harvesters was undertaken to define and quantify the symptom complex. The illness was correlated with cropping (picking) the tobacco while it was wet; the absorption of nicotine from the tobacco leaf is the probable cause. Cigarette smoking affords protection against the illness.[46]

SAFETY EDUCATION

Accidents are the fourth leading cause of death in the United States today, and are outranked only by heart, cancer, and cerebral hemorrhage fatalities. Accidents are the leading cause of death in children five to 14 years of age in the United States and 12 other countries in the Western Hemisphere.[47] They also account for about 100,000 deaths each year, and injure, disable, and cripple another 10 million persons.

Many parents are more concerned about the child's diet, a rash, or some mild disease than they are by the fact that accidents claim the lives of more than 15,000 children every year. Accidents kill more children each year than polio, cancer, heart disease, pneumonia, tuberculosis and kidney diseases combined. Approximately 40,000 to 50,000 children are permanently crippled by accidents in the United States each year.

During the bloody Second World War, the United States suffered an average of 65,330 combat dead and 149,077 combat wounded each year; during 1975 the accident toll was 100,000 dead and 10,000,000 injured. What other nation in history has managed to be more deadly at work and play than it has been at war? The number of Americans killed accidentally during 1975 was nearly triple the number of American fighting men killed during the entire Korean War.

If this is a normally "safe" week, 1800 Americans alive this morning will be dead in seven days from today. They will die in accidents, most of them avoidable. Another 173,000 will be hurt in avoidable accidents. During this average week, 11 hunters will either kill themselves by careless handling of their own guns or be shot to death by companions who mistake them for four-footed game; 31 other firearm deaths will include children between five and 14 years of age. Among the do-it-yourself handymen, 18 will be electrocuted doing home repair jobs because they forgot to turn off the current. Approximately 385 persons, most of whom are 65 and older, will suffer fatal falls on slippery pavements, in bathtubs, and on highly polished floors. Fires will claim another 121 lives, and many victims will be smokers who lit their last cigarette in bed just before falling asleep. About 50 will die from leaking gas or poisons taken by mistake. The leading accident killer, motor vehicles, will claim about 731 persons. Drownings, which claim about 6500 persons each year, will account for 138 fatalities during the average week. Varying only slightly from year to year, the annual accident toll amounts to approximately 150,000 fatalities and 10,050,000 injuries, 120,000 of which result in permanent disability.

Health department officials added accident prevention and safety education to their programs long ago. These programs include health education, epidemiological investigations, pilot studies, and research. Accidents can be prevented and the lives of many can thereby be prolonged.

Causes of Accidents

Although safety education is stressed in the public schools and in virtually all communities in the United States, many persons in our population have not learned common safety facts and attitudes. Many accidents are caused by individuals who perform skills beyond their ability, individuals who are emotionally disturbed, individuals who may have impaired vision and hearing, individuals who are fatigued, and individuals who are taking such drugs as antihistamines and tranquilizers. There seems to be no simple or single cure for accidents. Mechanical and personal failures, environmental hazards, inadequate knowledge, insufficient skills, improper attitudes, and bad habits are the prime causes of accidents.

Because of the importance of the human variables, the control of accidents falls within the province of preventive medicine and public health, as do the fields of industrial hygiene and other public health problems. In most instances, there is a causation in accidents, and attempts at control should involve consideration of the agent and the environment.

Physicians could help immensely with this problem by taking the initiative in identifying the causes of accidents leading to their occurrence and by indoctrinating patients with the principles of accident prevention while they are being treated.

In most work injury accidents, both an unsafe act and an unsafe condition are contributing factors in accidents. Congested working space, improperly stored materials, improper illumination, and improper safety devices on equipment contribute heavily to injuries. In schools, athletic coaches, physical education teachers, and recreation leaders should check equipment periodically to see that it is safe at all times for use in their programs.

HOME SAFETY

One person in 43 in the United States was disabled one or more days by injuries received in home accidents last year. Falls caused the most injuries (19,000), followed in order by fires and burns (7000), firearms (2600), poison (2500), machinery (2000), and poison gas (1700).

The state health departments are generally accepting the role of initiators and coordinators of statewide home safety efforts, especially in states having no state safety organization. In the majority of departments, current records of home accident fatalities in their state are maintained. Some state health departments conduct research studies in some phase of accident prevention.

Minnesota has been active in home safety as part of its public health activities. The safety program has been closely related to activities of state and local safety councils, the state and local departments of education and social welfare, the fire marshall's office, and the industrial commission. Accidents rank among the foremost causes of death and disability in Minnesota. Because of this, the Minnesota Department of Health has introduced a full force program against accidents, using its monthly bulletin, *Minnesota's Health,* radio broadcasts, stories of accidents from newspapers and radio stations, safety education in the schools, and pamphlets issued on accidents. There is convincing evidence that certain types of home accidents can be prevented through state and local health department programs.

Springfield, Oregon, conducted an accident study through the cooperation of the school district, the P.T.A., the Oregon traffic safety commission, and other local and state agencies. Thirteen elementary schools, three junior high schools, and two high schools with an enrollment of over 7200 students were included in the study. All accidents to school-age children were reported during the school year. Absenteeism, type of accident, and place of occurrence were checked. Sixty-five per cent occurred at school, 21 per cent at home, and 14 per cent in public places. Fifty-seven per cent of those occurring at school were associated with physical education and related sports.

SAFETY IN INDUSTRY

Eye Safety Available To All

The reduction of eye injuries in industry since the establishment of the National Bureau of Standards' Eye Protection Code in 1921 has brought eye injury rates in industry far below those of the general public. Yet the greatest danger is in home, recreational and automobile accidents—especially to children. The first decade of life yields more lost eyes than any subsequent decade, and almost one third of those losses are due to injuries which are largely preventable.

Since an economical means of prevention is readily available, it is tragic that a great many of the estimated 50 per cent of all Americans who wear spectacles are provided only with fragile glass, which upon impact often shatters into dangerous slivers to damage or destroy irreplaceable human vision. Millions more, who don't require spectacles, wear unsafe sunglasses.

The American Medical Association's Committee on the Medical Aspects of Automotive Safety points out that the same eye protection now enjoyed by industrial workers is available to the American public generally. This protection consists basically of a combination of heat-treated glass or impact-resistant plastic lenses with fire-retardant frames.

The use of safe spectacles is making some headway. The three military services are initiating a change to impact-resistant lenses for all service personnel. A number of states require safety lenses for personnel in all chemistry and vocational classes in school. Alaska became the first state to legislate safety lenses and fire-resistant frames for all glasses, and the National Highway Safety Bureau has footnoted its vehicle safety standards with an admonition that all drivers and passengers needing spectacles should have these prepared with safety materials.

With all this information at hand, American medicine with its allies in opticianry can hardly do less than encourage in the strongest fashion the

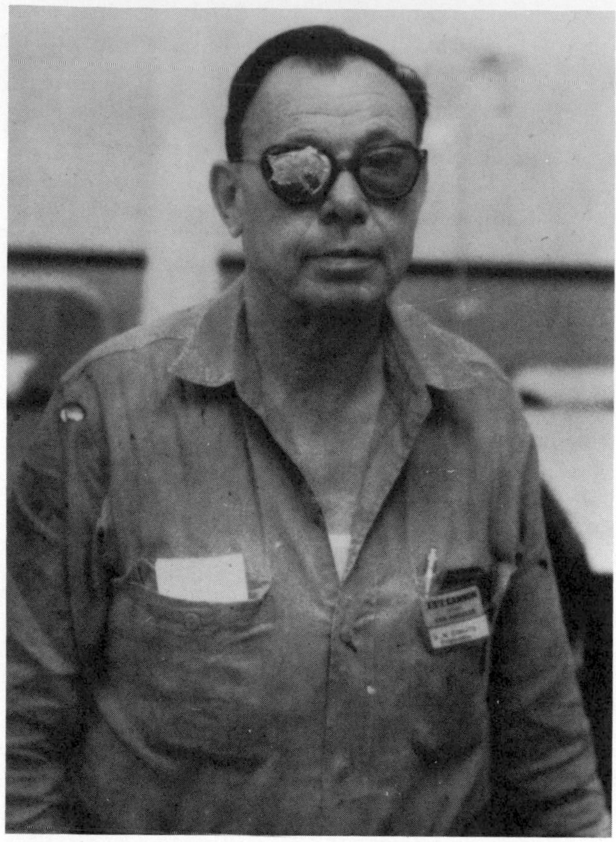

Figure 11–27 (Courtesy of Dr. Packard Thurber, Jr., and JAMA, *213*:1993, 1970. Copyright 1970 by the American Medical Association.)

replacement of all inferior spectacles and sunglasses with those which are truly protective shields.[48]

TRAFFIC SAFETY

The medical profession claims that accidents are our foremost public health problem. It is true that heart disease and cancer claim more lives than accidents, but then diseases take their heaviest toll in senior citizens. The auto, when it kills, takes more years of life. For example, it is the number one killer of the college-age group. Unfortunately, the interest of the average driver is for more horsepower, more speed, and new design, rather than for safety features.

The idea that driving a car is a vested right is diminishing. Instead it is becoming a sought-after privilege. Many states have tightened their licensing procedures and a few require medical examinations every few years. Most traffic experts recommend a four-pronged attack on the problem: increasing the number and quality of high school driver education courses and increasing traffic safety courses on the college level, encouraging parents to set good examples as drivers, making dangerous driving socially unacceptable among youngsters, and wherever possible, enforcing traffic rules through student government.

In spite of the gains made in traffic safety, the full potential of public education has not been fully exploited. It requires the efforts of the entire community—physicians, law enforcement officers, educators, lawyers, press and radio.

The American Medical Association, through its Committee on Automobile Crash Injuries and Deaths, has studied the problem with related interested industries. Year after year, approximately 40,000 Americans are killed in motor vehicle accidents. In the states where the accident rates have been decreasing, officials point to the rigid enforcement of the following safety measures:

1. Increasing the number of police patrols on the highways.
2. Suspension of licenses of motorists convicted of drunk driving.
3. Tougher examination for drivers' licenses and mandatory vehicle inspections.
4. Use of sheriff's deputies to reinforce regular highway police during peak travel periods.

5. Expansion of use of radar devices.
6. Establishing state speed limits where they are not already in force.

In addition to these measures, the energy crisis, which helped to reduce the speed limit to 55 miles per hour and lowered the number of miles many people drive as a result of increased gasoline costs, has probably helped to reduce auto fatalities to a significant extent.

Accident Prevention

Safety educators and safety engineers will continue to have a difficult time preventing accidents, saving lives, and extending the scope of safe living until the public is fully aroused. The organization of the Committee on Highway Safety of the National Governors' Conference shows great promise in striving for uniformity and promoting safety education. At the forty-eighth Conference of Governors, a committee of governors was appointed to undertake an immediate study to make recommendations for the adoption of:

1. A uniform set of motor-vehicle laws for the 50 states (including signs, speed limits, traffic lights, signals, etc.).
2. Uniform enforcement of motor vehicle laws.
3. Nationwide reciprocity in upholding convictions and penalties from the enforcement of motor vehicle laws.
4. The development of state and community-wide programs for safety education.

Various methods for studying this problem of motor vehicle accidents have been proposed; a few have been carried out. Many experts suggest that the epidemiological approach, so familiar to health departments in other programs, may be applied advantageously to studying causation and possible prevention of motor vehicle accidents. The epidemiological approach includes study of the host factors such as behavior and attitudes; motor and sensory defects; effects of fatigue, alcohol, and drugs on driver responses; and environmental factors, e.g., seasonal, geographic, climatic, and urban versus rural incidence.

Prevention of accidents can be grouped under the three E's—Education, Enforcement, and Engineering. The process of learning to live safely involves understanding the many hazards that one must encounter in his various daily activities, developing attitudes and behavior patterns that predispose one to adjust properly to his environment, and mastering skills that enable one to cope with particularly dangerous situations.

It is essential to motivate and educate people to assume the role of responsible citizens, to cooperate with authorities and others in upholding the law, and to make the home, school, community, factory, and highway safe places for all.

Safety Council

A school-community safety council can help prevent accidents and help develop social and civic responsibility. Perhaps no other phase of the school program offers students a greater opportunity to prepare for citizenship and "to learn by doing" than do these organizations. A school may organize a safety council to coordinate all safety matters brought to its attention, to coordinate the various school activities concerned with accident prevention, and to establish safety regulations regarding such matters as the use of bicycles and motor vehicles and safe conduct in and around the school. A school-community safety program should be concerned not only with teaching children and adults how to avoid accidents, but with eliminating the physical hazards that endanger them. All members and agencies in the community should cooperate and actively participate in promoting safety. The local safety and health council must maintain a continuous education program, and must find and eliminate safety hazards in an effort to prevent accidents.

RADIOLOGICAL HEALTH

One group of physical agents deserving separate attention today is the radiological agents. Examples of radiation or energy are all around us. The colors we see and the noises we hear depend upon the nature of these energy waves. A match, stove, and light bulb release heat and light while radio waves, infrared lights, and ultraviolet lights release wave light energy and heat. The sun, a magnificent example of heat and light, has available energy to start fires, burn our skins, and cause chemical explosions. These are all examples of electromagnetic or wave light radiations, and the lower-energy, long wave length radio waves cannot penetrate as far, and are therefore not as dangerous as the high-energy, short wave length gamma rays. The other type of radiation or energy is released by streams of atomic particles called protons, electrons, or alpha particles during chemical reactions. These are referred to as corpuscular radiations.

Types of Ionizing Radiation

All sources of radiation are effective because of ionization. Ionization is the property that enables radioactive particles or rays to interact with matter and split atoms and molecules into pairs of electrically charged fragments called ions. For example, in the electrolysis of water, H_2O or HOH, it ionizes into the H^+ ion, and the OH^- ion. Ionization of living matter results in tissue changes that may affect health. The extent of tissue ionization depends upon the composition of the tissue and the quantity, type, and energy of the radiation. Tissue damage caused by ionization is partially irreversible.

Alpha Particles

Alpha particles have tremendous ionizing power, 10,000 times that of gamma rays. However, the relatively large alpha particles have a low penetrating power and range and are easily stopped by a thick sheet of paper or the external layer of skin on the body. As a result, damage due to external exposure generally is not significant. If, on the other hand, an alpha-emitting substance is swallowed, absorbed, or inhaled, severe internal damage may result. Radium is a powerful alpha emitter, and, once inside the human body, its retention is practically permanent. Only traces leave the body, mostly in the form of radon gas in expired air, sweat, feces, and urine.

Beta Particles

As negatively charged electrons, beta particles have 100 times the ionizing power of gamma rays, but can travel only a few yards through the air. Ordinarily, they can be stopped by clothing and will penetrate only a fraction of an inch to the skin, affecting it very much like a burn. A thin sheet of plastic, such as Lucite, or of light metal, such as aluminum, will stop the beta particle. Beta particles are emitted along with gamma rays, generally. However, certain radioisotopes are pure beta emitters. Energetic beta particles are most dangerous following ingestion or inhalation.

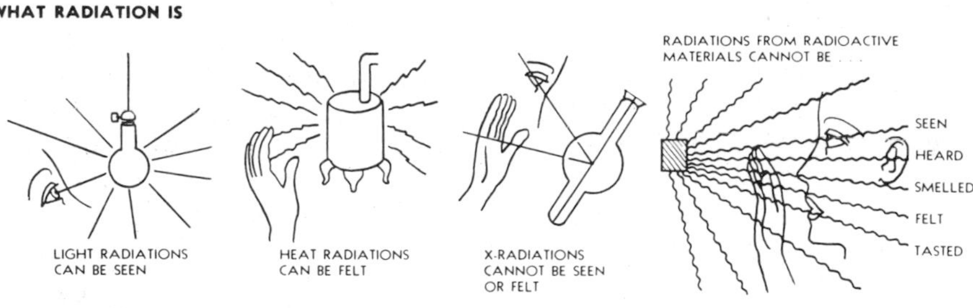

RADIOACTIVE RADIATIONS ARE STREAMS OF FAST-FLYING PARTICLES OR WAVES WHICH COME FROM UNSTABLE ATOMS

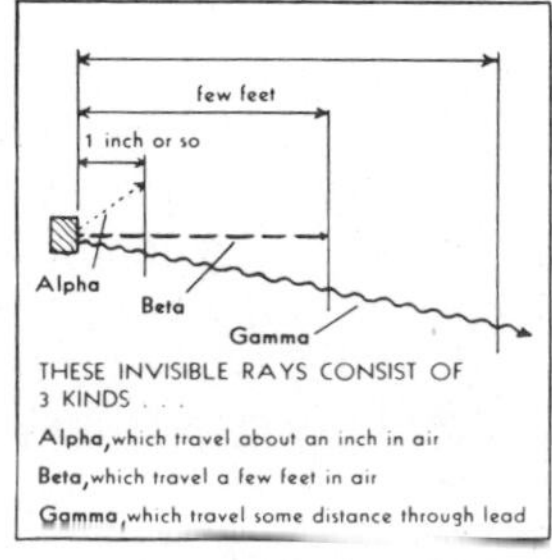

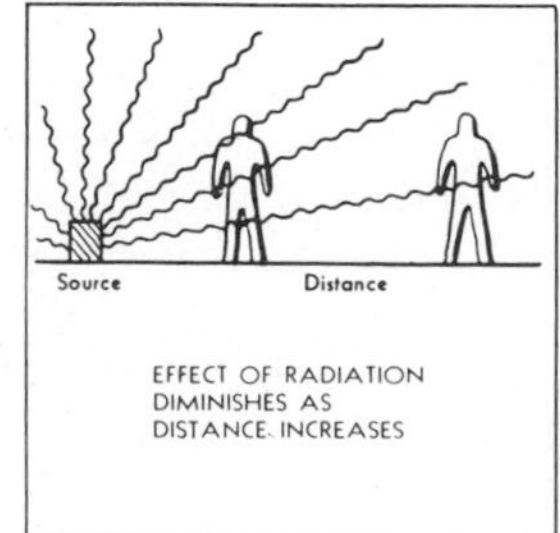

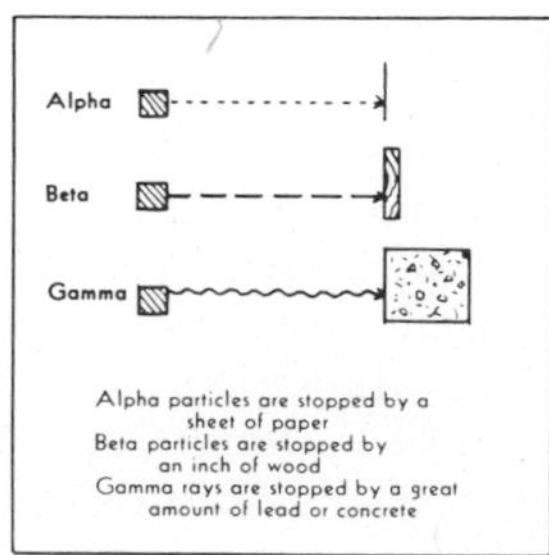

Figure 11–28 (From *You Can Understand the Atom*, U.S. Atomic Energy Commission.)

Gamma and X-rays

These have quite low specific ionization values, but characteristically are capable of penetrating matter. Lead, steel, and concrete are among those materials that are frequently used to reduce gamma or x-rays to harmless levels. As a group, gamma and x-ray radiations constitute the chief health hazard of external radiation. Only well-designed underground shelters could provide good protection from gamma radiation.

Neutrons

Neutrons are uncharged particles weighing about one-fourth as much as an alpha particle. They are incapable of causing ionization by themselves, but are able to impart sufficient energy to hydrogen atoms for them to cause ionization. Neutrons of high energy have a much greater biological effect than do low-energy neutrons. When an atom absorbs a neutron, it becomes radioactive, or emits gamma rays to get rid of the excess energy introduced by the captured neutron. High-energy neutrons are normally shielded with concrete, steel, water, or paraffin. Low-energy neutrons are readily absorbed by cadmium or boron. The major sources of neutrons are nuclear reactors.

Sources of Radioactivity

The application and frequency of use of radiation have increased tremendously in the past several years. This increase is not only the result of new developments in atomic pile–produced radioisotopes but also the result of an accelerated use of x-radiation and, in a more limited way, natural sources of gamma radiation, principally radium. It is not uncommon to find industrial plants, research laboratories, and hospitals where total exposure to radiation is the summation of the use of x-ray and fluoroscopic machines, radium, and radioisotopes.

The world is radioactive and will always remain so. The atoms of some elements, called the radioactive elements, undergo a spontaneous disintegration and release energy. Some of the common radioactive elements are uranium, thorium, actinium, polonium, and radium. The nuclei of these atoms are unstable and therefore explode. For example, after a series of disintegrations accompanied by radioactive energy, the radium atom finally becomes an isotope of lead, which is a stable element.

Nature

In the earth's crust are found large amounts of uranium, thorium, actinium, and their related elements. There is no portion of the earth's surface free from the radiation produced spontaneously by these materials. A square mile of surface soil 1 foot thick is conservatively estimated to contain an average of 1 gram of radium, 3 tons of uranium, and 6 tons of thorium, all of which are radioactive.[49] However, some natural places have subsoil that is rather free from radioactive elements and the earth's contribution to radioactivity is small there. Natural potassium has a radioactive isotope, potassium-40, the activity of which is appreciable. All natural potassium, whether in the earth's crust or as a component of living individuals, is thus radioactive and produces an appreciable increment in the total dose to which people are exposed. Likewise, the carbon which forms a large part of our bodies has a constant fraction, composed of the radioactive isotope of carbon of mass 14. This carbon is produced initially by the action of cosmic rays on the nitrogen of the atmosphere. Food, milk, and water, particularly water from wells and mineral springs, contain traces of radioactive substances detectable by modern, sensitive instruments. The air we breathe contains minute amounts of radon and thoron that are gaseous decay products of radium, uranium, and thorium from the earth.

It is interesting to note variations in background radiation. Total background radiation is least over the open ocean and greatest over granite. The weather, too, affects local conditions of atmospheric radioactivity. For example, radon, thoron, and their derivatives attach themselves to dust particles in the air; rainfall brings them down to the ground level; a snowfall prevents their escape from the ground into the air. Similarly, on a cloudy day there is less background radiation than on a clear day. Even man-made structures of wood, brick, or concrete emanate measurable quantities of radioactivity, and interior walls of plaster are sufficiently radioactive to affect the function of detecting instruments.

In Kerala, located at the southern tip of India, about 100,000 people live in fishing

TABLE 11–4 Types of Radiation

TYPE OF RADIATION	PHYSICAL NATURE	DISTANCE OF TRAVEL IN AIR	EFFECTIVE SHIELDING*	USUAL MEANS OF DETECTION	PRINCIPAL HAZARDS
ALPHA (α)	Heavy Particle, Helium nucleus, double positive charge–great ionizing power	Few inches maximum	Skin or thin layer of any solid material	Special laboratory instruments	Extreme hazard when taken into the body by inhalation, injestion, or through open wounds. Little external hazard.
BETA (β)	Light particle, electron, single negative charge	Few yards maximum	One-half inch of any solid material, clothing, Al	Geiger counter, film badge, dosimeter	Moderate internal and external hazards. Can cause skin burns.
GAMMA (γ)	Ray, similar to X-ray—low ionizing power—B particles usually emitted with γ rays	Very long	Lead, other heavy metals, concrete, tightly packed soil	Geiger counter, Ion chamber, Film badge, dosimeter	From sources external to the body—chief health hazard of external radiation.
NEUTRON (η)	Moderately heavy particle, neutral charge—high energy and low energy types	Very long	Water, steel, paraffin, concrete	Special laboratory instruments.	From sources external to the body.

*The best protection from *any* type of radiation is distance from the source of radiation (time and shielding are other factors). Gamma rays and neutrons are given off at the instant of detonation of an atomic bomb. This is termed *initial radiation.* Alpha, beta, and gamma radiating materials remain after the explosion. Radiation from this source is called *residual radiation.*

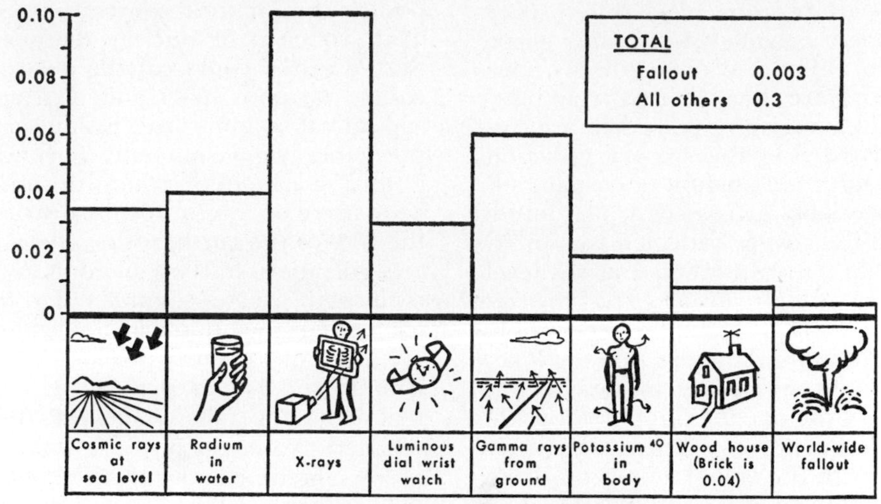

Figure 11–29 (From Teller, E., and Latter, A. L.: *Our Nuclear Future.* Criterion Books, New York, 1958.)

villages strung along 100 miles of a geological curiosity—an ocean beach whose black sands are radioactive. The people who live there have always lived in a radiation field about 10 times larger than the average radiation field in the United States. The incidence of babies born with Downs syndrome is 4 times higher in this area than in any other area in the world.

Cosmic Radiation

Cosmic radiation is that radiation coming from outside the earth, much of it from outside the solar system. Gamma rays of the very highest energy content are part of the complex nature of cosmic rays probably formed in the upper atmosphere

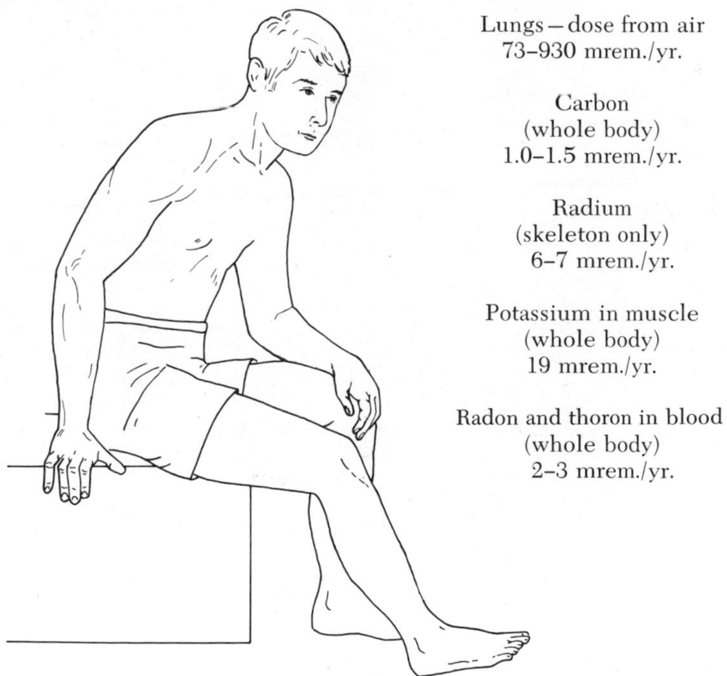

Figure 11–30 Distribution of radioactive substances in the human body.

by collisions of protons from outer space. They seemingly originate within our galaxy of stars—the Milky Way. Exceedingly energetic radiations are thus received from outer space, and all living things on earth are constantly bombarded by this celestial radiation. At high altitudes the amount of cosmic radiation is appreciably increased; at an altitude of 5000 feet the cosmic radiation is approximately double that experienced at sea level. Persons living at high altitudes are subjected to twice the natural radiation received by persons in nonmountainous areas. Pike's Peak has almost five times as much background radiation as does a point on the Pennsylvania Turnpike, which is designated as the place with the lowest amount of background radiation in the United States. Fortunately, however, the earth's atmosphere filters out most of the cosmic rays before they reach us. From all these natural sources of radioactivity, individuals may receive a total exposure in a lifetime of about 10 roentgens equivalent.

Weapons

In recent years there has been a man-made component added to the general exposure from natural sources of radioactivity. The sequence of nuclear detonations conducted in the course of the development of atomic weapons has resulted in addition of substantial amounts of fission products to the general environment. Through the action of stratospheric winds, this material has been more or less uniformly distributed over the face of the earth, with somewhat greater concentrations in the United States and generally with greater abundance in the Northern than in the Southern Hemisphere.[50] The mixture of fission products emits both gamma and beta radiations. It is estimated that from the fallout material thus far descended from earth there will be a total average lifetime exposure of about one-tenth of a roentgen equivalent.[51] This amounts to approximately 1 per cent of the lifetime exposure of people to natural radiation of the earth and cosmic sources.

Reactors

As nuclear reactors are constructed by private enterprise, there will be added to our responsibility a radioactive source of great potential danger. The potential harm is

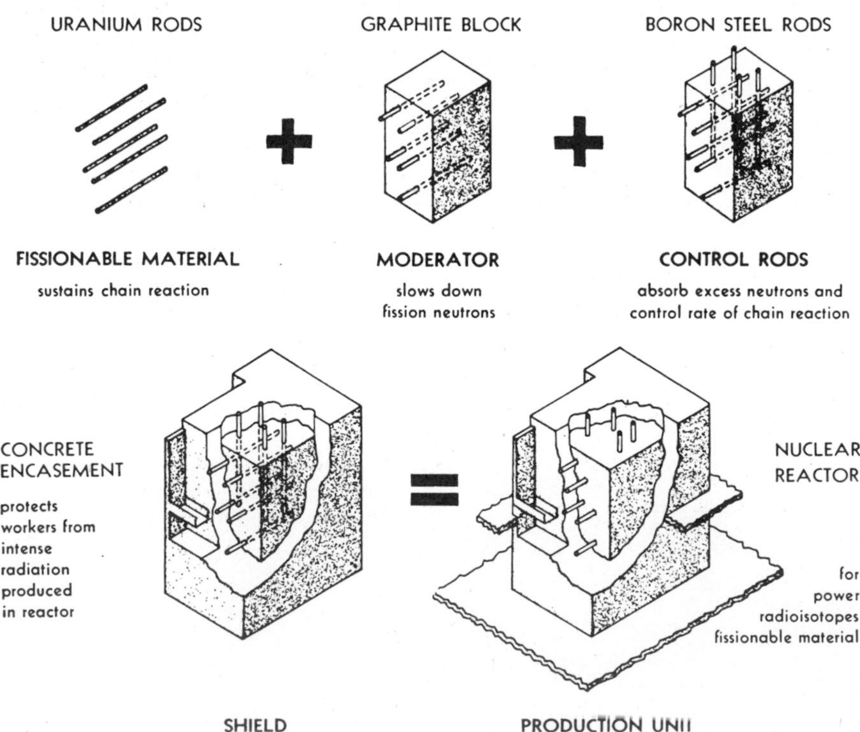

Figure 11–31 (From *You Can Understand the Atom.* U.S. Atomic Energy Commission.)

created by the large amount of radioactive fission products that accumulate in reactors under continuous operation. Nonetheless, the fact that reactors are potentially hazardous does not mean that they need to be so, or that we cannot learn to live with them in complete safety. Industry has learned how to control and live with many hazards.[52]

Medical Sources

Another source of radiation exposure is in the use of x-ray for various purposes. Essentially, these are diagnostic and therapeutic x-ray machines in hospitals and in offices of radiologists, physicians, dentists, chiropodists, chiropractors, and veterinarians. As far as the public is concerned, exposure to radiation is probably most common as a result of chest x-rays, dental x-rays, gastrointestinal series, and many other clinical procedures. Improperly shielded industrial x-ray equipment may cause exposure of operators; careless and incompetent operation of x-ray equipment may cause unnecessary exposure of the patient and of the operating technician. It has been estimated that the average individual exposure from such sources may amount to three or four roentgens during the reproductive lifetime.[53] Other common external sources include television tubes and watch dials.

Radiation Protection Rules

The Food and Drug Administration has established radiation protection standards for diagnostic x-ray machines and components. Under the standards, manufacturers must reduce patient and operator x-ray equipment produced after August 15, 1973. The standards will require that all types of equipment be capable of restricting beam size to that of the x-ray film or fluoroscope receptor. Beam restriction in general-purpose stationary x-ray machines would have to be automatic or the machines must be equipped with devices to prevent operation until the beam is restricted manually.

Roentgenographic equipment will have to incorporate features that will make possible a desired image quality at given settings for voltage, current, and time. The new standards also prescribe a limit—100 milliroentgens per hour at a distance of 1 meter from the tube assembly for leakage from x-ray tube assemblies. This limit reflects the recommendations of national and international authorities on radiation protection. Assemblers of roentgenographic equipment are regarded as manufacturers under the standard. They will be required to certify that the producers' instructions were followed, and that components are of the type required by the standard. Similar certifications must be made by radiologists, physicians and other users of x-ray equipment who install or replace components.

Color Television

The passage of the Radiation Control for Health and Safety Act (Public Law 90-602 in 1968) prompted both industry and government to take steps to reduce the radiation potential in color television sets manufactured after January 15, 1970. The federal standard limits x-ray emissions to 0.5 milliroentgen/hour. Every television receiver manufactured after this date must carry a label or tag certifying compliance with the federal standard. To assure that television sets meet the standard, the Bureau of Radiological Health of the Public Health Service reviews industry's quality control programs and enforces the standard. There should be no significant health hazard in viewing any color television set purchased after January 15, 1970, at a distance at which the image quality is satisfactory to the viewer. In purchasing a color television set, the buyer should check the back of the set for a label or tag certifying that it meets the federal standard.

Microwave Cataracts

Appleton has reported a connection between microwaves and cataracts:

> Microwaves in our environment and the possibility that they harm humans are facts of modern life. Microwaves are a form of nonionizing electromagnetic radiation, generally considered to include wavelengths from 1 millimeter to two meters long, which are common to radar devices used by commercial airlines and the federal government, line-of-sight telecommunication devices, "instant" cooking ovens, and diathermy treatment machines. Every American every day encounters microwaves. Experiments have shown that mam-

malian eyes can develop cataracts from exposure to microwaves. What is the risk of similar damage to man? Based on the available evidence, both clinical and experimental, the following conclusions appear reasonable:

1. Lens damage probably has not occurred in humans from cumulative exposure to low levels of microwave energy.

2. Lens damage probably could not occur in a human from acute exposure to microwave energy without associated severe facial burns.

It does appear that these microwave sources are safe to humans if existing standards of safety are observed, and there is an extremely wide margin of safety already built into these standards. It also appears that there is no justification for claims that cataracts occurring in individuals who have been casually or occupationally exposed to microwaves are the result of such exposure. Moreover, it is clear that litigation involving cataracts allegedly resulting from exceptional microwave exposure requires more scientific input.[54]

Measurement of Radiation

Roentgen or R. Quantity or dose of x-rays and gamma rays. Exact definition based on ionization produced in air by x-rays or gamma rays.

Roentgen Equivalent Man or rem. That quantity of any type of ionizing radiation which, when absorbed by man, produces an effect equivalent to the absorption by man of one roentgen of x- or gamma radiation.

Curie or c. A measure of the strength of the radioactive source in terms of atoms disintegrating per second.

Rad. A measure of the energy absorbed from radiation in a given amount of tissue. Roughly equivalent to a roentgen. (100 ergs absorbed per gram of tissue.)

Half-Life. The time required for radioactive elements to lose one-half their activity. For example, the half-life of one ounce of cobalt-60 is 5.3 years. Therefore, one ounce of cobalt-60 after 5.3 years becomes one-half ounce; after 5.3 more years it becomes one-quarter ounce; after 5.3 more years it becomes one-eighth ounce, etc. The half-life is important to us because it tells us how much of a radioactive element will remain after a given time, and how active the radioactivity is at any moment. The rays and half-life of various radioactive elements are listed below:

ELEMENT	RAYS	HALF-LIFE
Phosphorus-32	Beta	14 days
Iodine-131	Beta, gamma	8 days
Sulfur-35	Beta	87 days
Cobalt-60	Beta, gamma	5.3 years
Carbon-14	Beta	5000 years

Elements with a shorter half-life decay faster, and greater intensity is produced by the decay. The formula is:

$$\text{Half-life} = \frac{1}{\text{intensity}}$$

ELEMENT	HALF-LIFE
Radon	4 days
Strontium-90	28 years
Radium	1600 years
Uranium-238	10^9 years
Thorium	10^{14} years
Potassium	10^{20} years (in milk)

From the above list of elements, for example, we know that radon is the most dangerous. Internal and external human injury depends upon the half-life of the radioactive element.

Maximum Permissible Dose

The International Committee on Radiological Protection defined a maximum permissible weekly dose as a dose of radiation that, in the light of present knowledge, is not expected to cause appreciable bodily injury to any person at any time during his lifetime. This level has been steadily reduced, as shown below:

YEAR	MAXIMUM PERMISSIBLE DOSE
1928–1936	100 rads per year
1936–1947	35 rads per year
1947–1957	15 rads per year
1957–	5 rads per year

(It takes 50 normal chest x-rays per year to equal five rads.)

All recommendations as to permissible radiation exposures should be interpreted by recognizing the basic fact that any radiation exposure, except as required by medical necessity, is undesirable. There is a certain amount of background radiation present in our environment that is unavoidable. The only valid philosophy of radiation safety, based on present knowledge, is to reduce all radiation exposures above background levels to the lowest possible dose. Thus, maximum permissible exposures, such as those stated below, are to be used only as general guides.

It should not be considered that these are tolerable exposures, but rather that they represent upper limits and should be reached only infrequently, if ever. The latest recommendations of the National Committee on Radiation Protection as to maximum permissible exposures are:

1. The maximum permissible accumulated dose, in rems, at any age, is equal to 5 times the number of years beyond age 18, providing no annual increment exceeds 15 rems. Thus the accumulated maximum permissible dose equals 5(N–18) rems where N is the age and greater than 18. This applies to all critical organs except the skin, for which the value is double.

2. The maximum permissible weekly whole-body dose is 0.3 rem. Should the maximum permissible weekly dose be exceeded, no more than 3.0 rems should be accumulated in 13 weeks.

One of the most fundamental and at the same time most difficult problems is the determination of the degree of hazard associated with any particular radiation factor, and achieving a consensus as to what level of radiation should be considered acceptable in our present-day society.

The Irradiated Man

Radiation and radioactivity help us to date the age of the earth and other planets. The fact that certain radioactive elements, such as uranium, thorium, and potassium, which have accurately determined half-lives, are still found in nature today is a reliable indication that they could not have existed forever, and that they therefore had a beginning in time. The calculated time for the formation of these elements is approximately 4 billion years, which is taken as the age of the earth.

Of the 92 elements found in the earth's crust, the oceans. and the atmosphere, 16 (approximately one-sixth) are naturally radioactive. These radioisotopes, or radionuclides, are widely distributed in nature, in the food we eat, in the air we breathe, and in the liquids we drink. Man lives in a radioactive environment. He is radioactive and therefore is being irradiated from within as well as from external sources.

The radioactive elements in the body in sufficient concentration to be measured with our modern radiation detection instruments are potassium-40, carbon-14, and radium and its radioactive decay products. The radiation exposure received from these radionuclides which reside in the human body is called internal dose, and is proportional to the quantity of these elements present.

Cosmic radiation is that which is present in the universe as a whole, including earth. It originates in interstellar space and penetrates our atmosphere. We have been exposed to this radiation from conception. The earth and our buildings contain radioactive materials which emit radiation. The total radiation exposure contributed by nature is referred to as background radiation and varies with different locations on earth and in space.

Ultraviolet rays from sun or sunlamp are the chief cause of premature aging of the skin and of skin cancer. This was reported by the World Health Organization (WHO) in 1962 in their technical report series No. 248: "The only known natural source that is unequivocally carcinogenic is sunlight, largely or altogether in the ultraviolet wave lengths. Skin cancer has long been known to occur with greater frequency in persons, such as sailors and farmers, having high exposure to sunlight. The natural incidence of skin cancer is four times as high in the Southern as in the Northern parts of the United States (80/100,000 per year as compared to 20/100,000)."

It is well known that when the principle of radiation use—benefit versus risk—is applied to radiation in medical practice, radiation will continue to be used because the benefits outweigh the risk. Also, it is known that 90 to 95 per cent of the unnecessary radiation exposure to the general population is received from x-rays used in the healing arts. In a large survey made by the Public Health Service, it was stated that this genetically significant dose of 55 radiation units to the general public could be reduced to 19 radiation units by the proper use of x-ray beam restrictors to expose only the organs and tissues under investigation.

The radiation sources which contribute 95 per cent of our genetic dose are: medical, 53 per cent; background, 40 per cent; and occupational, about 2 per cent. Since the radiation used in medical application was the largest listed contributor, many health departments have begun a program of registration and inspection of all people who operate medical x-ray machines. The curtailment of unnecessary exposures of the general public to man-made x-radiation can reduce these exposures by an amount which is several times greater than the exposure received from nuclear-fueled electric power plants.

Plutonium

Of all issues relating to the present controversy concerning nuclear energy, the most important and urgent is that related to human health. Although nuclear plants will produce electrical energy, they will also unavoidably produce highly toxic radioactive wastes and substances such as plutonium, which is known to produce cancers and is used to make atomic weapons. Plutonium is an alpha particle emitter with a half-life of 24,000 years (therefore, biologically active for 480,000 years), and it is one of the most toxic substances man has ever known. Because of its extreme toxicity and tendency to burn spontaneously, it is customarily treated with a caution accorded few other substances. It is usually handled by remote control. When handled by hand, it is done so in sealed glass glove boxes using rubber gloves. Work areas are briskly ventilated and the air is thoroughly filtered. Air is regularly sampled for even the slightest contamination, and radiation monitors are stationed liberally about all areas. The maximum permissible body burden is set at 40 nanocuries, i.e., *40 billionths of a curie,* derived from a hypothesized near equivalence of plutonium to radium, which is known to produce human bone cancers. Reassurance is repeatedly given by many that such burdens or even higher amounts can be tolerated safely; others, with equal justification, say that most of the serious medical problems seen to date are most probably due to plutonium.

Health Aspects

General Considerations

There are four major considerations that we must consider in discussing the biological aspects of radiation. They include:

1. Type of ionization. For example, the alpha radiation, although possessed of considerable energy, is incapable of deep penetration. In striking contrast, gamma radiation is capable of deep penetration into tissues and is capable of traversing an appreciable thickness of material. Between these two extremes with respect to penetration, various energy levels of beta radiation are to be found that have appreciable penetrating power in tissue, although limited in depth of effective action.

	PENETRATION		IONIZATION
	Air	*Tissue*	
Alpha	0.1^1	0.01 centimeter	10,000
Beta	10^1	1.0 centimeter	100
Gamma	1000	10.0 centimeter	1

2. Intensity or energy of ionizing influence. This depends upon distance and amount and type of shielding between the source and the person.

3. Length of time a person is exposed to radiation.

4. Area of the body radiated. As indicated in the following discussion, proliferating cells are more sensitive to radioactivity. The whole body exposure to radiation is appreciably different from the irradiation of a single part. The tolerance of the entire individual to radiation is much less than that exhibited by any single organ or component of the body. Furthermore, there seems to be a great deal of variability among individuals to radiation.

Injury by Ionization of Water. Although there are several different physical forms of nuclear radiation, they all have similar biological effects. It appears that the chief mechanism of injury to living cells is the ionization of water, of which all living tissues are largely composed. Other cell destruction theories are that radiation (1) alters the permeability of cell membranes, (2) produces inherent toxic materials, (3) produces a change in intercellular relationships, or (4) produces a disturbance of enzyme systems.

In a very real sense, man is an aquatic animal. He not only is composed mostly of water, but he lives in an aqueous state, being dependent on foodstuffs that are themselves mostly water. Radiation, therefore, strikes at life through the medium of its most basic substance—water.[55] The ionization also creates a disturbance between the nucleus and cytoplasm of the cell.

In the interaction of ionizing radiation with water, several particularly toxic compounds are produced, which in turn have chemical effects upon the constituents of a living cell, especially the proteins. Amino acids, the building blocks of proteins, are excreted in the urine of a person exposed to too much radiation.

Influence of Number of Cells. Another principle involves the number of cells present in the organism. The more cells that are present, the less radiation is needed to kill the organism. For example:

ORGANISM	NUMBER OF ROENTGENS CAUSING DEATH
Mammals	200–1000
Frogs and goldfish	700
Tortoise	1500
Snail	10,000
Kissing bug	50,000
Fruit fiy	60,000
Paramecium	300,000
Virus	1,000,000

The above chart indicates that some species can survive a radiation dose many times greater than that which would kill an elephant or man. Cells are most susceptible to radiation damage when they are in the process of dividing. Since many insects, unlike humans, undergo no cell division during much of their lives, they are more highly resistant to radiation.

Influence of Level of Oxygen. The level of oxygen within a cell or organism at the time of radiation is also important. For example, oxygen deficiency slows the kissing bug's cell division, and when it molts, the bug shows two to three times less radiation damage than bugs that are irradiated in normal air. This indicates that less cell oxygen produces less cell damage, or conversely, more cell oxygen produces more cell damage. Since cells in humans are continually dividing, man may never hope to achieve an insect's resistance.[56]

Influence of Cell Proliferation. Proliferating cells, or the cells that grow the fastest, are most sensitive to radioactivity. A scale of *decreasing* cell sensitivity would be:

1. Lymphoid tissue—most sensitive of all tissue.
2. Bone marrow, leukocytes and other elements in the blood.
   (a) immature cells more sensitive than mature cells
   (b) red blood cells least sensitive component
3. Gonad, ovary, pancreas, kidney and other epithelial cells
4. Blood vessels and other endothelial cells (peritoneal tissue)
5. Connective tissue
6. Muscles
7. Bone
8. Nerve

QUESTIONS FOR DISCUSSION

1. What are the major sources of water in your community? State?
2. What diseases may be transmitted by water?
3. List four chemicals or elements that are added to the water, and explain why each is added.
4. List six criteria to consider when planning a safe community water supply.
5. (a) Discuss the water pollution problem in your community, state and nation.
   (b) How can water pollution be prevented?
6. Explain, step-by-step, the operation of a sewage treatment plant.
7. (a) What part does the local health department play in keeping water safe and pure,
   (b) State health department,
   (c) United States Public Health Service?
8. (a) Discuss the air pollution problem in your community, state, and nation.
   (b) How can air pollution be prevented and controlled?
9. Discuss the relationship between air and health.
10. What are the sources of air pollution?
11. (a) What part does the local health department play in preventing air pollution,
    (b) State health department,
    (c) United States Public Health Service?
12. What are the present concepts of occupational health?
13. (a) What part does the local health department play in occupational health programs,
    (b) State health department,
    (c) United States Public Health Service?
14. Briefly classify and discuss the environmental agents that may be harmful to health.
15. List nine easy rules for keeping food safe.
16. What germs and diseases may be transmitted by food?
17. (a) What part does the local health department play in food sanitation,
    (b) State health department,
    (c) United States Public Health Service?
18. Discuss: botulism, mussel poisoning, chemical poisoning.
19. Is it best to examine or educate food handlers? Explain.
20. Plan, organize, and outline a five hour program to educate food handlers.
21. (a) What part does the local health department play in milk sanitation,
    (b) State health department,
    (c) United States Public Health Service,
    (d) Department of Agriculture?
22. What diseases may be transmitted by milk?
23. "Pasteurization destroys certain vitamins and flavor, and is not necessary if milk is produced and handled under sanitary conditions." Discuss this statement.
24. List and briefly discuss five sanitary milk tests.

25. (a) What part does the local health department play in refuse disposal,
    (b) State health department?
26. (a) List five refuse disposal methods.
    (b) Which is considered best? Why?
27. Discuss the public health aspects of shellfish safety.
28. Discuss the public health aspects of botulism.
29. What is the function and scope of the Food and Drug Administration?
30. Discuss three recent trends in our society that have had a marked effect on the Food and Drug Administration.
31. How can the local health department provide assistance to the community in an effort to improve housing?
32. What are the major sources of your local water supply? Visit the plant and make a report on the trip.
33. Does the health department of the community in which you live advocate fluoridation of the public water supply? State the pros and cons of the issue.
34. List and briefly discuss the four types of ionizing radiation.
35. List and briefly discuss the sources of radiation.
36. What are the four major considerations involved in the biological aspects of radiation? Discuss.
37. Discuss the possible somatic and genetic effects of radiation.
38. Why is strontium-90 the most feared of all fallout isotopes?
39. Are x-rays necessary? Discuss.
40. List and briefly discuss the seven major preventive measures necessary to control community and personal radiation hazards and injury.
41. (a) List the major functions and activities of a radiological health division of a local health department.
    (b) State health department,
    (c) United States Public Health Service.
42. Briefly list and discuss major peaceful uses of atomic energy.
43. "Why should I build a fallout shelter? There won't be any survivors anyhow." Discuss this statement.
44. List the six steps for survival recommended by civil defense authorities.
45. How has the current increase in interest in environmental health in the U.S. come about?
46. What are the students at your school doing about the health of the environment?
47. Does your college swimming pool meet public health standards?
48. Who has charge of vector-borne diseases in your community and what are their duties?
49. What are your community's regulations regarding plumbing or septic tanks? What is its building code?
50. What are the qualifications of a sanitarian employed by the public health department? What courses must he have in college?
51. How can we prevent:
    (a) auto accidents,
    (b) home accidents,
    (c) school accidents?
52. What is the nature and function of a community safety countil?
53. List the characteristics of a good automobile driver. What skill should he possess?
54. What are the psychological factors involved in traffic accidents? How should psychosocial factors be handled in driver education courses?
55. Discuss alcohol and traffic accidents.
56. Discuss and report from the latest literature on the problems of drugs and operating a motor vehicle.
57. Interview the designated officials on the college campus or a local industry and find out what their safety program is. What are the good and weak points? How would you improve it?
58. In what age groups are accidents the leading cause of death in your community? What are the causes and what should be done about it?
59. Inspect some of the buildings on the campus for accident hazards. List and discuss ways for improvement.
60. What safety features for cars do experts recommend to reduce automobile accidents?
61. Investigate and check on the research on the following accident causes: skateboards, swimming, boating, glass doors, and motorcycles. Are these types of accidents a problem in your community?
62. Check with the Department of Motor Vehicles in your state and report on the status of auto accidents for the past year. Describe the administrative aspects of the Department.
63. Attend a traffic court session in your community and report the highlights to the class or group.
64. Contact the local police department in your community and gather information on the problem of alcohol and auto accidents.
65. Report on highlights from *Accident Facts,* published by the National Safety Council. Obtain the latest issue and compare statistics with those of the previous year.
66. Do the local public schools keep accident records? Contact the administrator for a copy of the accidents that have occurred for the past year. What are the causes of these accidents? Are the students insured?
67. Check the accident rate on a college campus. Are the students insured for accidents, sports, intramural activities, and off-campus activities? What research has been done on your campus regarding safety education?
68. Discuss the psychological tests used in driver education courses.

69. What safety materials do the following organizations distribute:
American Automobile Association, 1712 G St., N.W., Washington, D.C.; National Commissions on Safety Education, 1202 16 St., N.W., Washington, D.C.: The American Red Cross, 17 & D St., N.W., Washington, D.C.; and The National Safety Council, 427 North Michigan Ave., Chicago, Illinois?
70. What role do the police play in safety on the roads?
71. How many colleges in your state have safety committees? What are the functions of the committee?
72. List and briefly discuss the major causes of accidents.

QUESTIONS FOR REVIEW

1. List the major causes of injuries received in home accidents.
2. List six safety measures for the prevention of crash injuries and deaths.
3. What are the three E's for prevention of accidents?
4. List at least three general sources of water. How much water does the average American use daily? How much is the average American predicted to use by the year 2000?
5. What are the most common diseases contracted from polluted water?
6. What are the two names of the dye which can detect pollution in water?
7. What are the uses of both chlorine and copper sulphate?
8. What would be the purpose of adding 0.7 part per million to 1.5 parts per million of fluoride to a community's water supply?
9. List the eight types of water pollutants as classified by the Committee on Public Works.
10. Describe primary sewage treatment.
11. What are the three basic problems in using waste treatment plants?
12. What are three tests for the quality of water?
13. When is the annual mussel quarantine in effect because of shellfish poisoning?
14. What are the symptoms of shellfish poisoning?
15. What is the cause of the toxin in shellfish?
16. What are the potential effects of sulphate pollutants in the air? Of ozone pollutants?
17. What are the three general types of substances that are known to pollute the air?
18. What are the two major causes of air pollution?
19. Name at least eight of the toxic substances present in polluted air.
20. What is the name of the service that gathers scientific data on air pollution throughout the U.S.?
21. How are the pollutant samples collected by this service?
22. What three general kinds of knowledge must a community have before it can intelligently plan an air pollution control program?
23. What are the most important known effects of noise on psychological states?
24. What are some of the things we can do to reduce noise?
25. What are the general jobs of the local health department in protecting the public's health against food contamination?
26. What are symptoms of food poisoning?
27. What are the three specific purposes of a food-service sanitation program?
28. What is the least common and most highly lethal of bacteria food poisons in the U.S.?
29. How many years did it take before the attempts by Dr. Harvey W. Wiley and his associates to enact a Food and Drug Law succeeded? What was the catalyst that finally brought success?
30. What are two reasons why the efforts of the FDA have been hampered in the past?
31. What do the initials GRAS stand for in relation to food additives?
32. What are the four recommendations listed by the Committee on Meat and Poultry Inspection for improvement of all government food hygiene activities?
33. What are the seven sanitary milk tests?
34. What are the characteristics of the disease Q fever?
35. What are the three major components of a good waste handling program?
36. What are three present methods of ultimate disposal of waste? List six possible future methods of ultimate waste disposal.
37. What are the objectives of occupational health programs as defined by the AMA Council on Occupational Health?
38. Into what three categories can the local health department, in relation to occupational health, be divided?
39. List the three categories of environmental agents and give examples of each.
40. What is the major occupational disease in the U.S. in terms of disability and compensation costs?
41. What is the most common industrial health problem?
42. List the four types of ionizing radiation.
43. What are the major sources of neutrons?
44. What is the best protection from any type of radiation?
45. Where does cosmic radiation come from?
46. What are four man-made sources of radioactivity?
47. Define the following terms: roentgen or R; roentgen equivalent man or rem; curie or c; rad; half-life.

48. What is background radiation?
49. List the radiation sources that contribute 95 per cent of our genetic dose and the percentage of each.
50. What are the three radioactive elements in the body?
51. What is the only known natural source that is "unequivocally carcinogenic" according to the WHO?
52. What is the chief mechanism of injury to liver cells as a result of too much radiation?
53. When are cells most susceptible to radiation damage?
54. Briefly discuss plutonium and health.

REFERENCES

1. Trott, H.: West Coast report, water: What valid purpose? The Christian Science Monitor, May 20, 1964, p. 14.
2. Biancifiori, C., and Ribacchi, R.: Pulmonary tumours in mice induced by oral isoniazid and its metabolites. Nature (London), *194*:488, 1962.
3. Dubos, R.: The conflict between progress and safety. Arch. Environmental Health, *6*:449, 1963.
4. The Shattuck Report: *Report of Sanitary Commission of Massachusetts: 1850.* Reprinted by the American Health Association, New York, 1950.
5. Environmental health in community growth, an administrative guide to metropolitan area sanitation practices. Amer. J. Publ. Health, *53*:802, 821, 1963.
6. Scott, R. M., Seiz, D., Shaughnessy, H. J.: Rapid carbon test for coliform bacteria in water. Amer. J. Publ. Health, *54*:827, 1964.
7. Okun, D. A.: Planning for water supply development. Amer. J. Publ. Health, *54*:900, 1964.
8. Flanagan, J. E.: Physician's guide to water pollution. JAMA, *188*:1010, 1964.
9. Ibid.
10. *The Struggle for Clean Water.* Public Health Service Publication No. 958, United States Department of Health, Education and Welfare, 1962, p. 6.
11. *The Struggle for Clean Water,* Public Health Service Publication No. 958, United States Department of Health, Education and Welfare, 1962, pp. 6, 11.
12. How to fight air pollution. Washington, D.C., U.S. News and World Report, October, 1958, p. 81.
13. Rogers, S. M., and Edelman, S.: *A Digest of State Air Pollution Laws.* United States Department of Health, Education and Welfare, Public Health Service, Public Health Service Publication No. 711, 1963, p. vii.
14. JAMA, *228*:1653, 1974.
15. Second Report of the California State Department of Public Health: *Clean Air for California.* California State Department of Public Health, March, 1956, p. 5.
16. Initial Report of the Air Pollution Study Project: *Clean Air for California.* California State Department of Public Health, March, 1955, pp. 42, 47.
17. Noise pollution can harm circulatory system. JAMA, February 9, 1970.
18. Amer. J. Publ. Health, *63*(11): 982, 1973.
19. *Food Service Sanitation Manual, Including a Model, Food Service Sanitation Ordinance and Code, 1962 Recommendations of the Public Health Service.* United States Department of Health, Education and Welfare, Public Health Service Publication No. 934, 1963.
20. *You Can Prevent Foodborne Illness.* United States Department of Health, Education and Welfare, Public Health Service, Division of Environmental Engineering and Food Protection. Washington, D.C., Public Health Service Publication No. 1105, November, 1963.
21. Morbid. Mortal. Week Rep., *12*:311, 1963.
22. Downs, R.: Afterward from *The Jungle.* New York, New American Library of World Literature, 1956.
23. Committee on Meat and Poultry Inspection. Amer. J. Publ. Health, *60*:192, 1970.
24. *Training Course Manual, Milk Pasteurization Controls and Tests.* United States Department of Health, Education and Welfare, Public Health Service, Bureau of State Services, Division of Environmental Engineering and Food Protection, Robert A. Taft Sanitary Engineering Center, Cincinnati, Ohio, 1964.
25. Report of the Commissioner of Health: Guarding the health of Baltimore—1963. Baltimore Health News, *40*:11, 1964.
26. Harper, J. D.: The growing importance of industrial hygiene. Arch. Environment. Health, *6*:315, 1963.
27. Meigs, J. W.: Occupational health—talk or action? Amer. J. Publ. Health, *54*:519, 1964.
28. Connecticut State Medical Society: Guiding principles for occupational medicine. Adopted by House of Delegates, C.S.M.S., April 27, 1953.
29. *Slough Industrial Health Service, 14th and 15th Annual Reports, 1961–1962.* Windsor, England, Oxley & Son, Ltd.
30. Heimann, H., and Trasko, V. M.: Evolution of occupational health programs in state and local governments. Publ. Health Rep., *79*:945, 1964.
31. Siegel, G. S.: Neglect of occupational health in public planning. Pub. Health Rep., *79*:966, 1964.
32. The Council on Occupational Health, American Medical Association: Scope, objectives and functions of occupational health programs. JAMA, *174*:533, 1960.
33. Occupational Health Series I: *Dollars and Sense.* Santa Clara, Cal., County Health Department, Division of Occupational Health, 1958, p. 3.
34. *Santa Clara County Health Department Occupational Health Seminars.* California, Santa Clara County Health Department, 1959, p. 5.
35. *City of Baltimore, One Hundred and Forty-Eighth Annual Report of the Department of Health, 1962.* To the Mayor and City Council of Baltimore for the year ended December 31, 1962, p. 148.
36. Occupational health guidelines for Public Health nurses. California's Health, *21*:205, 1964.
37. Simmons, S. W.: DDT: The insecticide dichlorodiphenyltrichloroethane and its significance. *In* Muller, P. (ed.): *Human and Veterinary Medicine.* Vol. 2. Basel, Switzerland, Birkhauser Verlag Basel, 1959, p. 251.
38. Committee on Occupational Toxicology of the Council on Occupational Health: Evaluation of the present status of DDT with respect to man. JAMA, *212*:1055, 1970.

39. Occupational health notes. Publ. Health Rep., *78*:174, 1963.
40. Morbid. Mortal. Week. Rep., *11*:187, 1962.
41. Morbid. Mortal. Week. Rep., *13*:267, 1964.
42. Morbid. Mortal. Week. Rep., *13*:250, 1964.
43. Morbid. Mortal. Week. Rep., *14*:27, 1965.
44. Pierce, P. E., et al.: Alkyl mercury poisoning in humans. JAMA, *220* (11):1439, June 12, 1972.
45. Sokol, W. N., et al.: Meat-wrapper's asthma. JAMA, *226*: (6):639, November 5, 1973.
46. Gehlback, S. H., et al.: Green-tobacco sickness. JAMA, *229* (14):1880, September 30, 1974.
47. Goddard, J. L.: Accident prevention in childhood. Publ. Health Rep., *74*:523, 1959.
48. Safe spectacles and sunglasses for all. JAMA, September 21, 1970, p. 621.
49. Cowan, F. P.: Everyday radiation. Physics Today, *5*:18–20, 1952.
50. Eisenbud, M., and Harley, J. H.: Radioactive fallout in the United States. Science, *121*:677–80, 1955.
51. Commission on Atomic Energy: *Health and Safety Problems and Weather Effects Associated with Atomic Explosion.* Washington, D.C., U.S. Printing Office, 1955.
52. Davis, W. K.: *Industrial Power Reactors and Their Location.* Chicago, American Medical Association, 1955.
53. National Academy of Sciences: *The Biological Effects of Atomic Radiation.* Washington, D.C., National Academy of Sciences, 1956.
54. Appleton, B.: Microwave cataracts. JAMA, *229* (4):407, July 22, 1974.
55. Bugher, J. C.: Radiation and human health. Amer. J. Publ. Health, *47*:682, 1957.
56. Alexander, P.: *Atomic Radiation and Life* England, Pelican-Penguin Books, 1957, p. 85.

SUGGESTED READING

A Time to Choose: America's Energy Future (Report of the Ford Foundation Energy Policy Project). New York, Ballantine, 1974.

AMA film: *I Love You, Frank.* Available from AMA Film Library, or Radio, TV, and Motion Picture Department of AMA Headquarters, 535 N. Dearborn, Chicago, Ill.

American Mutual Insurance Alliance: *Handbook of Hazardous Materials.* Technical Guide No. 7, 1974.

Arena, J. M.: *Poisoning: Toxicology—Symptoms—Treatment.* Springfield, Ill., Charles C Thomas, 1974.

Boyd, E. M.: *Predictive Toxicometrics; Basic Methods for Estimating Poisonous Amounts of Foods, Drugs, and Other Agents.* Bristol, Pa., Scientechnica, 1972.

Brodeur, P.: *Expendable Americans.* New York, Viking, 1974.

Bushong, S. C.: *The Development of Radiation Protection in Diagnostic Radiology.* Cleveland, CRL Press, 1973.

Citizen's Guide: The National Debate on the Handling of Radioactive Wastes from Nuclear Power Plants. Natural Resources Defense Council, 664 Hamilton Ave., Palo Alto, Calif. 94301.

Clark, W.: Energy for Survival. New York, Anchor-Doubleday, 1975.

Commoner, B.: *The Closing Circle.* New York, Bantam Books, 1972.

Cralley, L. V. (ed.): *Industrial Environmental Health; the Worker and the Community.* New York, Academic Press, 1972.

Dagget, W.: *Health Protection of Radiation Workers.* Springfield, Ill., Charles C Thomas, 1975.

Daniels, F.: *Direct Use of the Sun's Energy.* New York, Ballantine Books, 1975.

DeBell, G. (ed.): *The Environmental Handbook.* New York, Ballantine Books, 1975.

Ehrlich, P. R.: *The Population Bomb.* New York, Ballantine Books, 1975.

Ehrlich, P. R., and Ehrlich, A. H.: *The End of Affluence.* New York, Ballantine Books, 1974.

Ehrlich, P. R., and Harriman, R. L.: *How To Be A Surviver.* New York, Ballantine Books, 1975.

Ehrlich, P. R., et al.: *Human Ecology: Problems and Solutions.* San Francisco, W. H. Freeman, 1973.

Eisenbud, M.: *Environmental Radioactivity.* 2nd ed. New York, Academic Press, 1973.

Environment Information Center: *Environment Information Access.* New York, 1974.

Finkel, A. J. (ed.): *Energy, the Environment, and Human Health.* Acton, Mass., Publishing Sciences Group, 1974.

Ford, D. F., et al.: *The Nuclear Fuel Cycle.* San Francisco, Friends of the Earth, 1974.

Ford Foundation: *A Time to Choose: America's Energy Future.* Final Report by the Energy Policy Project. Cambridge, Mass., Ballinger, 1975.

Foss, P. O. (ed.): *Politics and Ecology.* Belmont, Calif., Duxbury Press, 1975.

Freese, A. S.: *Protecting Your Family From Accidental Poisoning.* New York, Public Affairs Committee, 1974.

Gabree, J. (ed.): *Surviving the City.* New York, Ballantine Books, 1975.

Gilmore, C.: *Accident Prevention and Loss Control.* New York, American Management Association, 1970.

Greenwood, N. H., and Edwards, J. M. B.: *Human Environments and Natural Systems: A Conflict of Dominion.* Belmont, Calif., Duxbury Press, 1975.

Gubrium, J. F. (ed.): *Late Life: Communities and Environmental Policy.* Springfield, Ill., Charles C Thomas, 1975.

Hamilton, A., and Hardy, H. L.: *Industrial Toxicology.* 3rd ed. New York, Publishing Sciences Group, 1974.

Haskell, E. H., and Price, V. S.: *State Environmental Management: Case Study of Nine States.* New York, Praeger, 1973.

Hausler, W. J. (ed.): *Standard Methods for the Examination of Dairy Products.* 13th ed. Washington, D.C., American Public Health Association, 1974.

Kane, R., and Wistreich, G. A.: *Biology for Survival.* Beverly Hills, Calif., Glencoe Press, 1974.

Karger, S. (ed.): *Problems of Industrial Medicine in Ophthalmology.* Vols. 3 and 4. Chicago, Medical and Scientific Publishers, 1974.

Kiefer, H., and Manshort, R.: *Radiation Protection Measurements.* New York, Pergamon Press, 1972.

Leh, F. K. V., and Lak, R. K. C.: *Environment and Pollutions: Sources, Health Effects, Monitoring, and Control.* Springfield, Ill., Charles C Thomas, 1974.

Levine, N. D., et al.: *Human Ecology.* Belmont, Calif., Duxbury Press, 1975.

Mallino, D. L.: *Occupational Safety and Health.* Washington, D.C., Government Research Corp., 1973.

Marcus, M. G., and Detwyler, T. R.: *Urbanization and Environment: The Physical Geography of the City.* Belmont, Calif., 1975.

Marx, W.: *The Frail Ocean.* New York, Ballantine Books, 1975.

Mason, J. K., and Reals, W. J. (eds.): *Aerospace Pathology.* Washington, D.C., College of American Pathologists Foundation, 1973.

McKee, W. D. (ed.): *Environmental Problems in Medicine.* Springfield, Ill., Charles C Thomas, 1975.

Mesarovic, M., and Pestel, E.: *Mankind at the Turning Point: The Second Report to the Club of Rome.* New York, E. P. Dutton & Co., 1974.

Noble, J. H., et al. (eds.): *Emergency Medical Services.* New York, Behavioral Publications, 1973.

Ogden, E., et al.: *Manual for Sampling Airborne Pollen.* New York, Hafner, 1974.

Owen, D. F.: *Man's Environmental Predicament.* New York, Oxford University Press, 1974.

Polish Government, WHO, and USHEW: *Biological Effects and Health Hazards of Microwave Radiation.* Proceedings of an International Symposium, October, 1973. Warsaw, Polish Medical Publishers, 1974.

Pounds, E. T., and Stehney, V. A.: *Primary Pollution Packet.* Glenview, Ill., Scott, Foresman & Co., 1974.

Public Affairs Committee, New York: Pamphlets.

Rienow, L., and Rienow, R.: Moments in the Sun. New York, Ballantine Books, 1975.

Rockefeller, J. D., III: *The Second American Revolution.* New York, Harper & Row, 1973.

Russwurm, L. H., and Sommerville, E. (eds.): *Man's Natural Environment: A Systems Approach.* Belmont, Calif., Duxbury Press, 1975.

Rylander, R. (ed.): *Environmental Tobacco Smoke Effects on the Non-Smoker.* Paper, University of Geneva, 1974.

Salvato, J. A., Jr.: *Environmental Engineering and Sanitation.* 2nd ed. New York, Wiley-Interscience, 1972.

Scheele, R. V., and Wakley, J.: *Elements of Radiation Protection.* Springfield, Ill., Charles C Thomas, 1975.

Schilling, R. S. F.: *Occupational Health Practice.* London, Butterworth, 1973.

Schroeder, H. A.: *The Poisons Around Us. Toxic Metals in Food, Air, and Water.* Bloomington, Indiana University Press, 1974.

Schumacher, E. F.: *Small Is Beautiful: Economics As If People Mattered.* New York, Harper & Row, 1973.

Scott, R.: *Muscle and Blood.* New York, E. P. Dutton, 1974.

Sproul, C. W., and Mullanney, P. J. (eds.): *Emergency Care: Assessment and Intervention.* St. Louis, C. V. Mosby Co., 1974.

State Traffic Code and Driver's Handbook. (Obtainable from Motor Vehicle Department in each state.)

Steinhart, C., and Steinhart, J.: *Energy: Sources, Use and Role in Human Affairs.* Belmont, Calif., Duxbury Press, 1975.

Taras, M. J., et al. (eds.): *Standard Methods for the Examination of Water and Wastewater.* Washington, D.C., American Public Health Association, 1971.

U.S. Environmental Protection Agency, Office of Pesticide Programs: *Diagnosis and Treatment of Poisoning by Pesticides.* Washington, D.C., 1973.

Waldbott, G. L.: *Health Effects of Environmental Pollutants.* St. Louis, C. V. Mosby Co., 1973.

Waldron, H. A., and Stöfen, D.: *Sub-Clinical Lead Poisoning.* New York, Academic Press, 1974.

Willrich, M., and Taylor, T. B.: *Nuclear Theft: Risks and Safeguards. New York, Ballinger, 1974.*

Wilson, J. G.: *Environment and Birth Defects.* New York, Academic Press, 1973.

Xintaras, et al. (eds.): *Behavioral Toxicology: Early Detection of Occupational Hazards.* U.S. Department of Health, Education and Welfare, National Institute for Occupational Safety and Health, 1974.

APPENDICES

APPENDIX I

Your Career in Public Health

This section presents an overview of some of the many careers available in the public health field. For further information, contact your local or state health department.

Public Health Dental Hygienist

The Job

Dental hygienists are licensed auxiliary personnel in the dental profession. They are concerned primarily with dental health education and the preventive dental health services. The public health dental hygienist works under the general supervision of the public health dentist, helping health departments and school and community groups establish dental health programs. Some of her duties, for example, include giving classroom demonstrations of proper oral hygiene and techniques, advising school personnel and children about good dental health practices and nutrition as it relates to dental health, and providing oral prophylaxis and topical applications of fluoride. Often the dental hygienist participates in community dental surveys, including the inspection, recording, and interpretation of data which can lead to the organization of a community dental health program.

Requirements

I. Beginning position	
High school	College preparatory work emphasizing mathematics, science and English composition.
College	Two years in a curriculum for dental hygiene and a license to practice dental hygiene.
II. Advanced position Graduate work	Bachelor of Science degree in dental hygiene. Master of Public Health degree in public health education leads to work in the areas of supervisory and administrative work.

Food and Drug Inspector

The Job

The Food and Drug Inspector is responsible for protecting the health of the consumer. He inspects establishments producing and selling foods, drugs, cosmetics, and hazardous substances to insure compliance with state Food and Drug Laws. He inspects the ingredients and procedures used in food and drug manufacturing to safeguard against contamination or adulteration. He investigates labeling, advertising, and selling procedures and gathers evidence leading to the prosecution of any person who manufactures or sells adulterated, misbranded, or falsely advertised foods and drugs.

Requirements

I. Beginning position	Minimum requirement is Bachelor's degree with at least 30 semester hours in a biological or chemical science.
II. Advanced position	Requirements are one year of experience as a trainee with the Bureau of Food and Drug Inspections and supervisory and administrative experience for supervisory positions.

Public Health Administrator (Nonmedical)

The Job

The nonmedical administrator in a health department may serve as an administrative assistant to a program or to an assistant chief in charge of a program, such as chronic disease or maternal and child health; or he may be the chief of a nonmedical administrative unit, such as the Bureau of Personnel and Training. He is responsible for the fiscal administration of the unit. He determines work flow, has charge of forms and records, plans training programs for new staff members, and assists in programs development and the interpretation of the program to the public. In a local health department he may serve as an executive assistant to the local health officer involved in budget preparation, personnel management and training, accounting, and purchasing, as well as participating in program development.

Requirements

I. Beginning position	
College	Bachelor's degree in business administration or public health administration.
Graduate work	Hospital administration, public or public health administration or rehabilitation is desirable.
II. Advanced position	
Graduate work	Master's degree in public administration or Master's degree in public health administration is preferred.

Experience	Broad and extensive experience in the field. In some positions experience may be substituted for a portion of a graduate work. Certain jobs do not require a Master's degree.

Public Health Biologist (Vector Control)

The Job

Scientists who work in the field of vector control use medical entomology, parasitology, and vertebrate zoology to control and prevent diseases transmitted by insects, related invertebrates, small mammals, and certain other vertebrates. Most of the work is in the field of medical entomology, which is concerned with the relation of the insects and other arthropods to disease transmission. Opportunities exist in research, technical development, and consultation.

Requirements

I. Beginning position	Bachelor's degree in biology with specialization in medical entomology or vertebrate zoology.
II. Advanced position	Master of Science, Master of Public Health, Doctor of Science, or Doctor of Philosophy degree, with further training in parasitology, microbiology, virology, epidemiology, chemistry, toxicology, public health engineering, and public health administration.

Public Health Nurse

The Job

The public health nurse may work in a health department, a school system, a visiting nurse association, or industry. Always under the guidance of a physician, she is concerned with nursing care outside the hospital. She works with community groups and families in their homes and in clinics. She provides health counseling to promote physical and mental well-being, cares for the ill in their homes, and assists in the rehabilitation of the disabled.

There is no "typical" day for the public health nurse. She might begin by showing a mother how to bathe her new baby and how to make his formula. Then she might care for a bedridden grandmother who lives alone. Her third call may be teaching a mother how to give exercises to her crippled child and to arrange immunization for the rest of the family. That afternoon she might meet with the community health council or work with the doctor in the well-baby clinic.

Requirements

I. Beginning position	
College	Bachelor's degree from an institution approved for public health nursing by the National League for Nursing.

Other	Successful completion of State Board Nurse Examination for the Registered Nurse license. A State Public Health Nursing Certificate.
II. Advanced position	Master's degree in nursing administration, supervision or consultation; in maternal and child health; or in mental health, OR Master of Philosophy from a university approved by the American Public Health Association.

Public Health Nutritionist

The Job

The public health nutritionist works in a public health agency to promote better health through better nutrition. She serves as a consultant to professional colleagues—physicians, nurses, and the like—on current scientific findings on food and nutrition, and their application to the agency's programs and activities. She also interprets doctor's diet orders to patients, gives nutrition counseling to patients in clinics sponsored by the agency, provides assistance to nursing homes and small hospitals on administration of food service and management of diets, and helps school personnel with curriculum planning, nutrition activities, and appropriate resource materials. She provides current nutrition information to the public by articles and works with community leaders in planning nutrition programs. The nutritionist collects and interprets information about how people buy and select food, how they prepare their food, and what they eat. She works with others in exploring new fields relating to health.

Requirements

I. Beginning position	Bachelor's degree with specialization in foods and nutrition. Dietetic internship desirable.
II. Advanced position	Master of Philosophy or Master of Science degree in nutrition.

Public Health Sanitarian

The Job

A sanitarian has the responsibility of helping people understand the laws that protect their health; of providing technical advice and assistance so as to bring about voluntary compliance or, if necessary, enforcement of the laws.

A sanitarian may do all or specialize in the following jobs: survey and sample wells and community water supplies and work with the public health laboratory to assure safe water; approve subdivisions, make soil tests and supervise the installation of individual sewage disposal systems; conduct education courses in food surveys and work in housing improvement programs; investigate cases of rabies, food poisoning, typhoid fever and dysentery to find out what caused the cases, how the diseases were transmitted, and how other cases may be prevented; act in an advisory capacity to help the community if rodent or insect infestations are a problem and if so, to recommend the most feasible method for control and extermination. Some newer phases of work include air pollution control and radiological and occupational health.

Requirements

I. Beginning position	Sanitarians must obtain a license or a Certificate of Registration to practice in any state. There are three requirements for one to become eligible for registration: (1) college degree with a major in sanitation or sanitary engineering; (2) college degree and 16 semester units in public health courses; and (3) college degree including at least 30 semester hours of basic science and one year of full-time experience in a health department.
II. Advanced position	Three years of experience as a sanitarian in a public health agency, with at least one year spent in a supervisory capacity. Completion of one year of graduate study in public health in a recognized college may be substituted for one year of the required general experience.

Public Health Educator

The Job

The public health educator plans and carries out educational programs to increase public understanding about health so that people can resolve their own health problems and attain a state of physical, mental, and social well-being. The public health educator helps people solve health problems by stimulating local community leaders and groups to take appropriate health action. He often prepares news releases, provides audio-visual materials, and serves as a consultant to those who work to improve health conditions. He works closely with members of the health department staff, including health officers, nurses, and sanitarians.

Requirements

I. Beginning position	
College	Bachelor's degree with emphasis on psychology, sociology, anthropology, education, journalism, and biological sciences.
Graduate work	Master of Public Health degree with specialization in health education from an accredited school of public health.
II. Advanced position	Several years of experience with increasing responsibilities as a health educator.

Public Health Social Worker

The Job

The public health social worker is a member of the professional staff of the health department who assists in the prevention and alleviation of social distress which can cause or can result from ill health. The social worker may do family casework, serve as consultant to other health workers, or be involved in community organization, program planning, and research. There are now many job opportunities for social workers in the fields of chronic disease, mental health, alcoholism, crippled children services, and maternal and child health programs.

Requirements

I. Beginning position

College	Bachelor's degree in social welfare or one of the social sciences.
Graduate work	Completion of two years of graduate work leading to a Master's degree in an accredited school of social work.
Experience	Two years of supervised casework, group work or community organization.

II. Advanced position

Graduate work	Master's degree in social work. In addition, the Master's of Public Health is desirable.
Experience	One year of supervised casework, group work, or community organization, and one year of administration, supervision, or consultation.

Public Health Veterinarian

The Job

Veterinary public health is a specialty within the broad field of veterinary medicine. Veterinarians in public health carry on research, develop diagnostic and laboratory methods, give special training and advisory services, and conduct epidemiologic investigations and preventive medical programs concerned with diseases transmissible from animals to man. Over 100 of these diseases have been recognized and more than 20 are of significance in the United States. Prevention of these diseases in man depends upon the eradication or control of the diseases in animals. The armed forces employ many veterinarians as public health officers.

Many public health veterinarians are involved in studies of the effects on animals of conditions such as air pollution and radiation; research is being carried out in the area of organic disease, such as heart disease and cancer, with the hope that the findings can be used in preventing and curing diseases in man.

Requirements

I. Beginning position College	Pre-veterinary course or Bachelor's degree in one of the sciences.
Graduate work	Doctor of Veterinary Medicine degree from an accredited school of veterinary medicine.
II. Advanced position	Master of Public Health degree, subsequent to a degree in veterinary medicine. Work in a specialty leading to a Doctor of Public Health or Doctor of Philosophy degree is most desirable.

APPENDIX II

Planning a Program for Nutritional Health

Planning a Program for Nutritional Health*

FIELDS OF KNOWLEDGE	SOCIAL AND ECONOMIC FACTORS INVOLVED IN NUTRITIONAL STUDIES OF COMMUNITIES	IMPLICATIONS OF THESE STUDIES FOR TRAINING AND TEACHING*
I. The community and its culture.	1. The pattern of social grouping: family and kinship; status; work. 2. The pattern of adjustment to the environment.	1. The patterns of behavior between groups and individuals. 2. The patterns of authority in decision making and in leadership.
II. The food situation in general.	1. The use of local resources and the cultivation of foodstuffs. 2. The impact of local markets and the buying of food at stores. 3. The ritualistic use of food at feasts and ceremonies.	1. Attitudes toward economic activities and food production, both traditional and changing. 2. Ideas about food and its function and changing fashions in food.
III. Family diets, including snacks as well as habitual meals.	1. Varying standards of living. 2. The balance between using and selling available foodstuffs. 3. The fuel situation in relation to cooking. 4. The type of family units that make up cooking and eating groups.	1. Methods of household management. 2. Intelligence and ability applied to the housewives' tasks. 3. Time available for cooking, etc. 4. The demands of social obligations for hospitality, food exchange, etc.
IV. Nutritional state of the population in general, and of children.	1. Composition of selected households, including number of adults and children to be fed. 2. The food of the children. 3. The food of the adults, especially wage earners and pregnant women.	Health teaching in the community: 1. General principles of adequate diets. 2. Special needs of young children. 3. Meaning and evidences of malnutrition.

*From Read, M.: Background paper No. 8. In Burgess, A., and Dean, R. F. A. (eds.): *Malnutrition and Food Habits, Report of an International and Interprofessional Conference.* London, Tavistock, 1962, p. 60.

APPENDIX III

Improving Participation in Voluntary Action*

1. Do not expect to be able to gain much support from active youth for established or traditional middle class kinds of voluntary action, especially where it is controlled by conservative, traditional, or narrow viewpoints.

2. Expect most membership and participation in the usual kinds of voluntary action from people in the middle of the life cycle—from about age 30–60—where people tend to be married and have school or college-age children.

3. Expect most membership and participation in the usual kinds of voluntary action from middle and higher socioeconomic status persons.

4. Expect less voluntary organization membership and activity from people in poor physical or mental health (or who have close family members in poor physical or mental health), people who have especially extensive home and family responsibilities, people whose work or other major activity is very tiring physically, people who work long hours (at one or more jobs) or odd hours (night shift, rotating shifts, etc.), and people with disorderly or unstable career patterns (e.g., much job-hopping, frequent or prolonged unemployment, major changes in type of work, etc.).

5. Do not believe that traditional sex differences in voluntary action have to exist in the present or future.

6. Do not expect to change or improve the "ethnic/racial mix" of your voluntary organization or program unless you can and will do something about the "racism" embodied in your group, its members, goals, and activities.

7. Realize that there is nothing intrinsic to age, marital status, number of children, sex, race, ethnic background, socioeconomic status, physical or mental ability, or health that necessarily guarantees high or low voluntary activity.

8. Similarly, realize that there is nothing intrinsic to particular occupations, businesses, religious affiliations, political affiliations, school affiliations, or other institutional affiliations that guarantees high or low participation in voluntary action, even though some types of institutional or organizational affiliations are more conducive to voluntary action than others.

9. In recruiting people to voluntary action, always depend heavily on personal contact—presently active members asking their friends, relatives, acquaintances, etc. Voluntary action is people involving people, not just people helping people.

10. Within any voluntary organization or program, no matter how objective, concrete, and external its goal (e.g., helping certain people, accomplishing something in the political or economic realm, etc.), substantial provision should be made for the close personal interaction of its members. People need contact and appreciation from valued fellow members to encourage and renew their voluntary efforts, as well as to give them something to fall back on when their efforts go poorly.

---

*Reprinted from Smith, D. H., and Reddy, R. D.: Improving participation in voluntary action. Adult Leadership, January, 1972.

11. Do not ignore the mass media and good public relations even though they are not sufficient by themselves. The media are most helpful in making people *aware* of your goals, organization, and activities, rather than in making people get involved directly.

12. Since people who are active in one area are likely to be active in other areas (the "general activity syndrome"), your best chance of recruiting active members for your organization is to focus on people who are already active in other groups or areas of community life, even though this seems paradoxical.

13. In recruitment campaigns as well as in your attempts to motivate more and better participation by present volunteer members, try to develop the most favorable "attitudinal climate" or "atmosphere" for the organization in your publicity and orientation sessions or in your speeches and internal documents.

a. Emphasize moral, civic, and social obligations that can be fulfilled through your group's voluntary activity and through voluntary action in general.
b. Emphasize the aspects of voluntary action in general, and of your voluntary activity, that perform a social service and make a contribution to human betterment, rather than mere self-gratification; but don't overdo the "do-gooder" image!
c. Emphasize the contribution of voluntary action in general and of your organization in particular to your local community.
d. Emphasize that your organization tries to have just the amount of formality and official organizational rules and procedures that make for efficient functioning and accomplishing your goals.
e. Emphasize that voluntary organizations and programs in general can be very effective, even uniquely effective, in some vital areas when business and government services have failed to meet needs.
f. Try to overcome or counteract possible feelings of social isolation, powerlessness, alienation, apathy, etc., that people may be feeling, whether members or nonmembers.
g. Try to get each member's family, friends, and acquaintances to approve generally of your organization and participation in it.
h. Try to develop strong member loyalties to group goals and to the group itself.
i. Emphasize the attractiveness and worthwhile nature or worthwhile aspects of the group.
j. Emphasize a sense of "personal fit" between certain kinds of individuals and your organization.
k. Emphasize and develop the sense of fellowship, belonging, and "esprit de corps" of the group, on an interpersonal level quite apart from any objective goals or aims of the group.

14. Try to recruit members and develop new leadership from among people whose personalities are most conducive to high levels of voluntary action. Specifically, you should try to recruit or involve people characterized by the following:

a. Extraversion or an open, friendly, easy approach to other people.
b. Self-confidence and good psychic adjustment.
c. Dominance and assertiveness, a willingness to take charge and lead.
d. A desire to achieve, a sense of competence and efficacy.
e. Flexibility and adaptability.
f. Altruism and a sense of morality and justice.
g. More energy.

15. For most kinds of voluntary action, recruitment and promotion to leadership should be set up to favor people with more verbal intelligence and more social skills, in addition to any tasks or roles in the group.

16. Support and encourage an open, free society; work against repression and oppression of all kinds.

17. Try to help raise the overall economic level and organizational development level of your community if you wish to foster voluntary activity.

18. Don't exclude potential members you would like to have by excessively restrictive eligibility requirements.

19. One good way to obtain high participation (though usually lower nominal membership) in voluntary action groups or programs is to insist that all members play an active role or drop out.

20. Going beyond the level of a minimum participation requirement, try to give as many members as possible a meaningful

and (if possible) creative task or role to perform—through official positions, committees, task forces, etc.

21. Try to structure the benefits and rewards of group membership and participation so that more and better rewards of all kinds (tangible and intangible) go to those who are members (vs. nonmembers) and who participate more (vs. at a minimum level or not at all).

22. Avoid growing too large (e.g., over 100–200 members) in any one local chapter or branch.

23. Avoid letting your organization become "overformalized," with too many bureaucratic rules and regulations, too much hierarchy, etc. The extreme of this situation is a "top heavy" national organization where only the top elected officers and the paid staff (or perhaps only the latter) make all the basic decisions without participation of the broader membership. When this happens, there tends to be apathy or alienation at lower levels, and a consequent decline in relative efficiency and effectiveness.

24. Finally, try to build an effective evaluation system into all of your important organizational activities. No organization operates at top efficiency and effectiveness over long periods of time, even if the optimum may be approached during some special periods.

APPENDIX IV

What Bylaws Should Contain

Membership Provisions

Who can be a member
Types of membership
Methods of admitting new members
Method of dropping members
What constitutes "good standing"

Officers

Duties and powers
Provisions for filling unexpired terms
Rules for election
Procedure for recall

Dues

Amount for annual membership
When payable
Initiation fees
To whom all dues are payable

Amendments to Constitution and Bylaws

Notice to membership of proposed amendments
Type of notice required
Vote required to effect amendment
Procedure for proposing an amendment: petition, motion

Meetings

Types: regular and special
Procedure for calling special meetings
Quorum (designate a percentage of the membership)
Parliamentary authority
Provision for notification of membership if no regular meeting date is established
Who shall preside at special meetings

Board of Directors

Eligibility for membership to board
Duties
Frequency of meetings
Delegation of authority to act between regular meetings of the organization
Who is delegated to speak for the organization in emergencies
What constitutes a quorum (usually majority of members)
How to recall members
Authority to hire salaried staff

Standing Committees

Names (Finance, Membership, Constitution, Bylaws, etc.)
How selected or elected
Term of office
Quorum (usually majority of members)
Meetings (number and how called)

APPENDIX V

Risk Factors for Health Hazards of Women

RATE YOUR RISK FACTORS FOR THE MOST COMMON HEALTH HAZARDS OF WOMEN

	Yes	No
1. Do you travel in a car as a driver or passenger in excess of 10,000 miles a year?	_____	_____
2. When in a motor vehicle, do you wear a seat belt or a shoulder harness?	_____	_____
3. Do you now have or have you ever had feelings that life is not worth living?	_____	_____
4. Do you feel depressed ("blue") much of the time?	_____	_____
5. Has your mother or a sister had breast cancer?	_____	_____
6. Do you examine your breasts each month to detect lumps or changes?	_____	_____
7. Do you go to your doctor for a breast examination at least once a year?	_____	_____
8. Have you ever had elevated blood pressure?	_____	_____
9. Do you now smoke cigarettes?	_____	_____
10. Are you at present more than 10 per cent above your ideal weight?	_____	_____
11. Has your blood cholesterol ever been checked by a physician?	_____	_____
12. Have your natural parents, brothers, or sisters had diabetes (too much sugar in the blood)?	_____	_____
13. Have you ever been told that you have diabetes?	_____	_____
14. Have you had a Pap (cancer) smear within the past year?	_____	_____

15. Have you had unusual vaginal bleeding (not at your period)? ______ ______

16. Have you had a pelvic (female organ) examination within the past year? ______ ______

17. Do you drink alcoholic beverages (beer, wine, whisky, gin, vodka, etc.) in excess of seven drinks a week? ______ ______

18. Have you ever had rheumatic fever? ______ ______

19. Have you had a physical examination of your rectum by your doctor in the past year? ______ ______

20. Have you had an examination of your rectum or colon by your doctor with a lighted instrument (sigmoidoscope) in the past year? ______ ______

21. Have you had any bleeding from your rectum in the past six months? ______ ______

How You Rate: Any YES answers to Nos. 1, 3, 4, 5, 8, 9, 10, 12, 13, 15, 17, 18, or 21, or NO answers to 2, 6, 7, 11, 14, 16, 19, or 20 significantly increase your risk for one or more of the major health hazards of women.

All the risk factors indicated here are correctable by personal action.

Based on the health hazard appraisal of Life Extension Institute, New York City.

APPENDIX VI

Preventing Food Poisoning*

This bulletin has been prepared to meet the need for proper training and appropriate information for persons involved in the purchase, preparation, storage, and serving of food.

I. Personal Hygiene

A. The supervisor should check food handlers when they report to work for evidence or history of open sores, boils, infected hairs, hangnails, colds, sore throats, fever, or intestinal disorders. An employee who reports with any of the above should be excused from working with food and referred for appropriate medical attention.

B. Always wash hands before preparing, handling, or serving food and after use of toilet facilities. Keep fingernails trimmed and hands and forearms clean with soap and water. Bacteriological tests show that unwashed hands spread germs.

C. When sneezing and coughing, cover the nose and mouth with a handkerchief; after handling handkerchiefs and dirty rags, wash hands.

D. Keep fingers out of glasses and dishes and off bowls of spoons, tines or forks, and blades of knives.

II. Frozen Foods

A. Frozen foods should be held at 0° F. until thawed for use.

B. Thawing may be done by:

1. Removing from freezer and placing for required length of time in the refrigerator. This method permits thawing without excessive surface temperature.

2. By running cool, clean (potable) water over the food until thawed. The temperature of the water should not exceed 70° F.

3. Placing in the oven frozen and cooking for a proportionately longer time.

C. Employees should know the usual lowest temperature of their freezer and be governed accordingly by the length of time food is left in it unused. Studies by the United States Department of Agriculture show that the same amount of *frozen* food will keep in about the same way for the indicated length of time under the indicated temperatures:

DEGREES FAHRENHEIT	DAYS
30	5
25	10
20	21
15	42
10	91
5	180
0	365

A 5° rise in temperature approximately halves the potential storage life of most foods. *Prolonged thawing at room temperature is associated with food poisoning outbreaks.*

---

*From Preventing food poisoning. Trenton, N.J., Public Health News, *45*:66, March, 1964.

III. Other Foods

A. Foods easily susceptible to contamination—custards, pie fillings, salads, etc.—should be stored at a temperature below 45° F. or above 140° F. (On display shelves, such foods may be stored for short periods at 55° F., but these should be removed for consumption or returned to 45° F. storage after short intervals.)

B. Custards and cream fillings should be placed in shells, crusts, etc., either while hot (not less than 140° F.) or immediately following preparation if a cold process is used. Such fillings and puddings should be refrigerated at 45° F. or below in shallow pans immediately after cooking or preparation and held at that temperature until combined into pastries or served. Completed custard or cream-filled pastries, unless served immediately following filling, should be refrigerated at 45° F. or below promptly after preparation, and held at that temperature pending service.

C. Stuffings, poultry, and stuffed meats and poultry should be heated through to 165° F. with no interruption in the heating process. If this temperature cannot be maintained throughout (including the stuffing), the stuffing should be cooked separately and added to the meat or poultry before it is cooked.

D. Salads made of meat, poultry, seafood, potatoes, and eggs, and cream-filled products and similar foods should be prepared from chilled ingredients and held at or below 45° F. until served.

E. Pork and pork products should be cooked so that all parts of the meat reach a temperature not less than 150° F., as measured by a meat thermometer, unless such product has already been processed or treated to destroy trichinosis organisms.

F. Raw beef purchased as ground beef or hamburger should not be tasted or eaten raw or served undercooked.

G. Ideally, beef and pork products should be ground in separate grinders. If this is not possible, the grinder should be thoroughly cleaned before a different kind of meat is ground. There have been cases of trichinosis associated with eating what was believed to be rare ground beef hamburgers. Investigation has disclosed that in some instances beef was ground after pork, and that the grinder had not been thoroughly cleaned in the meantime.

H. All raw fruits and vegetables should be washed thoroughly before being cooked or served.

I. Foods highly susceptible to spoilage—cream-filled products, cream sauces, salads, etc.—should be used the day they are made if at all possible. Quantities should be planned accordingly.

J. Don't re-serve uneaten portions of food served to a customer.

K. If a food does not appear normal on inspection—odor, appearance, color—discard it. *Do not taste it.*

L. Obviously, utensils must be kept clean.

IV. Suggestions on Buying

A. For reasons indicated under III, be sure you get ground beef (unmixed with pork) when you order beef.

B. Buy only meats and poultry from establishments inspected under the federal or state meat inspection systems.

C. Buy milk and milk products from sources approved by the New Jersey State Department of Health.

D. Shellfish from sources approved by the New Jersey State Department of Health has identifying tags on the original shipment container.

E. If canned foods are to be used, they should have been processed in a commercial food processing establishment. Avoid canned goods processed in someone's home. Check canned goods and reject those with leaks, swelling, and excessive dents.

F. Check canned hams before purchase. If the container says "Keep under refrigeration," be sure it has been kept under refrigeration. (Some hams under three pounds need not be kept under refrigeration.)

V. Suggestions on Storage and Use

A. Even with a careful buying program, inspect all goods on receipt, especially if they have not been personally selected at time of purchase.

B. Make periodic checks of your refrigerator and freezer to make sure they are functioning properly. The refrigerator temperature should be below 45° F. The freezer temperature should be 0° F. or below. Keep in mind that large volumes put a greater strain on chilling capacity than small volumes do.

C. Allow for air circulation around foods in refrigerated areas. Do not cover open shelving. Do not store foods directly on the floor, in aisles, or against walls.

D. Rotate your foods so that the older foods, presumably purchased earlier, will be used before food purchased more recently.

E. On the basis of experience, use first those foods that are most perishable.

F. If frozen poultry wrapped in plastic is to be thawed, remove the plastic before transferring from freezer to refrigerator. If fresh poultry wrapped in plastic is to be stored in the refrigerator, remove the plastic wrapping before storage.

G. Wash thoroughly interior and exterior surfaces of poultry prior to use.

H. Hazardous chemicals and other materials used in cleaning the premises should be prominently labeled and stored in a separate area to avoid any possible confusion or unintentional substitution for condiments, seasonings, etc. If labels of such materials are lost or obliterated, discard them and get clearly identifiable materials.

Although the material in this pamphlet is intended primarily for persons who supervise or do the work or the purchasing for establishments that prepare food in large quantities—restaurants, cafeterias, caterers, those responsible for church dinners and other civic and charitable affairs—much of what is included may be useful information to the housewife or home manager who cooks for a single family.

For these people, there are some additional suggestions:

1. When shopping, purchase frozen and refrigerated foods last. Don't make long stops on the way home during which frozen or refrigerated foods could become soft or warm.

2. Using insulated bags helps to preserve the initial temperature of the product.

3. Select wisely in the first instance. Consistent freezing and refrigeration preserve the original quality of foods but cannot improve on the quality.

4. Milk and milk products should be refrigerated immediately on receipt. Room temperature storage of milk or milk products on tables or counters for extended periods should be avoided.

5. Flies, roaches, rodents, and other vermin are associated with the transmission of disease. All food handling premises should be kept free of such pests. Proper storage and handling of garbage and other wastes will assist in the control of vermin.

APPENDIX VII

State Health Department Inspection Forms

PRODUCER DAIRY INSPECTION FORM

TEXAS STATE DEPARTMENT OF HEALTH
and
U. S. PUBLIC HEALTH SERVICE

NAME

LOCATION

Gallons Sold Daily ....

Plant ....

....

SIR: An inspection of your dairy has this day been made, and you are notified of the violations marked below with a cross (X). Violation of the same requirement on two successive inspections calls for immediate degrading or permit suspension.

COWS

1. Cows, Health:
- Tuberculosis control according to Code ..... (a) .....
- Brucellosis control according to Code ..... (b) .....
- Evidence on file ..... (c) .....
- No extensive induration of udders ..... (d) .....
- No cows giving abnormal milk ..... (e) .....
- Other tests as required ..... (f) .....

MILKING BARN

2. Lighting:
- Adequate natural and/or artificial light properly distributed ..... (a) .....

3. Air Space and Ventilation:
- Well ventilated ..... (a) .....
- No overcrowding ..... (b) .....

4a. Floor Construction:
- Floor areas concrete or other impervious and easily cleaned material when required; in good repair ..... (a) .....
- Graded to drain ..... (b) .....
- Other barn portions separated ..... (c) .....

4b. Floor Cleanliness:
- Cleaned, as required ..... (a) .....
- No swine or fowl ..... (b) .....

5. Walls and Ceiling:
- Painted biennially or whitewashed annually or other satisfactory finish ..... (a) .....
- Clean; in good repair ..... (b) .....
- Ceiling tight if storage overhead ..... (c) .....
- Feed room or bins dust-tight with door or cover ..... (d) .....

6a. Cowyard, Grading and Draining:
- Graded to drain ..... (a) .....
- No pooled wastes ..... (b) .....

6b. Cowyard, Cleanliness:
- Cowyard clean and loose-housing areas properly maintained ..... (a) .....
- No swine ..... (b) .....

7. Manure Disposal:
- Fly breeding minimized by approved disposal methods ..... (a) .....
- Stored inaccessible to cows ..... (b) .....

MILK HOUSE

8a. Floors:
- Smooth; concrete or other impervious material; in good repair ..... (a) .....
- Graded to drain ..... (b) .....

8b. Walls and Ceiling:
- Approved material and finish ..... (a) .....
- Good repair ..... (b) .....

MILK HOUSE—Continued

8c. Lighting and Ventilation:
- Adequate natural and/or artificial light properly distributed ..... (a) .....
- Adequate ventilation ..... (b) .....
- Doors and windows closed during dusty weather ..... (c) .....

8d. Screening:
- All openings effectively screened and doors open outward and self-closing, unless flies otherwise kept out ..... (a) .....

8e. Miscellaneous Requirements:
- Used for milk-handling purposes only ..... (a) .....
- Milk house operations not conducted elsewhere ..... (b) .....
- No direct opening into living quarters or barn except as permitted by Code ..... (c) .....
- Adequate water-heating facilities ..... (d) .....
- 2-compartment stationary wash and rinse vats of adequate size ..... (e) .....
- Wastes properly disposed of ..... (f) .....

9. Cleanliness and Flies:
- Floors, walls, windows, shelves, tables, and equipment clean ..... (a) .....
- No trash or unnecessary articles ..... (b) .....
- Necessary fly-control measures used ..... (c) .....

TOILET AND WATER SUPPLY

10. Toilet:
- Provided; conveniently located ..... (a) .....
- Constructed and operated according to Code ..... (b) .....
- No evidence of human defecation or urination about premises ..... (c) .....
- Clean; no direct opening into milkroom ..... (d) .....

11. Water Supply:
- Safe sanitary quality (see Code) ..... (a) .....
- Adequate in quantity ..... (b) .....
- Easily accessible ..... (c) .....

UTENSILS AND EQUIPMENT

12. Construction:
- Smooth, heavy-gage material, non-corrodible, surface, non-absorbent, non-toxic, easily cleanable; joints and seams flush ..... (a) .....
- Good repair ..... (b) .....
- Straining, single-service pads used ..... (c) .....
- Small-mouth pails (seamless, if new) ..... (d) .....

13. Cleaning:
- Cleaned after each usage ..... (a) .....
- Must look and feel clean ..... (b) .....

14. Bactericidal Treatment:
- All milk containers and equipment subjected to approved bactericidal process (see Code) ..... (a) .....

UTENSILS AND EQUIPMENT—Continued

15. Storage:
- Left in treating chamber or bactericidal solution until used or stored properly above floor ..... (a) .....
- Single-service articles properly stored ..... (b) .....
- Equipment and utensils not exposed to toxic substances ..... (c) .....
- Returned milk cans promptly stored ..... (d) .....

16. Handling:
- No handling of milk-contact surfaces after bactericidal treatment ..... (a) .....

MILKING

17. Udders and Teats; Abnormal Milk:
- Milking done in barn or milking parlor ..... (a) .....
- Udders and teats clean ..... (b) .....
- Rinsed with bactericidal solution just prior to milking ..... (c) .....
- Abnormal milk excluded, and properly disposed of ..... (d) .....

18. Flanks:
- Flanks, bellies, and tails of cows clean at time of milking ..... (a) .....
- Brushing completed before milking begun ..... (b) .....
- Clipped when required ..... (c) .....

19. Milkers' Hands:
- No infections on hands or arms ..... (a) .....
- Washed; then rinsed with bactericidal solution before milking and upon recontamination ..... (b) .....
- Clean and dry while milking ..... (c) .....
- Hand-washing facilities, including soap, water, and individual clean towels convenient to milking operations ..... (d) .....

20. Clean Clothing:
- Clean outer garments ..... (a) .....

21. Milk Stools and Surcingles:
- Clean; stored above floor in clean place ..... (a) .....
- Stools of easily cleanable construction, no padding ..... (b) .....

22. Removal of Milk:
- Immediate removal to milk house or straining room when required ..... (a) .....
- Straining done in milk house or straining room, not in barn unless can protected by well-fitting cover and protected from manure and splash ..... (b) .....

23. Cooling:
- Milk either cooled to 50° F. or less, or delivered to plant within 2 hours after milking completed ..... (a) .....

24. Vehicles and Surroundings:
- Vehicles clean ..... (a) .....
- Constructed so as to protect milk ..... (b) .....
- No contaminating substances transported ..... (c) .....
- Surroundings clean, free from insect breeding and rodent harborages ..... (d) .....

Remarks:

5008

Date	Sanitarian

Note.—Item numbers correspond to item numbers for grade A raw milk for pasteurization in Milk Ordinance and Code—1953 Recommendations of the Public Health Service to which please refer.

IDAHO DEPARTMENT OF HEALTH
ENGINEERING AND SANITATION DIVISION

FOOD SANITATION REPORT Effective date — 7-1-63

Name			Address			Responsible person	
Type of Establishment	Program 20	Action taken	Activity or Service	Establishment Number		County Code	City Code
Date Time	Sanitarian's Number	Jurisdiction	Number of Employees	Number Served		Total Score	

Item No.

41—(1) **Floors** —2— Easily cleanable construction, smooth, good repair ( ); clean ( ); cleaned only after closing or between meals ( ), by dustless methods ( )

42—(2) **Walls and ceilings** —2— All: clean, good repair ( ); kitchen: light color ( ), walls smooth, washable to level of splash ( )

43—(3) **Doors and windows** —5— Outer openings with effective screens and outward-opening, self-closing doors, or fly-repellent fans, or flies absent ( )

44—(4) **Lighting** —2— Natural or artificial light equivalent to 10 foot-candles on working surfaces (except in dining room), 4 in storage rooms ( )

45—(5) **Ventilation** —2— All rooms (except cold storage) reasonably free of odors and condensation ( )

46—(6) **Toilet facilities** —5— Comply with plumbing code ( ); adequate, conveniently located for employees ( ); good repair, clean, no flies ( ); well lighted, outside ventilation ( ); in new establishments, no direct opening ( ); self-closing doors ( ); washing sign for employees ( ); privies, if used, comply State standards ( )

47—(7) **Water supply** —5— Running water accessible as required ( ); supply adequate ( ); safe, complies State standards ( )

48—(8) **Lavatory facilities** —5— Adequate, convenient ( ); hot and cold running water ( ); soap ( ); approved sanitary towels ( ); hands washed after toilet ( )

49—(9) **Construction of utensils and equipment** —5— Easily cleanable construction, self-draining, no corrosion ( ); good repair, no open seams, no chipped or cracked dishes ( ); no cadmium or lead utensils ( )

50—(10a) **Cleaning of equipment** —3— Clean cases, counters, shelves, tables, meat blocks, refrigerators, stoves, hoods ( ); clean cloths used by employees ( )

51—(10b) **Cleaning of utensils** —7— Single-service cups, plates, straws, caps used only once ( ); eating and drinking utensils thoroughly cleaned after each use ( ); other utensils cleaned each day ( ); suitable detergent used ( ); no cyanide or other poisonous compounds ( )

52—(10c) **Bactericidal treatment of eating and cooking utensils** —8— Approved bactericidal treatment after cleaning: Immersed 2 minutes in 170° F. water, or one-half minute in boiling water, or 2 minutes in approved chlorine rinse; or kept in steam cabinet 15 minutes at 170° F. or 5 minutes at 200° F.; or in hot air cabinet 20 minutes at 180° F. ( ); cabinets have thermometer in coldest zone ( ); large utensils adequately treated with live steam, boiling water, or chlorine spray or swab ( ); dishwashing machine properly operated Utensils comply bacterial standard ( ); drying cloths, if used, kept clean and used for no other purpose ( )

Item No.

53—(11) **Storage and handling of utensils** —4— Stored above floor in clean place protected from flies, splash, dust, etc., inverted or covered when practicable ( ); no handling of contact surfaces ( ); single-service cups, straws, etc., purchased in sanitary cartons, kept in clean dry place and properly handled ( ); dispensing spoons, dippers kept in hot or running water ( )

54—(12) **Disposal of wastes** —5— Liquid wastes into public sewer or as approved by State ( ); no back-siphonage into water supply from toilets, washing machines, sinks, etc. ( ); garbage stored in tight, non-absorbent, washable receptacles, covered pending removal ( ); removed frequently and receptacles washed to prevent nuisance ( )

55—(13) **Refrigeration** —6— Readily perishable foods (including cream-filled pastry, meats, milk, etc.) stored at 50° F. or less ( ); ice stored and handled in approved manner ( ); drip enters open trapped drain or pan ( )

56—(14a) **Wholesomeness of food** —6— Wholesome, clean, no spoilage ( ); prepared so safe for human consumption ( ); cream-filled pastry rebaked unless filling adequately cooked, and promptly cooled ( )

57—(14b) **Wholesomeness of milk products** —4— Milk, fluid milk products, frozen desserts from approved sources ( ); milk, etc., served in original individual bottles or from approved bulk dispenser ( )

58—(14c) **Wholesomeness of shellfish** —2— Shellfish from approved sources ( ); shucked shellfish kept in original containers ( )

59—(15a) **Storage of food and drink** —4— No contamination by overhead leakage or submerging ( ); not on floors subject to flooding from sewage backflow ( )

60—(15b) **Display and serving of food and drink** —6— Minimum manual contact with food and drink ( ); no open displays ( ); no animals or fowls ( ); flies, roaches, and rodents under control ( ); no uncolored poisonous insecticides or raticides ( )

61—(15c) **Ratproofing** —2— Structure ratproofed ( )

62—(16) **Cleanliness of employees** —5— Clean outer garments, used for no other purpose ( ); hands clean ( ); no spitting, no tobacco used where food prepared ( )

63—(17) **Miscellaneous** —2— Premises kept neat and clean ( ); no operations in living or sleeping rooms ( ); clean, adequate lockers for employees' clothing, not in kitchen ( ); soiled linens, coats, aprons kept in containers ( )

64-(Sec.9) **Disease control** —3— No person at work with any communicable disease, sores, or infected wounds ( ); Section 9 posted in all toilets ( ); employees' health certificates (if required locally) ( )

Remarks: ....

....

....

.... Sanitarian

Form DH 63320

STANDARD HOUSING ORDER FORM PROCEDURE*

NAME________________________________ LOCATION____________________

1. Repair, replace or provide foundation.
2. Repair or replace siding and trim where necessary.
3. Have exterior doors and sills made weathertight.
4. Repair or replace window sash, frames and glaze where necessary.
5. Replace broken window glass.
6. Repair or replace porch floor(s), steps, rail and roof supports where necessary.
7. Repair or replace roofing.
8. Repair chimney(s).
9. Repair or replace gutters, downspouts and downspout carry-offs.
10. Rehabilitate garage/shed/barn and render same ratproof or demolish same and remove from premises.
11. Have exterior stairways put in a good state of repair.
12. Repair or demolish rear lean-to addition.
13. Provide safe and unobstructed means of egress for each dwelling unit above the first floor.
14. Have interior stairways put in a good state of repair.
15. Repair walls and ceilings where necessary.
16. Re-cover worn flooring or satisfactorily repair.
17. Repair or replace sagging floor joists, posts and beams where necessary.
18. Remove and replace nonconforming wall and ceiling material.
19. Provide a water closet, tub or shower and kitchen sink for each dwelling unit.
20. Provide hot water service to lavatory, tub or shower and kitchen sink.
21. Have existing fixtures and appurtenances put in a good state of repair.
22. Remove sewage from basement and have all sewer lines put in operating condition.
23. Have electrical service, outlets, switches and fixtures put in a good state of repair.
24. Install additional circuits and outlets to provide adequate service to all habitable rooms.
25. Provide adequate light and ventilation for all habitable rooms.
26. Provide adequate lighting for public halls and stairways.
27. Limit occupancy of each dwelling unit to available floor space.
28. Have heating facilities put in a good state of repair.
29. Provide flue pipes, properly vented for hot water tank and all gas space heating equipment.
30. Provide a sufficient number of regulation metal garbage and rubbish containers with tight-fitting lids for each dwelling unit.
31. Remove all garbage, rubbish and debris from premises.
32. Eradicate rats on premises—begin extermination at once.
33. Exterminate all vermin.
34. Have supplied facilities put in a good state of repair.
35. Keep dwelling unit(s), (premises) vacant until above order is complied with.
36. In lieu of above mentioned order, vacate (or have vacated) premises for living quarters as said premises constitute a hazard to life and health and are not fit for human habitation.
37. Provide screens.
38. Provide adequate ceiling height.
39. Vacate garage/shed/barn/basement for living quarters.

DELETE THAT PART WHICH DOES NOT APPLY
TO ORDER BEING ISSUED.

DATE________________________

SANITARIAN__________________

*From Toledo's Health Annual Summary, 1963. Department of Public Health, Toledo, Ohio, 1963.

PHS-4006
4-62

INSPECTION REPORT
FOOD SERVICE ESTABLISHMENTS

Permit No. ____________
Type ____________ NSD ____________

CITY, COUNTY OR DISTRICT	NAME OF ESTABLISHMENT	ADDRESS	OWNER OR OPERATOR

Sir: Based on an inspection this day, the items marked below identify the violation in operation or facilities which must be corrected by the next routine inspection or such shorter period of time as may be specified in writing by the health authority. Failure to comply with this notice may result in immediate suspension of your permit (or downgrading of the establishment).* An opportunity for an appeal will be provided if a written request for a hearing is filed with the health authority within the period of time established in this notice for the correction of violations.

SECTION B. FOOD

1. FOOD SUPPLIES

Item		Specify:	Bakery products	Poultry and poultry products	Meat and meat products	Frozen desserts	Shellfish	Milk and milk products	Demerit points
1	Approved source								6
2	Wholesome - not adulterated								6
3	Not misbranded								2
4	Original container; properly identified								2
5	Approved dispenser								
6	Fluid milk and fluid milk products pasteurized								6
7	Low-acid and non-acid foods commercially canned								6

2. FOOD PROTECTION

Item		Preparation	Storage	Display	Service	Transportation	Demerit points
8	Protected from contamination						4
9	Adequate facilities for maintaining food at hot or cold temperatures						2
10	Suitable thermometers properly located						2
11	Perishable food at proper temperature						2
12	Potentially hazardous food at 45° F. or below, or 140° F. or above as required						6
13	Frozen food kept frozen; properly thawed						2
14	Handling of food minimized by use of suitable utensils						4
15	Hollandaise sauce of fresh ingredients; discarded after three hours						6
16	Food cooked to proper temperature						6
17	Fruits and vegetables washed thoroughly						2
18	Containers of food stored off floor on clean surfaces						2
19	No wet storage of packaged food						2
20	Display cases, counter protector devices or cabinets of approved type						2
21	Frozen dessert dippers properly stored						2
22	Sugar in closed dispensers or individual packages						2
23	Unwrapped and potentially hazardous food not re-served						4
24	Poisonous and toxic materials properly identified, colored, stored and used; poisonous polishes not present						6
25	Bactericides, cleaning and other compounds properly stored and non-toxic in use dilutions						

SECTION C. PERSONNEL

1. HEALTH AND DISEASE CONTROL

Item		Demerit points
26	Persons with boils, infected wounds, respiratory infections or other communicable disease properly restricted	6
27	Known or suspected communicable disease cases reported to health authority	6

2. CLEANLINESS

Item		Demerit points
28	Hands washed and clean	6
29	Clean outer garments; proper hair restraints used	2
30	Good hygienic practices	4

SECTION D. FOOD EQUIPMENT AND UTENSILS

1. SANITARY DESIGN, CONSTRUCTION AND INSTALLATION OF EQUIPMENT AND UTENSILS

Item		Good repair; no cracks	No chips, pits or open seams	Cleanable; smooth	Approved material	No corrosion	Proper construction	Accessible for cleaning and inspection	Demerit points
31	Food-contact surfaces of equipment								2
32	Utensils								2
33	Non-food-contact surfaces of equipment								2
34	Single-service articles of non-toxic materials								2
35	Equipment properly installed								2
36	Existing equipment capable of being cleaned, non-toxic, properly installed, and in good repair								2

2. CLEANLINESS OF EQUIPMENT AND UTENSILS

Item		Demerit points
37	Tableware clean to sight and touch	4
38	Kitchenware and food-contact surfaces of equipment clean to sight and touch	
39	Grills and similar cooking devices cleaned daily	
40	Non-food-contact surfaces of equipment kept clean	2
41	Detergents and abrasives rinsed off food-contact surfaces	2
42	Clean wiping cloths used; use properly restricted	2
43	Utensils and equipment pre-flushed, scraped or soaked	2
44	Tableware sanitized	4
45	Kitchenware and food-contact surfaces of equipment used for potentially hazardous food sanitized	
46	Facilities for washing and sanitizing equipment and utensils approved, adequate, properly constructed, maintained and operated	4
47	Wash and sanitizing water clean	2
48	Wash water at proper temperature	
49	Dish tables and drain boards provided, properly located and constructed	2
50	Adequate and suitable detergents used	2
51	Approved thermometers provided and used	2
52	Suitable dish baskets provided	
53	Proper gauge cocks provided	
54	Cleaned and cleaned and sanitized utensils and equipment properly stored and handled; utensils air-dried	2
55	Suitable facilities and areas provided for storing utensils and equipment	2
56	Single-service articles properly stored, dispensed and handled	2
57	Single-service articles used only once	6
58	Single-service articles used when approved washing and sanitizing facilities are not provided	

SECTION E. SANITARY FACILITIES AND CONTROLS

1. WATER SUPPLY

Item		Demerit points
59	From approved source; adequate; safe quality	6
60	Hot and cold running water provided	4
61	Transported water handled, stored; dispensed in a sanitary manner	6
62	Ice from approved source; made from potable water	6
63	Ice machines and facilities properly located, installed and maintained	2
64	Ice and ice handling utensils properly handled and stored; block ice rinsed	2
65	Ice-contact surfaces approved; proper material and construction	

*Applicable only where grading form of ordinance is in effect.

Page 2

Item	2. SEWAGE DISPOSAL	Demerit Points
66	Into public sewer, or approved private facilities	6
	3. PLUMBING	
67	Properly sized, installed and maintained	2
68	Non-potable water piping identified	1
69	No cross connections	6
70	No back siphonage possible	
71	Equipment properly drained	2
	4. TOILET FACILITIES	
72	Adequate, conveniently located, and accessible; properly designed and installed	6
73.	Toilet rooms completely enclosed, and equipped with self-closing, tight-fitting doors; doors kept closed	2
74	Toilet rooms, fixtures and vestibules kept clean, in good repair, and free from odors	2
75	Toilet tissue and proper waste receptacles provided; waste receptacles emptied as necessary	2
	5. HAND-WASHING FACILITIES	
76	Lavatories provided, adequate, properly located and installed	6
77	Provided with hot and cold or tempered running water through proper fixtures	4
78	Suitable hand cleanser and sanitary towels or approved hand-drying devices provided	2
79	Waste receptacles provided for disposable towels	2
80	Lavatory facilities clean and in good repair	2
	6. GARBAGE AND RUBBISH DISPOSAL	
81	Stored in approved containers; adequate in number	2
82	Containers cleaned when empty; brushes provided	2
83	When not in continuous use, covered with tight fitting lids, or in protective storage inaccessible to vermin	2
84	Storage areas adequate; clean; no nuisances; proper facilities provided	2
85	Disposed of in an approved manner, at an approved frequency	2
86	Garbage rooms or enclosures properly constructed; outside storage at proper height above ground or on concrete slab	2
87	Food waste grinders and incinerators properly installed, constructed and operated; incinerators areas clean	2
	7. VERMIN CONTROL	
88	Presence of rodents, flies, roaches and vermin minimized	4
89	Outer openings protected against flying insects as required; rodent-proofed	2
90	Harborage and feeding of vermin prevented	2

Item	SECTION F. OTHER FACILITIES 1. FLOORS, WALLS AND CEILINGS	Demerit Points
91	Floors kept clean; no sawdust used	2
92	Floors easily cleanable construction, in good repair, smooth, non-absorbent; carpeting in good repair	1
93	Floor graded and floor drains, as required	2
94	Exterior walking and driving surfaces clean; drained	2
95	Exterior walking and driving surfaces properly surfaced	1
96	Mats and duck boards cleanable, removable and clean	2
97	Floors and wall junctures properly constructed	2
98	Walls, ceilings and attached equipment clean	2
99	Walls and ceilings properly constructed and in good repair; coverings properly attached	1
100	Walls of light color; washable to level of splash	2
	2. LIGHTING	
101	20 foot-candles of light on working surfaces	2
102	10 foot-candles of light on food equipment, utensil-washing, hand-washing areas and toilet rooms	
103	5 foot-candles of light 30" from floor in all other areas	
104	Artificial light sources as required	2
	3. VENTILATION	
105	Rooms reasonably free from steam, condensation, smoke, etc.	2
106	Rooms and equipment vented to outside as required	2
107	Hoods properly designed; filters removable	2
108	Intake air ducts properly designed and maintained	1
109	Systems comply with fire prevention requirements; no nuisance created	2
	4. DRESSING ROOMS AND LOCKERS	
110	Dressing rooms or areas as required; properly located	1
111	Adequate lockers or other suitable facilities	1
112	Dressing rooms, areas and lockers kept clean	2
	5. HOUSEKEEPING	
113	Establishment and property clean, and free of litter	2
114	No operations in living or sleeping quarters	2
115	Floors and walls cleaned after closing or between meals by dustless methods	2
116	Laundered clothes and napkins stored in clean place	2
117	Soiled linen and clothing stored in proper containers	1
118	No live birds or animals other than guide dogs	2

DEMERIT SCORE OF THE ESTABLISHMENT ____________

REMARKS ____

____

____

____

____

Date ________________ Health Authority ______________________________

APPENDIX VIII

Student Semester Project

Choose a current major community health problem, research it, and discuss, using the following outline:

I. The Problem

1. Define the problem
2. Historical aspects
3. Compare the problem
   (a) local
   (b) state
   (c) nation
   (d) world
4. Where is the problem most acute?
5. Causes of the problem
6. Effect upon
   (a) infants
   (b) school age children
   (c) adults
   (d) old age

II. Statistical Analysis of the Problem

III. Factors Involved in the Problem

1. Sociological aspects
2. Psychological aspects
3. Economic aspects
4. Geographical aspects
5. Rural-urban aspects

IV. Prevention and Control

1. List the various agencies involved in prevention (local and state); services rendered; how financed
2. List the various agencies involved in control (local and state); services rendered; how financed
3. How is the program presently organized, administered, and financed?
4. Is the program coordinated? Does cooperation prevail?
5. How is the support of the public gained?
6. What is the role of the school, health department, voluntary agencies, and parents in attacking the problem?
7. Legislation—local and state
8. What health education methods, techniques, and materials are utilized?
9. Community organization for health

V. Current Research and the Future

1. What research is being done to combat this problem?
2. List the agencies giving research grants—amount of money allotted
3. Theory behind research
4. Writings in recent health journals
5. The future

VI. Evaluation, Interpretation, Analysis, and Recommendations

APPENDIX IX

Career Information

IF YOU ARE INTERESTED IN BEING:	LEVEL ON WHICH YOU MAY WORK		MINIMUM EDUCATION
	State	Local	
Administrator, Public Health (non-medical)	X	X	BA
Biologist, Public Health	X	X	BS
Cannery inspector	X	–	High school & experience
Chemist, Public Health	X	X	BS
Dental hygienist, Public Health		X	High school & technical training
Dentist, Public Health	X	X	DDS & license
Educator, Public Health	X	X	BA & MPH
Engineer, air sanitation	X	X	BS
Engineer, industrial hygiene	X	X	BS
Engineer, sanitary	X	X	BS
Engineering technician	X	–	High school & technical training
Food and drug inspector	X	–	BA
Food technology specialist	X	–	BA
Instrument technician, air sanitation	X	–	High school & experience
Laboratory assistant	X	X	High school
Meteorologist, air sanitation	X	X	BS
Microbiologist, Public Health	X	X	BS & registration
Nurse, Public Health	X	X	BS, RN, & PHN
Nutritionist, Public Health	X	X	BA
Occupational therapist	X	X	BA
Pharmacology specialist	X	–	BS & license
Physical therapist	X	X	BA
Physician, Public Health	X	X	MD & license
Physicist, Public Health	X	X	BS
Radiation protection specialist	X	–	High school & technical training
Sanitation Worker, Public Health	X	X	BS & license
Social Worker, Public Health	X	X	BA & MSW
Statistician, Public Health	X	X	BA
Veterinarian, Public Health	X	X	DVM & license

PUBLICATIONS AND ORGANIZATIONS THAT CAN HELP

Admission Requirements of American Dental Schools

Available from American Association of Dental Schools, 1625 Massachusetts Ave., N.W., Washington, D.C. 20036. $4.00.

A Career in Veterinary Medicine

Available from Bureau of Health Resources Development, Health Resources Administration, U.S. Department of Health, Education and Welfare, 9000 Rockville Pike, Bethesda, Md. 20014. Free.

College Costs Today

(Summary of costs of tuition, fees, room and board at most U.S. colleges and universities.) New York Life Insurance Co. Free. Available from any New York Life agent or local sales office.

Health Careers Guidebook, 3rd ed., 1972

Published jointly by the U.S. Department of Labor and the U.S. Department of Health, Education and Welfare. Available from the Superintendent of Documents, U.S. Government Printing Office, Washington, D.C. 20402, Stock Number 2900-0158. $2.25.

Health Professions Student Loan Program

Available from Bureau of Health Resources Development, Health Resources Administration, U.S. Department of Health, Education and Welfare, 9000 Rockville Pike, Bethesda, Md. 20014. Free.

How Medical Students Finance Their Education

Available from Bureau of Health Resources Development, Health Resources Administration, U.S. Department of Health, Education and Welfare, 9000 Rockville Pike, Bethesda, Md. 20014. Free.

Join the Life Corps

Available from Bureau of Health Resources Development, Health Resources Administration, U.S. Department of Health, Education and Welfare, 9000 Rockville Pike, Bethesda, Md. 20014. Free.

Need A Lift?

(Information on educational opportunities, careers, loans, scholarships, student employment.) Published by the American Legion Educational and Scholarship Program. Available from The American Legion, Dept. S, P.O. Box 1055, Indianapolis, Ind. 46206. 50 cents.

Nursing Student Loan Program

Available from Bureau of Health Resources Development, Health Resources Administration, U.S. Department of Health, Education and Welfare, 9000 Rockville Pike, Bethesda, Md. 20014. Free.

Pharmacy School Admission Requirements

(Includes information on pharmacy school requirements, tuition, fees, room, board, and expenses.) Available from American Association of Colleges of Pharmacy, Office of Student Affairs, 8121 Georgia Avenue, Silver Spring, Md. 20910. $4.00.

Where to Get Health Career Information

Available from National Health Council, Inc., 1740 Broadway, New York, N.Y. 10019. Single copies free.

Scholarships for American Indians

An informative booklet listing approximately 400 financial assistance opportunities for American Indians may be obtained through any Bureau of Indian Affairs scholarship office or from the Bureau of Indian Affairs Higher Education Program, P.O. Box 1788, Albuquerque, New Mexico 87102. Free.

SELECTED FILMS

Code Blue

Designed to motivate minority students to consider medical and health professions as a career.
Award winner, 1972. 26 min.

Galapagos: Laboratory for Evolution

Discusses why the Galapagos Islands, located on the equator 600 miles from the coast of Ecuador, have been a natural laboratory for evolution. EMC, 1971. 36 min.

Heart Attack

Examines the significant factors that cause or aggravate heart disease in Western societies. Emphasizes the importance of cholesterol levels in the blood. Concludes by demonstrating modern methods of treatment, including open-heart surgery. 1972. 25 min.

Old, Black and Alive

A film on the aged: "The only way to avoid getting old is to die young." 28 min.

Do No Harm

A film on the prescription drug industry. 46 min.

Man Made Man
A compact and well organized documentary on organ tissue transplants. CBS, 1967. 25 min.

Bolero
A thrilling sight and sound experience and a triumph of form and feeling. Zubin Mehta and the Los Angeles Philharmonic, 1973. 28 min.

A Right to Health
Explores community health centers in Watts (a suburb of Los Angeles) and other areas. 30 min.

Aquatic Locomotion
From Galapagos: Series. 20 min.

No Expectations
Their film is Real . . . Rocco, Irene, Tom, Bobby, and *Heroin.* 28 min.

Report on Acupuncture
Photographed in Taiwan, the film shows contemporary methods of training, practice and research. A normally painful tooth extraction is performed quickly and painlessly by using only acupuncture as the anesthetic. 28 min.

A Luta Continua
The latest film on the national liberation movement in Mozambique. Shows how Frelimo provides Health Education and Social Services to the people living in the liberated areas. 1971. 32 min.

The Pressure Is On
Explains what high blood pressure is, how the disease is detected, and what its implications are for black Americans. 25 min.

Future Shock
Imaginative documentation of the rapid social and technological changes now taking place and the illnesses and problems arising from difficulty in adapting to them. Narration by Orson Welles. Contemporary films, 1972. From the book by Alvin Toffler. 42 min.

Why Man Creates
Saul Bass's highly imaginative exploration of human creativity. Eight episodes. 28 min.

The Nuts and Bolts of Health Care Management—Communication
What good communication is and is not; how to achieve good communication. 30 min.

A Case of Neglect
Documentary of the myths and realities of health care for American children whose families often find it difficult to meet medical costs. The film evaluates Medicaid and its inadequacies. Color, 56 min.

The Unconquered Plague—Schistosomiasis
Filmed in St. Lucia, an island in the Caribbean. Illustrates cooperation and team effort by members of the community, showing how the people took pride in their projects. Emphasizes sociological and religious aspects, sanitation, innovative devices (foot bridges, swimming pools, hand laundry units), sanitation, snail control, and education.

INDEX

NOTE: Page numbers in *italics* refer to illustrations; page numbers followed by a (t) refer to tables.